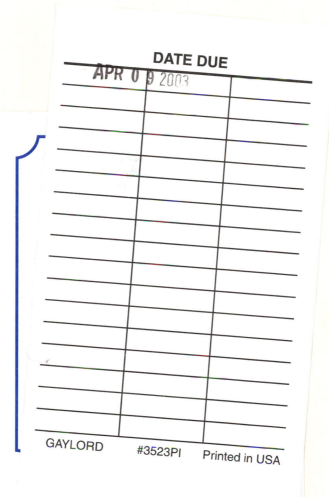

DATE DUE

APR 0 9 2003

GAYLORD   #3523PI   Printed in USA

POST ANESTHESIA CARE

POST ANESTHESIA CARE

JEFFERY S. VENDER, M.D., F.C.C.M.

Associate Professor of Clinical Anesthesiology
Northwestern University Medical School
Head of Anesthesiology
Director of Medical-Surgical Intensive Care
Evanston Hospital
Evanston, Illinois

BRUCE D. SPIESS, M.D.

Associate Professor and Chief
of Cardiothoracic Anesthesia
University of Washington
Seattle, Washington

W.B. SAUNDERS COMPANY
HARCOURT BRACE JOVANOVICH, INC.
Philadelphia / London / Toronto / Montreal / Sydney / Tokyo

W. B. SAUNDERS COMPANY
Harcourt Brace Jovanovich, Inc.

The Curtis Center
Independence Square West
Philadelphia, Pennsylvania 19106

Library of Congress Cataloging-in-Publication Data

Post anesthesia care / [edited by] Jeffery S. Vender, Bruce D. Spiess.
   p.   cm.
   ISBN 0-7216-5648-X
   1. Postoperative care.   2. Surgical intensive care.   I. Vender,
   Jeffrey S.   II. Spiess, Bruce D.
   [DNLM: 1. Anesthesia Recovery Period.   2. Postoperative Care.
   3. Postoperative Complications—prevention & control.   WO 183
   V452p]
   RD51.P63 1992   617′.919—dc20
   DNLM/DLC   91-46790

Editor: Richard Zorab

POST ANESTHESIA CARE   ISBN 0-7216-5648-X

Printed in Mexico

Last digit is the print number: 9   8   7   6   5   4   3   2   1

This work is dedicated with love to

Bobbie, Kim, and Todd Vender

and

Ann, Phillip, and Erica Spiess

We are forever grateful for their constant love and support which has contributed to this book's development.
JEFFERY S. VENDER, M.D.
BRUCE D. SPIESS, M.D.

Contributors

LEONARD C. BANDALA, M.D.

Associate in Clinical Anesthesia, Northwestern University Medical School, Chicago, Illinois
Respiratory Complications

LOREN A. BAUMAN, M.D.

Assistant Professor of Anesthesiology and Pediatrics, Bowman-Gray School of Medicine, Winston-Salem, North Carolina
Acute Perioperative Renal Dysfunction

RICHARD G. BELATTI, Jr., M.D.

Assistant Professor, Department of Anesthesiology, Creighton University School of Medicine, Omaha, Nebraska
Common Post Anesthetic Problems

KEITH H. BERGE, M.D.

Assistant Professor of Anesthesiology, Mayo Clinic and Mayo Medical School, Rochester, Minnesota
Problems after Head, Neck, and Maxillofacial Surgery

THOMAS W. FEELEY, M.D.

Professor of Anesthesia, Stanford University School of Medicine, Stanford, California
Postoperative Endocrine Problems

MARK L. FRANKLIN, M.D.

Fellow, Critical Care Medicine, Department of Anesthesia, Northwestern University Medical School, Chicago, Illinois
Pitfalls of Hemodynamic Monitoring

RICHARD E. GELFAND, M.D.

Clinical Associate, Northwestern University Medical School, Chicago, Illinois
Obstetric Patients in the PACU and ICU

HUGH C. GILBERT, M.D.

Assistant Clinical Professor, Northwestern University, Chicago, Illinois
Postoperative Pain Management

JAMES J. GORDON, M.D.

Assistant Professor of Medicine, Michigan State University, Ann Arbor, Michigan
Infectious Diseases

STEVEN C. HALL, M.D.

Associate Professor, Department of Anesthesiology, Northwestern University Medical School, Chicago, Illinois

Perioperative Pediatric Care

IRA J. ISAACSON, M.D.

Associate Professor of Anesthesiology, Emory University School of Medicine, Atlanta, Georgia

Postoperative Considerations After Major Vascular Surgery

JOHN KERCHBERGER, M.D.

Assistant Professor of Anesthesiology, Rush Medical College, Chicago, Illinois

Orthopedics

SALLY A. KRAFT, M.D.

Fellow, Pulmonary Medicine and Critical Care Medicine, Stanford University, Stanford, California

Postoperative Endocrine Problems

WILLIAM L. LANIER, M.D.

Assistant Professor of Anesthesiology, Mayo Clinic and Mayo Medical School, Rochester, Minnesota

Problems after Head, Neck, and Maxillofacial Surgery

JERROLD H. LEVY, M.D.

Associate Professor of Anesthesiology, Emory University School of Medicine, Atlanta, Georgia

Allergic and Transfusion Reactions

CHRISTINA M. CHOMKA LEYA, M.D.

Assistant Professor of Clinical Anesthesia, Northwestern University Medical School, Chicago, Illinois

Respiratory Complications

KIM LITWACK, Ph.D., R.N.

Associate Professor, Rush University School of Nursing, Chicago, Illinois

Immediate Postoperative Care: A Problem-Oriented Approach

JANE D. LOWDON, M.D.

Assistant Professor of Anesthesiology, Emory University School of Medicine, Atlanta, Georgia

Postoperative Considerations after Major Vascular Surgery

JESSE H. MARYMONT, III, M.D.

Associate in Clinical Anesthesia, Northwestern University Medical School, Chicago, Illinois

Postoperative Cardiovascular Complications

FREDERICK G. MIHM, M.D.

Associate Professor of Anesthesia, Stanford University School of Medicine, Stanford, California

Postoperative Endocrine Problems

R. FRANCIS NARBONE, C.R.N.A., M.B.A.

Chief Anesthetist, Department of Anesthesiology, Rush Presbyterian–St. Luke Medical Center, Chicago, Illinois
Quality Assurance in the Post Anesthesia Care Unit

ROBERT A. NATONSON, M.D.

Assistant Clinical Professor of Anesthesia, Northwestern University Medical School, Chicago, Illinois
Managing Perioperative Hypothermia and Hyperthermia

BRENT S. O'CONNOR, M.D.

Associate in Clinical Anesthesia, Northwestern University Medical School, Chicago, Illinois
Postoperative Cardiovascular Complications

SAMUEL M. PARNASS, M.D.

Assistant Professor of Anesthesiology, Rush Medical College, Chicago, Illinois
Problems of Ambulatory Surgery

WILLIAM T. PERUZZI, M.D.

Associate Professor, Division of Clinical Anesthesia, Northwestern University Medical School, Chicago, Illinois
Respiratory Care: Oxygenation, Bronchial Hygiene, and Mechanical Ventilation

DONALD S. PROUGH, M.D., F.C.C.M.

Professor of Anesthesia and Neurology, Bowman-Gray School of Medicine, Winston-Salem, North Carolina
Acute Perioperative Renal Dysfunction

KENNETH L. RODINO, M.D.

Associate in Clinical Anesthesia, Northwestern University Medical School, Chicago, Illinois
Pitfalls of Hemodynamic Monitoring

DAVID M. ROTHENBERG, M.D.

Assistant Professor of Anesthesiology. Rush University, Chicago, Illinois
Postoperative Acid-Base Disorders: Recognition and Management

TOD B. SLOAN, M.D., Ph.D.

Associate Professor, Director of Neuroanesthesia, University of Texas Health Science Center, San Antonio, Texas
Postoperative Central Nervous System Dysfunction

BRUCE D. SPIESS, M.D.

Chief, Division of Cardiothoracic Anesthesia, University of Washington School of Medicine, Seattle, Washington
Hemorrhagic Problems during the Immediate Postoperative Period

KENNETH J. TUMAN, M.D., F.C.C.M.

Associate Professor, Anesthesia and Critical Care, Rush Medical College, Chicago, Illinois

Fluid and Electrolyte Abnormalities and Management

JEFFERY S. VENDER, M.D., F.C.C.M.

Chief, Division of Anesthesia; Director, Medical/Surgical ICU, Evanston Hospital, Evanston, Illinois; Associate Professor, Clinical Anesthesia, Northwestern University Medical School, Chicago, Illinois

Respiratory Care: Oxygenation, Bronchial Hygiene, and Mechanical Ventilation

MICHAEL E. WEISS, M.D.

Assistant Professor, Clinical Medicine, University of Washington School of Medicine, Seattle, Washington

Allergic and Transfusion Reactions

GRANT O. WESTENFELDER, M.D.

Associate Professor, Clinical Medicine, Northwestern University Medical School, Chicago, Illinois

Infectious Diseases

Preface

Although pivotal in a patient's care, the intraoperative time period is short in the continuum of the hospitalization. The transition from operation to recovery is an important period. Recent data have shown that the majority of perioperative myocardial infarctions occur in the immediate postoperative period. Forty percent of untoward anesthesia events occur or are first detected in the postanesthesia care unit. Many complications of surgery may also be first manifested in that unit. Clearly a smooth transition through the early postoperative period is required for satisfactory patient outcome.

The focus of contemporary surgical and anesthetic techniques has been upon intraoperative care. Great expenditures of time, money and intellect have led to an expanded understanding of intraoperative pathophysiology. New surgical endeavors such as liver, heart and lung transplants are routinely undertaken at many centers. These surgeries were only dreams 25 years ago. Because of such success and other motivations, it is not surprising that a focus has been upon the intraoperative process.

This book is written to fulfill several purposes. It will provide an educational resource for health care providers involved in immediate postoperative patient care. As a compilation of recent information, it is hoped that this text will go beyond only providing information. Perhaps it will serve to further interest in a critical time period for patient care. Ultimately, surgical outcome will benefit from more interest, research and focus upon the immediate postoperative period.

Contents

IMMEDIATE POSTOPERATIVE CARE: A Problem-Oriented Approach

KIM LITWACK

As a result of anesthesia and surgery, patients admitted to the post anesthesia care unit (PACU) are subject to physiologic alterations. It is a well accepted fact that the immediate postoperative period is critical to the recovery of the patient; therefore attention to detail and skills in postoperative assessment and intervention are essential to prevent potential postoperative morbidity and mortality. Because anesthesia implies a transient alteration in perception and sensation, post anesthesia recovery implies that patients should return to their preoperative status or to the highest level of function of which they are capable postoperatively.

The role and responsibility of any PACU team is to assist the surgical patient to begin the process of reaching the highest potential postoperative level of function. An initial patient assessment must therefore be performed so an effective, individualized, realistic care plan can be developed for each patient. This chapter identifies the components of such a post anesthetic and postsurgical assessment.

After reading this chapter, the reader should be able to meet the following objectives.

1. Identify the components of an initial post anesthesia assessment
2. Understand the purpose and components of an effective anesthesia report
3. Discuss the benefits and limitations of currently utilized post anesthesia assessment approaches
4. Understand the purpose and components of a post anesthesia care plan
5. Use a "systems approach" to identify assessment criteria for recovery of the post anesthesia patient

6. Correlate assessed information into an acceptable care plan or scoring system that allows recovery tracking of the post anesthesia patient and suggests acceptable discharge or transfer criteria

ADMISSION TO THE PACU

The initial priority when admitting a patient to the PACU is evaluation of respiratory and circulatory adequacy. Immediate assessments should be made of the patient's airway patency and the rate and quality of respirations. If appropriate, oxygen therapy should be administered and ventilatory parameters set. Pulse oximetry monitoring should be initiated. [Although post anesthesia oximetry monitoring has not been a required "standard of care" in all states, the American Society of Anesthesiologists (ASA) Standards for Postanesthesia Care has required it as of January 1992.]

During this initial assessment, any signs of inadequate oxygenation (Table 1–1) and ventilation (Table 1–2) should be identified. Although many of the signs of respiratory inadequacy could have other, sometimes multifactorial explanations, the priority of assessing adequacy of oxygenation-ventilation dictates immediate assessment and assurance that respiratory insufficiency is not contributory.

The patient should have electrocardiographic (ECG) monitoring to determine cardiac rate and rhythm; however, ECG monitoring is not a substitute for auscultation of the heart. Blood pressure should be measured and

TABLE 1–1. SIGNS AND SYMPTOMS OF INADEQUATE OXYGENATION

Central nervous system
  Restlessness, agitation, confusion, coma
  Muscular twitches or seizures
Cardiovascular system
  Hypertension, tachycardia (sympathetic nervous system-mediated)
  Hypotension, bradycardia (direct hypoxic effect)
  Dysrhythmias
Skin
  Cyanosis (absent in severe anemia and vasoconstriction)
  Poor capillary refill
  Oximetry saturation less than 90%
Pulmonary system
  Increased to absent respiratory efforts
  Decreased PaO_2[a]

---

[a] Not standard practice to obtain during initial assessment.

TABLE 1–3. SIGNS OF ADEQUATE OXYGEN PERFUSION

Central nervous system
  Appropriate mentation
  Sensation, motor function, reflexes intact
  Electroencephalogram, evoked potential monitors appropriate for residual anesthetic exposure[a]
Cardiovascular system
  ECG, normal sinus rhythm without signs of ischemia
  Cardiac output appropriate for preload and metabolic activity[a]
  Skin warm, dry, with good color and capillary refill
Renal system
  Urine production >1 ml/kg/hr (of appropriate specific gravity and composition)[a]
  No evidence of osmotic diuresis
  No evidence of postobstructive diuresis
Pulmonary system
  Normal arterial blood gas[a]
  Normal intrapulmonary shunts[a]

---

[a] Not standard practice to obtain during initial assessment.

the adequacy of organ perfusion determined (Table 1–3).

The anesthesiologist should be an active participant in the patient's stabilization and

TABLE 1–2. SIGNS AND SYMPTOMS OF INADEQUATE VENTILATION

Spontaneous ventilation
  Increased or decreased respiratory frequency
  Nasal flaring
  Suprasternal or intercostal retractions
  Decreased to absent movement of air at mouth, nares, or endotracheal tube
  Abnormal airway sounds
  Decreased to absent breath sounds
  Diminished chest movement
  Diaphragmatic breathing
  Abnormal $ETCO_2$ or $PaCO_2$ values[a]
  Signs of inadequate oxygenation (Table 1–1)
Assisted or controlled ventilation
  Increased frequency of respiratory efforts
  Decreased chest expansion/contraction during ventilatory cycle
  Abnormally high inflation pressures
  Decreased to absent air movements in endotracheal tube
  Decreased to absent breath sounds
  Decreased air movement assessed by monitors (apnea, capnography)
  Abnormal $ETCO_2$ or $PaCO_2$ values[a]
  Signs of inadequate oxygenation (Table 1–1)

---

[a] Not standard practice to obtain during initial assessment.

transfer to the PACU. Initial assistance in applying supplemental oxygen, maintaining or verifying airway adequacy, and assessing circulatory status not only familiarizes PACU personnel with the patient but enhances a smooth transfer of care. Only after initial stabilization by attention to the "ABCs" of airway, breathing, and circulation can the anesthesiologist and the PACU nurse begin to communicate about other patient specifics, including any significant preoperative or intraoperative events.

ANESTHESIA REPORT

To ensure patient safety and continuity of care, the anesthesiologist must provide a verbal report to the PACU nurse, communicating specific information. Ideally, this report begins before the patient and anesthesiologist leave the operating room by making a telephone call to notify the PACU staff of estimated arrival time, patient condition, and anticipated needs (especially if nonroutine drugs, monitors, or procedures are contemplated). The importance of the anesthesia report is reflected in the ASA Standards for Postoperative Care:

Standard III: Upon arrival in the PACU, the patient shall be reevaluated and a verbal report pro-

**TABLE 1–4.
POST ANESTHESIA
ADMISSION REPORT:
COMPONENTS AND
SUGGESTED ORDER OF
REPORT**

General information
  Patient name
  Age
  Anesthesiologist/surgeon
  Procedure

Intraoperative management
  Components of anesthetic
  Total narcotics with time of last dose
  Muscle relaxants used (time of last dose)
  Muscle relaxant reversal used (doses and times)
  Other medications received (e.g., preoperative drugs, antibiotics, antiemetics, vasopressors)
  Extended blood loss
  Fluid/blood products administered
  Urine output

Intraoperative course
  Unexpected anesthetic effects and their management
  Unexpected surgical findings and their resolution
  Vitals and monitoring trends
  Results of laboratory tests

Patient history
  Acute (current episode and therapies through surgery)
  Chronic (medical history, medications, allergies)

PACU plan
  Potential and expected problems (with plan for interventions and resolution)
  Suggested PACU course (including need for nonstandard narcotics)
  Limits for acceptable/unacceptable laboratory tests, consults
  PACU discharge plan
  Planned therapeutics
  Responsible contact physician

vided to the responsible PACU nurse by the member of the anesthesia care team who accompanies the patient.

A complete report regarding the surgical/anesthetic course, preoperative conditions, and PACU treatment plan with therapeutic guidelines and endpoints is transmitted to the PACU nurse. A coherent order for the presentation of the information that should be included in the anesthesia report is presented in Table 1–4. The anesthesiologist should not leave the bedside until the PACU nurse accepts responsibility for the patient. Standard III-3 of the ASA Standards for Postanesthesia Care states:

The member of the anesthesia care team shall remain in the PACU until the PACU nurse accepts responsibility for the nursing care of the patient.

Ideally, the PACU nurse documents the anesthesia report in a record that allows rapid, efficient documentation. (A sample format is shown in Figure 1–1.)

INITIAL PACU ASSESSMENT

After the report is given and recorded, the PACU nurse performs a more complete postoperative assessment. The assessment should be thorough and targeted to the needs of the post anesthesia and postsurgical patient. The American Society of Post Anesthesia Nurses (ASPAN) includes the need for and components of an admission assessment in their Standards of Care.

Many post anesthesia assessment approaches (e.g., head-to-toe, major body systems, scoring systems) are currently utilized in PACUs. Each may have its own benefits and limitations, but any assessment approach should be able to do the following:

1. Determine the patient's physiologic status at the time of admission to the PACU
2. Allow periodic reexamination of the patient so physiologic trends become obvious
3. Establish the patient's baseline level so the effect of previous healthy conditions can be assessed and predicted as they affect current physiology
4. Assess ongoing status of the surgical site and its effect on any preexisting conditions and recovery
5. Assess recovery from anesthesia, noting residual effects
6. Allow compilation and trending of patient-specific characteristics that relate to discharge or transfer criteria

To accomplish these goals, a systematic approach must be coupled with an understanding of the various factors that affect a patient's recovery.

The "head-to-toe" assessment system utilized in some PACUs provides a comprehensive approach to physical assessment with its organization as its major benefit. The PACU nurse begins with an evaluation of neurologic status and then moves caudad, assessing respiratory, cardiovascular, gastrointestinal, and genitourinary function. Although this system is easily used to teach new practitioners in

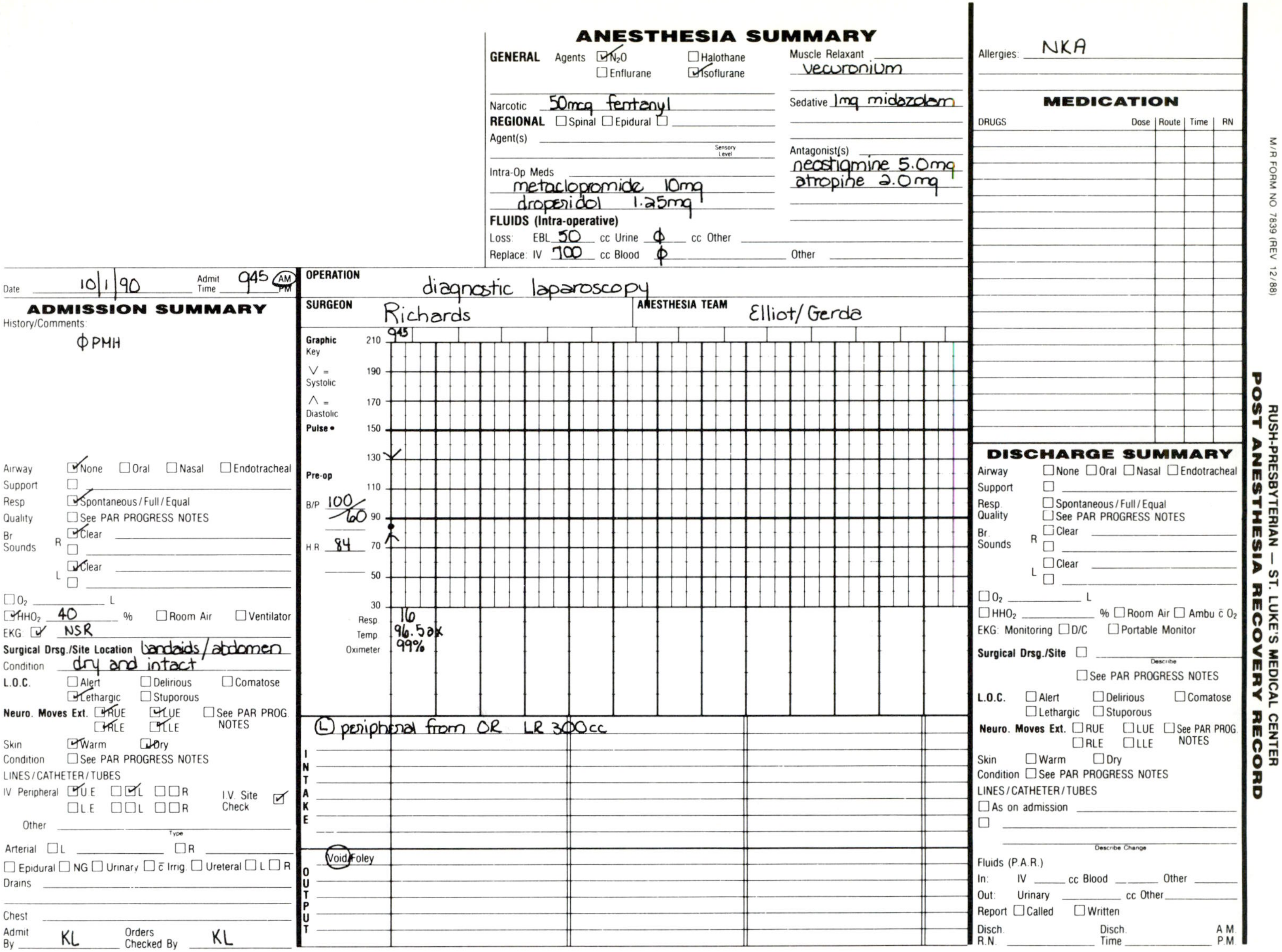

M/R FORM NO. 7839 (REV 12/88)

RUSH-PRESBYTERIAN — ST. LUKE'S MEDICAL CENTER
POST ANESTHESIA RECOVERY RECORD

MEDICATION

Allergies: NKA

DRUGS	Dose	Route	Time	RN

DISCHARGE SUMMARY

Airway: □None □Oral □Nasal □Endotracheal
Support: □ Spontaneous / Full / Equal
Resp Quality: □ See PAR PROGRESS NOTES
Br Sounds: R □ Clear   L □ Clear
□O₂ ___ % □Room Air □Ambu c̄ O₂
□HHO₂ ___ L □Portable Monitor
EKG: Monitoring □D/C
Surgical Drsg./Site ___ Describe ___
□ See PAR PROGRESS NOTES
L.O.C.: □Alert □Delirious □Comatose
□Lethargic □Stuporous
Neuro. Moves Ext. □RUE □LUE □See PAR PROGRESS NOTES
□RLE □LLE   NOTES
Skin: □Warm □Dry
Condition: □ See PAR PROGRESS NOTES
LINES/CATHETER/TUBES
□As on admission ___ Describe Change ___
Fluids (P.A.R.)
In: IV ___ cc Blood ___ Other ___
Out: Urinary ___ cc Other ___
Report □Called □Written
Disch R N ___ Disch Time ___ A M / P M

ANESTHESIA SUMMARY

GENERAL Agents ☑N₂O □Halothane ☑Isoflurane
□Enflurane

Muscle Relaxant: vecuronium
Sedative: 1mg midazolam

Narcotic: 50mg fentanyl
REGIONAL □Spinal □Epidural □
Agent(s) ___ Sensory Level ___

Antagonist(s): neostigmine 5.0mg
atropine 2.0mg

Intra-Op Meds: metaclopramide 10mg
droperidol 1.25mg

FLUIDS (Intra-operative)
Loss: EBL 50 cc Urine φ cc Blood φ cc Other ___
Replace: IV 700

ANESTHESIA TEAM: Elliot / Gerda

OPERATION	diagnostic laparoscopy
SURGEON	Richards

Graphic Key
∨ = Systolic
∧ = Diastolic
Pulse ●

Pre-op
B/P 100/60 90
H R 84

210 190 170 150 130 110 90 70 50 30
Resp Temp
Oximeter

96.5 ok
99%

(L) peripheral from OR   LR 300cc

Void / Foley

ADMISSION SUMMARY

Date 10/1/90   Admit Time 0945 AM/PM

History/Comments φ PHH

Airway: ☑None □Oral □Nasal □Endotracheal
Support: □Room Air □Ventilator
Resp Quality: ☑Spontaneous / Full / Equal
□ See PAR PROGRESS NOTES
Br Sounds: R ☑Clear   L ☑Clear
□O₂ ___ L ___ %
□HHO₂ 40
EKG ☑ NSR
Surgical Drsg./Site Location bandaids / abdomen
Condition dry and intact
L.O.C.: □Alert □Delirious □Comatose
□Lethargic □Stuporous
Neuro. Moves Ext. ☑RUE ☑LUE □See PAR PROG NOTES
☑RLE ☑LLE
Skin: ☑Warm ☑Dry
Condition: □ See PAR PROGRESS NOTES
LINES/CATHETER/TUBES
IV Peripheral ☑UE □UE R □ □ L ☑R IV Site Check ☑
□ LE □ LE □R □ □
Other ___
Arterial □L □R
□Epidural □NG □Urinary c̄ Irrig □Ureteral □L □R Type
Drains ___
Chest ___
Admit By KL   Orders Checked By KL

FIGURE 1-1. Postanesthesia record. (From Rush–Presbyterian–St. Luke's Medical Center; Chicago. With permission.)

the PACU, in that its organization provides a framework that encourages comprehensiveness, it has been criticized for being cumbersome and excessive. With the head-to-toe approach, significant time is required to complete the assessment, and practitioners may come to feel "locked in" to the order of assessment, becoming unable to "see" the entire patient. In addition, documentation of the head-to-toe assessment in lengthy if all findings are recorded.

After the respiratory assessment, the cardiovascular system is evaluated. The heart should be auscultated, noting any irregularities in rate or rhythm, the quality of the heart sounds, and the presence of any murmurs or extra sounds. Arterial pulses should be evaluated for strength and equality, and the status of the observable aspects of the venous system (with special emphasis on the jugular and peripheral veins) should be checked. An ECG admission strip should be obtained for a baseline and included in the postanesthesia chart. ECG rate and rhythm are noted. Blood pressure should be measured again and compared with preoperative, intraoperative, and first postoperative values in order to appreciate any initial trends. Body temperature, skin color, and condition should also be noted. All findings should be documented.

It is important to remember that the respiratory and cardiovascular admission assessments are by no means comprehensive; instead, they are designed to verify adequacy. If the surgery itself involved the thoracic region or was cardiac or vascular in nature, the assessment should be expanded during appraisal of the particular system affected by the surgery.

After respiratory and cardiovascular system assessment, the neurologic system is evaluated. Initial evaluation should include the patient's level of consciousness, degree of orientation, status of sensory and motor systems, pupillary size, equality and reaction to light, and any unusual posturing. The Glascow Coma Scale, although originally developed as a prognostic indicator for head injury, can be useful for assessing postoperative neurologic recovery. The presence and function of other neurologic monitors including dural bolts, external ventricular drains, or electroencephalopathy monitors would be evaluated at this time.

Renal system assessment focuses on fluid intake and output (blood, crystalloid, and col-

loid), as well as volume and electrolyte status. The anesthesiologist should provide all fluid totals in the verbal report, and the PACU nurse should note and record all intravenous lines, irrigation solutions, and infusions going into the patient. All drains, catheters, and tubes for output must also be noted and recorded, including the color and consistency of any drainage.

All data obtained in the admission assessment should be documented. Ideally the PACU record is organized in such a way as to facilitate that documentation (Fig. 1–1).

Many PACUs have incorporated a post anesthetic scoring system into their admission assessment. This numerical scoring system with objectively defined criteria provides consistent verification of patient status. The patient is usually scored (evaluated) on admission to the PACU and again at regular intervals until discharge.

The use of scoring systems to evaluate patient status began in 1953 with Apgar scoring to evaluate newborn infants.[1] In 1964 Carighan et al. proposed a post anesthetic scoring system that evaluated circulation, respiration, central nervous system, gastrointestinal, and renal function along a 6-point continuum[2] (Fig. 1–2). However, the Carighan scale's complexity coupled with its need to evaluate patients over an extended period prevented its becoming more widely used.

In 1970 Aldrete and Krovlik proposed a post anesthetic scoring system that utilized physiologic assessment data already being obtained or observed by the PACU nurse.[3] The Aldrete scoring system evaluates the patient's activity, respiration, circulation, consciousness, and color (Fig. 1–3). Patients receive a numerical score of 0, 1, or 2 in each area, with 2 representing the highest level of functioning. The Aldrete post anesthetic scoring system is the most widely used scoring system in PACUs today, although its predictive value in assessing recovery from anesthesia has never been studied prospectively.

Two criticisms of the Aldrete scoring system are its use of color and blood pressure as criteria reflecting post anesthetic recovery. Color is criticized as being a subjective finding, and blood pressure has been criticized as being unrelated to recovery from general anesthesia. In addition, as more and more surgery is being performed on an outpatient basis, only one preoperative (baseline) blood pres-

H.N.D. POSTANESTHETIC SCORING SYSTEM						
	0	**1**	**2**	**3**	**4**	**5**
Circ.	BP stable. Pulse always under 100	BP-change less than 30%. Pulse 100–120	Vasopressors OR Digitalis	BP under 100 in spite of treatment	Decompensated	Severe shock
Resp.	Rate under 15. Breath-holding more than 25 sec.	Rate 15–20. Productive cough	Rate over 20, rales OR temp. up to 100°	Temp. over 100°, partial atelectasis	Major atelectasis	Pneumonia
C.N.S.	Amnesic, satisfied	Confused OR recalls induction	Dissatisfied with anesthesia for any reason	Extrapyramidal signs	Major neurological complications	Coma
G.I.	Nothing	No more than 3 episodes of nausea	Nausea, vomited once only	Vomiting	Ileus	Evisceration OR perforation
Renal	Voids over 800 cc.	Over 800 cc. per catheter	Voids 500–800 cc.	500–800 cc. per catheter	Under 500 cc.	Anuria

FIGURE 1–2. Postanesthesia scoring system. (From Carighan G, Kerri-Szanto M, Lavelle J: Post-anesthetic scoring system. Anesthesiology 25:396–397, 1964. With permission.)

sure is often available. Furthermore, in a patient anticipating surgery, this blood pressure value may not be characteristic of the patient's normal blood pressure.

Steward[4] proposed a post anesthetic scoring system that evaluated only consciousness, airway, and movement. Robertson[5] modified the Steward scale to emphasize the importance of a clear airway and the awake state as being essential for patient safety (Fig. 1–4).

For any post anesthesia scoring system to be effective and useful, it must be simple to use. It should include routinely assessed parameters that do not make extra work for PACU practitioners. Criteria should be objective and applicable in all patient situations and should complement and support patient care. In addition, from a medicolegal standpoint, the objectivity of a post anesthesia scoring system may prove beneficial.

Study # _____

Name _____ Age _____ Sex _____ Hospital Number _____

Date _____ Preanesthetic Risk _____ Arrival Time to RR _____

Type of Surgery _____

Anesthetic Agents _____

Muscle relaxants other than for intubation _____

Anesthesia time _____ Anesthesiologist _____

		At Arrival	1 Hour	2 Hours	3 Hours
Able to move 4 extremities voluntarily or on command = 2 " " " 2 " " " " " = 1 " " " 0 " " " " " = 0	ACTIVITY				
Able to deep breathe & cough freely = 2 Dyspnea or limited breathing = 1 Apneic = 0	RESPIRATION				
BP ± 20% of Preanesthetic level = 2 BP ± 20–50% of Preanesthetic level = 1 BP ± 50% of Preanesthetic level = 0	CIRCULATION				
Fully awake = 2 Arousable on calling = 1 Not responding = 0	CONSCIOUSNESS				
Pink = 2 Pale, dusky, blotchy, jaundiced, other = 1 Cyanotic = 0	COLOR				
	TOTALS				

FIGURE 1–3. Aldrete scoring system. (From Aldrete AJ, Krovlik D: The postanesthetic recovery score. Anesth Analg 49:924–933, 1970. With permission.)

Consciousness	Score
Fully awake; eyes open; conversing	4
Lightly asleep; eyes open intermittently	3
Eyes open to command or in response to name	2
Responding to ear-pinching	1
Not responding	0
Airway	
Opening mouth or coughing or both, on command	3
No voluntary cough, but airway clear without support	2
Airway obstructed on neck flexion, but clear without support on extension	1
Airway obstructing without support	0
Activity	
Raising one arm on command	2
Non-purposeful movement	1
Not moving	0

FIGURE 1–4. Steward postanesthetic scoring system, as modified by Robertson. (From Robertson G, MacGregor D, Jones C: Evaluation of doxapram for arousal from general anesthesia in outpatients. Br J Anaesth *49*:133–139, 1977. With permission.)

ONGOING ASSESSMENT

After the PACU assessment is completed, the PACU nurse continues to apply the skills of ongoing assessment, diagnosis, and intervention. The patient's response to intervention is also assessed. The identification of an actual or potential alteration in function allows the PACU nurse to implement a plan based on the protocols for patient care developed and established by the medical director and nursing manager. After rendering any immediate care required, the anesthesiologist (and surgeon in the case of a surgical alteration) should be notified.

The development of patient care protocols and nursing diagnoses should be a high priority of PACU medical and nursing management, as they significantly affect the quality of care delivered to recovering patients. Patient care protocols that may be applied in the PACU include, but are not limited to, alterations in the following.

Ventilation
Cardiac output
Emergence
Thermoregulation
Coagulation
Fluid and electrolytes
Acid-base status
Comfort

Other chapters in this text detail the pathophysiology and management of patients experiencing the above alterations.

The establishment of patient care protocols not only facilitate management of the post anesthesia patient, but they can be used as indicators of readiness for discharge and as discharge criteria.

DISCHARGE FROM THE PACU

The patient leaving the PACU may be discharged to home, a 23-hour observation unit, an inpatient unit, or an intensive care unit. Clearly, the choice of discharge facility depends on patient need, patient acuity, and availability of resources. The level of care a patient receives in these varying facilities ranges from self-care, to supportive care, to total care. As a result, the criteria that must be met prior to discharge vary, depending on the facility to which the patient is discharged.

New standards of the Joint Commission for the Accreditation of Healthcare Organizations are requiring the use of outcome indicators as the basis of quality monitoring. Outcome indicators applied to discharge criteria require that criteria be stated in patient-centered statements, i.e., for discharge from the PACU, the patient will: [*specify requirements*]. Specific clinical criteria can be used to substantiate the clinician's judgment with objective data.

Table 1–5 provides an example of the use of outcome indicators for patient discharge. Outcome indicators should be established, be written, and be a part of PACU protocol. If the patient outcomes in Table 1–5 are not present, the patient should remain in the PACU until the criteria are met, be discharged only to an intensive care unit; or be evaluated by an anesthesiologist prior to discharge to a medical-surgical unit.

TABLE 1–5. DISCHARGE CRITERIA

Standard: To be discharged from the PACU, the patient must maintain effective ventilation and perfusion of the lungs, as evidenced by the following:

  Regular respiratory pattern
  Respiratory rate appropriate for age
  Clear bilateral breath sounds
  Absence of restlessness and confusion
  Vital signs within preoperative range
  Pulse oximetry >95% saturation
  Arterial blood gases within normal limits
  Ability to maintain a patent airway

SUMMARY

The initial patient assessment in the PACU centers on stabilization of the airway, breathing, and circulation and on determining the presence of a physiologic alteration. Once initial priorities have been attended to, the PACU care team can begin to establish discharge criteria for the patient and, more importantly, can implement interventions designed to move the patient toward discharge from the PACU.

References

1. Apgar V: A proposal for a new method of evaluation of the newborn infant. Anesth Analg 32:260–267, 1953.
2. Carighan G, Kerri-Szanto M, Lavelle J: Post-anesthetic scoring system. Anesthesiology 25:396–397, 1964.
3. Aldrete AJ, Krovlik D: The postanesthetic recovery score. Anesth Analg 49:924–933, 1970.
4. Steward D: A simplified scoring system for the postoperative recovery room. Can Anaesth Soc J 22:111, 1975.
5. Robertson G, MacGregor D, Jones C: Evaluation of doxapram for arousal from general anesthesia in outpatients. Br J Anaesth 49:133–139, 1977.

Bibliography

Aldrete J: Assessment of recovery from anesthesia. Curr Rev Recovery Room Nurs 1:163–167, 1980.
Beard K, Jick H, Walker A: Adverse respiratory events occurring in the recovery room after general anesthesia. Anesthesiology 64:269, 1986.
Israel J, Dekomfeld T (eds): Recovery Room Care. Chicago, Year Book Medical Publishers, 1987.
Smith J, Watkins J: Care of the Postoperative Surgical Patient. Boston, Butterworth, 1985.
Wetchler B: Postanesthesia scoring system: discharging ambulatory surgery patients. AORN J 41:382–384, 1985.
Yao F, Artusio J: Anesthesiology: Problem-Oriented Patient Management. Philadelphia, Lippincott, 1983.

COMMON POST ANESTHETIC PROBLEMS 2

RICHARD G. BELATTI, JR.

The appearance of problems or complications during the period immediately following surgery and anesthesia is one of the primary reasons the recovery room, as we know it today, has evolved. To most physicians the development of a complication means the advent of "an accidental condition or second disease occurring in the course of a primary disease."[1] To anesthesiologists, however, complications develop with such regularity that the word accidental usually does not apply. Anesthesiologists are more likely to view the development of a complication as an expected part of recovery care. It is essential, then, that anesthesiologists be aware of the most common immediate post anesthetic problems and know how to treat them.

FREQUENCY OF COMPLICATIONS

Zelcer and Wells prospectively studied 443 patients admitted to the recovery room of a university-affiliated hospital in Melbourne, Australia over a 1-month period. Complications developed in 133 patients for an incidence of 30 per cent. Some patients developed more than one complication. Most of the complications were central nervous system or cardiovascular in nature[2] (Table 2–1). This chapter deals with four of the most commonly seen immediate post anesthetic complications. Other common problems are dealt with in detail in other chapters.

DELAYED AROUSAL

Delayed awakening (Fig. 2–1 after general anesthesia is a common and often easily explained problem. The etiology can usually be attributed to 1) prolonged action of anesthetic drugs, 2) metabolic causes, or 3) neurologic injury.[3] In most cases the prolonged sedation is the result of residual general anesthetic. Hypoventilation due to high concentrations of inhaled anesthetic limits the exhalation of the agent and prolongs its elimination.[4] Narcotics used as adjuvants to inhalation agents may contribute to hypercarbia and sedation as well. Hypothermia, advanced age, hepatic dysfunction, and renal disease may contribute to prolonged recovery from anesthetics by heightening sensitivity, delaying elimination, or both. The use of premedication may also prolong recovery, especially if narcotics or benzodiazepines (particularly diazepam) are used.[5]

In addition to slowing elimination of potent inhalation anesthetics, hypoxia and hypercapnia may develop in the hypoventilating patient. The ensuing hypercapnia may cause significant narcosis as well as potentiate the depressive effects of anesthetics. In the diabetic patient, the administration of chlorpropamide or excessive insulin preoperatively may cause postoperative hypoglycemia, unconsciousness, or even coma.[6]

Severe electrolyte disturbances are most commonly seen following excessive water absorption during transurethral prostate surgery. The subsequent dilutional hyponatremia may manifest as sedation, coma, or hemiparesis.[3] Dilutional hyponatremia may also be seen following the inappropriate release of antidiuretic hormone. Hypocalcemia following parathyroid surgery may result in delayed awakening. High magnesium levels following the prolonged administration of magnesium sulfate to the eclamptic or preeclamptic parturient may also result in prolonged postoperative sedation as well as muscle weakness after a general anesthetic cesarean section.

Neurologic injury and subsequent unconsciousness may be the result of an unsuspected cerebrovascular accident. Intracranial hemorrhage may result from hypertensive re-

TABLE 2–1. COMPLICATIONS IN 133 PATIENTS

Complication	Frequency
Unable to arouse	41
Pain	39
Hypotension	33
Arrhythmia	32
Agitation/dysphoria	13
Hypertension	13
Vomiting	13
Nausea	11
Oliguria	5
Cyanosis	4
Hypoventilation	4
Laryngeal spasm	3
Cardiac ischemia	3
Hypothermia	1
Stridor	1
Hyperglycemia	1

After Zelcer J, Wells DG: Anaesthetic-related recovery room complications. Anaesth Intens Care *15*:168–174, 1987.

sponses to anesthetic or surgical manipulations, especially in the anticoagulated patient.[3] Paradoxical air emboli may cross a probe patent foramen ovale in the presence of a right-to-left shunt. Direct emboli from cardiac valves, intracardiac thrombi, and atherosclerotic vessels may also be a threat. Fat emboli may occur after massive long bone or tissue damage and may not present until during or after surgi-cal manipulation or reduction of the fractures.[7] Deliberate, induced hypotension in normal patients is not usually associated with neurologic damage. However, uncontrolled intraoperative hypotension may result in ischemia, especially in the patient with hypertension or carotid occlusive disease.[8]

TREATMENT

The successful treatment of delayed arousal depends on careful consideration of the differential diagnosis. Thorough review of the patient's preoperative medical condition and the intraoperative course of events, both surgical and anesthetic, usually points to an etiology. If the cause of the sedation is not immediately obvious, the first consideration should be assessing the patient's oxygenation and ensuring adequate gas exchange. Pulse oximetry, end-tidal carbon dioxide measurement, and arterial blood gases can give an estimate of any ventilatory depression and rule out ongoing hypoxia and hypercarbia as factors.

If the cause is thought to be residual inhalational anesthetic, maintaining adequate ventilation should be sufficient treatment. If available, mass spectrophotometry can provide an estimate of exhaled anesthetic concentrations and confirm the diagnosis. Residual narcotic

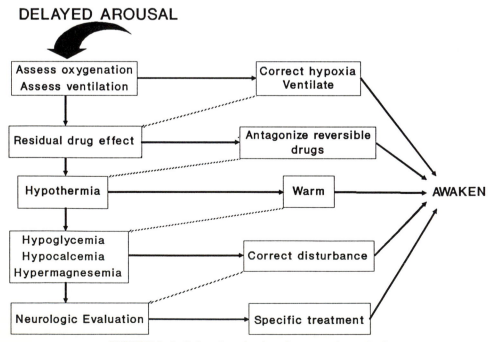

FIGURE 2–1. Delayed awakening after general anesthesia.

can be reversed by the specific antagonist naloxone, and anticholinergic central nervous system (CNS) depression can be reversed by physostigmine. Physostigmine has been reported to reverse sedation from other hypnotics and general anesthetics as well.[9,10]

The benzodiazepine antagonist flumazenil (Ro 15-1788; Hoffmann-La Roche) has been shown to directly antagonize the CNS sedative and amnestic effects of the benzodiazepines.[11] It has also been reported to partially reverse the cerebral effects of isoflurane in dogs.[12] Its duration of action is shorter than that of the longer-acting benzodiazepines (i.e., lorazepam, diazepam) but longer than that of midazolam.[11] Although still considered an investigational drug in the United States, flumazenil is already in clinical use in Europe. Aminophylline has also been reported to reverse benzodiazepine sedation, but the reports are less than conclusive in support of its use.[13,14]

Body temperature should be determined and warming instituted if hypothermia exists. Serum electrolytes, magnesium, and calcium should be checked if ion disturbance is suspected. Blood for a serum glucose assay may also be drawn, but the simple finger-stick glucose determination is faster and accurate enough to exclude hypoglycemia from consideration if normal. Other laboratory tests may be useful as well if hepatic or renal disease is under consideration.

Unless perioperative events point specifically to it, neurologic injury is usually a diagnosis of exclusion. If other causes of prolonged arousal have been excluded, a thorough neurologic consultation should be obtained.

AGITATION/DYSPHORIA

Immediate postoperative agitation or dysphoria (Fig. 2–2) is not a common problem but one that occurs frequently enough that anesthesiologists should be prepared to evaluate and treat it. Emergence excitement may be seen in as few as 0.4 per cent or as many as 13.0 per cent of patients.[2,15] However, it seems to be seen more frequently after tonsillectomy, thyroid surgery, circumcision, hysterectomy, and perineal and abdominal wall procedures.[15]

Hypoxia and resulting air hunger, as well as hypercarbia, may present as restlessness, disorientation, slurred speech, and agitation. Hyponatremia (as after prostate surgery), hypo-

chloremia, and acid-base changes can all be seen during the immediate postoperative period and can be the cause of mental confusion.[16] Pain is a common cause of restlessness and is frequently seen postoperatively.[17] The pain may be related to the surgery itself (i.e., incisional) or due to prolonged positioning on the operating table. Urinary bladder and gastric distension, which may cause considerable discomfort, are easily overlooked.

Drug reactions are commonly implicated as the cause of postoperative agitation. Such reactions are probably less common than they once were, as the use of offending drugs is less prevalent. The most frequently implicated drugs are the anticholinergics, most notably scopolamine and atropine. They have been shown to have CNS toxic effects that can include psychotic behavior, delirium, and motor disturbances.[18] Ketamine is also associated with a high incidence of unpleasant dreaming, which may result in delirium and agitation.[19] Neuroleptic drugs, e.g., droperidol, especially in high doses, may be associated with the development of dyskinesia and involuntary muscle activity as well as postoperative confusion.[20,21] The development of extrapyramidal reactions to even low doses of droperidol has also been reported.[22] Eckenhoff et al. found a fairly high incidence of postoperative excitement with diethyl ether and cyclopropane, but a very low incidence with halothane or thiopental with nitrous oxide.[15] Prolonged administration of the modern agents alone has not been associated with any appreciable incidence of emergence excitement, although delayed mental impairment was common.[23]

The patient's state of apprehension or anxiety can have a marked effect on the appearance of emergence agitation. Especially apprehensive patients and, conversely, those seemingly unconcerned about forthcoming major surgery may show significant anxiety upon emergence. Young patients tend to have an increased incidence of postoperative excitation as do patients undergoing emergency procedures.[15,24] Several psychiatric factors have been shown to increase the incidence of postoperative delirium. A history of alcoholism, insomnia, depression, and debility statistically increases the chances of emergence phenomenon.[24]

TREATMENT

The goals of the treatment of postoperative agitation include 1) determining an etiology, 2)

AGITATION/DYSPHORIA

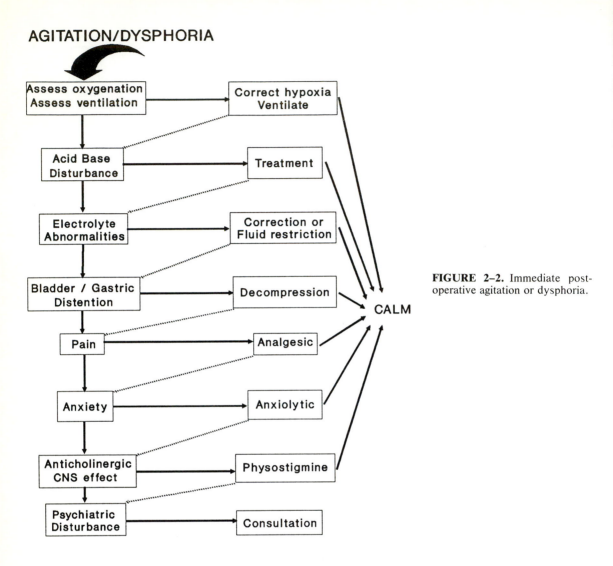

FIGURE 2–2. Immediate postoperative agitation or dysphoria.

initiating specific therapy, and 3) protecting patients from injuring themselves.[25] When one encounters a restless, confused postoperative patient, the first efforts must be addressed to ensuring that the agitation is not the result of hypoxia. Presuming pain to be the cause of agitation in a hypoxic patient and treating the excitement with narcotics or sedatives may have disastrous consequences. Hypoxia should be quickly excluded from the differential diagnosis by pulse oximetry, arterial blood gas determination, or both. The practice of relying on the appearance of cyanosis to indicate hypoxia is fraught with danger. Cyanosis may not be present until at least 5 gm/dl of blood becomes desaturated, at which point significant hypoxia may already be present. Moreover, the observation of cyanosis may be hindered by lighting, pigmentation, anemia, and

observer bias.[26] A high recovery room score may not even ensure adequate oxygenation. In children, at least, wakefulness has been shown to bear no correlation with oxygen saturation during the immediate postoperative period.[27] All postoperative patients who undergo any form of general anesthetic or sedation should receive supplemental oxygen via a mask or nasal cannula. If pulse oximetry is available, continuous monitoring in the recovery room is ideal.

Hyponatremia may be suspected in the confused postprostate surgery patient, especially if the surgery was prolonged. A serum electrolyte determination can confirm the diagnosis. The treatment usually consists of fluid restriction and, rarely, hypertonic saline administration. Severe acid-base disturbances can be diagnosed and therapy directed by arterial blood gas determination. If pain appears to be the diagnosis after the exclusion of hypoxia, intravenous narcotics may be administered in small increments. Regional anesthesia, intrathecal and epidural opioids, and local anesthetic infiltration can also be successful in treating the pain. The intramuscular route of administration of narcotics can be unpredictable in onset, uptake, duration, and effect and has no place in modern recovery room care. Gastric distension may be relieved by nasogastric aspiration, and urinary bladder distension is easily treated by in-and-out catheterization.

The CNS effects of the anticholinergics are usually dramatically reversed by the administration of physostigmine.[9,18] The duration of the CNS effects of the anticholinergics may be longer than the action of the physostigmine owing to its rapid metabolism. As a result, repeated doses may be required if delirium reappears.[18] There are reports that physostigmine might be effective for reversing the CNS effects of droperidol and some general anesthetics as well.[9,10,28] The incidence of hallucinations with ketamine may be decreased by benzodiazepine or droperidol administration.[29]

When dealing with perioperative anxiety, the best treatment is prevention. The frequency of postoperative anxiety can be reduced by a thorough and informative preanesthetic visit.[30] Discussions about the type of anesthesia and its risks, as well as explanations of the routines, both preoperative and postoperative, can allay anxiety and reduce recovery room confusion. Some patients need reassurance that they will not experience intraoperative awareness and will receive pain medications, if needed, upon awakening. If postoperative endotracheal intubation or mechanical ventilation is anticipated, the patient should be informed and the reasons fully discussed. Patients should be told that they will be unable to talk so long as the endotracheal tube is in place and that every effort will be made to make them comfortable until it is removed.

Occasionally, one is faced with a restless postoperative patient who does not seem to be getting relief from narcotic administration. Assuming that the other possible diagnoses are excluded, the agitation may be the manifestation of anxiety. The sedation resulting from the accumulation of the continued doses of narcotics may eventually quiet the patient, although small intravenous doses of a short-acting benzodiazepine such as midazolam may be warranted. The anxiolytics should be administered in reduced doses, as their respiratory depressant effects may be additive with existing narcotics, sedatives, or residual general anesthetics. If overt psychotic behavior is apparent, despite adequate treatment, psychiatric consultation should be obtained.

NAUSEA/VOMITING

Nausea and vomiting (Fig. 2–3), though usually not life-threatening, are probably the most unpleasant and lasting memories many patients have of their anesthetic. In fact, most patients judge our proficiency at administering anesthesia by their perioperative experiences. Although the incidence has decreased in recent years, nausea and vomiting still result in significant postoperative morbidity and patient discomfort.[2,31,32] *Nausea* is described as a subjective, unpleasant mental experience, usually leading to vomiting. *Retching* is the rhythmic muscular activity that usually precedes vomiting. *Vomiting* is defined as the forceful expulsion of gastrointestinal contents through the mouth.[33]

The act of vomiting is controlled by the bilateral vomiting center. It is located in the medulla near the tractus solitarius in close proximity to the dorsal motor nucleus of the vagus and other nuclei responsible for the physiologic processes involved in vomiting. Once stimulated, the vomiting center sends efferent impulses via the fifth, seventh, ninth, tenth, and twelfth cranial nerves, the phrenic nerves, and the spinal nerves to the esophagus, stomach, and diaphragm. This diverse efferent output is responsible for the considerable physiologic response accompanying emesis.

The vomiting center receives input from four major routes (Fig. 2–4): 1) Irritative stimuli can arise directly from the gastrointestinal tract. Irritation or distension of the stomach and initial portion of the duodenum seem to provide the strongest stimulation. 2) Input from the chemoreceptor trigger zone (CTZ) is responsible for most drug-related nausea and vomiting. The CTZ is a bilateral area located on the floor of the fourth ventricle above the area postrema. Stimulation of the CTZ by certain drugs and metabolic disorders results in triggering of the vomiting center and subsequent emesis. 3) Stimulation of the labyrinthine apparatus (motion sickness) can result in afferent impulses being transmitted by the vestibular nuclei to the cerebellum. From

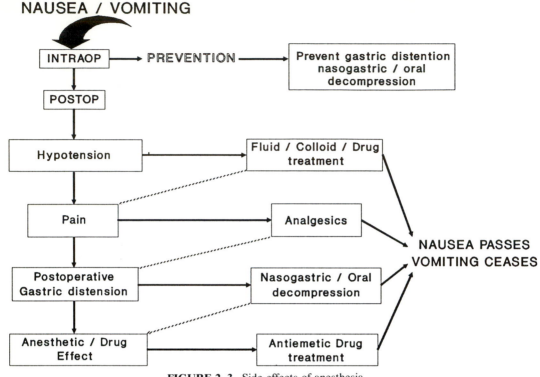

FIGURE 2–3. Side-effects of anesthesia.

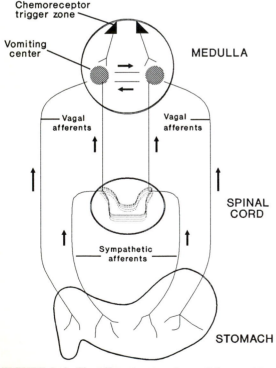

FIGURE 2–4. The afferent connections of the vomiting center. (After Guyton AC: Textbook of Medical Physiology. 6th ed., Philadelphia, Saunders, 1981, pp. 832–834. With permission.)

there the signal is believed to be passed to the chemoreceptor trigger zone and on to the vomiting center. 4) Various visual and cortical (psychic) input, e.g., disquieting scenes, noisome odors, can directly stimulate the vomiting center, as well.[34]

Decidedly unpleasant, vomiting can also be dangerous. The physical exertion may increase postoperative bleeding and disrupt delicate suture lines. Tearing or rupture of the esophagus is probably rare but must be a concern in patients with a history of esophageal pathology. Aspiration of emesis is a life-threatening complication in the patient whose airway protective reflexes are blunted by residual anesthetic or sedative drugs or damaged by surgical activity. If the vomiting is protracted, dangerous hypokalemia, hypochloremia, hyponatremia, and dehydration may develop. Nausea and vomiting are leading causes of unexpected hospitalization following surgery.[35]

Though blamed by many suffering patients as the cause of their nausea and vomiting, the newer general anesthetics have generally resulted in less nausea and vomiting than their predecessors. Interestingly, halothane in sub-anesthetic doses may even be antiemetic.[36]

Whereas ether and cyclopropane had nausea and vomiting associated with their use as much as 56 per cent of the time,[31] the newer agents appear to trigger these complaints somewhat less frequently. The authors of a review of the subject estimated that the incidence of emetic problems accompanying anesthesia is still around 30 percent, however.[37]

The contribution of nitrous oxide to postoperative nausea and vomiting is a sharply debated subject. Some investigators have suggested that nitrous oxide causes an increased incidence of emetic sequelae.[38,39] The use of nitrous oxide is said to cause nausea and vomiting by gastric distension, sympathetic stimulation, and changes in middle ear pressure. Not all investigators have been able to prove an association between the use of nitrous oxide and the development of postoperative nausea and vomiting, however.[40]

Adjuvant drugs given preoperatively or in conjunction with the inhalation anesthetics may themselves be suspected of contributing to the high rate of emetic sequelae accompanying modern anesthesia. The opioids, when given as premedicants, may contribute to nausea and vomiting. Premedication with morphine sulfate is known to increase the incidence of postoperative emetic problems.[41] Meperidine has also been shown to cause nausea and vomiting when administered as a premedication.[42] There is disagreement as to which of the two narcotics causes the highest incidence of emetic sequelae.[40] At least one review has indicated that meperidine may even be antiemetic at doses less than 1 mg/kg.[43]

When administered alone or in conjunction with the narcotics, the anticholinergics can act as potent antiemetics.[41] Of the available anticholinergics, scopolamine (hyoscine) appears to be slightly more effective than atropine,[44] and glycopyrrolate appears to have no antiemetic effect, presumably owing to its inability to cross the blood-brain barrier.[45]

Muscle relaxants are thought not to influence postoperative vomiting.[37] The reversal of the muscle relaxants may contribute, however. Neostigmine has potent muscarinic effects and may increase intestinal peristalsis and may even trigger spasm.[46] King et al. reported an increased incidence of postoperative nausea and vomiting in patients whose muscle relaxant was reversed with neostigmine, even though atropine was administered at the same time.[46]

Spinal anesthesia has long been known to trigger a significant incidence of nausea and vomiting. Bonica et al. found a 21 per cent incidence of emesis accompanying spinal anesthesia and only an 8.8 per cent incidence accompanying peripheral nerve block.[32] During spinal anesthesia, a systolic blood pressure below 80 mm Hg results in a significant increase in emesis. The administration of 100 per cent oxygen to patients with hypotension of less than 80 mm Hg significantly decreases the development of emesis. Based on these data, Ratra et al. theorized that vomiting center hypoxia is responsible for the emesis seen with hypotensive spinal anesthesia.[47]

Gastric distension or irritation causes nausea and vomiting by direct stimulation of the vomiting center.[34] The stomach may be most commonly distended during anesthesia by manual insufflation via mask ventilation. The swallowing of air or blood may also result in significant stomach irritation.[37] Approximately 10 per cent of patients swallow air perioperatively.[48] Nitrous oxide diffusion into the stomach and bowel may also contribute to distension, especially in the presence of swallowed air.[48]

The site of the surgery may influence the development of postoperative nausea and vomiting. In the pediatric population, strabismus surgery and orchiopexy have been associated with a significant incidence of nausea and vomiting.[35] In adults, gastrointestinal procedures have a high frequency of postoperative emesis, whereas the incidence is low with abdominal wall procedures.[32] Laparoscopic procedures may be associated with postoperative nausea and vomiting as well,[35] and a high incidence has been associated with ophthalmic and otologic procedures.[36,49] The duration of the procedure may also affect the frequency of postoperative nausea and vomiting. Generally, the longer the procedure, the higher the incidence of postoperative emetic complications.[32,37] The presence of postoperative pain triggers nausea and vomiting in many patients. Thus relieving postoperative pain often relieves the nausea as well.[50]

Certain patient characteristics may be associated with postoperative nausea and vomiting. Patients with a history of motion sickness or those who have had previous episodes of postoperative vomiting are most likely to experience postoperative emetic sequelae with each subsequent anesthetic.[51] A certain number of patients experience nausea after a period of fasting, even prior to the administration of any drugs.[37] Early postoperative ambulation may also increase postoperative emesis.[52] Many patients develop nausea upon their first movement and thus may have emesis during transport from a postanesthesia care unit.[40]

The female gender is said to be associated with a high incidence of postoperative emesis. Summarizing several studies, Palazzo and Strunin stated that "emetic episodes are two to three times more common among females."[37] A study by Muir et al. at the Mayo Clinic confirmed an association between female gender and postoperative nausea and vomiting.[40]

The incidence of nausea and vomiting tends to decrease with advancing age and may be twice as high in children as in adults.[37,40] Obesity has been said to increase the frequency of emesis as well.[48] However, some investigators have been unable to associate any increase in emesis with obesity.[40]

Other circumstances may act to increase the likelihood of postoperative emesis in any given patient. Patients with a full stomach from either a recent meal or swallowed blood are likely to vomit on induction of or emergence from anesthesia. Intoxication with alcohol or illicit drugs may also increase the frequency of emesis. Acute appendicitis or bowel obstruction is notoriously associated with pre- and postoperative emesis. In neurosurgical patients, especially those with closed head injury, increased intracranial pressure may trigger nausea and vomiting.[37]

Treatment

The most effective treatment for postoperative emetic sequelae is prevention of their occurrence. Several maneuvers merit mention as being fairly simple to perform and effective in their usefulness. Avoidance of gastric insufflation is paramount. As mentioned above, gastric distension is a common cause of nausea, and because prevention is easier than treatment avoidance of manual ventilation except via an endotracheal tube minimizes the chance of inflating the stomach with anesthetic gases. The stomach can be distended with other substances during anesthesia. The most common and preventable factor is the swallowing of blood during oral, pharyngeal, or nasal surgery. In addition to irritation caused by direct distension, blood is a gastric irritant.[37] Packing the pharynx and the active use of suctioning in such situations can reduce the volume of in-

gested blood. If distension of the stomach is suspected, it should be decompressed intraoperatively. One should be vigilant for unrecognized nasal bleeding postoperatively as a cause of late-occurring nausea as well.

A nasogastric suctioning tube may be useful for emptying fluids or gases from the stomach. Unfortunately, its presence in the patient emerging from anesthesia may trigger gagging and subsequent vomiting.[53] An oral airway may elicit much the same response in a partially conscious patient. In an extubated patient, such an airway must be removed at the first signs of gagging in order to prevent vomiting and subsequent aspiration. Vigorous nasal or oropharyngeal suctioning can also elicit a strong gag reflex and trigger vomiting. If extensive suctioning is to be performed, it is best taken care of while the patient is still anesthetized or while the airway is protected by an endotracheal tube.

Early movement during the postoperative period is associated with nausea.[40,54] Although early ambulation is often a goal of outpatient, same-day surgery, it may be prudent to limit movement in patients prone to nausea.

Many drugs have been shown to possess antiemetic qualities. Some are most effective when given prophylactically. Many of the drugs are associated with a significant incidence of negative or undesirable side effects. As a result, many investigators consider prophylactic administration unjustified,[55] whereas others consider their prophylactic use justified in specific cases or circumstances.[54] Included in this list of circumstances are patients at higher risk than average because of personal characteristics or the surgical site.

The available antiemetics can be divided into five major groups: anticholinergics, phenothiazines, antihistamines, butyrophenones, and antidopaminergics.

The *anticholinergics* have long been known to have antiemetic qualities. The three most common drugs in this class are atropine, scopolamine (hyoscine), and glycopyrrolate. Glycopyrrolate has no apparent antiemetic properties. Unlike atropine and scopolamine, it is a quaternary ammonium compound and has no central effects, presumably because it cannot cross the blood-brain border.[56] Atropine and scopolamine are tertiary amines and do possess central effects. Both drugs act directly on the vomiting center. Of the two, scopolamine appears to be more sedating.[54] Atropine was first described as an antiemetic in 1883.[57] It has been shown to decrease nausea and vomiting by up to 50 per cent with or without the concomitant administration of morphine.[41] Unfortunately, it can cause considerable tachycardia, and thus its use is limited to those tolerant of any increase in heart rate. Scopolamine appears to be a slightly more effective antiemetic.[44] It usually causes no increase in heart rate. The anticholinergics are seldom used for their antiemetic effects, however. They can cause dry mouth, sedation, disorientation, agitation, and hallucinations, especially in the elderly. As a result, their usefulness is severely limited. Scopolamine is an effective prophylactic for motion sickness when given via a transdermal patch. Unfortunately, the patch has thus far not shown great efficacy for the treatment of perioperative emesis.[58,59]

The *phenothiazines* are also effective antiemetics. For the most part, the clinically useful ones also possess antidopaminergic, anticholinergic, and antihistaminic activity. They are broadly broken down into two groups, dimethylamino phenothiazines (promethazine and chlorpromazine) and the piperazines (prochlorperazine and perphenazine). The dimethylamino drugs are less antiemetic and more sedating. Conversely, the piperazines cause less sedation and are better antiemetics.

Chlorpromazine (Thorazine) is an effective prophylactic antiemetic. However, it can cause hypotension and sedation, which limits its postoperative usefulness.[60] It is also ineffective for treating motion sickness.[54] Promethazine (Phenergan), frequently used as a premedication, is an effective prophylactic antiemetic. It is also antihistaminic and anticholinergic and has been suggested as useful in asthmatic patients. It may cause delayed postoperative arousal and sedation. It is effective against motion sickness and, as such, is particularly useful in ear surgery patients.[54]

Prochlorperazine (Compazine) possesses antidopaminergic activity and increases lower esophageal sphincter tone.[61] It may depress the cough reflex, so close guard of the airway must be maintained until the effects of sedatives and anesthetics have worn off.[35] Perphenazine is antidopaminergic as well but causes more sedation than prochlorperazine. Though the piperazines are excellent antiemetics, they frequently cause extrapyramidal side effects,[62] which may be seen after relatively small doses and may arise up to 24 hours after administration. The first line of treatment of these dangerous side effects is intravenous promethazine.[54]

The *antihistamines* can be effective antiemetic agents. They appear to function on the vomiting center and the vestibular pathways. They are especially effective for treating motion sickness. They can all cause sedation, a side effect that may limit their universal use. They do appear to have fewer side effects than the phenothiazines, however, and some choose them as their first line drug.[54] The most commonly used drugs in this group include cyclizine (Marezine), promethazine (Phenergan), diphenhydramine (benadryl), and dimenhydrinate (Dramamine).

The *butyrophenones* function as antiemetics owing to their strong antidopamine activity. They act at the chemoreceptor emetic trigger zone.[63] The two commercially available drugs in this category are haloperidol (Haldol) and droperidol (Inapsine). Although both possess antiemetic activities, droperidol has been used more extensively. It appears to be effective when given at almost any time perioperatively.[64] It is effective when given by the oral,[65] intramuscular, and intravenous[64] routes. It has a half-life of 2.3 hours after intravenous administration and a duration of action of 3 to 6 hours.[35,66] Many studies have proved its efficacy as a prophylactic antiemetic in small doses (0.005 to 0.070 mg/kg), and some investigators have advocated its use as the drug of choice for prophylaxis.[54] It appears to be as effective in small doses (0.25 mg/70 kg) as it is in large doses.[67] The butyrophenones do have side effects associated with their use that must be kept in mind. They possess mild α-adrenergic blocking activity, which may result in vasodilation and hypotension.[35] They may also cause drowsiness.[59] Extrapyramidal reactions, including acute dystonia, parkinsonism, and akathisia may occur. The symptoms may manifest soon after drug administration, or they may not occur until several hours later, long after many ambulatory patients have already been discharged to home. For the most part, the side effects are considered to be dose-dependent, although extrapyramidal reactions after doses as low as 0.65 mg have been reported.[22] Dysphoric-type reactions have also been reported when the drug has been given preoperatively. Some patients have even refused to undergo surgery after receiving droperidol preoperatively.[64]

The *antidopaminergics* domperidone and metoclopramide (Reglan) do not possess antihistaminic properties and are not phenothiazines.[54] These drugs appear to be gastrointestinal system stimulants. They increase lower esophageal sphincter tone and decrease gastric emptying time.[35,54] Metoclopramide has both central and peripheral activity.[66] Both drugs have few side effects associated with their use at the usual clinical doses. Because metoclopramide can cross the blood-brain barrier, it may cause sedation, dysphoric reactions, and extrapyramidal symptoms in higher doses, however.[68] Metoclopramide is used extensively in the United States in doses of 5 to 20 mg IM or IV for both prophylaxis and treatment of nausea and vomiting. It has a half-life of 2.76 hours after intravenous administration and a duration of action of 1 to 2 hours after intramuscular or intravenous injection.[35,66] Domperidone is a newer antiemetic with activity similar to that of metoclopramide. Domperidone cannot cross the blood-brain barrier as easily and so affects only the CTZ that is outside the barrier.[54] It can be given by the intravenous or intramuscular route but is currently unavailable for clinical use in the United States. When compared to metoclopramide, it has been said to be more suited for treatment than for prophylaxis of nausea and vomiting.[54]

Other treatments have been suggested as well, but none has gained widespread acceptance. The active compound in marijuana smoke, Δ^9-tetrahydrocannabinol, and a synthetic cannabinoid, nabilone, have been shown to possess antiemetic properties. The high incidence of undesirable side effects associated with these substances makes it unlikely that their clinical use will ever be realized.[54] Intravenous lidocaine has been reported to decrease the incidence of postoperative vomiting in children after strabismus surgery.[69] However, in a comparison study, intravenous droperidol was significantly more

effective than lidocaine at reducing postoperative vomiting without prolonging recovery time.[70] Acupuncture and acupressure have been shown to decrease postoperative emesis under certain conditions.[71,72] However, many of these techniques are not widely known, and their effectiveness has not been firmly established in Western medicine.[73]

Along with the above-mentioned medications and maneuvers, it is important to remember the supportive care of the nauseated or vomiting patient. If vomiting is severe, electrolyte replacement should be considered. Prolonged vomiting may result in hypovolemia. Intravenous fluid infusions may need to be increased to compensate. Narcotics should never be withheld from nauseated patients complaining of pain. Pain itself may cause vomiting.[50]

[*Editor's note:* Further discussion of nausea and vomiting as it pertains to outpatient recovery may be found in Chapter 20.]

SHIVERING

Postanesthetic shivering (Fig. 2–5) was first described in 1950.[74] It has been seen after virtually all currently used anesthetics including halothane, enflurane, isoflurane, and narcotic–nitrous oxide.[75] Shivering is usually attributed to intraoperative hypothermia and, in fact, is usually thought of as a thermoregulatory function. In physiologic terms, a *shiver* is defined as an involuntary tremor in homeotherms induced by cooling, the effect of which is production of body heat.[76]

Postanesthetic shivering may be seen after general anesthesia in 22 to 50 per cent of cases.[77] The incidence seems to be increased

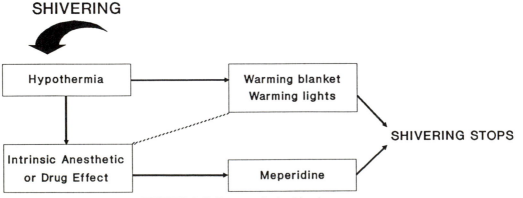

FIGURE 2–5. Postanesthetic shivering.

in prolonged cases and in those involving large amounts of blood loss, fluid administration, or both. Area of surgery, type of premedication, type of anesthesia, and sex appear to have no effect on the frequency of postanesthetic shivering, whereas advancing age is associated with a decreasing incidence.[78]

Shivering may be seen after regional anesthesia as well. It is commonly associated with epidural anesthesia, a fact well witnessed by those practicing obstetric anesthesia. The incidence associated with epidural anesthesia has been noted to be 45 to 64 per cent, although shivering is seen to accompany labor and delivery in approximately 23 per cent of normal parturients not receiving epidural anesthesia.[79]

Shivering is associated with several undesirable physiologic effects. Oxygen consumption, carbon dioxide production, and metabolic rate may increase as much as 500 per cent above baseline levels during postanesthetic shivering.[80–82] It may be an added stress not well tolerated by patients with cardiac, pulmonary, or vascular disease. Indeed, reports of myocardial infarction attributed to this stress have been recorded.[83] Wound dehiscence, dental damage, and increased intraocular pressure may also develop and are of concern.[75,84]

The shivering seen postoperatively has traditionally been viewed as a thermodynamic response to the hypothermia that may develop during modern anesthesia and surgery in air-conditioned operating rooms.[77] Indeed, body temperatures predictably fall with exposure in the operating room.[85] Unfortunately, many studies show no correlation between patients who shiver and the fall in body temperature. Many patients become hypothermic and show no signs of shivering. Furthermore, abolishing the shivering with medication does not usually increase body temperature.[77]

Other researchers have attributed the postanesthetic tremor not to hypothermia but to adrenal suppression, respiratory alkalosis, pyrogen release, or decreased sympathetic activity.[84] More intriguingly, however, it has been suggested that shivering is the result of the recovery of spinal cord activity before the upper motor neurons have recovered from the effects of the general anesthetic.[84,86,87] Investigators have discovered that the postanesthetic "shiver" electromyographic (EMG) pattern is unlike that associated with pure hypothermia.[84,88] Hypothermic shivering appears to be characterized by a low-amplitude modulated "waxing and waning" EMG signal of four to eight cycles per minute that does not include prolonged clonic activity. The EMG obtained during postanesthetic "shivering" is strikingly different, however. During recovery from isoflurane anesthesia, the EMG appears to show poorly defined bursts ranging from 5 to 15 Hz as well as pronounced clonus-like signals at 6 Hz.[84,88] Sessler et al. found no correlation between rectal temperature and EMG or clinical muscle activity. There was correlation, however, between all types of muscular activity and an end-tidal isoflurane concentration range of 0.10 to 0.19 per cent. They interpreted their findings to indicate that the postanesthetic tremor was actually spinal reflex hyperactivity caused by the inhibition of descending cortical control by residual anesthetic rather than thermoregulatory activity.[84] In an editorial published in the same journal, Hammel suggested that the abnormal postanesthetic tremor may still be a thermodynamic response to hypothermia, with the residual anesthetic interfering with normal activity in the responding muscles.[89]

TREATMENT

It has been suggested that prevention of intraoperative cooling might lessen postoperative shivering. In laparoscopy patients, the intraoperative use of an active airway heater/humidifier in the anesthesia gas circuit appears to lessen patient cooling significantly. Conahan et al.[90] found that patients were significantly warmer upon arrival in the recovery room, tended to shiver less, and, on average, were discharged 31 per cent sooner than control patients not receiving airway warming. However, passive heat and moisture exchangers used in a similar group of patients resulted in no preservation of body temperature, nor did their use shorten recovery time.[91]

In a group of children weighing between 5 and 30 kg, a passive heat and moisture exchanger appeared to retard temperature loss, and an active airway heater-humidifier increased body temperature during its use on the same patient population.[92]

Numerous interventions have been suggested as treatment for post anesthetic shivering. The most common and traditional are concerned with warming the patient in some fashion. The most successful appear to involve surface warming. Sharkey et al. were able to halt shivering in 22 of 30 post anesthetic patients by applying radiant heat from three 250 watt infrared heatlamps to the anterior thorax through a lightweight gown or sheet. The patients ceased shivering within 60 seconds of infrared heat application and resumed shivering within 42 seconds when the heat was removed.[93] The study indicated that peripheral warming alone, without changing the core temperatures, inhibited or stopped post anesthetic shivering.

Sessler and Moayeri[94] compared the use of heating lamps, a thermal warmer, a circulating-water blanket, and a Bair Hugger forced-air warmer on healthy, unanesthetized volunteers. They found that when set on "medium" the Bair Hugger was more effective than the radiant devices and as effective as the circulating-water blanket at heat transfer. When set on "high," the forced-air warmer transferred enough heat to increase mean body temperature approximately 1.5°C/hr. Lennon et al.[95] were able to reduce postoperative shivering and shorten recovery room time significantly by the use of the Bair Hugger forced-air warmer on a group of 30 postoperative patients.

Several drugs have been suggested as treatment for post anesthetic shivering as well. Magnesium sulfate and methylphenidate (Ritalin) have shown some effectiveness.[77,86] Paralysis with neuromuscular blocking drugs and high dose morphine sulfate infusions effectively suppress shivering and its metabolic consequences, but they require prolonged ventilatory support and extend the period required for rewarming.[96] The most effective drug treatment appears to be small intravenous doses of meperidine (Demerol). Doses as small as 12.5 mg suppressed shivering in 67 per cent of patients in one study, and 50 mg stopped post anesthetic shivering in 100 per cent in another.[80,97] The small doses of meperidine also lessened the increases in oxygen consumption, carbon dioxide production, and minute ventilation associated with shivering.[80] Although the role of preoperative drugs in the development of post anesthetic shivering has not been thoroughly investigated, one study has indicated that patients on chronic propranolol therapy have a greatly reduced incidence of post anesthetic shivering.[78]

The shivering associated with epidural anesthesia has been attributed to the cold temperature of the crystalloid infusion or local anesthetic. Unfortunately, warming the crystalloid or epidural solution has had conflicting results. Some investigators have successfully prevented shivering by warming the infusing crystalloid or the epidural anesthetic solution.[98,99] On the other hand, some have observed no change in the incidence of shivering or even an increased incidence when warming solutions.[100,101] Harris et al. showed that the shivering was not the result of toxic levels of lidocaine or excessive catecholamine levels as has been suggested.[100] Once the shivering has developed, the epidural administration of narcotics has been shown to be an effective treatment.[102] Pretreatment with meperidine prior to the blockade does not appear to prevent shivering, however.[100]

References

1. Jones HW, Hoerr NL, Osol A: Blakiston's New Gould Medical Dictionary, 1st ed. New York, Blakiston, 1949.
2. Zelcer J, Wells DG: Anaesthetic-related recovery room complications. Anaesth Intens Care *15*:168–174, 1987.

Delayed Arousal
3. Denlinger JK: Prolonged emergence and failure to regain consciousness. *In* Orkin FK, Cooperman LH, eds: Complications in Anesthesiology. Philadelphia, Lippincott, 1983, pp. 368–380.
4. Stoelting RK, Eger EI II: The effects of ventilation and anesthetic solubility on recovery from anesthesia: an in vivo and analog analysis before and after equilibrium. Anesthesiology *30*:290–296, 1969.
5. Korttila K: Postanesthetic cognitive and psychomotor impairment. Int Anesthesiol Clin *24*(4):59–74, 1986.
6. Schen RJ, Khazzam AS: Postoperative hypoglycemic coma associated with chlorpropamide. Br J Anaesth *47*:899–900, 1975.
7. Patrick RT, Devloo RA: Embolic phenomena of the operative and postoperative period. Anesthesiology *22*:751–758, 1961.
8. Strandgaard S: Autoregulation of cerebral blood flow in hypertensive patients. Circulation *53*:720–727, 1976.
9. Rosenberg H: Physostigmine reversal of sedative drugs. JAMA *299*:1168, 1973.
10. Artru AA, Hui GS: Physostigmine reversal of general anesthesia for intraoperative testing: associated EEG changes. Anesth Analg *65*:1059–1062, 1986.
11. Klotz U, Kanto J: Pharmacokinetics and clinical use of flumazenil (Ro 15-1788). Clin Pharmacokinet *14*:1–12, 1988.
12. Roald OK, Forsman M, Steen PA: Partial reversal of the cerebral effects of isoflurane in the dog by the benzodiazepine antagonist flumazenil. Acta Anaesthesiol Scand *32*:209–212, 1988.
13. Wangler MA, Kilpatrick DS: Aminophylline is an antagonist of lorazepam. Anesth Analg *64*:834–836, 1985.
14. Sleigh JW: Failure of aminiphylline to antagonize midazolam sedation. Anesth Analg *65*:540, 1986.

Agitation/Dysphoria

15. Eckenhoff JE, Kneale DH, Dripps RD: The incidence and etiology of post-anesthetic excitement. Anesthesiology 22:667–673, 1961.
16. Kaufer C: Etiology of consciousness disturbances in surgery. Minn Med 51:1509–1515, 1968.
17. Donovan M, Dillon P, McGuire L: Incidence and characteristics of pain in a sample of medical-surgical inpatients. Pain 30:69–78, 1985.
18. Ketchum JS, Sidell FR Jr, Crowell EB, et al: Atropine, scopolamine, and ditran: comparative pharmacology and antagonists in man. Psychopharmacology 28:121–145, 1973.
19. Katz NM, Agle DP, DePalma RG, et al: Delirium in surgical patients under intensive care. Arch Surg 104:310–313, 1972.
20. Black JL, Richelson E, Richardson JW: Antipsychotic agents: a clinical update. Mayo Clin Proc 60:777–789, 1985.
21. Korttila K, Linnoilla M: Skills related to driving after intravenous diazepam, flunitrazepam, or droperidol. Br J Anaesth 46:961–969, 1974.
22. Melnick BM: Extrapyramidal reactions to low-dose droperidol. Anesthesiology 69:424–426, 1988.
23. Davidson LA, Steinhelber JC, Eger EI II, et al: Psychological effects of halothane and isoflurane anesthesia. Anesthesiology 43:313–324, 1975.
24. Morse RM, Litin EM: Postoperative delirium: a study of etiologic factors. Am J Psychiatry 126:388–395, 1969.
25. McCammon RL: Management of Postanesthesia Complications in the Recovery Room. 1987 Review Course Lectures. Lake Buena Vista, Florida, International Anesthesia Research Society, 1987, pp. 90–97.
26. Comroe JH, Botelho S: The unreliability of cyanosis in the recognition of arterial anoxemia. Am J Med Sci 214:1–6, 1947.
27. Soliman IE, Patel RI, Ehrenpreis MB, Hannallah RS: Recovery scores do not correlate with postoperative hypoxemia in children. Anesth Analg 67:53–56, 1988.
28. Bidwai AV, Cornelius LR, Stanley TH: Reversal of Innovar-induced postanesthetic somnolence and disorientation with physostigmine. Anesthesiology 44:249–252, 1976.
29. Sadove MS, Hartano D, Redlin T, et al: Clinical study of droperidol in the prevention of the side effects of ketamine anesthesia: a progress report. Anesth Analg 50:526–532, 1971.
30. Rosenberg H: Postoperative emotional responses. In Orkin FK, Cooperman LH (eds): Complications in Anesthesiology. Philadelphia, Lippincott, 1983, pp. 355–367.

Nausea/Vomiting

31. Waters RM: The present status of cyclopropane. Br Med J 2:1013–1017, 1936.
32. Bonica JJ, Creps W, Monk B, et al: Postoperative nausea, retching and vomiting. Anesthesiology 19:532–540, 1958.
33. Borison HL, Wang SC: Physiology and pharmacology of vomiting. Pharmacol Rev 5:192–230, 1953.
34. Guyton AC: Textbook of Medical Physiology, 6th ed. Philadelphia, Saunders, 1981, pp. 832–834.
35. Litwack K, Parnass S: Practical points in the management of postoperative nausea and vomiting. J Post Anesth Nurs 3:275–277, 1988.
36. Haumann J, Foster P: The antiemetic effect of halothane. Br J Anaesth 35:114–117, 1963.
37. Palazzo MGA, Strunin L: Anesthesia and emesis. I. Etiology. Can Anaesth Soc J 31:178–187, 1984.
38. Alexander GD, Skupski JN, Brown EM: The role of nitrous oxide in postoperative nausea and vomiting. Anesth Analg 63:175, 1984.
39. Lonie DS, Harper NJN: Nitrous oxide and vomiting. Anaesthesia 41:703–707, 1986.
40. Muir JM, Warner MA, Offord KP, et al: Role of nitrous oxide and other factors in postoperative nausea and vomiting: a randomized and blinded prospective study. Anesthesiology 66:513–518, 1987.
41. Riding JE: Post-operative vomiting. Proc R Soc Med 53:671–677, 1960.
42. Didier EP, Barila TG, Slocum HC, et al: An evaluation of antiemetic drugs in the control of postoperative vomiting. Surg Forum 5:707–712, 1954.
43. Bellville JW: Postanesthetic nausea and vomiting. Anesthesiology 22:773–780, 1961.
44. Clarke SJ, Dundee JW, Love WJ: Studies of drugs given before anaesthesia. VIII. Morphine 10 mg alone and with atropine or hyoscine. Br J Anaesth 34:523–526, 1962.
45. Mirakhur RK, Dundee JW: Lack of anti-emetic effect of glycopyrrolate. Anaesthesia 36:819–820, 1981.
46. King MJ, Milazkiewicz R, Carli F, Deacock AR: Influence of neostigmine on postoperative vomiting. Br J Anaesth 61:403–406, 1988.
47. Ratra CK, Badola RP, Bhargava KP: A study of the factors concerned in emesis during spinal anesthesia. Br J Anaesth 44:1208–1211, 1972.
48. Eger EI II: Anesthetic Uptake and Action. Baltimore, Williams & Wilkins, 1974, p. 174.
49. Smessaert A, Schehr C, Artusio J: Nausea and vomiting in the immediate postanesthetic period. JAMA 170:2072–2076, 1959.
50. Anderson R, Krohg K: Pain as a major cause of postoperative nausea. Can Anaesth Soc J 23:366–369, 1976.
51. Purkis IE: Factors that influence postoperative vomiting. Can Anaesth Soc J 11:335–353, 1964.
52. Madej TH, Simpson KH: Comparison of the use of domperidone, droperidol and metoclopramide in the prevention of nausea and vomiting following gynaecological surgery in day cases. Br J Anaesth 58:879–883, 1986.
53. Holmes C: Postoperative vomiting after ether/air anaesthesia. Anaesthesia 20:199–206, 1965.
54. Palazzo MGA, Strunin L: Anaesthesia and emesis. II. Prevention and management. Can Anaesth Soc J 31:407–415, 1984.
55. Adriana J, Summers FW, Anthony SO: Is the prophylactic use of antiemetics in surgical patients justified? JAMA 175:666–671, 1961.
56. Mirakhur RK, Dundee JW: Lack of antiemetic effect of glycopyrrolate. Anaesthesia 36:819–20, 1981.
57. Burtles R, Peckett BW: Post-operative vomiting. Br J Anaesth 29:114–123, 1957.
58. Aronson JK, Sear JW: Transdermal hyoscine (scopolamine) and postoperative vomiting. Anaesthesia 41:1–3, 1986 (editorial).
59. Tigerstedt I, Salmela L, Aromaa U: Double-blind comparison of transdermal scopolamine, droperidol and placebo against postoperative nausea and vomiting. Acta Anaesthesiol Scand 32:454–457, 1988.
60. Knapp MR, Beecher HK: Postanesthetic nausea, vomiting and retching. JAMA 160:376–385, 1956.

61. Brock-Utne JG, Rubin J, Welman S, et al: The action of commonly used antiemetics on the lower oesophageal sphincter. Br J Anaesth 50:295–298, 1978.
62. Ayd J Jr: A survey of drug induced extrapyramidal reactions. JAMA 175:1054–1060, 1961.
63. Peroutka SJ, Snyder SH: Antiemetics: neurotransmitter receptor binding predicts therapeutic actions. Lancet 1:658–659, 1982.
64. Verhasselt L, Troch E, Verheecke G: Dehydrobenzperidol as preoperative anti-emetic: most effective administration time. Acta Anasthesiol Belg 39:43–48, 1988.
65. Nicolson SC, Kaya KM, Betts EK: The effect of preoperative oral droperidol on the incidence of postoperative emesis after paediatric strabismus surgery. Can J Anaesth 35:364–367, 1988.
66. Van Den Berg AA, Lambourne A, Yazji NS, Laghari NA: Vomiting after ophthalmic surgery. Anaesthesia 42:270–276, 1987.
67. Millar JM, Hall PJ: Nausea and vomiting after prostaglandins in day case termination of pregnancy. Anaesthesia 42:613–618, 1987.
68. Gilman AG, Goodman LS, Rall TW, Murad F: Goodman and Gillman's The Pharmacological Basis of Therapeutics, 7th ed. New York, Macmillan, 1985, p. 108.
69. Warner LO, Rogers GL, Martino JD, et al: Intravenous lidocaine reduces the incidence of vomiting in children after surgery to correct strabismus. Anesthesiology 68:618–621, 1988.
70. Christensen S, Farrow-Gillespie A, Lerman J: Incidence of emesis and postanaesthetic recovery after strabismus surgery in children: a comparison of droperidol and lidocaine. Anesthesiology 70:251–254, 1989.
71. Ghaly RG, Fitzpatrick KTJ, Dundee JW: Antiemetic studies with traditional Chinese acupuncture. Anaesthesia 42:1108–1110, 1987.
72. Fry ENS: Acupressure and postoperative vomiting. Anaesthesia 41:661–662, 1986.
73. Weightman WM, Zacharias M, Herbison P: Traditional Chinese acupuncture as an antiemetic. Br Med J [Clin Res] 295:1379–1380, 1987.

Shivering

74. Bastien J: Quelques remarques sur les anesthesies intra-veineuses prolongees. Anesth Analg 7:161–165, 1950.
75. Mahajan RP, Grover VK, Sharma SL, et al: Intraocular pressure changes during muscular hyperactivity after general anesthesia. Anesthesiology 66:419–421, 1987.
76. Stuart DG, Kawamura Y, Hemingway A: Activation and suppression of shivering during septal and hypothalamic stimulation. Exp Neurol 4:485–506, 1961.
77. Liem ST, Aldrete JA: Control of post-anesthetic shivering. Can Anaesth Soc J 21:506–510, 1974.
78. Lee SL, Shaffer MJ: Low incidence of shivering with chronic propranolol therapy. Lancet 86:500, 1986.
79. Chan VW, Morley-Forster PK, Vosu HA: Temperature changes and shivering after epidural anesthesia for cesarean section. Reg Anaesth 14:48–52, 1989.
80. Macintyre PE, Pavlin EG, Dwersteg JF: Effect of meperidine on oxygen consumption, carbon dioxide production, and respiratory gas exchange in postanesthetic shivering. Anesth Analg 66:751–755, 1987.
81. Jones HD, McLaren CAB: Postoperative shivering and hypoxaemia after halothane, nitrous oxide and oxygen anesthesia. Br J Anaesth 37:35–41, 1965.
82. Bay J, Nunn JF, Prys-Roberts C: Factors influencing arterial PO_2 during recovery room anaesthesia. Br J Anaesth 40:398–406, 1968.
83. Gonzales ER: Stopping postop shivers eases rewarming. JAMA 28:2802, 1982.
84. Sessler DI, Israel D, Pozos RS, et al: Spontaneous post-anesthetic tremor does not resemble thermoregulatory shivering. Anesthesiology 68:843–850, 1988.
85. Roe CF, Goldberg MJ, Blair CS, et al: The influence of body temperature on early postoperative oxygen consumption. Surgery 60:85–92, 1966.
86. Brichard G, Johnstone M: The effect of methylphenidate (Ritalin) on post-halothane muscular spasticity. Br J Anaesth 42:718–721, 1970.
87. Soliman MG, Gillies DMM: Muscular hyperactivity after general anesthesia. Can Anaesth Soc J 19:529–535, 1972.
88. Pozos RS, Israel D, McCutcheon R, et al: Human studies concerning thermal-induced shivering, postoperative "shivering," and cold-induced vasodilation. Ann Emerg Med 16:1037–1041, 1987.
89. Hammel HT: Anesthetics and body temperature regulation. Anesthesiology 68:833–835, 1988 (editorial).
90. Conahan TJ, Williams GD, Apfelbaum JL, Lecky JH: Airway heating reduces recovery time (cost) in outpatients. Anesthesiology 67:128–130, 1987.
91. Goldberg ME, Jan R, Gregg CE, et al: The heat and moisture exchanger does not preserve body temperature or reduce recovery time in outpatients undergoing surgery and anesthesia. Anesthesiology 68:122–123, 1988.
92. Bissonnette B, Sessler DI, LaFlamme P: Passive and active inspired gas humidification in infants and children. Anesthesiology 71:350–354, 1989.
93. Sharkey A, Lipton JM, Murphy MT, Giesecke AH: Inhibition of postanesthetic shivering with radiant heat. Anesthesiology 66:249–252, 1987.
94. Sessler AI, Moayeri A: Skin-surface warming: heat flux and central temperature. Anesthesiology 73:218–224, 1990.
95. Lennon RL, Hosking MP, Conover MA, Perkins WJ: Evaluation of a forced-air system for warming hypothermic postoperative patients. Anesth Analg 70:424–427, 1990.
96. Zwischenberger JB, Kirsh MM, Dechert RE, et al: Suppression of shivering decreases oxygen consumption and improves hemodynamic stability during postoperative rewarming. Ann Thorac Surg 43:428–431, 1987.
97. Claybon LE, Hirsh RA: Meperidine arrests postanesthetic shivering. Anesthesiology 53:S180, 1980.
98. Workhoven MN: Intravenous fluid temperature, shivering, and the parturient. Anesth Analg 65:496–498, 1986.
99. Ponte J, Collett BJ, Walmsley A: Anesthetic temperature and shivering in epidural anaesthesia. Acta Anaesthesiol Scand 30:584–587, 1986.
100. Harris MM, Lawson D, Cooper CM, Ellis J: Treatment of shivering after epidural lidocaine. Reg Anaesth 14:13–18, 1989.
101. McCarroll SM, Cartwright P, Weeks SK, Donati F: Warming intravenous fluids and the incidence of shivering during caesarean sections under epidural anaesthesia. Can Anaesth Soc J 33:S72–S73, 1986.
102. Brownridge P: Shivering related to epidural blockade with bupivacaine in labour, and the influence of epidural pethidine. Anaesth Intens Care 14:412–417, 1986.

POSTOPERATIVE CARDIOVASCULAR COMPLICATIONS

3

JESSE H. MARYMONT, III
and BRENT S. O'CONNOR

There are a wide variety of potential cardiovascular complications following anesthesia and surgery. The purpose of this chapter is to address the more common adverse cardiovascular events experienced by the postoperative patient: hypertension, hypotension, chest pain, and cardiac arrhythmias.

Coordinated efforts of the post anesthesia care unit (PACU) team are essential for early recognition, proper evaluation, accurate diagnosis, and effective treatment of these complications. Results of any intervention should be noted and carefully reviewed, as they are often helpful in identifying the etiology of the problem.

PHYSIOLOGY OF BLOOD PRESSURE

Blood flow (Q) through all vessels depends on only two factors[1]: 1) the pressure differential between the two ends of the vessel (ΔP); and 2) the resistance to blood flow through the vessel (R). This relation is described by the equation

$$Q = \Delta P/R \quad or \quad CO = (MAP - CVP)/SVR$$

where Q = blood flow or cardiac output (CO); ΔP = the pressure drop across the systemic circulation (MAP − CVP), where MAP = mean arterial pressure, CVP = central venous pressure; R = the systemic vascular resistance (SVR).

Note that the pressure within the vessel does not directly reflect the flow through that vessel. When resistance to flow is high and pressure across the vessel merely adequate, flow could be dangerously low. Until we look at the patient and make a determination of the adequacy of organ perfusion (e.g., urinary output, mental status), all we have is a number, "once removed." Anytime a patient is evaluated because of abnormal vital signs, care must be taken to compare and contrast the examination of the patient with the "numbers."

CONTROL OF BLOOD PRESSURE

Control of systemic blood pressure consists of rapidly acting nervous and slower humeral (hormonal) mechanisms.

Nervous system
  Carotid sinus
Humeral system
  Epinephrine, norepinephrine
  Renin, angiotensin, aldosterone
  Vasopressin (antidiuretic hormone, ADH)

Neural control of moment-to-moment blood pressure rests within the carotid sinus baroreceptor. At blood pressures above 60 mm Hg, efferent activity from the baroreceptor increases, reaching a maximum level at 180 mm Hg. These impulses are rapidly responsive to blood pressure changes. The rate of impulse generation varies with the normal pressure fluctuations of the cardiac cycle, increasing during systole and decreasing with diastole.[2] Furthermore, efferent activity changes most rapidly above and below the pressure of 90 to 100 mm Hg, the normal mean arterial pressure.

Carotid sinus impulses are carried through Hering's nerve via the glossopharyngeal nerve to inhibit the vasoconstrictor center and excite the vagal center of the medulla. The resulting vasodilatation, decreased contractility, and lowered heart rate serve to lower blood pressure. Decreases in pressure lower efferent nervous output with opposite effects.

Humeral control of blood pressure effects changes over hours to days, though it becomes activated within minutes of a change in blood pressure. The three blood-borne mediators of blood pressure are vasopressin, epinephrine/norepinephrine, and the renin-angiotensin-aldosterone system.

Vasopressin, or antidiuretic hormone (ADH), is stored in the posterior pituitary gland. Release of ADH may be triggered by a decrease in blood pressure. In addition to a direct vasoconstricting action, ADH causes increased absorption of water by the renal tubules, which tends to increase blood volume and restore blood pressure toward normal[3] as it concentrates the urine.

Epinephrine and norepinephrine are stored in the adrenal medulla and released into the circulation in response to stress (blood loss, hypotension, emotion, fright, fight, or flight). The net effect of these hormones is to increase venous return, cardiac output, and SVR, thereby raising arterial blood pressure.[4]

Renin is an enzyme released by the kidney in response to decreased renal blood flow, which usually accompanies hypotension.[5] It acts on a circulating protein (angiotensinogen, an α_2-globulin) to form angiotensin I, which is then converted to angiotensin II, a powerful vasoconstrictor that raises blood pressure by causing an increase in venous return (which increases cardiac output) and by increasing SVR. In addition to its vascular effects, angiotensin II stimulates the release of aldosterone from the adrenal cortex. Aldosterone causes the kidney to resorb sodium and water from the renal tubules,[6] which increases the blood volume and restores blood pressure toward normal.

MEASUREMENT OF BLOOD PRESSURE

Blood pressure is defined as the force exerted by the blood against a unit area of the vessel wall.[1] This pressure is most often measured in clinical practice by use of a stethoscope and a blood pressure cuff connected to a mercury or aneroid manometer. This indirect method makes use of a cuff that circles an extremity and is inflated to a pressure sufficient to occlude the arterial inflow. Pressure is then slowly released while the examiner auscultates the artery distal to the cuff. The appearance, character, and disappearance of the resulting Korotkoff sounds serves to define the systolic and diastolic blood pressures.[7]

In addition to the manual measurement of blood pressure, other noninvasive methods exist, all of which rely on the use of an encircling cuff and inflatable bladder but differ in the method used to detect blood flow under and distal to the deflating cuff. These methods include manual or photoelectric detection of a distal pulse, measurement of the oscillations in cuff pressure induced by arterial pulsations, and photoplethysmographic measurements of blood pressure that rely on digital blood volume and the cuff pressure needed to keep it constant.[7]

Indirect measurements of blood pressure are subject to the variability of cuff size, which can substantially affect the result; for example, too narrow a cuff results in falsely elevated blood pressure measurements, while a cuff too large for the extremity may result in a value lower than the actual pressure.[8] Standards relating arm circumference to bladder dimensions have been reported elsewhere.[9] In addition to erroneous blood pressure measurements caused by improper cuff size, patients with severe atherosclerosis may have falsely high pressures when measured with a cuff. This "pseudohypertension" arises when the sclerotic arterial wall is too stiff to be compressed by the blood pressure cuff.[10] Patients in shock with elevated systemic vascular resistance have a falsely low systolic blood pressure when measured with a cuff.[11]

Whenever the clinical situation warrants, direct intraarterial blood pressure measurement provides instant, continuous systemic blood pressures. The pressure in the cannulated artery is transmitted via noncompliant tubing to a pressure transducer, where it impinges on a strain gauge. Transducers connected to an arterial line allow beat-to-beat evaluation of blood pressure and access for repeated arterial blood sampling but are not without their pitfalls[7,11] (see Chapter 4). Catheter "fling," air bubbles, misplaced transducers, improper transducer calibration, failure to flush after aspiration of arterial blood, equipment failure, and the like can lead to erroneous readings. Before a decision is made to treat a patient with an abnormal blood pressure reading, the accuracy of the measurement should be verified. The transducer should be zeroed at the level of the patient's heart and secured at that height. Any change in patient position should prompt rezeroing of the transducer at the new height. To diagnose kinking, the waveform of the arterial trace on the oscilloscope should then be examined while extending the patient's wrist and manipulating the dressing over the arterial catheter. The flush tubing should be inspected for air bubbles or blood, aspirated, and then flushed clean.

Kinking of the catheter can be reduced by placing the arterial line more proximally in the radial artery, avoiding the wrist joint and thereby minimizing movement that could kink the catheter as it enters the skin. Accidental disconnection, a potentially life-threatening event when unrecognized, can be reduced by drying the skin and catheter after placement and connection of the flush tubing, spraying the area lightly with tincture of benzoin, and then tightening the flush tubing on the catheter hub using a hemostat or clamp to hold the catheter hub immobile prior to taping.

Complications of arterial line insertion range from the frequent and mild (e.g., arterial thrombosis, asymptomatic in 96 per cent of patients) to the rare and significant (e.g., neurologic deficit due to catheter flushing-induced cerebral embolus).[11] Duration of cannulation, catheter size and shape, location and method of cannulation, frequency of flush and tubing change, and the site of the arterial line contribute to the incidence and type of complications.[7,11]

HYPERTENSION

Systemic arterial hypertension (Htn) can be defined as a blood pressure greater than 160/95 mm Hg[12] or 20 per cent higher than the patient's baseline level. Using these definitions, Htn is a common occurrence during the early postoperative period. Studies have shown an increased level of circulating catecholamines in these patients,[13,14] suggesting an autonomic cause. The increased blood pressure may result from an elevated cardiac output, increased SVR, or both.[15,16]

SIGNIFICANCE OF POSTOPERATIVE HYPERTENSION

Asymptomatic Htn during the postoperative period is usually benign and short-lived, and may be viewed as a reactive event to a variety of noxious stimuli including pain, excitement, shivering, and mild hypothermia. More than 50 per cent of patients admitted to the recovery room with at least two consecutive blood pressure measurements higher than 190/100 mm Hg have a history of Htn. Conservative management with treatment of the cause of Htn (analgesics, warming, and observation) is usually effective.[17]

Elevated blood pressure increases ventricular wall tension, afterload, and myocardial work,[15] which could precipitate myocardial ischemia or infarction in the patient with significant coronary artery disease. There are studies that show a greater incidence of postoperative mortality or morbidity, including myocardial infarction (MI), in the hypertensive population,[18–20] whereas one large prospective study[21] found no increased risk for patients with preoperative Htn. In the patient with congestive heart failure or impaired ventricular function, the increase in SVR and impedance to ejection of blood from the left ventricle could reduce cardiac output and provoke pulmonary edema. In patients with compromised cardiac reserve, benign, reactive Htn could have serious sequelae if not treated.

Severe Htn may be defined as a diastolic blood pressure (BP) greater than 120 mm Hg.[15] The significance of this value depends on several factors: baseline BP, presence of signs or symptoms of end-organ damage, and the site of surgery. At any level of arterial Htn the risk of complications is greater for those patients with acute increases in pressure than it is for the chronic hypertensive.[22] Severe Htn is a cause for concern, as it carries with it the risk of serious complications, including MI, arrhythmia, acute renal failure, congestive heart failure, and subarachnoid or cerebral hemorrhage.[15]

Evidence of end-organ damage associated with severe Htn defines a hypertensive emergency.[15,22] Headache, mental status changes, and a variety of neurologic signs (nystagmus, weakness, Babinski) may be present; it may be difficult to distinguish them from the effects of residual anesthetic agents. Rales, tachycardia with an S_3 gallop, and jugular venous distension suggest acute left ventricular failure, whereas substernal pain or heaviness suggests myocardial ischemia or infarction.

Hypertension may also cause postoperative bleeding from vessels that would not leak at normal pressures.[15] In the patient with recent intracranial, cardiac, or major vessel surgery, even mild increases in blood pressure can have deleterious effects; and early treatment may be necessary to minimize the risk of bleeding or anastomotic leak. Increases in mean arterial pressure may contribute to postoperative cerebral edema in the neurosurgical patient, and the incidence of neurologic deficit following carotid endarterectomy is greater in those patients who are either hypertensive or hypotensive during the postoperative period.[23,24]

ETIOLOGY OF HYPERTENSION

Some of the causes of Htn during the early postoperative period are listed in Table 3–1. The most common cause of hypertension during the early postoperative period is pain; hypoxemia, hypercarbia, fluid overload, delirium, and reaction to presence of an endotracheal tube are also frequently seen.[17,25,26] Relative hypervolemia may exist and cause hypertension when the patient, who is volume-loaded during spinal or epidural anesthesia, recovers from sympathetic blockade. Percussion of the lower abdomen and a review of the patient's recent input and output occasionally reveal a distended bladder as the cause of hypertension.[17]

Treatment of pain is essential to the successful management of the postoperative patient and warrants a thorough discussion (see Chapter 19). Delirium during emergence from general anesthesia is most common in the young when inadequate analgesia is present. Intravenous narcotics in small, repeated doses comprise appropriate treatment once hypoxemia, hypercarbia, and cerebral ischemia have been ruled out.[26] Emergence delirium is more common when scopolamine premedication has been used, especially in the absence of narcotic analgesia[27]; physostigmine in 1- to 3-mg IV doses has been successful in reversing scopolamine-related delirium.[28]

Respiratory disturbances are discussed elsewhere in this book (see Chapter 5). The assessment of oxygenation and ventilation should be part of the initial evaluation of the hypertensive patient.

More than half of the patients with pheochromocytoma have a history of hypertensive crisis.[29] Although paroxysmal hypertension may be a feature of this disease, 60 per cent of patients have consistent hypertension.[30] Postoperative management of the patient with pheochromocytoma is complex and challenging; mainstays of treatment include preoperative drug therapy with α- and possibly β-adrenergic blockers, the tyrosine hydroxylase inhibitor α-methyl-p-tyrosine,[29] volume repletion and maintenance, and careful monitoring.

Despite convincing evidence that withdrawal of antihypertensive medication before surgery is potentially dangerous,[31] some patients experience exacerbation of their chronic Htn because of drug withdrawal. Antihypertensive medication should be continued up to and including the day of surgery.[32] Rebound Htn, with plasma catecholamine levels as high as those found in pheochromocytoma, has been described following withdrawal of clonidine.[33] Cessation of β-blocker therapy has been associated with tachycardia, diaphoresis, anxiety, unstable angina, malignant arrhythmias, myocardial infarction, and sudden death.[29] These patients should be restarted on the antihypertensive medications as soon as possible; interim control of blood pressure with parenteral agents may be necessary.

In addition to the causes listed in Table 3–1, the type of surgery may predispose to postoperative Htn. For example, 30 to 60 per cent of patients undergoing coronary artery bypass surgery were found to be hypertensive within the first 3 hours after operation.[34] Surgery in the area of the carotid sinus is also associated with postoperative Htn; 10 per cent of patients who underwent radical neck dissection were hypertensive during the first 2 hours, whereas the incidence of Htn following carotid endarterectomy varies from 19 to 38 per cent.[35] Htn

TABLE 3–1. ETIOLOGY OF HYPERTENSION DURING THE EARLY POSTOPERATIVE PERIOD

Respiratory problems
  Hypoxemia
  Hypercarbia
Drug-induced conditions
  Antihypertensive withdrawal
  Delirium
Metabolic abnormalities
  Pheochromocytoma
  Cushing syndrome
  Primary hyperaldosteronism
  Renovascular hypertension
Miscellaneous etiologies
  Pain
  Anxiety
  Fluid overload
  Distended bladder
  Factitious hypertension
  Hypothermia
  Tight cast
  Toxemia of pregnancy (preeclampsia)

in this setting is particularly dangerous, as it can cause localized bleeding, hematoma formation, and resultant deformation of the upper airway, leading to obstruction.

TREATMENT

Most cases of "reactive" Htn can be successfully treated with adequate analgesia, warming, and observation.[17] Symptomatic or severe Htn unresponsive to conservative therapy warrants specific treatment. Before deciding to treat, one must be assured that the BP measurement is accurate; postoperative values should be interpreted in the light of the patient's preoperative baseline measurement. In previously normotensive patients, damage to the central nervous system can occur with diastolic pressures as low as 110 mm Hg, whereas the chronically hypertensive patient may be asymptomatic with a diastolic blood pressure of 120 mm Hg or higher.[36]

Ideal therapy for the severely hypertensive patient with evidence of end-organ damage should consist of a fast-acting, titratable, rapidly reversible, efficacious drug with no side effects. It must always be borne in mind that sudden decreases in blood pressure accompanying treatment of Htn can have catastrophic results; seizures, cerebrovascular accidents, acute myocardial infarction, renal failure, and death have been reported.[15]

Antihypertensive drugs (Table 3–2) can be classified into seven groups: 1) direct-acting vascular smooth muscle relaxants (vasodilators, e.g., sodium nitroprusside, nitroglycerine); 2) adrenergic antagonists that block the effects of sympathetic nervous stimulation (α-blockers attenuate vasoconstriction, whereas β-blockers decrease the heart rate, the force of contraction, and cardiac output); 3) angiotensin-converting enzyme inhibitors (e.g., captopril), which act primarily by preventing production of angiotensin II; 4) ganglionic

TABLE 3–2. PHARMACOLOGIC ANTIHYPERTENSIVE THERAPY

Vasodilators
Adrenergic blockers
Angiotensin converting enzyme inhibitors
Ganglionic blockers
Calcium channel blockers
Diuretics
Norepinephrine depleting agents, including α_2-agonists

blocking drugs (e.g., trimethaphan), which inhibit the entire autonomic (sympathetic and parasympathetic) nervous system; 5) calcium channel blockers (e.g., nifedipine, verapamil), which decrease myocardial contractility and relax vascular smooth muscle; 6) diuretics (e.g., hydrochlorothiazide), which cause water and sodium loss and vasodilation; and 7) inhibitors of norepinephrine formation, storage, and release, a group that includes the α_2-agonists clonidine and α-methyldopa as well as the less popular depleting-type drugs reserpine and guanethidine. Excluded are other drugs (e.g., tricyclic antidepressants, narcotics, sedatives, and monoamine oxidase inhibitors) that may lower blood pressure as a side effect.

The prolonged-onset time and variable bioavailability of oral agents as well as their longer half-life make them ineffective or inappropriate for the immediate postoperative setting. Variable muscle blood flow and inability to "reverse" the action of intramuscularly injected agents also makes this route suboptimal. Intravenous injection and infusion provide more precise dosage and better control of antihypertensive therapy, and our discussion is limited to those agents.

Drug doses used in this chapter are broad and are meant as general guidelines only. Drug doses should *always* be individualized because of the great variability in patient response, body weight, organ (dys)function, and underlying sympathetic tone. When in doubt, err on the side of underdosage and modify as needed.

Nitroprusside

Although nitroprusside is not without side effects, it approaches being the ideal drug for management of severe Htn in the critical care environment. Sodium nitroprusside (SNP) is a potent, titratable, direct-acting vasodilator with rapid onset, short half-life, and few side effects; it is probably the drug of choice for treatment of acute, severe Htn.[29,36,37] As with any vasodilating drug, caution must be exercised when treating any patient with known or suspected aortic stenosis.

Sodium nitroprusside should be given intravenously by infusion pump, as it is potent (starting dose is 0.1 μg/kg/min); ideally, the patient's blood pressure response is continuously assessed. With its direct vasodilating action on arterioles and veins, a decrease in SVR and preload are the most consistent effects of SNP; changes in cardiac output and heart rate are variable. Generally, cardiac output increases in the hypertensive patient with heart failure (owing to the decrease in impedance as SVR is lowered) and decreases in patients with normal or low preload as venodilation causes a drop in venous return; the head-up position augments this venous pooling and enhances the hypotensive action of SNP.[37] Most patients respond to SNP with a reflex tachycardia, but the patient in heart failure or pulmonary edema may experience a lowering of the heart rate as pulmonary pressures decrease and cardiac output rises.

Cyanide is released as SNP is metabolized; the final metabolite is thiocyanate. Although cyanide toxicity is possible with prolonged use of SNP, it is uncommon.[37] Thiocyanate is renally excreted with a half-life of 4 days; when renal failure exists, this half-life is prolonged. Hypoxia, nausea, disorientation, psychosis, tinnitus, and muscle spasms are signs of thiocyanate toxicity (blood level >10 mg/dl). Reduction in arterial oxygen tension with SNP and other direct-acting vasodilators may occur, presumably as a result of the decrease in hypoxic pulmonary vasoconstriction. Application of positive end-expiratory pressure may attenuate the reduction in PaO_2.[38]

Reflex tachycardia and the potential for a sudden hypotensive response to the initiation of SNP therapy could serve to increase myocardial oxygen demand while simultaneously decreasing its supply. In addition, SNP has been associated with the coronary steal phenomenon.[39,40]

Nitroglycerine

In the setting of Htn with myocardial ischemia, nitroglycerine (NTG) may be the preferable vasodilator.[41] NTG is a vasodilating drug with dose-dependent effects. At low doses (blood levels of 1 to 2 ng/ml), as with sublingual or transdermal application, venodilatation and decreased preload are the predominant effects.[40,42] The higher blood levels (>3 ng/ml) seen with intravenous NTG (1 to 3 μg/kg/min) are associated with decreased SVR and lowered blood pressure as both venous and arterial beds dilate.[43] Low dose NTG also increases the size of epicardial coronary arteries and enhances collateral flow to ischemic myocardium.[40]

This dosage-mediated selectivity of action makes NTG a versatile drug, effective for treatment of angina in low doses, congestive

heart failure and pulmonary edema in low to moderate doses, and systemic hypertension in higher doses.[40,44] NTG is, however, first and foremost a venodilator. For a given amount of reduction in blood pressure, NTG produces a greater reduction in preload than does SNP.[40] Reductions in preload and cardiac output with resultant hypotension can occur with NTG, especially in the patient with unsuspected hypovolemia. The intravenous half-life of 2 minutes and the dose-dependent hypotensive effects allow for precise titration of blood pressure with NTG, although there are patients in whom the more potent arteriolar dilator SNP is needed to control Htn.[40]

Labetalol

Labetalol hydrochloride is a combined selective α_1- and nonselective β-blocker that has proved useful for the management of postoperative Htn.[45] It also blocks reuptake of norepinephrine into nerve terminals.[46] The α/β-blockade ratio is 1:7 when the drug is given intravenously.[40] In contrast to pure α-blockers, which tend to cause a reflex tachycardia as they lower SVR, and pure β-blockers, which tend to cause bradycardia and a drop in cardiac output with an increased SVR, labetalol causes primarily a reduction in SVR, with variable effects on contractility and cardiac output.[16,46] Heart rate either decreases slightly or shows little change. These hemodynamic effects are especially desirable in the hypertensive with coronary artery disease. With a decreased afterload, slower heart rate, and a less hyperdynamic ventricle, a reduction in myocardial work and improvement of the oxygen demand/supply ratio would result. As with any β-blocker, its benefit in the patient with bronchospastic disease or heart failure must be weighed against the risk of bronchoconstriction and negative inotropic effects.[9] Labetalol may cause less bronchoconstriction than the other nonselective β-blockers, however, as it appears to have some intrinsic β_2-agonistic effects.[46]

After a test dose of 2.5 to 5.0 mg IV, the dose may be increased to 20 to 80 mg. Labetalol may also be given by an infusion of 2 mg/min until a total of 300 mg has been given or blood pressure has been controlled.[47] With a half-life of 2 to 4 hours, labetalol lacks the rapid "offset" (5 to 10 minutes) of the ideal antihypertensive; nevertheless it is a useful and predictable drug for managing postoperative Htn.

Hydralazine

Hydralazine is a direct-acting arteriolar vasodilator with minimal effects on preload. After an intravenous bolus, blood pressure decreases over 10 to 20 minutes with variable response.[47] Reflex tachycardia and increased contractility are common and limit the drug's usefulness in patients with coronary artery disease, as angina or myocardial ischemia may ensue. Propranolol administered in small doses with hydralazine can attenuate the heart rate increase; if the patient is taking β-blockers and has an effective level when given hydralazine, there may be less of a tachycardiac response. Diastolic blood pressure may be lowered more than systolic pressure.[48]

The dosage of hydralazine is 5 to 20 mg IV, and its duration of action is 3 to 4 hours. With its variable response and relatively long half-life, the cautious physician might err on the side of lower dosage; therefore repeat or increase the dose if the response within 10 to 20 minutes is inadequate. Despite these drawbacks, hydralazine has stood the test of time and remains an effective drug for the treatment of moderate increases in blood pressure during the postoperative period.

Verapamil

Verapamil is discussed elsewhere as an antiarrhythmic agent. The drug also has a blood pressure-lowering effect mediated by arteriolar vasodilation and myocardial depression. Intravenous verapamil can cause hypotension, especially in the patient with preexisting ventricular dysfunction, and concurrent administration of a β-blocking drug may result in atrioventricular (AV) block.[49]

Nifedipine

Nifedipine, another calcium entry blocker, has more usefulness as an antihypertensive drug. With greater peripheral vasodilating effects than verapamil, nifedipine frequently causes a reflex tachycardia as the baroreceptor responds to the decrease in blood pressure with an increased sympathetic outflow.[49] With a half-life of 4 to 6 hours and an onset time of 20 minutes after sublingual or oral dosage, the drug is less controllable than those given by infusion.

HYPOTENSION

ETIOLOGY

Hypotension was the most common complication during the immediate postoperative period in a series of 112,000 patients given anesthetics in a large teaching hospital.[50] Hypotension can have serious sequelae, including ischemia of the various organ systems (myocardial infarction, stroke, acute renal failure), all of which depend on an adequate blood pressure to maintain oxygen and substrate delivery. Table 3–3 lists some of the causes of hypotension in the postoperative setting.

Examination of the equation

$$CO = (MAP - CVP)/SVR$$

reveals that hypotension must result whenever cardiac output or systemic vascular resistance falls. Of these two causes, a drop in cardiac output secondary to hypovolemia is probably the more common. Decreases in cardiac output may result from any number of specific causes, although most fall into one of two categories: hypovolemia or myocardial dysfunction (pump failure).

Hypovolemia is a decrease in the circulating blood volume. With less volume in the vascular space, there is a decrease in venous return and a lower preload (CVP or PCW). This situation causes decreased ventricular filling and a

TABLE 3–3. ETIOLOGY OF HYPOTENSION DURING THE EARLY POSTOPERATIVE PERIOD

Absolute hypovolemia
    Blood loss
    Inadequate fluid replacement
    Bowel preparation
    Ongoing occult bleeding
Relative hypovolemia
    Diuretics
    Antihypertensives
    Decreased sympathetic tone
Other causes
    Arrhythmia
    Tension pneumothorax
    Pulmonary embolus
    Decreased myocardial contractility
    Sepsis
    Addisonian crisis
    Cardiac tamponade
    Histamine release
    Anaphylaxis

lower stroke volume and cardiac output. Increases in venous capacitance in the patient with a normal blood volume defines relative hypovolemia. A decrease in venous tone results in peripheral pooling of blood, decreased venous return, and low cardiac output. Compensatory mechanisms associated with an intact sympathetic nervous system (tachycardia, increased venous and arteriolar tone) are normally able to sustain blood pressure in the face of a volume deficit of less than 10 to 20 per cent.[51] However, the residual effects of many anesthetic drugs are likely to attenuate the normal physiologic responses to hypovolemia, leading to hypotension as an early manifestation of hypovolemia.[52]

In the nonmedicated patient, hypotension is associated with signs and symptoms that may not be apparent in the patient recovering from general or regional anesthesia.[25] The typical pale, gray, clammy patient with obvious confusion or syncope and tachycardia is a rarity among hypotensive patients during the immediate postoperative period. Cerebral ischemia presenting as confusion, disorientation, combativeness, or loss of consciousness may be masked by residual anesthetic effects. Tachycardia may not occur in the patient with significant sympathetic block from regional anesthesia and may be blunted by the cardiovascular effects of anesthetic drugs (e.g., narcotics, anticholinesterases). Likewise, cutaneous manifestations such as diaphoresis and the characteristic cold, clammy extremity of the hypotensive patient are often absent in the patient with a sympathetic nervous system depressed by narcotics or residual anesthetic drugs.

The hypotensive effect of hypovolemia arising from intraoperative blood and fluid losses may be masked by the sympathetic stimulating effects of surgery while in the operating room; once surgery ends and the patient is relatively unstimulated, this hypovolemia frequently results in hypotension.

Hypovolemia may be absolute, as in the patient with occult surgical bleeding or poorly compensated "third space" and evaporative fluid losses, or it may be relative. Relative hypovolemia may occur in the treated hypertensive, in whom chronic diuretic use has resulted in volume contraction, or in the patient with regional anesthetic-induced sympathectomy, in whom a normal intravascular volume is now contained in an increased vascular space. Mild hypothermia (defined as a core body temperature of 32° to 35°C) can result in venoconstriction[51] with normal or even elevated blood pressures. During rewarming, peripheral vasodilation can unmask the hypovolemia, producing hypotension responsive to volume infusion.[53]

The second cause of low cardiac output hypotension is *myocardial pump failure*. Most patients with hypotension caused by ventricular dysfunction have cardiac disease present preoperatively and depend on increased sympathetic tone and high filling pressures to maintain cardiac output.[51] Brought on by residual anesthetic-induced myocardial depression, arrhythmia, or ischemic dysfunction, pump failure is more likely in the patient with preexisting coronary artery disease, recent myocardial infarction, ventricular dysfunction, or valvular heart disease. Large fluid loads, common in the operative setting, may be well tolerated by the patient while spinal or epidural conduction block exists with its attendant increase in venous pooling. As the block wears off and vascular tone returns to normal, fluid overload may manifest as respiratory distress, myocardial ischemia, or overt pulmonary edema. Similarly, the patient anesthetized with general anesthesia and positive pressure ventilation (which decreases venous return) may tolerate a large fluid load only to develop signs of volume excess when awake and breathing spontaneously, perhaps vasoconstricted as a result of pain and sympathetic discharge.

Myocardial infarction in the postoperative patient is more likely to be painless (25 to 61 per cent) than in the nonsurgical patient (10 to 15 per cent).[18] Residual anesthetic agents and analgesic drugs probably account for the increased number of clinically asymptomatic infarcts.[54] Increases in myocardial oxygen demand or decreases in supply associated with hypotension and tachycardia may produce ischemia in the patient with significant coronary artery disease (Table 3–4). To minimize the risk of perioperative ischemia in these patients, great care should be taken to avoid any precipitating causes. Invasive monitoring of pulmonary artery pressures, scrutiny of the electrocardiogram (ECG) with attention to the ST-T wave complex, and aggressive treatment of contributory factors can hopefully detect myocardial ischemia before hypotension appears.

Decrease in SVR is the third cause of hypotension in the postoperative patient. Antihypertensive medications with vasodilating mechanisms, anesthetic drugs that release histamine or have α-blocking capability (bu-

TABLE 3–4. PERIOPERATIVE MYOCARDIAL ISCHEMIA: COMMON CAUSES

Increased O_2 demand
    Tachycardia (pain, anxiety, hypoxemia, acidemia, hypovolemia, drug effect)
    Hypertension
    Increased myocardial contractility (pain, anxiety, "hyperdynamic circulation")
    Shivering
    Fluid overload

Decreased O_2 supply
    Tachycardia (decreased coronary perfusion time)
    Hypotension
    Hypoxemia
    Anemia
    Fluid overload

tyrophenones, phenothiazines), and anaphylactoid reactions to drugs or blood products can decrease SVR and venous tone.[51] Excluding iatrogenic causes (vasodilator overdose, rapid antibiotic administration) and chronic liver failure, the most likely cause of lowered SVR is sepsis (see Chapter 21).

Patients with malnutrition, malignancy, immunosuppressive drug therapy,[55] known infections, or major burns and trauma patients[56] are at increased risk for sepsis. Those with ischemic or infarcted bowel, genitourinary surgery,[52] or abscess manipulation and drainage may also be at greater risk. Patients at the extremes of age (under 1 year or over 65 years) and those with chronic illnesses (diabetes, alcoholism, drug abuse) are at increased risk for septic shock.[57]

Less common causes of hypotension (Table 3–3) include massive pulmonary embolism and cardiac tamponade. *Massive pulmonary embolism* may present with tachypnea, chest pain, and dyspnea. Tachycardia and dyspnea are the most consistent findings.[58] Arterial blood gas analysis usually shows low or normal PCO_2 (despite a minute ventilation two to three times normal) and hypoxemia. Increased deadspace accounts for the relatively higher than expected PCO_2; and release of vasoconstricting-bronchoconstricting substances, causing mismatch of ventilation and perfusion, accounts for the hypoxemia. Hypotension is caused by a mechanical block of right heart output and acute cor pulmonale. Pulmonary embolism is estimated to be fatal in fewer than 10 per cent of cases[58]; however, an embolism massive enough to result in hypotension is frequently fatal.

Cardiac tamponade is most commonly seen after cardiac surgery or trauma (including iatrogenic trauma) and results from bleeding into the pericardial space. Anticoagulation in the setting of tuberculosis, tumor with chest involvement, postradiation pericarditis, or renal failure with dialysis may also cause acute tamponade.[59] The typical clinical picture of rising venous pressure, falling blood pressure, and quiet heart (Beck's triad) may not develop if tamponade results from slow accumulation of fluid or blood; more commonly, symptoms of congestive heart failure (orthopnea, dyspnea, jugular venous distension) are seen.[59] Examination of the ECG may show diffuse low voltage or ST changes; rarely, electrical alternans is present. If a pulmonary artery catheter is in place or inserted, equalization of the right atrial, right ventricular diastolic, pulmonary artery diastolic, and pulmonary artery occlusion pressures is strong support for the diagnosis.[60] Therapy with isoproterenol and fluids may support the patient pending definitive surgical treatment; pericardiocentesis is both diagnostic and therapeutic but carries the risks of pneumothorax, coronary artery laceration, and myocardial puncture.[61]

TREATMENT

Treatment of hypotension should begin immediately, while the etiology is being determined (Table 3–5). Intravenous replacement-type fluids should be rapidly infused and

TABLE 3–5. TREATMENT OF HYPOTENSION

1. Administer oxygen.
2. Administer fluid bolus.
3. Stop drug infusions (e.g., antibiotics, vasodilators).
4. Check heart rate, treat bradycardia or other arrhythmia.
5. Elevate legs.
6. Perform physical examination: auscultate chest, inspect wound, search for bleeding.
7. Do a rapid chart review.
8. Communicate with surgeon.
9. Obtain relevant laboratory studies.
10. If there is no response to volume loading: invade with pulmonary artery catheter, evaluate and treat myocardial pump dysfunction or low systemic vascular resistance.
11. If needed administer vasopressor or inotrope pending data.

supplemental oxygen given. All nonessential drug infusions (e.g., antibiotics) and vasodilating drugs should be stopped and the immediate drug history reviewed. The ECG monitor can quickly reveal any rhythm disturbance. After ruling out an erroneous value due to an oversized cuff, an elevated transducer, or some other cause, the legs should be elevated and an intravenous bolus of replacement-type fluid administered. When the legs are flexed at the pelvis and elevated, an "autotransfusion" of approximately 2 U of blood occurs[25] Improvement in the subsequent BP readings supports the diagnosis of hypovolemia, as does the finding of oliguria responsive to fluids. After administration of a fluid bolus, a decrease in tachycardia associated with an increase in the blood pressure toward normal is a strong indication that the patient is hypovolemic. A quick review of the anesthetic record and the patient's chart may reveal useful information, e.g., bowel preparation, history of congestive heart failure, blood loss and replacement.

The physical examination should include inspection of the wound for evidence of bleeding. Occult surgical bleeding must be considered when hypotension transiently responds to a fluid bolus only to recur shortly thereafter, especially in the patient with known altered coagulation status or at risk for disseminated intravascular coagulation (DIC). Retroperitoneal bleeding after periaortic surgical dissection, pelvic or hip fractures, or open prostate surgery and the postpartum patient with retained products of conception are infamous examples.

The chest should be examined for symmetric expansion and breath sounds, especially in the patient receiving positive pressure ventilation and patients at risk for pneumothorax (e.g., surgical site, recent central venous cannulation). Tension pneumothorax is a life-threatening complication of mechanical ventilation and must be considered anytime hypotension occurs in a patient receiving positive airway pressure therapy.

A hematocrit and any other indicated laboratory work (chest roentgenogram, arterial blood gas analysis, ECG) are ordered; sometimes the first clue to septic shock as the etiology of hypotension is when the blood gas assay reveals a mixed metabolic acidosis and respiratory alkalosis.[57]

Communication with the surgeon should take place early during evaluation of the hypotensive patient, especially when there is minimal response to volume infusion. Diagnosis of the etiology of the hypotension should be constantly reevaluated; frequently discussion with the surgeon is helpful, as each approaches the problem from a different perspective and area of expertise. The surgeon will want to examine the wound and will make the final decision as to whether exploration for bleeding is necessary.

A negative response to elevating the legs and rapid infusion (5 to 15 minutes) of 250 to 500 ml of fluid should raise the suspicion that the etiology of hypotension may not be hypovolemia. Any patient not responding to fluid resuscitation should undergo preload, afterload, and ventricular function assessment with either a central venous pressure (CVP) line or pulmonary artery catheter.[62] Low SVR or pump failure must be considered and are best investigated by placement of a pulmonary artery catheter and thermodilution cardiac output measurement. CVP measurements probably reflect left ventricular filling pressures in the patient with normal biventricular function in the absence of significant pulmonary disease. Treatment with a vasopressor or inotrope to support blood pressure while invasive monitors are being inserted may be indicated. Table 3–6 relates pulmonary artery catheter measurements with likely etiologies.

Treatment of ventricular dysfunction not caused by ischemia is aimed at increasing contractility and ejection fraction. Positive inotropes (dopamine, dobutamine, epinephrine) increase contractility, whereas vasodilators decrease SVR and increase the ejection fraction and cardiac output. Ischemic dysfunction improves when the underlying cause (e.g., tachycardia, hypoxemia) is corrected.

Low filling pressures suggest hypovolemia, whereas elevation of the pulmonary artery occlusion pressure with a low cardiac output indicates decreased myocardial contractility and the need for inotropic support. Low filling pressures with elevated or normal cardiac out-

TABLE 3–6. EVALUATION OF PULMONARY ARTERY CATHETER DATA

Cardiac Output	Low PAOP	High PAOP
Low	Hypovolemia	Pump failure
High	Sepsis	Poor data
	Drug effect	Sepsis
		Fluid overload

put and low SVR suggest sepsis as a likely etiology.

CHEST PAIN

Chest pain is a subjective sensation experienced by the patient. A specific pain may have one of several unrelated etiologies (Table 3–7). The importance of chest pain during the perioperative period is directly related to its etiology. Myocardial ischemia and myocardial infarction may lead to significant morbidity and mortality. However, not all chest pain experienced by postoperative patients is so ominous.

The primary and immediate goal is to identify and treat those patients with serious underlying diseases. The patient who has experienced chest pain in the PACU may be transferred to an intensive care unit (ICU) or to the regular nursing floor. This decision is important and takes into account the suspected etiology of the chest pain. Of the cardiac etiologies of chest pain, only myocardial ischemia and acute myocardial infarction are discussed here. Other cardiac etiologies of chest pain are seen much less commonly during the acute postoperative period.

TABLE 3–7. ETIOLOGY OF CHEST PAIN

Pulmonary/cardiovascular pain
    Myocardial ischemia or infarction
    Hypertrophic cardiomyopathy
    Mitral valve prolapse
    Systemic hypertension
    Pulmonary hypertension
    Pulmonary embolus
    Pneumothorax
    Pneumomediastinum
    Pneumonia
    Pericarditis
Esophageal/visceral pain
    Reflux esophagitis
    Esophageal dysmotility
    Esophageal perforation
    Peptic ulcer
    Pancreatitis
    Small bowel obstruction
    Diverticulitis
    Biliary colic
    Renal colic
    Neoplasm
Musculoskeletal pain
    Sternoclavicular joint inflammation
    Thoracic outlet syndrome
    Cervical spinal disease

CARDIOVASCULAR ETIOLOGIES

Cardiovascular etiologies are of primary importance in the differential diagnosis of perioperative chest pain. In a patient with a history of coronary artery disease or a history of risk factors for development of coronary artery disease, chest pain implies myocardial ischemia or acute myocardial infarction until proved otherwise. Myocardial ischemia occurs when myocardial oxygen demand is greater than myocardial oxygen supply (Table 3–4). Factors that constitute myocardial oxygen demand include the heart rate, preload, afterload, and contractile state of the myocardium. Factors that determine myocardial oxygen supply are the oxygen content of the arterial blood and the amount of coronary blood flow.

During the intraoperative and postoperative periods, there are physiologic alterations that may lead to myocardial ischemia. Anesthesia and surgery influence oxygen supply and demand. Postoperatively, the complaint of chest pain may not be spontaneously offered by the patient. Treatment of surgical pain with narcotics and depression of the mental status due to residual anesthetic agents serve to mask the usual discomfort of myocardial ischemia. In addition, chest pain may be misinterpreted as being exclusively due to recent surgical manipulation, and so no other cause is investigated.

The pain associated with myocardial ischemia is classically described by the patient as a heavy pressure or a squeezing or constricting sensation in the chest. This pain may also originate in or radiate to the arms, shoulders, neck, or palate. The pain of myocardial infarction is typically more intense, of longer duration, and associated with more nausea and diaphoresis than is the pain of myocardial ischemia. However, even with a fully awake patient, ECG-documented myocardial ischemia or myocardial infarction may occur without the subjective sensation of any chest pain or discomfort. In this case it is called ''silent'' myocardial ischemia or myocardial infarction.[63–65]

The most common etiology of angina is atherosclerotic narrowing of the coronary arteries. Because of this narrowing there is an inability to increase oxygen delivery to the perioperative heart stressed by anesthesia, surgery, pain, hypoxemia, or anxiety. Other pathology involving the coronary arteries can limit coronary artery blood flow as well, including coronary artery thrombosis and coronary artery spasm. When an increase in oxygen demand occurs (increased heart rate, preload, afterload, contractility), the inability to increase oxygen delivery (owing to fixed or dynamic stenosis of the coronary arteries) leads to ischemia. With fixed stenosis (atherosclerosis) of the coronary arteries, an increase in heart rate or blood pressure occurs prior to the onset of chest pain and causes the imbalance in myocardial oxygen supply and demand. With dynamic lesions due to coronary artery spasm, a decrease in the oxygen supply occurs, and tissue ischemia may occur without an increase in the oxygen demand of the myocardium. With a decrease in the oxygen supply to the myocardium, an increase in heart rate or blood pressure may not occur prior to the onset of chest pain. The chest pain occurs first, with tachycardia and hypertension representing responses to ischemia and not etiologic factors.

Patients with chest pain in the PACU should have their heart rhythm and rate monitored continuously. In addition, a 12-lead hard copy ECG tracing should be obtained to document any myocardial ischemia or infarction and serve as a comparison to other ECGs. An imbalance of myocardial oxygen supply and demand may be present without abnormal ECG changes. A normal ECG, even if obtained during a period of chest pain, does not completely exclude a cardiac origin for the pain.[66] An ECG tracing obtained during chest pain should be compared with the preoperative ECG to determine if new changes are present. Arrhythmias may also be associated with myocardial ischemia or infarction (see section on arrhythmias in this chapter).

Continuous ECG monitoring is useful in the patient at risk for myocardial ischemia. An early study involving exercise treadmill tests revealed that 89 per cent of all ischemic changes detected using a 12-lead ECG system were found using lead V_5.[67] A more recent study in patients undergoing noncardiac surgery under general anesthesia confirmed that V_5 is the most sensitive (75 per cent) of the 12 leads for the detection of ischemia.[68] Continuous ECG is also useful for detecting arrhythmias that may develop during myocardial ischemia or acute myocardial infarction.

Myocardial ischemia due to atherosclerotic coronary artery disease or coronary artery spasm may lead to different types of ECG change. If ischemia occurs because of atherosclerotic narrowing of coronary arteries, with an increase in myocardial oxygen demand the ECG frequently reveals ST segment depression or T wave inversion. If ischemia occurs because of coronary artery spasm, ST segment elevation, which is evidence of transmural myocardial ischemia, may be found on the ECG. With coronary artery spasm, nitroglycerin or nifedipine may reverse the spasm and quickly lead to normalization of the ST segments. If chest pain occurs because of acute myocardial infarction, there are several ECG possibilities: The T waves are tall and peaked, the ST segments are depressed, the T waves are inverted, the ST segments are elevated (and may not normalize with nitroglycerin or nifedipine), or Q waves develop.

There is no blood test that can acutely diagnose myocardial ischemia or acute myocardial infarction. The levels of serum glutamic oxaloacetic transaminase (SGOT), lactic dehydrogenase (LDH), creatine kinase (CK), and myocardial creatine kinase (MB-CK) are useful markers for myocardial infarction (cell death). However, these laboratory tests require significant time to perform and may be done only once a day in the hospital. The tests do not reveal myocardial ischemia, and the heart releases these enzymes into the blood several hours (not immediately) after symptoms of acute myocardial infarction occur. To complicate matters further, the trauma of surgery itself may lead to increased blood levels of these enzymes from tissues other than the heart.

The treatment of myocardial ischemia and acute myocardial infarction involves reversal of the underlying imbalance between myocardial oxygen supply and demand. The goal is to increase the amount of oxygen delivered to the myocardium and decrease the amount of oxygen required by the myocardium (Table 3–8).

Morphine sulfate is one of several drugs that may be used to treat the pain of myocardial ischemia or infarction. Morphine should be administered intravenously, in 1- to 3-mg increments, with careful patient assessment between each dose. Respiratory depression and hypotension may occur. Proper equipment for ventilatory resuscitation, as well as naloxone hydrochloride (a narcotic antagonist), should be immediately available. Hypotension is usually caused by a decreased venous and arterial vascular tone, with decreased preload and afterload. Appropriate intravenous access to al-

TABLE 3–8. POSTOPERATIVE TREATMENT OF MYOCARDIAL ISCHEMIA AND ACUTE MYOCARDIAL INFARCTION

1. Reverse the underlying cause of the imbalance between myocardial oxygen supply and demand.
2. Reassure the patient.
3. Administer supplemental oxygen.
4. Ensure good intravenous access.
5. Treat clinically significant hypotension, hypertension, and anemia.
6. Give morphine sulfate for analgesia.
7. Monitor the ECG continuously for ischemia/infarction as well as for arrhythmias.
8. Obtain a 12-lead hard copy ECG tracing.
9. Evaluate the need for antiarrhythmic therapy.
10. Perform frequent clinical assessments.
11. Give pharmacologic therapy (nitrates, β-blockers, calcium channel blockers).
12. Evaluate the need for an intensive care unit bed postoperatively.
13. Consider a cardiology consultation.

low for rapid intravenous fluid administration should be in place before morphine is administered.

Nitrates are commonly the first-line drugs used to treat chest pain of ischemic origin. Nitrates are venous and arterial dilators, primarily dilating the systemic veins and thus reducing left ventricular filling volume (preload) and myocardial oxygen demand. The systemic arterial vasculature may also be dilated, reducing afterload. The arterial system is much less sensitive to the effects of nitroglycerin than is the venous system. The coronary arteries are dilated by nitrates, leading to increased collateral blood flow and more blood (oxygen) delivered to the ischemic myocardium.

There are many nitrate preparations. Nitroglycerin sublingual tablets (0.3 to 0.6 mg) have an onset of action within 1 minute and a duration of action up to 30 minutes. Nitroglycerin sublingual tablets are readily available, are easy to administer, and act quickly. If chest pain is relieved by sublingual nitroglycerin, nitroglycerin ointment (1 to 3 inches) may be applied to the patient's skin. The onset of effect of topical nitroglycerin ointment is usually within 1 hour after application. However, its action is not as predictable, as the absorption of drug through the skin is not reliable, especially in the "cold," or vasoconstricted, postoperative patient. Orally administered nitrate preparations, as with other oral intake, may

not be appropriate during the acute postoperative period.

If chest pain is not relieved by sublingual nitroglycerin, an intravenous nitroglycerin infusion may be started. A low starting dose is recommended (0.5 to 1.5 μg/kg/min); the dose may be increased slowly until the chest pain is relieved or the patient's blood pressure drops significantly. Intravenous nitroglycerin begins to take effect immediately, and when discontinued its actions are terminated within minutes. Monitoring the postoperative patient who requires large doses of intravenous nitroglycerin may involve insertion of an arterial line to monitor systemic blood pressure continuously as well as insertion of a pulmonary artery catheter to monitor ventricular filling pressure, cardiac output, and mixed venous oxygen saturation. Administration of intravenous nitroglycerin may decrease morbidity and mortality associated with acute myocardial infarction.[69–71] Sublingual nitroglycerin tablets as well as intravenous nitroglycerin are reported to relieve coronary artery spasm.[72]

Hemodynamically, adverse effects of nitroglycerin administration include systemic hypotension and reflex tachycardia. Systemic hypotension occurs because of the relaxant effects of nitroglycerin on the vascular smooth muscle of the capacitance vessels of the body. Peripheral pooling results in decreased venous return and low cardiac output. Frequent blood pressure measurement is mandatory in the patient receiving nitroglycerin. A large intravenous line, especially in the hypovolemic postoperative patient, is needed to rapidly infuse fluid to treat the hypotension. If significant hypotension occurs, the nitroglycerin infusion should be terminated until the blood pressure stabilizes. A reflex tachycardia due to vascular relaxation can occur. Treatment of the tachycardia with a β-blocker may be appropriate in patients with good left ventricular function.

Another class of drugs used to treat chest pain of cardiac origin is the β-adrenergic blockers. β-Adrenergic receptors exist on the membranes of cardiac (β_1) as well as peripheral vascular and bronchial (β_2) smooth muscle. β-Blockers compete with the endogenous β-receptor agonists norepinephrine and epinephrine for attachment to the β-receptors on the cell membranes. A β-antagonist is labeled as β_1-selective if low doses inhibit cardiac β_1-activity with much less influence on the β_2-activity of the peripheral vascular and bronchial smooth muscle. However, in higher doses the β_1-specific antagonists also block the β_2-activity.

During the acute postoperative period, rapid onset of β-blockade requires the use of intravenous drugs. Currently available intravenous β-blockers include propranolol, metoprolol, esmolol, and labetalol. Intravenous β-blockers are titrated to lower the heart rate and blood pressure and to alleviate the symptoms of angina. The dosages used to treat myocardial ischemia are similar to those used to treat arrhythmias. (Refer to the arrhythmia section in this chapter.)

The value of β-blockers is thought to be in their ability to decrease myocardial oxygen demand. β_1-Blockade of the heart decreases the patient's heart rate and myocardial force of contraction. Patients with chest pain due to myocardial ischemia with coronary artery atherosclerosis and an increased heart rate or force of ventricular contraction may benefit from the reduced heart rate and contractility. The combination of β-blockers and nitrates has been previously discussed. Intravenous β-blockers given to patients with myocardial ischemia may lessen the chance of progression to an acute myocardial infarction.[73,74] Myocardial ischemia due to coronary artery spasm is not improved, and may be worsened, by the administration of a β-blocker.[75] With β-blockade, there is an unopposed vasoconstriction (α) effect on the coronary vessels.

Treatment of evolving acute myocardial infarction with β-blockers is controversial.[76–80] Nitrates are the initial drugs of choice for acute myocardial infarction, but β-blockers may decrease the extent of myocardial injury. Postoperative patients with high sympathetic tone, causing tachycardia and increased ventricular contractility, may benefit from β-blockade. β-Blockers titrated slowly to decrease the heart rate not only decrease myocardial oxygen demand but increase oxygen supply by lengthening diastolic left ventricular filling time.[73,74,81,82] Left ventricular perfusion occurs mostly during diastole. With the use of intravenous β-blocking drugs, caution must be observed. Of primary importance is the continuous display of the ECG (heart rhythm and rate). Bradycardia and heart block may occur. Sick sinus syndrome, second degree heart block, and third degree heart block are contraindications to the use of intravenous β-blockers. Heart failure may be precipitated in patients with poor left ventricular function. Bronchoconstriction may occur by blocking

β_2-mediated bronchodilation in patients with pulmonary disease. Caution should be used when β-blockers are given to a patient taking verapamil, as advanced heart block or severe hypotension may develop.

The calcium channel blockers (antagonists) are another class of drugs used to treat chest pain of cardiac origin. Calcium influx into cells is necessary for many processes: coronary artery spasm, peripheral vasoconstriction, myocardial contraction, and cardiac electrical activity. By inhibiting the flow of calcium through specific calcium ion channels in the cell membranes, calcium channel blockers have diverse cardiovascular effects.

For the treatment of chest pain due to coronary artery spasm, the calcium channel blockers are effective.[83,84] The constriction of coronary artery and peripheral arterial smooth muscle is dependent on the extracellular to intracellular movement of calcium. The flux of calcium into cells is necessary for coronary artery and peripheral vascular contraction to occur. Consequently, the administration of calcium channel blockers, by restricting the movement of extracellular calcium into the cells, dilates the coronary arteries and peripheral arterial beds. This finding is in contrast to that in cardiac muscle cells, which have a large reserve of intracellular calcium: Thus low doses of calcium channel blockers usually have little effect on normal cardiac muscle cell contraction.[85,86] With larger doses of calcium channel blockers, inhibition of normal myocardial contraction does occur. This specific effect of calcium channel blockers dilates a "spastic" coronary artery in such a dose that myocardial contractility is usually not significantly hampered.

During the acute postoperative period, immediate treatment of coronary artery spasm is needed. If the angina is not precipitated (preceded) by an increase in heart rate or blood pressure, and acute ST segment elevation is noted on ECG, coronary artery spasm is a potential diagnosis. In this setting, treatment involves intravenously, sublingually, or buccally administered drugs. Orally administered calcium channel blockers, even assuming normal gastrointestinal absorption in the postoperative patient, do not take effect acutely. The beneficial use of nitrates to treat coronary artery spasm have been discussed, as have the potentially harmful effects of β-blocking agents. Intravenous verapamil and sublingual or buccal nifedipine are useful to treat coronary artery spasm acutely. These preparations are readily available, quick in onset, and easy to administer. Intravenous verapamil should be given in incremental doses of 0.075 to 0.150 mg/kg, given slowly over 1 to 2 minutes. Peak effect is achieved within 5 minutes. The total intravenous dose of verapamil should not exceed 10 mg. This dosing schedule is similar to that used when verapamil is administered to treat arrhythmias. Nifedipine is not generally available in an intravenous preparation. However, nifedipine may be given by puncturing the 10 mg capsule and depositing the capsule's contents either under the tongue (sublingual) or between the gum and cheek (buccal). Nifedipine is then detected in the patient's serum within 3 minutes.[87] Nifedipine acts to dilate the spastic coronary artery and the systemic arterial beds and to lower afterload (decrease myocardial oxygen demand) if hypertension occurs as a result of the coronary artery spasm-induced myocardial ischemia.

Because of their diverse effects on the cardiovascular system, caution should be used when administering calcium channel blockers. Verapamil may decrease heart rate, decrease cardiac conduction, decrease myocardial contractility, and dilate the peripheral arterial vasculature (leading to hypotension). Verapamil should be used with caution in patients with poor left ventricular function and in those taking β-blockers or who have preexisting cardiac conduction defects. The primary adverse effect of nifedipine is due to peripheral arterial vasodilation. Hypotension with its associated reflex tachycardia can result in further imbalance of myocardial oxygen supply and demand.

PULMONARY ETIOLOGIES

Pulmonary Embolus

Disorders of the pulmonary system may lead to chest pain during the postoperative period. Pulmonary emboli may be associated with a sharp, pleuritic type of chest pain that may be confused with the pain of myocardial ischemia and infarction. Small pulmonary emboli are usually asymptomatic, whereas large pulmonary emboli may cause chest pain in addition to dyspnea, tachypnea, and cyanosis. Sudden cardiovascular collapse may be the presenting sign of massive pulmonary emboli. Pulmonary emboli are more common in the immobile postoperative patient, the postpar-

tum patient, and the patient with poor ventricular function or thrombophlebitis; it is also common in women taking birth control pills. Hemoptysis may be present. A tachypneic patient with clear lungs on chest auscultation and a negative chest roentgenogram is suspect for having pulmonary emboli.

Owing to occlusion of the pulmonary artery, the ECG may show signs of right ventricular strain (a rightward shift of the QRS axis and T wave inversion in the right precordial leads). New-onset sinus tachycardia or atrial fibrillation may occur. The chest film is usually normal but may reveal a peripheral wedge-shaped area of pulmonary infarction. Arterial blood gas assays usually demonstrate a low arterial oxygen level (hypoxemia) or carbon dioxide (hypocarbia) tension. Nuclear medicine ventilation-perfusion lung scans are screening procedures. However, the definitive diagnostic procedure is the pulmonary angiogram.

Acute therapy for pulmonary emboli involves systemic anticoagulation with a bolus of intravenous heparin followed by a continuous heparin infusion. The goal is to obtain a partial thromboplastin time (PTT) 1.5 to 2.0 times control.[88] Supplemental oxygen should be administered. In severe cases supportive therapy with positive inotropic and pulmonary vasodilator drugs may be needed. Intubation of the trachea and mechanical ventilation to decrease the work of breathing are also therapeutic options. If systemic anticoagulation is contraindicated for fear of excessive bleeding in the postoperative patient, then placement of an inferior vena cava filter (umbrella) should be considered. This type of filter prevents pelvic and lower extremity venous thrombi (blood clots) from traveling to the pulmonary artery circulation.

Pneumothorax

Pneumothorax during the postoperative period is frequently associated with ipsilateral chest pain. A pneumothorax may occur because of rupture of a pulmonary bleb or needle instrumentation of the parietal and visceral pleura. Rupture of a pulmonary bleb may be spontaneous or due to positive pressure ventilation (especially with positive end-expiratory pressure). The process of percutaneous internal jugular or subclavian vein cannulation, certain methods of brachial plexus local anesthesia blockade, and surgical procedures involving invasion of the chest may lead to a postoperative pneumothorax. The patient with a pneumothorax may complain of sharp chest pain and dyspnea. Physical examination varies with the extent of the pneumothorax. A small pneumothorax may reveal only a slight decrease in breath sounds on the ipsilateral side. A large pneumothorax reveals a marked decrease in breath sounds and hyperresonance on the ipsilateral side. A chest roentgenogram shows the degree of lung collapse. Treatment varies depending on the situation. A small pneumothorax (less than 20 per cent) in an otherwise healthy, spontaneously breathing patient may be observed, with no immediate intervention needed. A larger pneumothorax, especially in a patient with poor cardiopulmonary reserve, requires chest tube placement.

If positive pressure ventilation is administered to a patient with a pneumothorax, a tension pneumothorax may occur. In such cases the lung acts as a one-way valve and allows gas to enter the pleural space during inspiration but does not allow it to escape during expiration. The continued collection of gas within the pleural space then compresses the ipsilateral lung and shifts the mediastinal structures to the contralateral side. A decrease in venous return, hypoxemia, hypotension, and cardiovascular collapse may result. Tension pneumothorax is a medical emergency. It is potentially life-threatening, and decompression of the pleural space is mandatory.

GASTROINTESTINAL ETIOLOGIES

Gastrointestinal disturbances may cause chest pain[89] and may be difficult to distinguish from myocardial ischemia. History, physical examination, and some laboratory examinations (ECG, chest film, abdominal film, blood tests) can be accomplished during the immediate postoperative period. However, more complicated testing in the radiology department is not always easily performed, especially in the patient having chest pain in the PACU. For many gastrointestinal problems, involved radiologic procedures are needed to make the definitive diagnosis, further complicating patient management. When in doubt as to the etiology of pain, the conservative approach is to treat the patient as if myocardial ischemia is present until proved otherwise.

Reflux esophagitis is the regurgitation of gastric contents into the esophagus, causing inflammation of the esophageal mucosa. Regurgitation is due to an incompetent lower esophageal sphincter (a physiologic barrier), which may in turn be associated with a hiatus hernia. However, reflux esophagitis may occur in a patient without a hiatus hernia, and not all individuals with a hiatus hernia have reflux esophagitis. The patient complains of heartburn, indigestion, or gas. The symptom of retrosternal "burning" is also consistent with reflux esophagitis.

Lower esophageal sphincter spasm causes retrosternal chest pain that may radiate to the neck, arms, or back. A squeezing sensation may also be present. To make the distinction between esophageal spasm and myocardial ischemia even more confusing, the pain of each is relieved by nitrates[90,91] and nifedipine.[92,93] Nitrates and nifedipine cause relaxation of the lower esophageal sphincter.

Rupture of the esophagus is most commonly secondary to instrumentation or manipulation of the esophagus. Thus patients during the postoperative period who have undergone surgical procedures involving the esophagus should be followed closely. The patient may complain of radiating chest pain, and an upright chest film may reveal a pleural effusion or air in the mediastinum. Esophageal rupture may cause shock and lead to death.

Gastrointestinal causes of chest pain, apart from those of esophageal etiology, may be cholecystitis, peptic ulcer, or pancreatitis. Gallstones may lead to inflammation of the gallbladder wall, with resulting right upper quadrant or epigastric pain. The pain may radiate to the back and shoulders. Nausea, vomiting, fever, and chills may occur. Right upper quadrant tenderness is present. The pain of peptic ulcer disease is epigastric. It is relieved by milk or antacids. Perforation of a peptic ulcer leads to upper abdominal pain and muscle spasm. Free air under the diaphragm is found on an upright abdominal roentgenogram. Acute pancreatitis causes upper abdominal pain with radiation to the back. Fever and abdominal tenderness may be present. Laboratory examination reveals an elevated white blood cell count and amylase level.

ARRHYTHMIAS

Arrhythmias are a common occurrence during the acute postoperative period. Their successful treatment necessitates recognition, evaluation, and management of the patient, not just of the specific arrhythmia. An arrhythmia noted preoperatively may also be seen intraoperatively and postoperatively.

INCIDENCE

There are few studies documenting the incidence of arrhythmias during the acute postoperative period. Cohen et al.[94] followed 112,721 adults given anesthetics (general, regional and local) over two time periods. Time period I consisted of 52,197 anesthetics (1975–1978), and time period II consisted of 60,524 anesthetics (1979–1983). Overall, during time period I arrhythmias occurred intraoperatively in 3.6 per cent of the anesthetics, and for time period II it was 4.3 per cent. In the PACU after surgery, the incidence of arrhythmias for these same patient populations was 0.56 and 0.76 per cent, respectively, for the first and second time periods.

Cohen et al. found that the incidence of arrhythmias in the PACU was less than that in the operating room. However, there were certain limitations to this study. Not all patients were included; specifically, obstetric and pediatric patients were excluded. Of the patients studied, an ECG oscilloscope was used, but a permanent ECG record was not obtained. Thus some arrhythmias may have not been detected by the PACU staff.

MECHANISMS

Cardiac arrhythmias occur because of two mechanisms. The first involves a disorder of impulse formation and the second a disorder of impulse conduction. In addition, a combination of these two mechanisms may occur and result in an arrhythmia.[95]

Impulse formation is due to diastolic depolarization during phase IV of the action potential. Pacemaker cells are able to depolarize spontaneously (called automaticity). Normally, the cells of the sinus node are the first cells of the heart to achieve diastolic depolarization and initiate an action potential, which is conducted through the heart. Disorders of impulse formation include discharge rates of the sinus node that are too slow or too fast. Discharge from an ectopic pacemaker, which is usually suppressed by the sinus node activity, is also a disorder of impulse formation. Another example is an ectopic pacemaker that inappropriately increases its rate of discharge and thus steals, or captures, cardiac rhythm away from the sinus node.

Disorders of impulse conduction include atrioventricular (AV) conduction block and reentry. Once an impulse is initiated within the sinoatrial (SA) node, normal propagation of the impulse is through the internodal pathways within the atria to the AV node. From the AV node, the impulse is conducted through the bundle of His, then the left and right bundle branches to the Purkinje network and cardiac muscle fibers. A conduction block is either a delay in or a complete lack of conduction of an impulse from the SA node throughout the heart. Reentry is a manifestation of altered conduction. Reentry may occur in the sinus node, atrium, AV junction, or ventricular conduction system.[96]

The combination of abnormal impulse formation and conduction is also of concern. A premature ventricular contraction, initiated by abnormal automaticity, may then become ventricular tachycardia sustained by reentry.

It is useful to understand the possible mechanisms for an arrhythmia. However, it is not possible to determine the exact electrophysiologic mechanism for all arrhythmias. ECG examination does not with certainty determine whether an arrhythmia is due to a disorder of impulse formation, impulse conduction, or a combination of the two. Nonetheless, for purposes of patient management, one can postulate that a particular arrhythmia is more likely to have a particular mechanism.

CLINICAL PRESENTATION

The significance of a particular arrhythmia is based on the clinical evaluation of the patient (Table 3–9). Two major complications of arrhythmias are a decrease in the myocardial oxygen supply/demand ratio and a decrease in cardiac output. With tachycardia and the resultant reduced diastolic time, myocardial oxygen supply may decrease owing to reduced coronary artery blood flow. In addition, myocardial oxygen demand increases with the increased heart rate. Tachycardia, bradycardia, conduction block, or loss of rhythmic atrial and ventricular contraction may decrease the blood flow through the coronary arteries and brain owing to a reduction in cardiac output. Angina, a symptom of myocardial ischemia, may not be present in the PACU.

The decision to treat an arrhythmia must be made on an individual basis. A young woman

TABLE 3–9. CLINICAL CONSEQUENCES OF ARRHYTHMIAS

Symptoms
  Palpitations
  Chest pain
  Nausea
  Lethargy
  Dyspnea

Signs
  Slow, fast, irregular, or absent pulse and heart sounds
  Hypotension
  Mental status changes (including syncope)
  Apnea
  Pulmonary rales
  Diaphoresis
  "Cardiopulmonary arrest"

with a supraventricular tachycardia associated with mitral valve prolapse may tolerate the event better than an elderly man with coronary artery disease and cerebral vascular disease. Even if a patient may seem clinically "stable," an arrhythmia may deteriorate rapidly and require active resuscitation of the patient. Anticipation of such events is essential.

ECG Monitoring

The specific diagnosis of an arrhythmia during the acute postoperative period is commonly based on continuous ECG monitoring. Some patients are transported from the oper-ating room suite to the PACU room with ECG monitoring continued during transport. If not monitored during transport, ECG monitoring should be initiated as soon as the patient arrives in the PACU.

The five-electrode or three-electrode ECG system may be used. The five-electrode system, specifically the V_5 lead, is useful for monitoring anterolateral myocardial ischemia (Fig. 3–1). Inferior wall ischemia is monitored by lead II. As described by Kaplan and King,[97] the five-electrode system can monitor ECG leads I, II, III, aVR, aVL, aVF, and V_5. Leads V_5 and II can be monitored simultaneously to aid with ischemia and arrhythmia detection.

However, the ECG leads that are the most appropriate for monitoring for ischemia are not necessarily the most useful for monitoring for rhythm disturbances. Use of the ECG for arrhythmia recognition focuses on the observation of the P wave and QRS complex.[98] P wave analysis and awareness of the P wave and QRS complex relation are poorly accomplished by lead V_5. Lead II and its modifications are useful for the analysis of arrhythmias. Lead II easily identifies P waves because it is parallel to the P wave vector.

Many PACUs utilize a three-electrode ECG system. A modified V_5 lead system can be accomplished by placing the left arm lead in the V_5 position (fifth intercostal space at the anterior axillary line) and the right arm lead under the right clavicle or just to the right of the manubrium of the sternum.[99] If the oscilloscope is set to lead I, a modified V_5 lead is produced. The left leg lead may be placed in its usual position; and if the oscilloscope is set

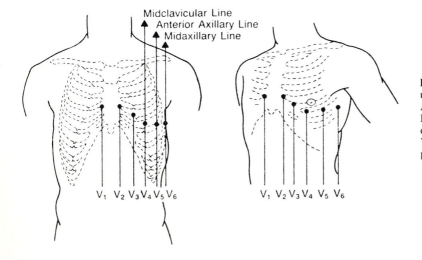

Midclavicular Line
Anterior Axillary Line
Midaxillary Line

V_1 V_2 V_3 V_4 V_5 V_6

V_1 V_2 V_3 V_4 V_5 V_6

FIGURE 3–1. Locations of the unipolar precordial leads. (From Atlee JL: Perioperative Cardiac Dysrhythmias: Mechanisms, Recognition, Management. Chicago, Year Book, 1985, p. 103. With permission.)

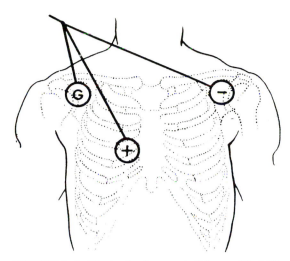

FIGURE 3–2. Electrode placement of the modified CL_1 lead (MCL_1). (From Marriott HJL: Practical Electrocardiography, 8th ed. Baltimore, Williams & Wilkins, 1988, p. 120. With permission.)

TABLE 3–10. ETIOLOGY OF POSTOPERATIVE ARRHYTHMIAS

Catecholamine release (sympathetic discharge)
    Pain
    Anxiety
    Surgical stress
    Hypovolemia
Primary cardiac origin
    Preexisting arrhythmia
    Myocardial ischemia and infarction
    Heart failure
Inhalation anesthetics
    Halothane
    Enflurane
    Isoflurane
    Nitrous oxide
Intravenous anesthetics
    Ketamine
    Narcotics (morphine, fentanyl, sufentanil)
Reversal of neuromuscular blockade
    Anticholinesterase agents
    Anticholinergic agents
Regional anesthesia
Electrolyte and acid-base disorders
    Hyperkalemia
    Hypokalemia
    Hypercarbia
    Hypoxemia
    Alkalosis
    Acidosis
Hypothermia

to lead II, enhanced inferior wall arrhythmia and ischemia detection is possible.

Another useful lead for monitoring arrhythmias is the MCL_1 lead (modified central lead) (Fig. 3–2). Here the left arm electrode is placed under the outer left clavicle, and the left leg electrode is placed in the V_1 position (fourth intercostal space to the right of the sternum). The right arm electrode is placed in its usual position, and the oscilloscope is set to lead III.

The 12-lead ECG is the standard to which other arrhythmia detection systems are compared. A printed copy of all 12 leads is easy to obtain during the acute postoperative period. An esophageal ECG, intracardiac electrogram, or endotracheal ECG is at times also useful.[97] Discussion of these techniques is beyond the scope of this chapter.

ETIOLOGY

There are many potential etiologies for postoperative arrhythmias (Table 3–10). Although the exact determination of a specific etiology is not always possible, a working differential diagnosis may more effectively guide patient management. If possible, one should treat the cause of an arrhythmia. Frequently, review of the patient's preoperative, intraoperative, and postoperative course yields needed information. Assessment of the airway and physical examination of the respiratory system are mandatory. Oxygenation and ventilation should be immediately assessed. However, one should never delay treatment of hemodynamically significant arrhythmias while waiting for results to return from the laboratory.

Increased catecholamine release (sympathetic discharge) is probably the most common cause of the benign arrhythmias during the acute postoperative period. Pain, anxiety, and surgical stress lead to sinus tachycardia and premature ventricular complexes. Hypovolemia leads to a compensatory tachycardia.

Primary cardiac disease causes arrhythmias, and preexisting arrhythmias may persist. Sick sinus syndrome, conduction block, and various atrial or ventricular arrhythmias may be more frequent after the physiologic alterations that occur postoperatively. Myocardial ischemia and infarction are commonly associated with arrhythmias, e.g., premature ventricular complexes, ventricular tachycardia, ventricular fibrillation, and bradycardias. Heart failure may lead to a tachycardia in order to support cardiac output with a decreased stroke volume.

The potent inhalation agents (halothane, enflurane, isoflurane) as well as nitrous oxide[100] have been associated with intraoperative arrhythmias. However, at the end of the surgical procedure, when the anesthetic gases are discontinued, ventilation acts to excrete almost all of these agents from the body. During the acute postoperative period, there is usually minimal inhalation agent remaining in the body. Postoperative hypoxemia, hypercarbia, pain, anxiety, and resultant catecholamine release are the more common causes of arrhythmia.

The effects of intravenous anesthetic agents may continue into the postoperative period. Ketamine is associated with an increased heart rate owing to central sympathetic stimulation and decreased reuptake of norepinephrine. However, aside from an increased heart rate, ketamine is not usually associated with other rhythm disturbances. With the exception of meperidine,[101] the use of narcotics (morphine, fentanyl, sufentanil, alfentanil) may cause bradycardia. Bradycardia occurs because of central vagal stimulation.

The reversal of muscle relaxants frequently alters heart rate. Administration of an anticholinesterase (neostigmine, pyridostigmine, edrophonium) can lead to bradycardia. The anticholinesterase agents antagonize nondepolarizing neuromuscular blockade by inhibiting acetylcholinesterase at the neuromuscular junction. Thus acetylcholine at the neuromuscular junction is increased and the competitive effects of the nondepolarizing neuromuscular blockade are reversed. Acetylcholinesterase agents increase acetylcholine not only at the skeletal muscle but throughout the rest of the body. Specifically, an increase in acetylcholine at the heart (muscarinic effect) causes bradycardia. To prevent such bradycardia, which would occur in the operating room or the PACU, the anticholinesterase agent is administered with an anticholinergic agent (atropine, glycopyrrolate).

Regional anesthesia may lead to postoperative arrhythmias. If spinal or epidural anesthesia involves thoracic levels 1 through 4, the sympathetic fibers responsible for cardiac acceleration stimulation are blocked. Bradycardia may result from parasympathetic (vagal) predominance. This point is especially important when the patient is moved from the operating room to the PACU. With sympathetic blockade, the cardiovascular system is not able to compensate for the redistribution of the blood volume that occurs during patient movement. Bradycardia, hypotension, and cardiovascular collapse may occur. In addition, direct intravascular administration or overdosage of local anesthetic agents may lead to arrhythmias and cardiovascular collapse.

Electrolyte and acid-base disorders may cause arrhythmias. Potassium plays a major role in determining the resting membrane potential of the specialized conduction cells within the heart. Hyperkalemia at a serum potassium level of 6.5 mEq/L causes narrowed and peaked T waves. At a level of 7.0 to 8.0 mEq/L, the QRS complex widens, the PR interval increases, and the P wave disappears. A serum potassium level higher than 10.0 mEq/L may produce a sine wave pattern on ECG, ventricular asystole, or ventricular fibrillation.

Various authors have discussed the potential risks of hypokalemia.[102–104] ECG changes of hypokalemia include ST segment abnormalities, T wave flattening, and U waves. Specifically, the role of hypokalemia as the etiologic agent of arrhythmias during the acute postoperative period has not been well studied. Only a few studies have evaluated preoperative potassium levels in relation to intraoperative arrhythmias.[105,106] Areas of debate include whether to postpone elective surgical procedures in the hypokalemic noncardiac patient as well as the hypokalemic cardiac patient. Limiting the discussion to the postoperative period, hypokalemia is certainly a potential cause of arrhythmias. However, there are limited data at this time to imply that patients with a potassium level of 3.0 to 3.5 mEq/L are more likely to experience postoperative arrhythmias. Nonetheless, potassium replacement is appropriate in the postoperative hypokalemic patient who is having an arrhythmia. In addition, other causes of the arrhythmia should be excluded.

Hypercarbia and hypoxemia may occur postoperatively and lead to arrhythmias. Immediately postoperatively, all patients should be given supplemental oxygen after a general anesthetic. Ventilation and oxygenation must frequently be assessed, with intubation and mechanical ventilation initiated if needed. Hypercarbia leads to acidosis, with an increase in sympathetic nervous system activity. Metabolic factors may also cause significant acidosis. Hypoxemia not only stimulates catecholamine secretion, it leads to myocardial ischemia. Hypocarbia, most commonly due to excessive mechanical ventilation, results in alkalosis and potassium shifts into cells (hypo-kalemia).

Hypothermia[107,108] causes a decreased heart rate, T wave inversion, and a decrease in cardiac conduction. Prolongation of the PR interval, QT interval, and QRS duration may result. Elevation of the ST segment, called an Osborn or J wave, may be confused with the ST segment changes of myocardial ischemia. If the rectal temperature drops to below 30°C, ventricular fibrillation may occur.

TREATMENT

Once the decision has been made to treat an arrhythmia, there are usually several options available (Table 3–11). First, if the clinical circumstances allow, the cause of an arrhythmia should be evaluated and reversed. Second, the various methods of available treatment should be considered: pharmacologic, pacemaker, synchronized cardioversion, and defibrillation. Pharmacologic treatment of an arrhythmia involves intravenously administered agents.

Atropine blocks acetylcholine at cardiac muscarinic receptors. Vagolytic action increases SA node automaticity and AV conduction. Atropine is the drug of choice for several types of bradycardia. The dosage is 0.5 mg IV, which may be repeated to a total of 2.0 mg. This total dose provides maximal vagolytic action.[109]

Isoproterenol is a nonspecific β-adrenergic agonist, i.e., both β_1- and β_2-receptors are stimulated. When atropine is ineffective, isoproterenol is used as a temporary measure to treat bradycardia and heart block. It is administered as a continuous infusion of 2 to 10 μg/min and titrated to obtain a ventricular response of more than 60 beats/min. However, isoproterenol therapy has its disadvantages, and it is used only to support the patient until more definitive therapy with a pacemaker can be undertaken. β_1 Activity leads not only to an increased heart rate but also to increased myocardial contractility and automaticity, with the potential for inducing tachyarrhythmias. β_2 Activity leads to systemic vasodilation and the possibility of decreased blood pressure, which may lower coronary artery perfusion. Caution is needed when administering isoproterenol to any patient but especially to one with coronary artery disease.

Lidocaine decreases automaticity by reducing the slope of phase IV diastolic depolarization.[110] It may also decrease conduction through reentry pathways by transforming a unidirectional block into a bidirectional block.[111] Indications for lidocaine include treatment of premature ventricular complexes and ventricular tachycardia, and it is used as an adjunct to the management of ventricular fibrillation. Lidocaine should be administered as an intravenous bolus, followed by a continuous infusion. A bolus of 1.0 to 1.5 mg/kg with an infusion rate of 1 to 4 mg/min (15 to 60 μg/kg/min) is usually adequate. Because of rapid peripheral distribution, the serum half-life of a lidocaine bolus is 15 minutes. One hour is required to achieve a steady-state level from an infusion. To avoid central nervous system toxicity, the dosage should be decreased in the elderly as well as in patients with decreased cardiac output or hepatic dysfunction.

Procainamide is used when lidocaine is not effective against ventricular arrhythmias. It reduces automaticity by decreasing phase IV diastolic depolarization. Intraventricular conduction is also slowed. There are two methods for administering a loading dose of procainamide. Continuous ECG monitoring and careful blood pressure monitoring should be followed for both. With the first method,[112] 100 mg of procainamide (1.5 mg/kg) is given over a 2-minute period and repeated every 5 minutes until one of the following occurs: 1) the arrhythmia is abolished; 2) a total of 1 g of drug (15 mg/kg) is given; 3) untoward drug effects appear, i.e., hypotension or AV or intraventricular conduction disturbances. The second method[113] is to administer a loading

TABLE 3–11. TREATMENT OF ARRHYTHMIAS

1. Clinical evaluation of the patient, with reversal of any suspected underlying cause for the arrhythmia (if time permits)
2. Cardiopulmonary resuscitation if needed
3. Oxygen therapy
4. Pharmacologic therapy
   a. Atropine
   b. Isoproterenol
   c. Lidocaine
   d. Procainamide
   e. Bretylium
   f. Digoxin
   g. β-Blockers (propranolol, metoprolol, esmolol, labetalol)
   h. Calcium channel blockers (verapamil)
5. Pacemaker
6. Synchronized cardioversion
7. Defibrillation

dose of procainamide (17 mg/kg) over 1 hour, also looking for any untoward effects. After either loading dose method, a maintenance infusion of 20 to 80 μg/kg/min should be started. In patients with heart failure or renal dysfunction, the loading and maintenance doses of procainamide may need to be decreased.

Bretylium[96] is used to treat ventricular tachycardia and ventricular fibrillation refractory to other forms of therapy (lidocaine, procainamide, synchronized cardioversion, defibrillation). Initially, bretylium releases norepinephrine from peripheral adrenergic nerve terminals, which results in transient (about 20 minutes) hypertension and tachycardia. After initially causing norepinephrine release, bretylium then prevents norepinephrine release from sympathetic nerve terminals without depressing preganglionic or postganglionic sympathetic nerve conduction, impairing conduction across sympathetic ganglia, depleting the adrenergic neuron of norepinephrine, or decreasing the responsiveness of adrenergic receptors.[114] By inhibiting norepinephrine release from peripheral adrenergic nerve terminals, bretylium may cause hypotension. Bretylium increases the ventricular fibrillation threshold. The reason bretylium is an antiarrhythmic agent has not been determined (i.e., sympathectomy-like state or an electrophysiologic action).[115] With ventricular fibrillation and pulseless ventricular tachycardia, bretylium is given as an initial bolus of 5 mg/kg IV with repeated boluses of 10 mg/kg every 15 to 30 minutes. The maximum total dose is 30 mg/kg. For ventricular tachycardia with a pulse, a dilute bretylium infusion of 5 to 10 mg/kg is given over 10 minutes. If needed, the maintenance bretylium infusion is 2 mg/min in a 70 kg patient.

Digoxin, by decreasing the rate of conduction through the AV node, controls the ventricular rate in patients with atrial fibrillation or atrial flutter. Decreased conduction through the AV node may be due either to a vagal effect of digoxin or to a more direct extravagal effect on the cells.[116] Larger doses of digoxin may be needed to control ventricular rates in patients with atrial fibrillation and atrial flutter, compared to when it is used as a positive inotropic agent. Digoxin has been replaced by verapamil as the drug of choice for the treatment of paroxysmal supraventricular tachycardia. In a normal adult, the intravenous loading dose of digoxin is 0.5 to 1.0 mg (0.25 to 0.50 mg given initially followed by 0.25 mg q6h for two or three doses). Maintenance dosage is 0.125–0.500 mg IV daily. Initial effects are seen within 30 minutes of intravenous digoxin, with peak effect at about 2 hours. This delay in onset of action makes digoxin an inappropriate initial treatment for arrhythmias (atrial fibrillation, atrial flutter, paroxysmal supraventricular tachycardia) if hemodynamic compromise is present. Smaller doses should be used in the elderly and in patients with renal dysfunction. Digoxin toxicity may lead to numerous cardiac arrhythmias.

Propranolol is the most commonly used β-blocking agent. It blocks the ability of catecholamines to attach to the β-receptors. Propranolol is nonselective in its action, i.e., blocks both the β_1- and β_2-receptors. Propranolol decreases the rate of spontaneous phase IV depolarization in the SA node and decreases conduction through the AV node. Clinically, propranolol should be used to treat catecholamine- or myocardial ischemia-induced arrhythmias of either supraventricular or ventricular origin, especially if other treatments fail. By decreasing AV node conduction, reentry at the AV node during paroxysmal supraventricular tachycardia may be abolished. Also, the ventricular response during atrial fibrillation or atrial flutter may be decreased. Propranolol should be given in increments of 0.1 to 0.5 mg IV every 5 minutes, with the total dose not to exceed 0.1 mg/kg. It has a plasma half-life of 4 hours. Hypotension, congestive heart failure, bronchospasm, and masking of hypoglycemia-related signs are adverse effects of propranolol.

Metoprolol is a β_1 cardioselective receptor antagonist. Metoprolol in smaller doses does not effect β_2-receptors as much as propranolol. The indications and precautions with metoprolol are similar to those of propranolol. The dosage of metoprolol is also similar to that of propranolol, with increments of 0.25 to 0.50 mg IV every 5 minutes, with the total dose not to exceed 0.1 mg/kg. It has a plasma half-life of 4 hours.

Esmolol is a β_1 cardioselective receptor antagonist with an elimination half-life of about 9 minutes. It is administered as an initial intravenous bolus of up to 500 μg/kg followed by a continuous infusion starting at 50 μg/kg/min. Dosage is titrated to effect. If needed, one may repeat the bolus and increase the rate of infusion. Larger bolus doses may subsequently be used. Indications for esmolol therapy are similar to those of propranolol. The β_1 cardioselective blockade of esmolol, as well as its short duration of action, may make its use advantageous compared to propranolol or metoprolol.

Labetalol combines α_1-receptor blockade and nonselective β-blockade. Given intravenously, the ratio of α/β blockade is $1:7$. Initial bolus doses should be 2.5 to 10.0 mg. Administration of twice the previously administered bolus may be repeated every 5 to 10 minutes. Dosage is titrated to effect. During the acute postoperative period, labetalol is most often used to treat catecholamine-induced sinus tachycardia and associated hypertension.

Verapamil is a calcium channel blocker that decreases conduction and increases refractoriness through the AV node. Verapamil is used to treat paroxysmal supraventricular tachycardia, atrial fibrillation, and atrial flutter. Because paroxysmal supraventricular tachycardia involves reentery at the AV node, verapamil terminates this rhythm 90 per cent of the time. With atrial fibrillation and atrial flutter, verapamil successfully reduces the ventricular rate. Verapamil can be given as 0.075 to 0.150 mg/kg IV over 1 to minutes. Peak therapeutic effects occur within 5 minutes. Repeat doses of up to 0.15 mg/kg may be given 30 minutes later. No single dose should exceed 10 mg. Untoward effects due to verapamil may include hypotension secondary to peripheral vasodilatation and decreased ventricular function. Verapamil should not be used with AV block or in the presence of sick sinus syndrome unless a pacemaker is present. In addition, caution should be used when treating patients with verapamil who are already taking β-blockers.

Specific Arrhythmias

There are numerous arrhythmias. Specific ones are listed in Table 3–12.

Sinus Tachycardia

Sinus tachycardia results from an increased discharge rate of the sinus node (Fig. 3–3). The rhythm is regular, with a heart rate of usually 100 to 160 beats/min. The QRS complex is normal (narrow), as is the P wave morphology. Common causes of sinus tachycardia include pain, anxiety, hypoxemia, hypercarbia, fever, hypovolemia, and congestive heart failure. In patients with coronary artery disease or valvular heart disease, the following may occur: hypotension, myocardial ischemia or a decreased cardiac output. Once the pri-

TABLE 3–12. SPECIFIC ARRHYTHMIAS

Sinus tachycardia
Atrial flutter
Atrial fibrillation
Paroxysmal supraventricular tachycardia (PSVT)
Sinus bradycardia
First degree atrioventricular (AV) block
Second degree AV block: type I, type II
Third degree AV block (complete heart block)
Premature atrial contractions (PACs)
Premature ventricular contractions (PVCs)
Ventricular tachycardia
Torsades de pointes (twisting of the points)
Ventricular fibrillation
Ventricular asystole
Electromechanical dissociation (EMD)
Wolff-Parkinson-White syndrome: reentry supraventricular tachycardia, atrial fibrillation

mary cause of sinus tachycardia has been treated. β-blockers may then be used (if heart failure is not present) to lower the heart rate.

Atrial Flutter

Atrial flutter is characterized by a regular rapid atrial rate of 250 to 350 beats/min. It is thought to result from reentry within the atrium. At the AV node there are varying degrees of conduction block, with the ventricular rate usually half the atrial rate. The ECG reveals "sawtooth" flutter waves in leads II, III, and aVf. The QRS complex is usually normal, but with a conduction defect it widens. Ischemic heart disease, mitral valvular disease, hypertensive heart disease, cor

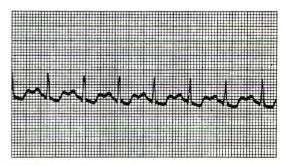

FIGURE 3–3. Sinus tachycardia. Note regular rhythm at the rate of 121 beats/min. Each QRS is preceded by an upright P wave in lead 2. (From Textbook of Advanced Cardiac Life Support, 2nd ed. New York, American Heart Association, 1987, p. 68. With permission.)

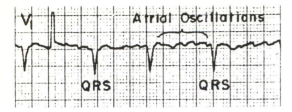

FIGURE 3–4. Atrial fibrillation. Irregular fibrillatory waves are seen interrupting the baseline. The ventricular response is 75 to 88 beats/min. (From Shoemaker WC: Textbook of Critical Care, 2nd ed. Philadelphia, Saunders, 1989, p. 370. With permission.)

pulmonale, cardiomyopathy, pericarditis, postcardiac surgery, and hyperthyroidism are the most common cause of atrial flutter.[117] Myocardial ischemia or congestive heart failure may develop because of the atrial flutter. Pharmacologic treatment is with digoxin, β-blockers, or verapamil, all of which decrease the ventricular rate. However, the therapy of choice for atrial flutter with a rapid ventricular rate and hemodynamic instability is synchronized cardioversion. Low energy levels, usually 50 to 100 joules, may convert new-onset atrial flutter to sinus rhythm.

Atrial Fibrillation

Atrial fibrillation is characterized by irregular atrial activity that occurs from 300 to 600 beats/min (Fig. 3–4). There is no organized atrial contraction, so distinct P waves are not present. An irregular ventricular rhythm usually results. The QRS is normal unless a conduction defect exists. The ventricular rate is 150 to 200 beats/min. Associated conditions include chronic cardiac or pulmonary disease, pulmonary embolus, and hyperthyroidism. As with atrial flutter, myocardial ischemia and congestive heart failure may occur. Atrial fibrillation may appear after cardiac or other

thoracic procedures. Prophylactic digitalization has been recommended for certain thoracic procedures.[118,119] Pharmacologic therapy of atrial fibrillation includes digoxin, β-blockers, and verapamil. The goal is to decrease the ventricular rate, preferably to fewer than 100 beats/min. When a rapid ventricular response and hemodynamic instability exist, the treatment of choice is synchronized cardioversion. Normal sinus rhythm may be restored if atrial fibrillation is not chronic. Low energy levels, starting with 50 joules, are utilized.

Paroxysmal Supraventricular Tachycardia

Paroxysmal supraventricular tachycardia (PSVT) is usually an AV nodal reentrant tachycardia (Fig. 3–5). The heart rate is regular at 150 to 250 beats/min. The QRS is normal unless a conduction defect exists. The onset of PSVT is usually sudden, following a premature atrial complex. The termination is also sudden. PSVT may occur in otherwise normal, as well as diseased, hearts. A healthy patient may tolerate the tachycardia well. However, as with other tachyarrhythmias, the presence of preexisting heart disease may lead to myocardial ischemia or congestive heart failure. Carotid sinus massage may be used in the stable patient unless cerebrovascular disease is present. Carotid sinus massage may lead to conversion of PSVT to normal sinus rhythm or to a decreased rate of the tachycardia (while the massage is taking place). Pharmacologic therapy involves verapamil (the drug of choice), which may convert the patient to sinus rhythm (Fig. 3–6). Digoxin and propranolol may also be used to treat PSVT; however, there is less chance of conversion to sinus rhythm than with verapamil. For the unstable patient, synchronized cardioversion, initially with 75 to 100 joules, is the treatment of choice.

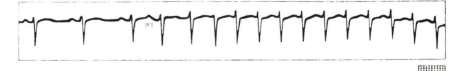

FIGURE 3–5. Paroxysmal supraventricular tachycardia (PSVT) initiated by a premature atrial beat (bracketed P). Note that the RR interval during PSVT shortens over the first three beats of the tachycardia. The established rate for the tachycardia is 188 beats/min. (From Atlee JL: Perioperative Cardiac Dysrhythmias: Mechanisms, Recognition, Management. Chicago, Year Book, 1985, p. 239. With permission.)

FIGURE 3–6. Paroxysmal supraventricular tachycardia (PSVT). This sequence was developed to assist teaching how to treat a broad range of patients with sustained PSVT. Some patients require care not specified herein. This algorithm should not be construed as prohibiting such flexibility. Flow of the algorithm presumes PSVT is continuing. (From Textbook of Advanced Cardiac Life Support, 2nd ed. New York, American Heart Association, 1987, p. 244. With permission.)

Unstable	Stable
↓	↓
Synchronous Cardioversion 75–100 Joules	Vagal Maneuvers
↓	↓
Synchronous Cardioversion 200 Joules	Verapamil, 5 mg IV
↓	↓
Synchronous Cardioversion 360 Joules	Verapamil, 10 mg IV (in 15–20 min)
↓	↓
Correct Underlying Abnormalities	Cardioversion, Digoxin, β-Blockers, Pacing as Indicated (see Text)
↓	
Pharmacological Therapy + Cardioversion	

If conversion occurs but PSVT recurs, repeated electrical cardioversion is *not* indicated. Sedation should be used as time permits.

Sinus Bradycardia

Sinus bradycardia implies a heart rate of fewer than 60 beats/min. There is otherwise normal electrical activity of the heart, with the origin of the impulse at the SA node (Fig. 3–7). Conduction through the AV node, bundle of His, and Purkinje fibers results in a normal P wave preceding each QRS complex, which is followed by a T wave. The QRS complex is usually narrow. Sinus bradycardia may be seen in athletes and patients with sinus node dysfunction. In the postoperative patient, sinus bradycardia has many potential etiologies (Table 3–13). Treatment is needed if myocardial ischemia, hypotension, an escape rhythm, or low cardiac output occurs. The underlying cause should be treated. Additional therapy includes atropine in 0.5 mg increments up to a total of 2.0 mg. If atropine therapy is ineffective, as a temporary measure an isoproterenol infusion administered at a dose of 2 to 10 μg/min can be used. Isoproterenol should be used cautiously because of its ability

TABLE 3–13. ETIOLOGIES OF SINUS BRADYCARDIA

Drug-induced bradycardia
    β-Blockade
    Calcium channel blockade
    Reversal of neuromuscular blockade
    Narcotics
Hypoxemia
Carotid sinus dysfunction
Hypothermia
Reflex activity due to hypertension
"High" spinal or epidural blockade
Increased intracranial pressure
Acute inferior wall myocardial infarction
Distended bladder
Mesenteric stimulation
Oculocardiac reflex
Carotid sinus reflex
Airway suctioning

to induce ventricular arrhythmias. As more definitive therapy, placement of a transvenous pacemaker is indicated, rather than persisting with atropine or isoproterenol.

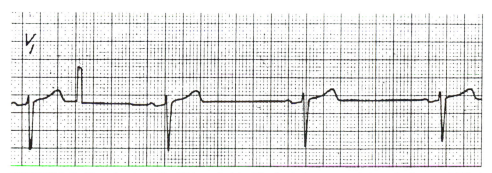

FIGURE 3–7. Sinus bradycardia (38 beats/min). All criteria for a normal sinus rhythm are fulfilled except the rate, which is less than 60 beats/min. (From Shoemaker WC: Textbook of Critical Care, 2nd ed. Philadelphia, Saunders, 1989, p. 373. With permission.)

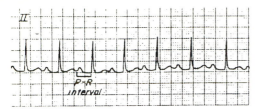

FIGURE 3–8. First degree AV block. The PR interval is prolonged at 0.26 second. (From Shoemaker WC: Textbook of Critical Care, 2nd ed. Philadelphia, Saunders, 1989, p. 375. With permission.)

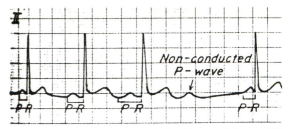

FIGURE 3–9. Mobitz I (Wenckebach) second degree AV block. Gradual prolongation of the PR interval is followed by a nonconducted P wave. The following complex shows a shortened PR interval, and the cycle is resumed. (From Shoemaker WC: Textbook of Critical Care, 2nd ed. Philadelphia, Saunders, 1989, p. 375. With permission.)

Atrioventricular Block

Atrioventricular blocks are divided into three categories: first, second, and third degree. The diagnosis of each may be made by the surface ECG. With first degree AV block, every P wave is followed by a QRS complex. With this block, the PR interval is prolonged (0.21 second or more). With first degree AV block, the conduction delay may be located within the AV node or the His-Purkinje system. Causes of first degree AV block include increased vagal tone or AV node dysfunction (Fig. 3–8). With a normal heart rate, no treatment is needed. However, new-onset first degree AV block may progress to a higher degree of AV block, and thus further observation is required during the acute postoperative period.

Second degree AV block is divided into two types. With each type, some atrial impulses are conducted to the ventricles and others are not. Type I second degree AV block, also called Mobitz type I or Wenckebach, usually occurs at the level of the AV node (Fig. 3–9). It appears when the PR interval gradually increases, revealing decreased conduction through the AV node. The P wave may not be conducted to the ventricles. Increased vagal tone, or drug effects on the AV node (verapamil, digoxin, propranolol), may cause the block. Inferior wall myocardial infarction may also cause type I block.

Type II second degree AV block, also called Mobitz type II, usually occurs below the level of the AV node, at the bundle branch level (Fig. 3–10). Unlike type I AV block, with type II AV block the PR interval does not increase prior to a nonconducted beat. A complete block of either the right or left bundle branch, in addition to an intermittent block in the contralateral bundle branch, is needed for type II AV block to occur. Vagal predominance and drug effects do not cause type II AV block. Anterior wall myocardial infarction may result in type II AV block. There is a worse prognosis associated with type II than with type I AV block.

Third degree AV block, also called com-

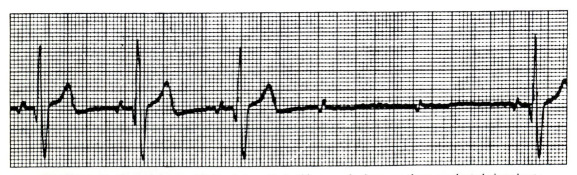

FIGURE 3–10. Second degree AV block type II. In this example there are three conducted sinus beats followed by two nonconducted P waves. The PR interval of conducted beats remains constant, and the QRS is wide. (From Textbook of Advanced Cardiac Life Support, 2nd ed. New York, American Heart Association, 1987, p. 82. With permission.)

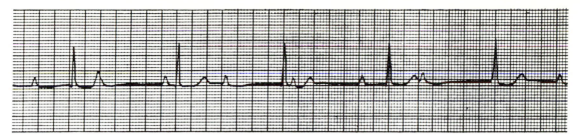

FIGURE 3–11. Third degree AV block occurring at the level of the AV node. Atrial rhythm is slightly irregular due to the presence of sinus arrhythmia. Ventricular rhythm is regular at a slower rate (44 beats/ min). There is no constant PR interval. The QRS complexes are narrow, indicating supraventricular origin below the level of the block. (From Textbook of Advanced Cardiac Life Support, 2nd ed. New York, American Heart Association, 1987, p. 83. With permission.)

plete heart block, illustrates the absence of any conduction between the atria and ventricles (Fig. 3–11). The atria and ventricles beat independently, with ventricular contraction initiated by intrinsic pacemakers either high or low in the ventricles. The ventricular rate is usually less than 60 beats/min, although the exact rate depends on the site of the ventricular pacemaker. The QRS complex may be narrow or wide, also depending on the site of the ventricular pacemaker. Causes of third degree heart block include drug effects as well as both inferior and anterior wall myocardial infarctions.

Clinically, the concern is that AV blocks may progress in severity to reduce cardiac output. Myocardial ischemia, dyspnea, and mental status changes may occur. Drug therapy, which may temporarily increase heart rate, includes atropine and isoproterenol (Fig. 3–12). Treatment of AV blocks is similar to that for sinus bradycardia. Atropine 0.5 mg IV given up to a total of 2.0 mg may acutely increase the heart rate. Isoproterenol infusion of 2 to 10 μg/minute is useful as a temporary measure. Pacemaker placement is the definitive therapy for clinically significant disease. First degree AV block and second degree type I AV block rarely require pacemaker placement. Second degree type II AV block and third degree AV block warrant serious consideration of pacemaker placement.

Premature Atrial Contractions

Premature atrial contractions (PACs) arise early from an ectopic atrial focus, i.e., a focus other than the SA node (Fig. 3–13). This premature depolarization results in a premature and abnormally shaped P wave. The P wave may be upright or inverted, depending on the

origin of the beat and the spread through the atria. If the AV node is partially refractory to this early electrical activity, the PR interval may be increased. Rarely is the P wave not conducted through the AV node and into the ventricles. Usually, the QRS complex during a PAC is normal, which is one distinguishing factor between a PAC and a premature ventricular complex (PVC). However, during a PAC, a right (more common) or left (less common) bundle branch block may occur, with a resulting widened QRS complex. The early atrial activity depolarizes and resets the SA node. Thus the duration from the PAC to the following sinus beat is one full cycle length. This feature is also used to distinguish a PAC from a PVC. The interval between the normal sinus node P waves before and after the PAC is less than twice the normal PP interval (called a noncompensatory pause). PACs may occur without apparent cause. However, sympathetic stimulation, hypoxemia, hypercarbia, myocardial ischemia, and digitalis toxicity may be factors. If an underlying cause is found, it should be treated. PACs do not usually need further treatment; however, propranolol, verapamil, or digoxin may be used if needed. Progression of PACs to other tachyarrhythmias is possible, which should be remembered when evaluating patients.

Premature Ventricular Contractions

Premature ventricular contractions (PVCs) are early beats of ventricular origin (Fig. 3–14). A PVC may result from either an increase in ventricular automaticity or reentry. The PVC is usually not preceded by a P wave. Because the origin of the PVC is in the ventricle, the QRS complex is wide (0.12 second or

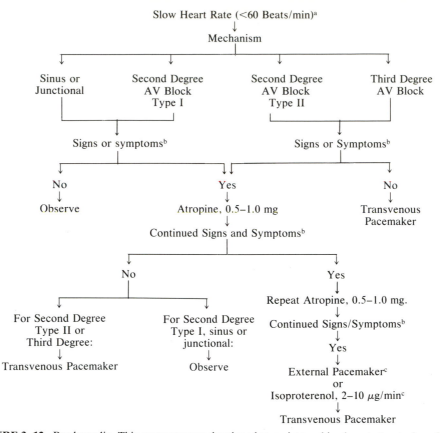

Slow Heart Rate (<60 Beats/min)[a]
↓
Mechanism

| Sinus or Junctional | Second Degree AV Block Type I | Second Degree AV Block Type II | Third Degree AV Block |

Signs or symptoms[b]   Signs or Symptoms[b]

No   Yes   No
↓   ↓   ↓
Observe   Atropine, 0.5–1.0 mg   Transvenous Pacemaker
            ↓
            Continued Signs and Symptoms[b]

No   Yes
↓   ↓
                                      Repeat Atropine, 0.5–1.0 mg.
                                      ↓
For Second Degree   For Second Degree   Continued Signs/Symptoms[b]
Type II or   Type I, sinus or   ↓
Third Degree: junctional: Yes
↓   ↓   ↓
Transvenous Pacemaker   Observe   External Pacemaker[c]
                                         or
                                         Isoproterenol, 2–10 μg/min[c]
                                         ↓
                                         Transvenous Pacemaker

FIGURE 3–12. Bradycardia. This sequence was developed to assist teaching how to treat a broad range of patients with bradycardia. Some patients require care not specified herein. This algorithm should not be construed to prohibit such flexibility. AV = atrioventricular.

[a] A solitary chest thump or cough may stimulate cardiac electrical activity and result in improved cardiac output and may be used at this point.

[b] Hypotension (blood pressure <90 mm Hg), premature ventricular contractions, altered mental status or symptoms (e.g., chest pain or dyspnea), ischemia, or infarction.

[c] Temporizing therapy.

(From Textbook of Advanced Cardiac Life Support, 2nd ed. New York, American Heart Association, 1987, p. 242. With permission.)

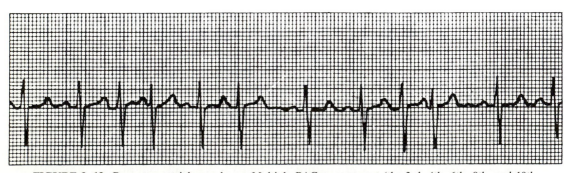

FIGURE 3–13. Premature atrial complexes. Multiple PACs are present (the 3rd, 4th, 6th, 9th, and 10th complexes) resulting in an irregular rhythm. (From Textbook of Advanced Cardiac Life Support, 2nd ed. New York, American Heart Association, 1987, p. 69. With permission.)

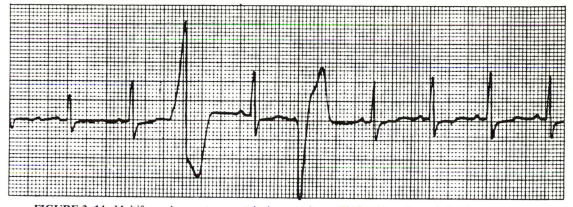

FIGURE 3–14. Multiformed premature ventricular complexes (PVCs). Note the variation in morphology and in the coupling interval of the PVCs. (From Textbook of Advanced Cardiac Life Support, 2nd ed. New York, American Heart Association, 1987, p. 75. With permission.)

Assess for Need for
Acute Suppressive Therapy
↓

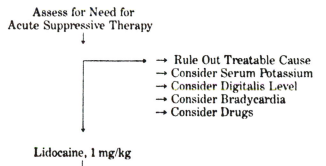

→ Rule Out Treatable Cause
→ Consider Serum Potassium
→ Consider Digitalis Level
→ Consider Bradycardia
→ Consider Drugs

Lidocaine, 1 mg/kg
↓
If Not Suppressed,
Repeat Lidocaine, 0.5 mg/kg Every 2-5 min,
Until No Ectopy, or up to 3 mg/kg Given
↓
If Not Suppressed,
Procainamide 20 mg/min
Until No Ectopy, or up to 1,000 mg Given
↓
If Not Suppressed,
and Not Contraindicated,
Bretylium, 5-10 mg/kg Over 8-10 min
↓
If Not Suppressed,
Consider Overdrive Pacing

Once Ectopy Resolved, Maintain as Follows:
After Lidocaine, 1 mg/kg ... Lidocaine Drip, 2 mg/min
After Lidocaine, 1-2 mg/kg ... Lidocaine Drip, 3 mg/min
After Lidocaine, 2-3 mg/kg ... Lidocaine Drip, 4 mg/min
After Procainamide ... Procainamide drip, 1-4 mg/min (Check Blood Level)
After Bretylium .... Bretylium Drip, 2 mg/min

FIGURE 3–15. Ventricular ectopy: acute suppressive therapy. This sequence was developed to assist teaching how to treat a broad range of patients with ventricular ectopy. Some patients require therapy not specified herein. This algorithm should not be construed as prohibiting such flexibility. (From Textbook of Advanced Cardiac Life Support, 2nd ed. New York, American Heart Association, 1987, p. 243. With permission.)

longer) and abnormal in appearance. The QRS complex is opposite in polarity (direction) from the ST segment and T wave. During a PVC, the SA node fires, and the underlying rhythm of the sinus node is not disturbed. As a result, a fully compensated pause occurs because the next discharge from the SA node is normal. The time between the QRS complex preceding the PVC and the QRS complex following the PVC is twice the time interval of a normal cycle for that patient. The etiology of PVCs include underlying myocardial ischemia, myocardial infarction, heart failure, electrolyte abnormalities, hypoxemia, hypercarbia, acid-base disturbances, and digitalis toxicity. When possible these underlying causes should be reversed. Not all PVCs need to be treated. PVCs occur in healthy people during normal daily activity. For example, healthy teenage boys,[120] young women,[121] military personnel,[122] and actively employed men[123] have been found to have PVCs. Elderly patients with normal maximum exercise test and thallium scintigraphy were found to have unifocal PVCs (80 per cent), multifocal PVCs (35 per cent), and couplets (11 per cent).[124]

However, if PVCs occur in postoperative patients suspected of having myocardial ischemia or acute myocardial infarction, they should be treated (Fig. 3–15). Drugs to improve the balance between myocardial oxygen supply and demand need to be administered (nitroglycerin, morphine, β-blockers, calcium channel blockers, oxygen). The use of lidocaine in this setting is controversial. Commonly, lidocaine is administered in the presence of 1) six or more PVCs per minute, 2) PVCs that are closely coupled (QR/QT less than 0.85), 3) PVCs that fall on the T wave of the preceding beat (R-on-T phenomenon), 4) PVCs that occur in pairs (couplets) plus in runs (ventricular tachycardia), or 5) PVCs that are multiformed.[96] PVCs in the presence of myocardial ischemia or infarction may be associated with an increased incidence of ventricular fibrillation. The PVCs themselves may not be the cause of ventricular fibrillation after acute myocardial infarction; they may simply be a marker that identifies a patient as being at increased risk for ventricular fibrillation.[125] If lidocaine is unsuccessful in treating the PVCs, procainamide or bretylium may be used.

Ventricular Tachycardia

Ventricular tachycardia is defined as three or more premature ventricular beats in succes-

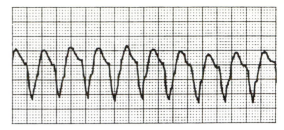

FIGURE 3–16. Ventricular tachycardia. The rhythm is regular at a rate of 158 beats/min. The QRS is wide. No evidence of atrial depolarization is seen. (From Textbook of Advanced Cardiac Life Support, 2nd ed. New York, American Heart Association, 1987, p. 78. With permission.)

sion (Fig. 3–16). Usually the heart rate in ventricular tachycardia is at least 100 beats/min. The QRS complex is widened, being more than 0.12 second in duration. With an ectopic ventricular pacemaker or ventricular reentrant conduction, there is AV dissociation. The SA node depolarizes the atria, and the ventricles contract independently. The P waves, which have no constant relation to the QRS complexes, are sometimes seen on the ECG. The distinction between ventricular tachycardia and supraventricular tachycardia with aberrant ventricular conduction may be difficult. However, in the presence of a tachycardia with a wide QRS complex, it should be treated as ventricular tachycardia until proved otherwise. Ventricular tachycardia may progress to ventricular fibrillation. Myocardial ischemia, electrolyte abnormalities, and hypoxemia are common causes of ventricular tachycardia. If possible, the cause of ventricular tachycardia should be evaluated while treatment is undertaken. Treatment depends on whether the patient has a pulse or is pulseless and if he or she is stable or unstable. Oxygen, lidocaine, procainamide, and synchronized cardioversion are used to treat patients with ventricular tachycardia and a pulse (Fig. 3–17). If pulseless ventricular tachycardia is present, treatment should be the same as for ventricular fibrillation.

Torsades de Pointes

Torsades de pointes (twisting of the points) is a specific form of ventricular tachycardia in which the QRS complexes appear to twist around the isoelectric line of the ECG (Fig. 3–18). Torsades is associated with a prolonged QT interval; and prolongation of the QT interval involves delayed repolarization.[126] Al-

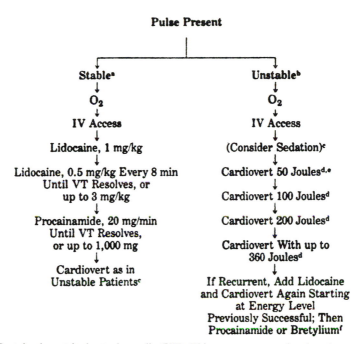

```
No Pulse                              Pulse Present
   ↓                                       |
Treat as VF                                |
                          ┌────────────────┴────────────────┐
                          ↓                                  ↓
                       Stableᵃ                           Unstableᵇ
                          ↓                                  ↓
                         O₂                                 O₂
                          ↓                                  ↓
                      IV Access                          IV Access
                          ↓                                  ↓
                  Lidocaine, 1 mg/kg              (Consider Sedation)ᶜ
                          ↓                                  ↓
              Lidocaine, 0.5 mg/kg Every 8 min    Cardiovert 50 Joulesᵈ·ᵉ
                  Until VT Resolves, or                     ↓
                     up to 3 mg/kg                Cardiovert 100 Joulesᵈ
                          ↓                                  ↓
                Procainamide, 20 mg/min           Cardiovert 200 Joulesᵈ
                  Until VT Resolves,                        ↓
                   or up to 1,000 mg              Cardiovert With up to
                          ↓                            360 Joulesᵈ
                   Cardiovert as in                        ↓
                  Unstable Patientsᶜ           If Recurrent, Add Lidocaine
                                               and Cardiovert Again Starting
                                                    at Energy Level
                                               Previously Successful; Then
                                               Procainamide or Bretyliumᶠ
```

FIGURE 3–17. Sustained ventricular tachycardia (VT). This sequence was developed to assist teaching how to treat a broad range of patients with sustained VT. Some patients require care not specified herein. This algorithm should not be construed as prohibiting such flexibility. Flow of the algorithm presumes that VT is continuing. VF = ventricular fibrillation.

ᵃ If patient becomes unstable (see footnote b for definition) at any time, move to ''Unstable'' arm of the algorithm.

ᵇ Unstable indicates symptoms (e.g., chest pain or dyspnea), hypotension (systolic blood pressure <90 mm Hg), congestive heart failure, ischemia, or infarction.

ᶜ Sedation should be considered for all patients, including those defined in footnote b as unstable, except those who are hemodynamically unstable (e.g., hypotensive, in pulmonary edema, or unconscious).

ᵈ If hypotension, pulmonary edema, or unconsciousness is present, unsynchronized cardioversion should be performed to avoid delay associated with synchronization.

ᵉ In the absence of hypotension, pulmonary edema, or unconsciousness, a precordial thump may be employed prior to cardioversion.

ᶠ Once VT has resolved, begin intravenous (IV) infusion of antiarrhythmic agent that has aided resolution of VT. If hypotension, pulmonary edema, or unconsciousness is present, use lidocaine if cardioversion alone is unsuccessful, followed by bretylium. In all other patients the recommended order of therapy is lidocaine, procainamide, and then bretylium. (From Textbook of Advanced Cardiac Life Support, 2nd ed. New York, American Heart Association, 1987, p. 241. With permission.)

though the mechanism for torsades is not fully understood, it is thought to involve reentry. Prolongation of the QT interval may be caused by drugs, electrolyte imbalance, or congenital abnormalities. If possible, treatment should reverse any underlying cause. Drugs that increase the QT interval, e.g., quinidine and procainamide, should be discontinued. β-

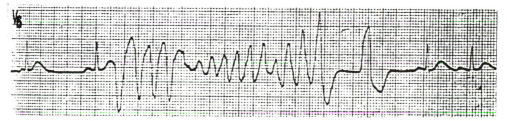

FIGURE 3–18. Torsades de pointes initiated by an R-on-T ventricular extrasystole. (From Marriott HJL: Practical Electrocardiography: Mechanisms, Recognition, Management, 8th ed. Baltimore, Williams & Wilkins, 1988, p. 227. With permission.)

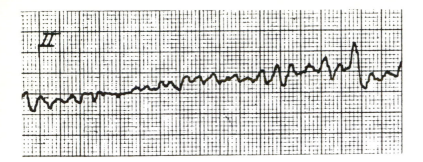

FIGURE 3–19. Ventricular fibrillation. Coarse, irregular complexes are seen. There are no identifiable P waves or QRS complexes. (From Shoemaker WC: Textbook of Critical Care, 2nd ed. Philadelphia, Saunders, 1989, p. 372. With permission.)

Blocking drugs have been recommended preoperatively for patients with the prolonged QT interval syndrome.[127] Other therapy for torsades includes atrial or ventricular overdrive pacing, cardioversion, and isoproterenol infusion (increases the heart rate and shortens the PR interval).

Ventricular Fibrillation

Ventricular fibrillation involves disorganized activity of the ventricles (Fig. 3–19). The ECG illustrates the chaotic electrical activity, in which no P waves, QRS complexes, or T waves are seen. Irregular waveforms of changing size and shape occur. Ventricular fibrillation results from myocardial ischemia, myocardial infarction, electrolyte imbalance, hypoxemia, or hypothermia. There is no cardiac output, and the patient is pulseless and unconscious. Treatment of ventricular fibrillation is the same as that for pulseless ventricular tachycardia. Early electrical defibrillation is the treatment of choice (Fig. 3–20). Other important therapy includes support of the patient with cardiopulmonary resuscitation as

well as epinephrine, lidocaine, and bretylium. Early administration of lidocaine has been recommended as prophylactic therapy to decrease the incidence of ventricular fibrillation associated with acute myocardial infarction.[128]

Ventricular Asystole

Ventricular asystole occurs when no ventricular electrical activity is present (Fig. 3–21). Without electrical activity, there is no ventricular contraction or cardiac output. The approach to a "flat line" ECG involves not only examination of the patient but also checking that the ECG leads are attached to the patient correctly. Occasionally, P waves are present on the ECG. To make the diagnosis of ventricular asystole, more than one ECG lead should be viewed. If there is any question that ventricular fibrillation may be present, treatment should be as ventricular fibrillation and not as ventricular asystole. The prognosis of ventricular asystole is poor, whereas ventricular fibrillation may be treatable with defibrillation. As with other emergency situations, CPR should be started. Epi-

---

FIGURE 3–20. Ventricular fibrillation (and pulseless ventricular tachycardia).[a] This sequence was developed to assist teaching how to treat a broad range of patients with ventricular fibrillation (VF) or pulseless ventricular tachycardia (VT). Some patients require care not specified herein. This algorithm should not be construed as prohibiting such flexibility. Flow of algorithm presumes that VF is continuing. CPR = cardiopulmonary resuscitation.

[a] Pulseless VT should be treated identically to VF.

[b] Check pulse and rhythm after each shock. If VF recurs after transiently converting (rather than persists without ever converting), use whatever energy level has previously been successful for defibrillation.

[c] Epinephrine should be repeated every five minutes.

[d] Intubation is preferable. If it can be accompanied simultaneously with other techniques, then the earlier the better. However, defibrillation and epinephrine are more important initially if the patient can be ventilated without intubation.

[e] Some may prefer repeated doses of lidocaine, which may be given in 0.5 mg/kg boluses every 8 minutes to a total dose of 3 mg/kg.

[f] Value of sodium bicarbonate is questionable during cardiac arrest, and it is not recommended for routine cardiac arrest sequence. Consideration of its use in a dose of 1 mEq/kg is appropriate at this point. Half of original dose may be repeated every 10 minutes if it is used.

(From Textbook of Advanced Cardiac Life Support, 2nd ed. New York, American Heart Association, 1987, p. 238. With permission.)

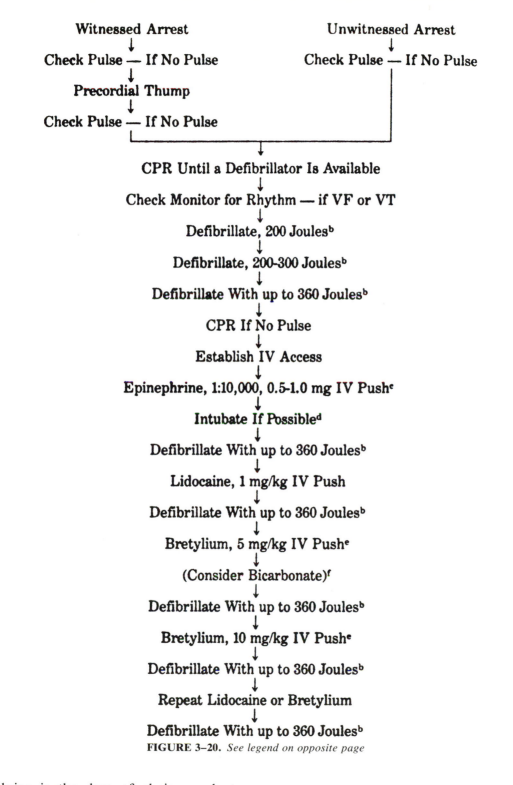

Witnessed Arrest

↓

Check Pulse — If No Pulse

↓

Precordial Thump

↓

Check Pulse — If No Pulse

Unwitnessed Arrest

↓

Check Pulse — If No Pulse

CPR Until a Defibrillator Is Available

↓

Check Monitor for Rhythm — if VF or VT

↓

Defibrillate, 200 Joules[b]

↓

Defibrillate, 200-300 Joules[b]

↓

Defibrillate With up to 360 Joules[b]

↓

CPR If No Pulse

↓

Establish IV Access

↓

Epinephrine, 1:10,000, 0.5-1.0 mg IV Push[c]

↓

Intubate If Possible[d]

↓

Defibrillate With up to 360 Joules[b]

↓

Lidocaine, 1 mg/kg IV Push

↓

Defibrillate With up to 360 Joules[b]

↓

Bretylium, 5 mg/kg IV Push[e]

↓

(Consider Bicarbonate)[f]

↓

Defibrillate With up to 360 Joules[b]

↓

Bretylium, 10 mg/kg IV Push[e]

↓

Defibrillate With up to 360 Joules[b]

↓

Repeat Lidocaine or Bretylium

↓

Defibrillate With up to 360 Joules[b]

FIGURE 3–20. *See legend on opposite page*

nephrine is the drug of choice, and atropine may also be used (Fig. 3–22). Transvenous pacemaker placement or external pacing may be effective treatment of ventricular asystole.

Electromechanical Dissociation

Electromechanical dissociation (EMD) is characterized by adequate electrical activity of the heart, with an absence of systemic per-

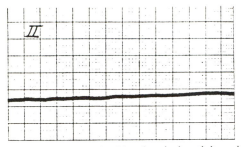

FIGURE 3–21. Asystole. No electrical activity, either atrial or ventricular, can be seen. (From Shoemaker WC: Textbook of Critical Care, 2nd ed. Philadelphia, Saunders, 1989, p. 374. With permission.)

fusion. No palpable pulse is present.[129] Identification and treatment of the underlying cause is the key to successful therapy. Causes of EMD include hypovolemia, cardiac tamponade, tension pneumothorax, hypoxemia, acidosis, massive myocardiac damage from infarction, prolonged ischemia during resuscitation, and pulmonary embolism.[96] Treatment of

If Rhythm Is Unclear and Possibly Ventricular
Fibrillation, Defibrillate as for VF. If Asystole is Present[a]
↓
Continue CPR
↓
Establish IV Access
↓
Epinephrine, 1:10,000, 0.5 - 1.0 mg IV Push[b]
↓
Intubate When Possible[c]
↓
Atropine, 1.0 mg IV Push (Repeated in 5 min)
↓
(Consider Bicarbonate)[d]
↓
Consider Pacing

FIGURE 3–22. Asystole (cardiac standstill). This sequence was developed to assist teaching how to treat a broad range of patients with asystole. Some patients may require care not specified herein. This algorithm should not be construed to prohibit such flexibility. Flow of the algorithm presumes asystole is continuing. VF = ventricular fibrillation; IV = intravenous.

[a] Asystole should be confirmed in two leads.

[b] Epinephrine should be repeated every 5 minutes.

[c] Intubation is preferable; if it can be accomplished simultaneously with other techniques, the earlier the better. However, cardiopulmonary resuscitation (CPR) and use of epinephrine are more important initially if the patient can be ventilated without intubation. (Endotracheal epinephrine may be used.)

[d] Value of sodium bicarbonate is questionable during cardiac arrest, and it is not recommended for the routine cardiac arrest sequence. Consideration of its use in a dose of 1 mEq/kg is appropriate at this point. Half of the original dose may be repeated every 10 minutes if it is used.

(From Textbook of Advanced Cardiac Life Support, 2nd ed. New York, American Heart Association, 1987, p. 239. With permission.)

Continue CPR
↓
Establish IV Access
↓
Epinephrine, 1:10,000, 0.5 - 1.0 mg IV Push[a]
↓
Intubate When Possible[b]
↓
(Consider Bicarbonate)[c]
↓
Consider Hypovolemia,
Cardiac Tamponade,
Tension Pneumothorax,
Hypoxemia,
Acidosis,
Pulmonary Embolism

FIGURE 3–23. Electromechanical dissociation. This sequence was developed to assist teaching how to treat a broad range of patients with electromechanical dissociation. Some patients require care not specified herein. This algorithm should not be construed to prohibit such flexibility. Flow of algorithm presumes that electromechanical dissociation is continuing. CPR = cardiopulmonary resuscitation; IV = intravenous.

[a] Epinephrine should be repeated every 5 minutes.

[b] Intubation is preferable. If it can be accomplished simultaneously with other techniques, the earlier the better. However, epinephrine is more important initially if the patient can be ventilated without intubation.

[c] Value of sodium bicarbonate is questionable during cardiac arrest, and it is not recommended for routine cardiac arrest sequence. Consideration of its use in a dose of 1 mEq/kg is appropriate at this point. Half of the original dose may be repeated every 10 minutes if it is used.

(From Textbook of Advanced Cardiac Life Support, 2nd ed. New York, American Heart Association, 1987, p. 240. With permission.)

the underlying cause should be undertaken. Cardiopulmonary resuscitation with the use of epinephrine 0.5 to 1.0 mg IV, repeated every 5 minutes, is needed (Fig. 3–23).

Wolff-Parkinson-White Syndrome

The Wolff-Parkinson-White (WPW) syndrome is the most common preexcitation syndrome. An abnormal accessory AV conduction pathway (Kent bundles) exists, and the ventricular myocardium is prematurely depolarized. The accessory conduction pathway bypasses the normal AV node and the His bundle-Purkinje system. The usual conduction delay through the AV node is bypassed. The QRS complex is a fusion beat, with an initial delta wave due to early conduction through the accessory pathway, in combination with the normal conduction system of the heart (Fig. 3–24). The ECG characteristics of the WPW syndrome usually, but not always, in-

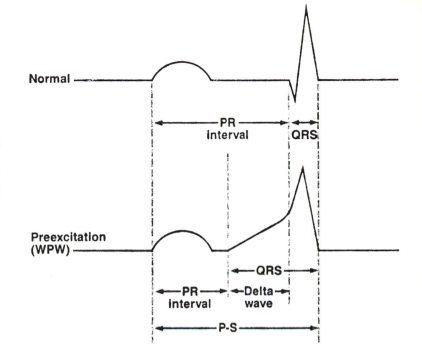

FIGURE 3–24. WPW syndrome is a form of accelerated conduction (preexcitation) due to the presence of an anomalous conducting tract between the atria and ventricles (usually a bundle of Kent). The syndrome is defined electrocardiographically by a shortened PR interval and a pathognomonic prolongation of the initial portion of the QRS complex (delta wave). (From Wyndham, CRC: Wolff-Parkinson-White syndrome. Hosp Med *20*:137, 1984. With permission.)

clude the delta wave, a short PR interval (0.12 second or less), and a broad QRS complex.[130] There are two arrhythmias that commonly occur in patients with the WPW syndrome: reentry supraventricular tachycardia and atrial fibrillation.[131] These arrhythmias are of special concern in these patients because their management is different when associated with the WPW syndrome.

The reentry supraventricular tachycardia in patients with WPW syndrome most commonly utilizes the normal AV node conduction system for the anterograde (forward) conduction and the accessory pathway for the retrograde (backward) conduction. The QRS complex is normal, not widened. Because the pharmacologic goal in this instance is to prolong conduction time and refractoriness in the AV node, appropriate drug therapy includes verapamil, propranolol, and digitalis.[132] In addition, vagal maneuvers, intravenous edrophonium chloride, intravenous phenylephrine hydrochloride, or overdrive pacing may be useful. If hemodynamic compromise is present, cardioversion should be performed immediately.

Atrial fibrillation in patients with the WPW syndrome is a life-threatening arrhythmia. If the impulses are conducted down the accessory pathway, there is no conduction delay as would occur in the AV node. The QRS complexes are widened, and the ventricular rate

may be up to 400 beats/min. Ventricular fibrillation may result.[133–135] The pharmacologic goal for atrial fibrillation is to decrease the speed of conduction in the accessory pathway. Procainamide is useful because it prolongs the refractory period in the accessory pathway.[136] Digitalis and verapamil are contraindicated, as they may increase the ventricular response.[137–139] Cardioversion should be considered early in the management of atrial fibrillation in the presence of WPW syndrome.

References

1. Physics of blood, blood flow and pressure: hemodynamics. *In* Guyton AC (ed): Textbook of Medical Physiology, Philadelphia, Saunders, 1981, pp. 206–218.
2. Short term regulation of mean arterial blood pressure. *In* Guyton AC (ed): Textbook of Medical Physiology. Philadelphia, Saunders, 1981, pp. 246–258.
3. Reitan JA: Control of the systemic circulation. *In* Scurr C, Feldman S (eds): Scientific Foundations of Anaesthesia. London, Heineman, 1982, pp. 132–144.
4. Weiner N: Norepinephrine, epinephrine, and the sympathomimetic amines. *In* Goodman LS, Gilman A (eds): The Pharmacological Basis of Therapeutics, 6th ed. New York, Macmillan, 1980, pp. 138–175.
5. Azer S: Management of postoperative hypertension and hypotension in the recovery room. Mt Sinai J Med *48*:365–368, 1981.
6. Hayes RC, Murad F: Adrenocortical steroids and

their synthetic analogs. *In* Goodman LS, Gilman A (eds): The Pharmacological Basis of Therapeutics, 6th ed. New York, Macmillan, 1980, pp. 1466–1496.

7. Carrol GC: Blood pressure monitoring. Crit Care Clin *4*:411–434, 1988.

8. Sibai BM: Pitfalls in diagnosis and management of preeclampsia. Am J Obstet Gynecol *159*:1–5, 1988.

9. Kirkendall WM, Feinleib M, Freis ED, et al: Recommendations for human blood pressure determinations of sphygmomanometers: subcommittee of the AHA postgraduate education committee. *News from the American Heart Association* AHA reprint booklet 70-019-B, 1981, pp. 1146A–1155A.

10. Messerli F, Ventura H, Amodeo C: Osler's maneuver and pseudohypertension. N Engl J Med *312*:1548, 1985.

11. Clark C, Harman E: Hemodynamic monitoring: arterial catheters. *In* Civetta JM, Taylor RW, Kirby, RR (eds): Critical Care. Philadelphia, Lippincott, 1988, pp. 289–302.

12. Miller ED: Antihypertensive therapy. *In* Kaplan JA (ed): Cardiac Anesthesia. Orlando: Grune & Stratton, 1987, pp. 393–409.

13. Prys-Roberts C, Greene LT, Meloche R, Foex P: Studies of anesthesia in relation to hypertension. II. Haemodynamic consequences of induction and endotracheal intubation. Br J Anaesth *43*:531–541, 1971.

14. Wallach R, Karp RB, Reves JG, et al: Pathogenesis of paroxysmal hypertension developing during and after coronary bypass surgery: a study of hemodynamic and humeral factors. Am J Cardiol *46*:559–565, 1980.

15. Houston MC: Hypertensive urgencies and emergencies: pathophysiology, clinical aspects and treatment. *In* Chernow B, Shoemaker WC (eds): Critical Care, State of the Art, Vol. 7. Fullerton, CA, Society of Critical Care Medicine, 1986, pp. 151–241.

16. Chauvin M, Deriaz H, Viars P: Continuous I.V. infusion of labetalol for postoperative hypertension. Br J Anaesth *59*:1250–1256, 1987.

17. Gal TJ, Cooperman LH: Hypertension in the immediate postoperative period. Br J Anaesth *47*:70–74, 1975.

18. Von Knorring J: Postoperative myocardial infarction: a prospective study in a risk group of surgical patients. Surgery *90*:55–60, 1981.

19. Steen PA, Tinker JH, Tarhan S: Myocardial reinfarction after anesthesia and surgery. JAMA *239*:2566–2570, 1978.

20. Tinker JH: Perioperative myocardial infarction. Semin Anesth *1*:253–263, 1982.

21. Goldman L, Caldera DL, et al: Multifactorial index of cardiac risk in noncardiac surgical procedures. N Engl J Med *303*:897–902, 1980.

22. Koch-Wesler J: Hypertensive emergencies. N Engl J Med *290*:211–214, 1974.

23. Asiddao CB, et al: Factors associated with perioperative complications during carotid endarterectomy. Anesth Analg *61*:631, 1982.

24. Owens ML, Wilson SE: Prevention of neurologic complications of carotid endarterectomy. Arch Surg *117*:551, 1982.

25. Cullen DJ: Recovery room complications. AORN J *26*:746–763, 1977.

26. Cullen DJ, Cullen BL: Postanesthetic complications. Surg Clin North Am *55*:978–998, 1975.

27. Eckenhoff JE, Kneale DH, Dripps RD: The incidence and etiology of post anesthetic excitement. Anesthesiology *22*:667–673, 1961.

28. Smiler BG, Bartholomew EG, et al: Physostigmine reversal of scopolamine delirium in obstetric patients. Am J Obstet Gynecol *116*:326–329, 1973.

29. Martin DE, Kammerer WS: The hypertensive surgical patient: controversies in management. Surg Clin North Am *63*:1017–1033, 1983.

30. Herman H, Mornex R: Human tumors secreting catecholamines: cardiovascular manifestations. New York, Macmillan, 1964, pp. 1–14.

31. Prys-Roberts C, Meloche R, Foex P: Studies of hypertension in relation to anesthesia. I. Cardiovascular responses of treated and untreated patients. Br J Anaesth *43*:122–137, 1971.

32. Prys-Roberts C: Hypertension and anesthesia—fifty years on. Anesthesiology *50*:281–284, 1979.

33. Hart GR, Anderson RJ: Withdrawal syndromes and the cessation of antihypertensive therapy. Arch Intern Med *141*:1125–1127, 1981.

34. Fremes SE, et al: Effects of postoperative hypertension and its treatment. J Thorac Cardiovasc Surg *86*:47–56, 1983.

35. McGuirt WF, May JS: Postoperative hypertension associated with radical neck dissection. Arch Otolaryngol Head Neck Surg *113*:1098–1100, 1987.

36. Cash JM, Dellinger RP: Hypertensive emergencies and urgencies. *In* Civetta JM, Taylor RW, Kirby, RR (eds): Critical Care. Philadelphia, Lippincott, 1988, pp. 1011–1019.

37. Blashke TF, Melmon KL: Antihypertensive agents and the drug therapy of hypertension. *In* Goodman LS, Gilman A (eds): The Pharmacological Basis of Therapeutics, 6th ed. New York, Macmillan, 1980, pp. 793–818.

38. Stoelting RK: Peripheral vasodilators. *In* Stoelting RK (ed): Pharmacology and Physiology in Anesthetic Practice. Philadelphia, Lippincott, 1987, pp. 307–321.

39. Lowenstein E, Reiz S: Effects of inhalation anesthetics on systemic hemodynamics and the coronary circulation. *In* Kaplan JA (ed): Cardiac Anesthesia. Orlando, Grune & Stratton, 1987, pp. 3–35.

40. Kates RA: Antianginal drug therapy. *In* Kaplan JA (ed): Cardiac Anesthesia. Orlando, Grune & Stratton, 1987, pp. 451–517.

41. O'Connor JP, Wynands JE: Anesthesia for myocardial revascularization. *In* Kaplan JA (ed): Cardiac Anesthesia. Orlando, Grune & Stratton, 1987, pp. 551–588.

42. Gerson H, Allen FB, Seitzer JL, et al: Arterial and venous dilation by nitroprusside and nitroglycerine—is there a difference? Anesth Analg *61*:256–260, 1982.

43. Armstrong PW, Armstrong JA, Marks GS: Pharmacokinetic-hemodynamic studies of intravenous nitroglycerine in congestive heart failure. Circulation *62*:160–166, 1980.

44. Needleman P, Johnson EM: Vasodilators and the treatment of angina. *In* Goodman LS, Gilman A (eds): The Pharmacological Basis of Therapeutics, 6th ed. New York, Macmillan, 1980, pp. 819–833.

45. Leslie JB, Kalayjian RW, et al: Intravenous labetalol for treatment of postoperative hypertension. Anesthesiology *67*:413–416, 1987.

46. Weiner N: Drugs that inhibit adrenergic nerves and block adrenergic receptors. *In* Goodman LS, Rall TW, Murad F (eds): The Pharmacological Basis of

Therapeutics, 7th ed. New York, Macmillan, 1985, pp. 176–210.

47. Ziegler MG: Antihypertensive therapy. *In* Chernow B (ed): The Pharmacologic Approach to the Critically Ill Patient, 2nd ed. Baltimore, William & Wilkins, 1988, pp. 365–388.

48. Stoelting RK: Antihypertensive drugs. *In* Stoelting RK (ed): Pharmacology and Physiology in Anesthetic Practice. Philadelphia, Lippincott, 1987, pp. 294–306.

49. Stoelting RK: Calcium entry blockers. *In* Stoelting RK (ed): Pharmacology and Physiology in Anesthetic Practice. Philadelphia, Lippincott, 1987, pp. 335–346.

50. Cohen MM, Duncan PG, Pope WDB, Wolkenstein C: A survey of 112,000 anesthetics at one teaching hospital. Can Anesth Soc J *33*:1:22–31, 1986.

51. Mecca RS: Postanesthesia recovery. *In* Barash PG, Cullen BF, Stoelting RK (eds): Clinical Anesthesia. Philadelphia, Lippincott, 1989, pp. 1397–1425.

52. Stoelting RK, Miller RD: Basics of Anesthesia. New York, Churchill Livingstone, 1984, pp. 419–432.

53. Farmer JC: Temperature-related injuries. *In* Civetta JM, Taylor RW, Kirby RR (eds): Critical Care. Philadelphia, Lippincott, 1988, pp. 693–700.

54. Mauney FM, Ebert PA, Sabiston DC: Postoperative myocardial infarction: a study of predisposing factors, diagnosis and mortality in a high risk group of patients. Ann Surg *172*:497–502, 1970.

55. Luce JM: Pathogenesis and management of septic shock. Chest *91*:883–888, 1987.

56. Wilson RW: Sepsis prophylaxis in the surgical patient at risk. *In* Sibbald WJ, Sprung CL (eds): Perspectives on Sepsis and Septic Shock. Fullerton, CA, The Society of Critical Care Medicine, 1986, pp. 301–337.

57. Wahl SC: Septic shock. Nursing *89*:52–59, 1989.

58. Moser KM: Pulmonary thromboembolism. *In* Petersdorf RG, Adams RD, Braunwald E, et al (eds): Harrison's Principles of Internal Medicine. New York, McGraw-Hill, 1983, pp. 1561–1567.

59. Braunwald E: Pericardial disease. *In* Petersdorf RG, Adams RD, Braunwald E, et al (eds): Harrison's Principles of Internal Medicine. New York, McGraw-Hill, 1983, pp. 1458–1465.

60. McKiernan TL: The pericardium. *In* Civetta JM, Taylor RW, Kirby RR (eds): Critical Care. Philadelphia, Lippincott, 1988, pp. 1003–1009.

61. Sladen RA: Management of the adult cardiac patient in the intensive care unit. *In* Ream AK, Fogdall RP (eds): Acute Cardiovascular Management. Philadelphia, Lippincott, 1982, pp. 481–548.

62. Feely TW: The recovery room. *In* Miller RD (ed): Anesthesia. New York, Churchill Livingstone, 1986, pp. 1921–1945.

63. Lindsey HE, Cohn PF: "Silent" myocardial ischemia during and after exercise testing in patients with coronary artery disease. Am Heart J *95*:441–447, 1978.

64. Chierchia S, Lazzari M, Freedman B, et al: Impairment of myocardial perfusion and function during painless myocardial ischemia. J Am Coll Cardiol *1*:924–930, 1983.

65. Cecchi AC, Dovellini EV, Marchi F, et al: Silent myocardial ischemia during ambulatory electrocardiographic monitoring in patients with effort angina. J Am Coll Cardiol *1*:934–939, 1983.

66. Haiat R, Desoutter P, Stoltz J-P: Angina pectoris

without ST-T changes in patients with documented coronary disease. Am Heart J *105*:883–884, 1983.

67. Blackburn H, Katigbak R: What electrocardiographic leads to take after exercise? Am Heart J *67*:184–185, 1964.

68. London MJ, Hollenberg M, Wong MG, et al: Intraoperative myocardial ischemia: localization by continuous 12-lead electrocardiography. Anesthesiology *69*:232–241, 1988.

69. Flaherty JT, Becker LC, Bulkley BH, et al: A randomized prospective trial of intravenous nitroglycerin in patients with acute myocardial infarction. Circulation *68*:576–588, 1983.

70. Jugdutt BL, Becker LC, Hutchins GM, et al: Effect of intravenous nitroglycerin on collateral blood flow and infarct size in the conscious dog. Circulation *63*:17–28, 1981.

71. Bussmann WD, Passek D, Seidel W, Kaltenbach M: Reduction of CK and CK-MB indexes of infarct size by intravenous nitroglycerin. Circulation *63*:615–622, 1981.

72. Hopkins DG, Harrison DC: Coronary artery spasm. *In* Hurst JW (ed): The Heart, 6th ed. New York, McGraw-Hill, 1986, p. 1014.

73. Peter T, Norris RM, Clarke ED, et al: Reduction of enzyme levels by propranolol after acute myocardial infarction. Circulation *57*:1091–1095, 1978.

74. Herlitz J, Elmfeldt D, Hjalmarson A, et al: Effect of metoprolol on indirect signs of the size and severity of acute myocardial infarction. Am J Cardiol *51*:1282–1288, 1983.

75. Robertson RM, Wood AJJ, Vaughn WK, Robertson D: Exacerbation of vasospastic angina pectoris by propranolol. Circulation *65*:281–285, 1982.

76. Frishman WH, Furberg CD, Friedewald WT: Beta adrenergic blockade for survivors of acute myocardial infarction. N Engl J Med *310*:830–837, 1984.

77. Braunwald E: Treatment of the patient after myocardial infarction. N Engl J Med *302*:290–293, 1980.

78. Hjalmarson A, Ehnfeldt D, Herlitz J, et al: Effect on mortality of metoprolol in acute myocardial infarction. Lancet *2*:823, 1981.

79. Muller J, Roberts R, Stone P, et al: Failure of propranolol administration to limit infarct size in patients with acute myocardial infarction. Circulation *68*(suppl III):294, 1983 (abstract).

80. International Collaborative Study Group: Reduction of infarct size with the early use of timolol in acute myocardial infarction. N Engl J Med *310*:9–15, 1984.

81. Yusuf S, Peto R, Bennett D, et al: Early intravenous atenolol treatment in suspected acute myocardial infarction. Lancet *2*:273–276, 1980.

82. Roberts R, Croft C, Gold HK, et al: Effect of propranolol on myocardial-infarct size in a randomized blinded multicenter trial. N Engl J Med *311*:218–225, 1984.

83. Johnson SM, Mauritson DR, Willerson JT, Hillis DL: Comparison of verapamil and nifedipine in the treatment of variant angina pectoris—preliminary observations in 10 patients. Am J Cardiol *47*:1295–1300, 1981.

84. Stone PH, Antman EM, Muller JE, Braunwald E: Calcium channel blocking agents in the treatment of cardiovascular disorders. II. Hemodynamic effects and clinical applications. Ann Intern Med *93*:886–904, 1980.

85. Braunwald E: Mechanism of action of calcium-chan-

nel blocking agents. N Engl J Med *307*:1618–1627, 1982.

86. Braunwald E: Calcium-channel blockers: pharmacologic considerations. Am Heart J *104*:665–671, 1982.

87. Rutherford JD, Braunwald E, Cohn PF: Chronic ischemic heart disease. *In* Braunwald E (ed): Heart Disease: A Textbook of Cardiovascular Medicine, 3rd ed. Philadelphia, Saunders, 1988, p. 1332.

88. Senior RM: Pulmonary embolism. *In* Wyngaarden JB, Smith LD (eds): Cecil, Textbook of Medicine, 18th ed. Philadelphia, Saunders, pp. 442–450.

89. Long WB, Cohen S: The digestive tract as a cause of chest pain. Am Heart J *100*:567–572, 1980.

90. Rozen P, Gelfond M, Salzman S, et al: Radionuclide confirmation of the therapeutic value of isosorbide dinitrate in relieving the dysphagia in achalasia. J Clin Gastroenterol *4*:17–22, 1982.

91. Gelford M, Rozen P, Gilat T: Isosorbide dinitrate and nifedipine treatment of achalasia: a clinical manometric and radionuclide evaluation. Gastroenterology *83*:963–969, 1982.

92. Berger K, McCallum RW: Nifedipine in the treatment of achalasia. Ann Intern Med *96*:61–62, 1982.

93. Traube M, Hongo M, Magyar L, McCallum RW: Effects of nifedipine in achalasia and in patients with high-amplitude peristaltic esophageal contractions. JAMA *252*:1733–1736, 1984.

94. Cohen MM, Duncan PG, Pope WBD, Wolkenstein C: A survey of 112,000 anaesthetics at one teaching hospital (1975–1983). Can Anaesth J *33*:22–31, 1986.

95. Hoffman BF, Rosen MR: Cellular mechanisms for cardiac arrhythmias. Circ Res *49*:1–15, 1981.

96. Textbook of Advanced Cardiac Life Support, 2nd ed. Dallas, American Heart Association, 1987, pp. 13, 47–49, 104–106, 240–241.

97. Kaplan JA, King SB: The precordial electrocardiographic lead (V₅) in patients who have coronary-artery disease. Anesthesiology *45*:570–574, 1976.

98. Rogers MC: Diagnosis and treatment of intraoperative cardiac dysrhythmias. *In* Miller RD (ed): Anesthesia, 2nd ed, Vol. 1. New York, Churchill Livingstone, 1986, pp. 499–521.

99. Blitt CD: Monitoring for outpatient anesthesia. *In* Blitt CD (ed): Monitoring in Anesthesia and Critical Care Medicine. New York, Churchill Livingstone, 1985, pp. 685–690.

100. Roizen MF, Plummer GO, Lichtor JL: Nitrous oxide and dysrhythmias. Anesthesiology *66*:427–431, 1987.

101. Sebel PS, Bovill JG: Opioid analgesics in cardiac anesthesia. *In* Kaplan JA (ed): Cardiac Anesthesia, 2nd ed, Vol. 1. Orlando, Grune & Stratton, 1987, p. 74.

102. Kaplan NM: Our appropriate concern about hypokalemia. Am J Med *77*:1–4, 1984.

103. Harrington JT, Isner JM, Kassirer JP: Our national obsession with potassium. Am J Med *73*:155–159, 1982.

104. Wong KC: Hypokalemia and dysrhythmias. J Cardiothorac Anesth *3*:529–531, 1989.

105. Vitez TS, Soper LE, Wong KC, Soper P: Chronic hypokalemia and intraoperative dysrhythmias. Anesthesiology *63*:130–133, 1985.

106. Hirsch IA, Tomlinson DL, Slogoff S, Keats AS: The overstated risk of preoperative hypokalemia. Anesth Analg *67*:131–136, 1988.

107. Emslie-Smith D, Sladden GE, Stirling GR: The significance of changes in the electrocardiogram in hypothermia. Br Heart J *21*:343–351, 1959.

108. Trevino A, Razi B, Beller BM: The characteristic ECG of accidental hypothermia. Arch Intern Med *127*:470–473, 1971.

109. O'Rourke GW, Greene NM: Autonomic blockade and the resting heart rate in man. Am Heart J *80*:469–474, 1970.

110. Collinsworth KA, Kalman SM, Harrison DC: The clinical pharmacology of lidocaine as an antiarrhythmic drug. Circulation *50*:1217–1230, 1974.

111. ElSherif N, Scherlag BJ, Lazzara R, Hope RR: Reentrant ventricular arrhythmias in the late myocardial infarction period. IV. Mechanism of action of lidocaine. Circulation *56*:395–402, 1977.

112. Giardina EG, Heissenbuttel RH, Bigger JT Jr: Intermittent intravenous procainamide to treat ventricular arrhythmias. Ann Intern Med *78*:183–193, 1973.

113. Lima JJ, Conti DR, Goldfarb AL, et al: Safety and efficacy of procainamide infusions. Am J Cardiol *43*:98–105, 1979.

114. Zipes DP: Management of cardiac arrhythmias: pharmacological, electrical, and surgical techniques. *In* Braunwald E (ed): Heart Disease, A Textbook of Cardiovascular Medicine, 3rd ed. Philadelphia, Saunders, 1988, p. 635.

115. Euler DE, Scanlon PJ: Mechanisms of the effect of bretylium on the ventricular fibrillation threshold in dogs. Am J Cardiol *55*:1396–1401, 1085.

116. Fisch C: Electrocardiography and vectorcardiography. *In* Braunwald E (ed): Heart Disease, A Textbook of Cardiovascular Medicine, 3rd ed. Philadelphia, Saunders, 1988, p. 219.

117. Rakita L, Vrobel TR: Electrocardiography in critical care medicine. *In* Shoemaker WC (ed): Textbook of Critical Care, 2nd ed. Philadelphia, Saunders, 1989, p. 369.

118. Shields TW, Ujiki G: Digitalization for prevention of arrhythmias following pulmonary surgery. Surg Gynecol Obstet *126*:743–746, 1968.

119. Mowry F, Reynolds E: Cardiac rhythm disturbances complicating resectional surgery of the lung. Ann Intern Med *61*:688–695, 1964.

120. Dickinson DF, Scott O: Ambulatory electrocardiographic monitoring in 100 healthy teenage boys. Br Heart J *51*:179–183, 1984.

121. Sabotka PA, Mayer JH, Bauernfeind RA, et al: Arrhythmias documented by 24-hour continuous ambulatory electrocardiographic monitoring in young women without apparent heart disease. Am Heart J *101*:753–759, 1981.

122. Hiss RG, Lamb LE: Electrocardiographic findings in 122,043 individuals. Circulation *25*:947–961, 1962.

123. Hinkle LE, Carver ST, Stevens M: The frequency of asymptomatic disturbances of cardiac rhythm and conduction in middle-aged men. Am J Cardiol *24*:629–650, 1969.

124. Fleg JL, Kennedy HL: Cardiac arrhythmias in a healthy elderly population: detection by 24-hour ambulatory electrocardiography. Chest *81*:302–307, 1982.

125. Zipes DP, Noble RJ: Assessment of electrical abnormalities. *In* Hurst JW (ed): The Heart, 6th ed. New York, McGraw-Hill, 1986, p. 284.

126. Reynolds EW, Vander Ark CR: Quinidine syncope and the delayed repolarization syndromes. Mod Concepts Cardiovasc Dis *45*:117–122, 1976

127. Galloway PA, Glass PSA: Anesthetic implications of prolonged QT interval syndromes. Anesth Analg *64*:612–620, 1985.

128. Koster RW, Dunning AJ: Intramuscular lidocaine

for the prevention of lethal arrhythmias in the pre-hospitalization phase of acute myocardial infarction. N Engl J Med *313*:1105–1110, 1985.

129. Vincent JL, Thijs L, Weil MH, et al: Clinical and experimental studies on electromechanical dissociation. Circulation *64*:18–27, 1981.

130. Sherf L, Neufeld MN: The Pre-excitation Syndrome: Facts and Theories. New York, Yorke Medical Books, 1978.

131. Wellens HJJ: Wolff-Parkinson-White syndrome. I. Diagnosis, arrhythmias and identification of the high risk patient. Mod Concepts Cardiovasc Dis *52*:53–56, 1983.

132. Wellens HJJ: Wolff-Parkinson-White syndrome. II. Treatment. Mod Concepts Cardiovasc Dis *52*:57–59, 1983.

133. Sellers TD, Campbell RWF, Bashore TM, Gallagher JJ: Effects of procainamide and quinidine sulfate in the Wolff-Parkinson-White syndrome. Circulation *55*:15–22, 1977.

134. Sellers TD, Bashore TM, Gallagher JJ: Digitalis in the pre-excitation syndrome: analysis during atrial fibrillation. Circulation *56*:260–267, 1977.

135. Gallagher JJ, Pritchett ELC, Sealy WC, et al: The pre-excitation syndromes. Prog Cardiovasc Dis *20*:285–327, 1978.

136. Bashore TM, Sellers TD, Gallagher JJ, Wallace AG: Ventricular fibrillation in the Wolff-Parkinson-White syndrome. Circulation *2*:187, 1976.

137. Cosio FG, Benson DW, Anderson RW, et al: Onset of atrial fibrillation during antidromic tachycardia: association with sudden cardiac arrest and ventricular fibrillation in a patient with Wolff-Parkinson-White syndrome. Am J Cardiol *50*:353–359, 1982.

138. Sellers TD, Bashore TM, Gallagher JJ: Digitalis in the pre-excitation syndrome: analysis during atrial fibrillation. Circulation *56*:260–267, 1977.

139. Gulamhusein S, Ko P, Carruthers SG, Klein GJ: Acceleration of the ventricular response during atrial fibrillation in the Wolff-Parkinson-White syndrome after verapamil. Circulation *65*:348–354, 1982.

4 PITFALLS OF HEMODYNAMIC MONITORING

MARK L. FRANKLIN and KENNETH L. RODINO

As medical technology has advanced, so has our ability to monitor patients. Many factors play a role in the acquisition and application of the data, but most important is accurate interpretation of obtained data and integrating it with appropriate clinical judgment. Utilization of derived data without regard to how accurately it reflects the system from which it comes may lead to improper conclusions and subsequent adverse outcomes. In order for our interpretations to be appropriate, an understanding of data acquisition processes and their limitations becomes imperative. In this chapter, we focus the discussion on the pitfalls of data interpretation and its utilization as it applies to the care of anesthetized and surgical patients. Complications may also arise from the use of monitoring equipment and procedures, e.g., pulmonary artery rupture with pulmonary artery catheterization. These complications are addressed where appropriate.

NONINVASIVE BLOOD PRESSURE MONITORING

Since 1903, when Cushing[1] first recommended routine blood pressure monitoring for surgical patients, frequent blood pressure measurement has become standard care for these patients, especially those anesthetized and critically ill. Blood pressure measurement reflects organ perfusion, in that blood flow is proportional to blood pressure and inversely proportional to resistance ($Q = P/R$). Vascular tone, the resistance to flow, must therefore also be considered for blood pressure to be a reflection of tissue perfusion. For instance, a high blood pressure with intense vasoconstriction is likely to represent poor tissue perfusion. Because blood pressure also varies in a complex way during each cardiac and respiratory cycle, a significant variation exists both within and between techniques of measurement.[2] The configuration of the arterial tree (consisting of multiple divisions and an ever decreasing luminal diameter), the autoregulation of regional blood flow, and the dynamics of pulsatile waves all influence blood pressure measurement. These multiple variables make blood pressure monitoring a function of the site and technique of the measurement.[3]

Commonly employed techniques for indirect blood pressure measurement fall into two basic categories—auscultation and oscillometry—i.e., detection by manual or automatic methods. Manual methods, most commonly involving Riva-Rocci sphygmomanometers and auscultation of Korotkoff sounds, rely on the sounds produced by turbulent blood flow, the instability of the arterial wall, and shock wave formation as external pressure on a major artery is reduced.[4] External pressure is supplied via a cuff encircling the artery and the surrounding compressible tissue. The slow release of suprasystolic cuff pressure and auscultation over a major artery, most commonly the brachial, produce characteristic sounds of the various blood pressure components. Some of the occluding cuff pressure is lost owing to tissue compression, the loss being greater with narrow cuffs.[1] Blood pressure measured with a too narrow cuff results in an erroneously elevated measurement. Measurement with too wide a cuff underestimates the actual blood pressure. Cuff width should therefore be 30 to 40 per cent of limb circumference. Other factors that affect tissue compliance surrounding the limb influence the blood pressure measurement. Shivering, which decreases limb compliance, artificially elevates blood pressure.[4]

The rate of cuff deflation is important because Korotkoff sounds may be missed with

KOROTKOFF SOUNDS

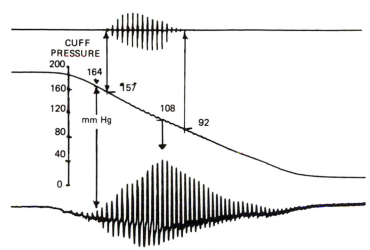

FIGURE 4–1. Oscillations as detected by automated blood pressure cuffs and their relation to auscultation of Korotkoff sounds. Note that oscillations begin before the appearance of Korotkoff sounds. (From Geddes LA: Cardiovascular Devices and Their Applications. New York, John Wiley & Sons, 1984.

OSCILLATIONS IN CUFF PRESSURE

rapid deflation. A rate of deflation of 3 mm Hg/s limits this source of error. Coupling the heart rate to the rate of deflation (2 mm Hg/beat) also increases accuracy.[5] Because sound generation is dependent on blood flow, low flow states (e.g., cardiogenic shock or intense vasoconstriction) can cause underestimation of the blood pressure.[6] Impairment of sound transmission due to loose tubing or poor hearing may also lead to errors in the blood pressure measurement.

Automated blood pressure devices most commonly rely on the oscillometric principle. These devices measure the oscillations produced by arterial pulsations within the encircling cuff (Fig. 4–1). As the cuff pressure is gradually reduced, maximal impulses are sensed by the device and recorded as the mean arterial pressure (MAP). The computer then assigns the systolic blood pressure (SBP) as a per cent of maximal oscillation, usually 50 per cent of the maximum. The diastolic blood pressure (DBP) is assigned as a point from the maximal pulsation, usually 80 per cent of the peak.[4,8] Alternatively, the device averages successive pairs of oscillations, placing the SBP as the point of maximal rise in cuff pressure produced by oscillations and the DBP at the point of maximal decline in cuff pressure[8] (Fig. 4–2). As with manual methods, similar problems with cuff size and measurement hold true. Automated oscillometric devices tend to be sensitive to motion artifact because motion produces oscillation. Variations of blood pressure due to the effects of ventilation also influence the measurement. This source or error is

diminished by signal averaging the oscillations over a period of time. Studies have shown a favorable correlation of automated methods with direct invasive methods.[2,10,11]

Complications from prolonged cuff inflation have been reported, e.g., compartment syndrome, ulnar paresthesia, and thrombophlebitis.[12] Time for perfusion must be adequate, especially in limbs with poor perfusion, i.e., vasoconstriction and peripheral vascular disease.

PRESSURE MONITORING SYSTEMS

Direct pressure monitoring can be accomplished by converting the intravascular pressure to an electrical signal via a pressure transducer. Accessing the vascular tree with an indwelling catheter and connecting it with fluid-filled tubing and stopcocks to a fluid-filled pressure-sensing diaphragm permits this conversion. In order to appropriately assess the data derived from pressure monitoring, a basic comprehension of the mechanical characteristics of the transducer systems is necessary. The many interrelated physical features of transducers are complex, and so only a brief discussion is undertaken here. Other sources are available for an in-depth analysis of these systems.[4,13,14]

Transducing systems consist of an electromechanical strain gauge, or pressure transducer, that ideally is displaced proportionally to the pressure applied, creating an equivalent

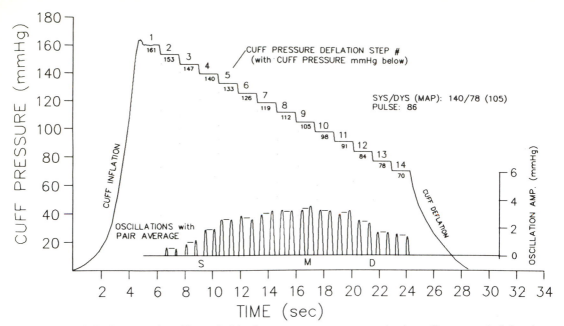

FIGURE 4–2. Automated oscillometric blood pressure measurements. As the cuff pressure is inflated above systolic and slowly deflated, the device measures oscillations produced by arterial pulses. The device assigns the systolic pressure to the point of maximal increase in oscillations (S) and the diastolic as the point of maximal decline oscillations (D). It can also be noted that by averaging successive oscillations the artifact due to respiration and motion can be minimized. (From Ramsey M: Blood pressure monitoring: automated oscillometric devices. J Clin Monit 7:161, 1991. With permission.)

output voltage. This system is analogous to a harmonic oscillator. In this analogy, the mass is the fluid within the transducing system from the catheter to the transducer. Three forces act on this mass: 1) the external driving force; 2) the spring force; and 3) the damping force. The spring force is proportional to the displacement from equilibrium and represents the response of the fluid and the diaphragm to compression. The damping force is proportional to the velocity and represents the viscous forces of the fluid. The spring and damping forces are restoring forces. The external driving force is the blood pressure applied.[15] An output energy proportional to the driving force is created. This electrical signal is then filtered, amplified, and displayed on an oscillometer. The physical characteristics of the fluid-filled tubing and diaphragm influence the output of the electrical signal.

The mechanical properties that most affect the dynamic responsiveness of the transducer system are the natural frequency (f_n) and the damping coefficient. Natural or resonant frequency refers to the frequency at which the system resonates or rings. If the frequency to be measured is near the f_n, the signal is amplified ("overshoot"). To minimize the effects of the f_n of the system on blood pressure mea-

surement the connecting tubing should be short, noncompliant, contain as few stopcocks as possible, and be connected to a large-bore catheter. It is not always feasible to meet these conditions and still have the system functional for blood sampling, flushing, and easy cannulation.

The damping coefficient describes the forces that tend to restore the system to its baseline. These extinguishing frictional and viscous forces of the fluid-filled tubing and diaphragm blunt the responsiveness of the transducer. The damping coefficient can be calculated from the following equation.[16]

$$D = \frac{16n}{d^3} \sqrt{\frac{3LVd}{\pi\rho}}$$

where
  n = viscosity of the fluid
  ρ = density of the fluid
  d = diameter of the catheter
  L = length of the catheter
  Vd = transducer volume displacement

A signal may be: 1) overdampened; 2) underdampened; or 3) optimally dampened (Fig. 4–3). With an overdampened signal, the response of the system is blunted; and with an underdampened signal the response tends to

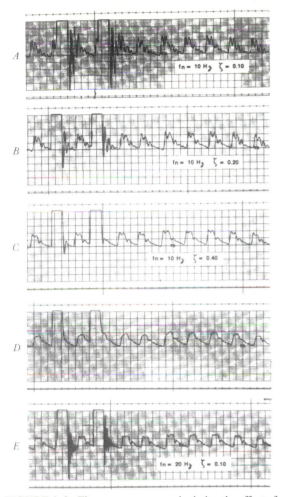

FIGURE 4–3. Five pressure traces depicting the effect of damping on the trace. **A.** Trace has a low f_n and a damping coefficient of 0.1. Note the overshoot and ringing in the trace. **B.** The damping coefficient has been increased to 0.2 with the f_n remaining the same. The ringing after flushing is attenuated. **C.** This trace represents near-optimal damping with a coefficient of 0.4. **D.** An overdampened signal is represented, as no ringing is noted after flushing. **E.** By shortening the length of tubing the f_n is increased and the damping coefficient remains low, with little distortion of the waveform. (From Gardner RM: Direct blood pressure measurement—dynamic response requirements. Anesthesiology 54:227, 1981. With permission.)

Hz (1 Hz = 60 cycles/s) would be sufficient to measure pulse waveforms occurring at 1 to 2 Hz and impart little amplification to the waveform. It would be sufficient if the pulse were a simple sine wave. In reality, the pulse wave is a series of sine waves (Fourier series) with frequency components of approximately 20 Hz.[4] Consequently, as the frequency components of blood pressure approach the f_n, the pressure trace is amplified, especially as the heart rate approaches the f_n.

To evaluate the dynamic response of the system one can perform a snap or pop test (Fig. 4–5). By snapping the flush valve rapidly and recording the pressure trace on a strip recorder, the system briefly rings at its natural frequency. The f_n can be calculated as the cycles per second before returning to the pressure trace. Excessive ringing may be diminished by increasing the damping coefficient, i.e., by introducing a small air bubble into the pressure tubing.[17] The damping coefficient can be calculated as the difference in amplitude between successive peaks in the "ringing" pattern. The ideal system would oscillate minimally (approximately three times) before quickly returning to baseline.

Equally important in the use of transducer systems is the appropriate calibration and zero referencing of the system. The calibration of the monitoring system is accomplished by connecting the system to a known pressure, often a mercury manometer. Most of the monitors used currently do not require frequent calibration of the internal electronic components: preamplifier, amplifier, and filter. To zero reference (or simply "zero") the transducing system, the pressure of the system is exposed to air, as atmospheric pressure acts equally on the patient and the system. The point in the line where it is opened to air is the zero reference, not necessarily the level of the transducer. To prevent the problem of transducer drift, the transducer system must be periodically re-zeroed.

Although most monitoring systems provide a numeric readout of blood pressure, these numbers may not be an accurate reflection of the blood pressure. The electronic monitor is programmed to report the high and low readings of the pressure waveform as the systolic and diastolic pressures, respectively. Artifacts, under- and overdampened traces, and effects of the ventilatory cycle influence the high and low portions of the displayed waveform.

resonate or overshoot. An optimally dampened signal accurately displays the blood pressure. The natural frequency and damping coefficient are inversely related: As one goes up, the other goes down (Fig. 4–4). For example, a damping coefficient of 0.2 will cause a reduction of the f_n by 20 per cent.

Most transducing systems have a natural frequency of 10 to 20 Hz and a damping coefficient of 0.2 to 0.3.[17] One may think an f_n of 10

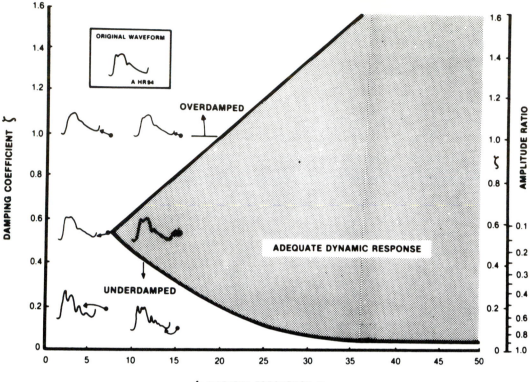

FIGURE 4-4. Typical dynamic response plot. The shaded area represents an adequate response for that heart rate and waveform characteristics. (From Gardner RM: Direct blood pressure measurement—dynamic response requirements. Anesthesiology *54*:227, 1981. With permission.)

INVASIVE BLOOD PRESSURE MONITORING

Considerable controversy has developed as to the "best" way to measure blood pressure: invasive versus noninvasive methods. Nonin- vasive techniques tend to correlate well with each other; but there is not necessarily a cor- relation between invasive and noninvasive techniques.[3] Although many believe that inva- sive pressure monitoring is the "gold stan- dard," it has limitations. Whereas invasive

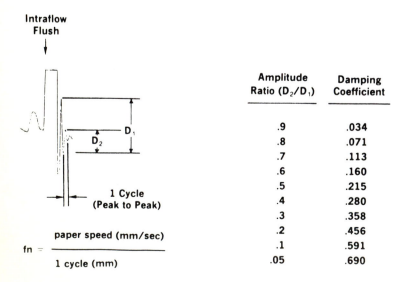

Amplitude Ratio (D_2/D_1)	Damping Coefficient
.9	.034
.8	.071
.7	.113
.6	.160
.5	.215
.4	.280
.3	.358
.2	.456
.1	.591
.05	.690

FIGURE 4-5. Snap test wave- form allowing calculation of the damping coefficient and the natu- ral frequency. The f_n is the cycles per second in the ring pattern. The damping coefficient can be obtained from the chart on the right. (From Bedford RF: Inva- sive blood pressure monitoring. *In* Blitt CD (ed): Monitoring in Anesthesia and Critical Care Medicine, 2nd ed. New York, Churchill Livingstone, 1990, p. 93. With permission.)

methods measure pressure directly, noninvasive methods rely on flow or volume changes for measurement. Invasive methods tend to yield a higher measurement, possibly secondary to natural amplification and reflected waves.

The configuration of the arterial tree creates a natural amplification of the pressure waveform as it moves distally from the heart (Fig. 4–6). As the intraluminal diameter narrows, there is confinement of the pulsed energy with a resultant more rapid rise of the pressure wave and subsequent higher systolic peak. Atherosclerosis and aging, which diminish the elasticity of the vessel walls, also result in systolic amplification. The diastolic pressure is consequently lower, as there is less elastic compliance of the narrower artery. The net effect of these changes, as the waveform propagates distally, is a small change in mean arterial pressure. During the postcardiopulmonary bypass period, the opposite holds true: The radial artery pressure is lower than the central arterial pressure, presumably owing to changes in vascular resistance.

As the pulse wave is propagated distally, it may be reflected and added or subtracted from the displayed waveform (Fig. 4–7). Bifurcations and arteriole–artery junctions are considered to be the principal site of reflection.[3] Vasoconstriction and thrombosis also accentuate reflection.[13]

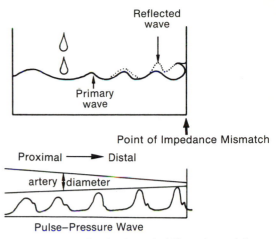

FIGURE 4–7. Reflection from the bifurcation and the arterial-arteriole junction also contributes to the arterial waveform. The closer to the aorta the pressure is measured, the less these changes affect the waveform. The effects of decreasing arterial lumen diameter on the pulse waveform is also shown. (From Bedford RF: Invasive blood pressure monitoring. *In* Blitt CD (ed): Monitoring in Anesthesia and Critical Care Medicine, 2nd ed. New York, Churchill Livingstone, 1990, p. 93. With permission.)

Complications of arterial cannulation include thrombosis, distal ischemia, hematoma, and infection. Arterial cannulation is usually performed at a site with collateral blood flow, thereby minimizing the potential for distal ischemia. The Allen test has been advocated as a way of assessing the collateral flow with mixed results.[18,19] Hematoma formation and catheter site infection can be minimized by meticulous attention to the technique of insertion and care.

PULMONARY ARTERY PRESSURE MONITORING

Development of the flow-directed, balloon flotation pulmonary artery catheter (PAC) has allowed the clinician to further evaluate left ventricular preload and function. In addition to measuring intracardiac pressure, the PAC allows one to: 1) sample intracardiac and mixed venous blood and make calculations based on these samples; 2) determine cardiac output, most frequently by thermodilution; 3) aid in the diagnosis of various intracardiac lesions; 4) assess volume via fluid challenge; 5) diagnose myocardial ischemia; and 6) differentiate cardiac from noncardiac pulmonary edema. Optimal PAC utilization depends on proper application of reliable data and an understanding of the factors that alter the validity of measured and calculated data.[20]

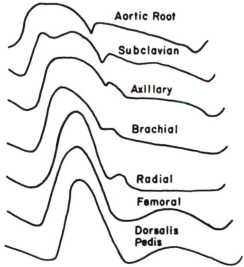

FIGURE 4–6. Changes in the arterial pressure waveform as it propagates distally, produced by the natural amplification. This amplification is a consequence of a narrowing arterial lumen and a decrease in elastance of the smaller vessels. (From Bedford RF: Invasive blood pressure monitoring. *In* Blitt CD (ed): Monitoring in Anesthesia and Critical Care Medicine, 2nd ed. New York, Churchill Livingstone, 1990, p. 93. With permission.)

Studies have shown that right heart pressures provide an unreliable estimate of left ventricular filling pressures. In certain patients the CVP, in fact, varies inversely.[21–23] The pulmonary artery catheter allows for closer assessment of left ventricular filling pressures. As the PAC balloon is inflated, the catheter "wedges" in an arterial segment, creating a static column of fluid from the catheter tip to the left ventricle at end-diastole. In the absence of a pressure gradient, imparted by internal or external forces, the pressure measured at the tip of the PAC reflects left ventricular end-diastolic pressure (LVEDP) (Fig. 4–8). Many factors can interfere with this static column and alter this relation. The following discussion focuses on these factors.

The pressure–volume relation of the left ventricle at end-diastole is dependent on ventricular compliance, as described by Frank-Starling curves (Fig. 4–9). Many factors have been identified that alter compliance and, sub-

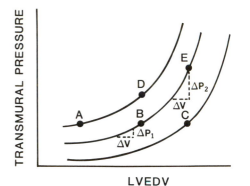

FIGURE 4–9. Typical ventricular compliance curves. As volume increases along each curve, there is a progressive increase in pressure with that change, moving from point B to point E. The compliance of the ventricle may also change; i.e., as the compliance decreases, the pressure is higher at the same volume, moving from B to D. (From Tuman KJ, Carroll GC, Ivankovich AD: Pitfalls in interpretation of pulmonary artery catheter data. J Cardiothorac Anesth 3:625, 1989. With permission.)

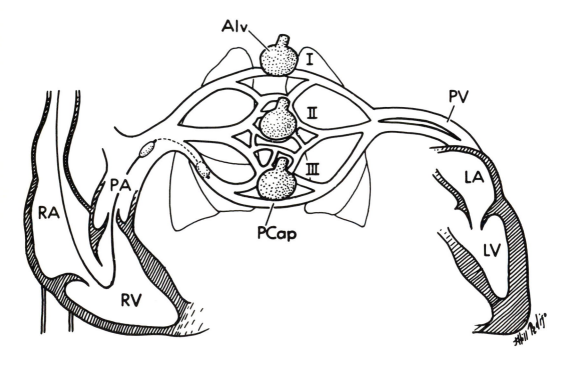

PAEDP ⟷ PWP ⟷ PVP ⟷ LAP ⟷ LVEDP

FIGURE 4–8. Pulmonary artery pressure measure at the tip of the flow-directed catheter. Note the various influencing factors affecting the relation of the pressure measured at the tip of the pulmonary artery catheter and the left ventricular end-diastolic pressure. CVP, central venous pressure; RA, right atrium; RV, right ventricle; PA, pulmonary artery; PAEDP, pulmonary artery end-diastolic pressure; PAOP, pulmonary artery occlusive pressure; Alv, alveolar pressure; I, II, III, lung zones as described by West; PVP, pulmonary venous pressure. PCap, pulmonary capillary pressure; PV, pulmonary vein; LA, left atrium; LV, left ventricle; LVEDP, left ventricular end-diastolic pressure; LVEDV, left ventricular end-diastolic volume. (From Vender JS: Invasive cardiac monitoring. *In* Vender JS (ed): Intensive Care Monitoring. Philadelphia, Saunders, 1988, p. 468. With permission.)

TABLE 4–1. FACTORS AFFECTING VENTRICULAR COMPLIANCE

Decreased ventricular compliance
    Myocardial ischemia
    Restrictive cardiomyopathies
    Aortic stenosis
    Cardiac tamponade
    Positive end-expiratory pressure
    Inotropes

Increased ventricular compliance
    Vasodilators (nitroglycerin, nitroprusside)
    Congestive cardiomyopathies
    Aortic regurgitation
    Mitral regurgitation

sequently, the pressure-volume relation (Table 4–1).

Left atrial pressure (LAP) usually equals LVEDP. Alterations in left ventricular compliance and the presence of cardiac valvular disease can affect this relation. Valvular disease exaggerates the disparity between LAP and LVEDP. Mitral regurgitation may cause "cannon v-waves," leading to a misinterpretation that the PAC is not in the "wedge" position[25] (Fig. 4–10). A decrease in ventricular compliance, such as with ischemia and cardiomyopathies, causes the LVEDP to rise more with atrial contraction than the LAP.[27]

Normally the pulmonary artery occlusive pressure (PAOP) approximates the left atrial pressure if the catheter tip is appropriately in West's zone III.[28,29] If the PAC is instead located in either of West's lung zones I or II, the PAOP may reflect alveolar pressure and not LAP.[30] Fortunately, because pulmonary artery catheters are flow-directed, they most often are placed in West's zone III. Airway pressure therapy and pulmonary venous disease further interfere with this relation, so the pressure is measured at end-expiration.

The effects of ventilation and intrathoracic pressure need to be examined. The changes imparted by ventilation and airway pressure therapy influence the measurement of central venous and pulmonary artery pressures as well. Intrathoracic pressure changes throughout each ventilatory cycle, increasing with spontaneous exhalation and decreasing with spontaneous inhalation. With positive pressure ventilation the opposite occurs; the intrathoracic pressure increases with inspiration and decreases with expiration. These changes in intrathoracic pressure are reflected (central venous and pulmonary artery) waveforms. To minimize these effects, the pulmonary artery pressure is measured at end-expiration, when the respiratory musculature is resting and the intrathoracic pressure is stable (Fig. 4–11).

Changes in intrathoracic pressure from transmitted positive end-expiratory pressure (PEEP) therapy are likewise reflected in the pressure waveforms. Depending on the compliance of the lung and thorax, a portion of the additional pressure from PEEP therapy impedes extrathoracic venous return,[32] often resulting in an elevated CVP/PAP measurement, dependent on the lung compliance. Measuring intrapleural pressure, which can be cumbersome, and subtracting it from the CVP/PAP (transmural pressure) eliminates this effect. Although removing PEEP during pressure measurements may seem like an attractive solution, it is not recommended. The beneficial effects of PEEP are quickly lost and may lead to hypoxemia. Sudden removal of PEEP's impedance to venous return may result in an acute volume overload. If PEEP therapy is to be reinstituted after the measurement, the pressure, measured without PEEP, does not adequately reflect the patient's current cardiovascular status.[33]

The pulmonary artery diastolic (PAD) pres-

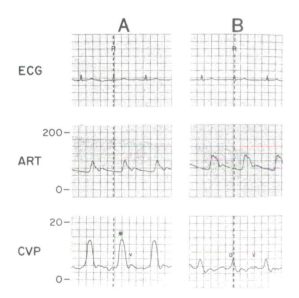

FIGURE 4–10. Effects of ventilation on a pulmonary artery trace. With spontaneous ventilation the end-expiratory pressure is the higher pressure of the trace. The trace on the left is an example of this effect. A, spontaneous breath. Positive pressure ventilation causes the end-expiratory pressure to be the lower pressure of the trace. The right hand trace is of a mechanically ventilated patient, where the breath is indicated by A. (From Schmitt EA, Brantigen CO: Common artifacts of pulmonary artery wedge pressure: recognition and interpretation. J Clin Monit 2:44, 1986. With permission.)

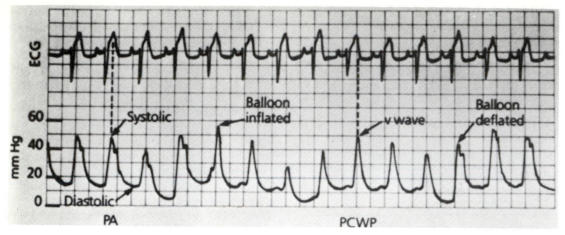

FIGURE 4–11. Cannon v-waves with acute mitral regurgitation. Note the difference between the PA and PAOP trace: slower rise in the peak, lack of c-wave, v-wave occurring later in relation to the QRS, and narrower spike of the PAOP trace with v-waves. (From Amin DA, Shah PK, Swan HJC: The Swan-Ganz catheter: indications for insertion. J Crit Illness *1*:54, 1986. With permission.)

sure provides an approximation of the PAOP. The usual difference between PAD and PAOP is 1 to 4 mm Hg.[34,35] Changes in pulmonary vascular resistance alter this relation. Pulmonary hypertension causes the PAD to be exaggerated. Tachycardia may also widen the difference, likely related to the decrease in the diastolic filling time.[36] In the absence of right heart dysfunction, the CVP can be used as an estimate of PAD.

"Overwedging" is also a problem encountered in the measurement of pulmonary artery occlusive pressures. As the balloon is inflated the tracing increases continually, as continuous-flush fluid accumulates between the tip and the vessel, without appropriate waveform characteristics (Fig. 4–12). This reaction is thought to be due to balloon herniation over the tip of the PAC or the tip of the catheter lying against the vessel wall. Overwedging has been identified as a potential risk factor in pul-

monary artery rupture.[36] Pulmonary artery rupture risks may be minimized by: 1) appropriate patient selection, especially among elderly patients; 2) utilizing pulmonary artery diastolic pressures or minimizing balloon tip inflations; 3) slow, progressive inflation of the balloon tip; 4) preinsertion confirmation of balloon shape and function; and 5) using the appropriate volume of air only.[20] If pulmonary artery rupture occurs, therapy is directed at supportive measures, maintenance of volume status, and coagulation. Separation and isolation of the lungs with a double-lumen endotracheal tube may allow adequate gas exchange. Occasionally, surgical intervention is necessary.

The fluid challenge involves rapid infusion of a volume, usually 50 to 250 ml of crystalloid solution, and observing the change in measured pulmonary artery or central venous pressures. A normal change in the pressure

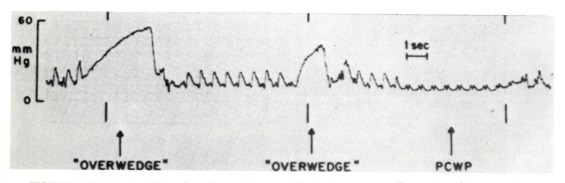

FIGURE 4–12. Overwedging of a pulmonary artery catheter trace may predispose to pulmonary artery rupture. (From Barash PG, Nardi D, Hammond G, et al: Catheter-induced pulmonary artery perforation: mechanisms, management, and modifications. J Thorac Cardiovasc Surg *82*:5, 1981. With permission.)

would be 2 to 4 mm Hg followed by a return to baseline within 15 minutes. A lesser change would imply reduced preload, whereas a dramatic increase would indicate near-maximal capacitance. This measurement allows the clinician to further define the cardiovascular status and make appropriate interventions. The fluid challenge is also applicable when using a pulmonary artery catheter and following pulmonary artery occlusive pressures as well as cardiac output.

CENTRAL VENOUS PRESSURE MONITORING

Accessing the central circulation for pressure monitoring, blood sampling, and fluid infusion can lead to complications. These complications can be grouped into three basic categories (Table 4–2): 1) those related to cannulation or insertion; 2) those related to catheter passage or advancement; and 3) those related to the presence of the catheter.

Central venous pressure (CVP) measurement can provide a useful evaluation of the right ventricular function.[37,38] CVP is a useful evaluation of venous return because it is measured at the junction of the heart and the venous system. CVP measurement can aid in the

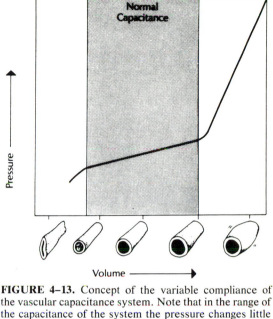

FIGURE 4–13. Concept of the variable compliance of the vascular capacitance system. Note that in the range of the capacitance of the system the pressure changes little with a change in volume. (From Shapiro BA, et al: Circulation and perfusion. *In* Clinical Application of Respiratory Care, 4th ed. St. Louis, Mosby Year Book, 1991, p. 209. With permission.)

diagnosis of cardiac tamponade by the equalization of diastolic filling pressures (CVP = PAOP = PAD).[39] Although CVP measurement provides considerable hemodynamic information, it has limitations. Evaluations must be done in the context of overall cardiac function, as well as the changes with relation to time and intervention.

Central venous pressure measurement provides an indication of venous return. The ventricular preload is primarily dependent on venous return. The venous system can be characterized as a variable compliance system[33] (Fig. 4–13). In the shaded area of Figure 4–13 the venous system is compliant, and addition of further volume results in little increase in pressure. When the capacitance of the venous system is reached, it becomes noncompliant, and further increases in volume result in large increases in pressure.[26] One must remember that venous tone and vascular reflexes play an important role in venous return.

The preload is defined as the length of the myocardial fibers at rest, or end-diastolic ventricular volume. Because we cannot directly measure end-diastolic volume at the bedside but pressure measurements are readily available, we commonly use CVP to predict end-

TABLE 4–2. COMPLICATIONS DUE TO VARIOUS FACTORS

Central venous cannulation
  Arterial puncture
  Pneumothorax, hemothorax
  Nerve injury
  Air embolization
  Horner syndrome
  Mediastinal/pleural effusion
  Chylothorax
  Catheter embolization

Catheter passage
  Arrhythmias/heart block
  Knotting/kinking
  Valvular damage
  Perforation of the vessel

Catheter presence
  Thrombosis
  Pulmonary artery rupture
  Sepsis/infection
  Endocarditis
  Arrhythmias
  Pulmonary infarction
  Hematologic abnormalities
  Valve damage
  Thromboembolism

From Vender,[20] with permission.

diastolic volume. This assumption is not valid, as the pressure-volume relation of the vascular system is not linear, as discussed above. Manipulation of preload by fluid volume challenge (see above) and following the subsequent changes in pressure allow the clinician to evaluate the adequacy of venous return and volume status.

Analysis of the CVP waveform yields additional information about the cardiovascular system. The typical waveform consists of an a-wave (atrial contraction), c-wave (tricuspid valve protruding into the atria), and v-wave (venous return with the tricuspid valve closed).[40] Tachycardia causes fusion of the waveform components, thereby limiting the utility of the waveform. Loss of the a-wave is likely related to loss of the atrial contraction, i.e., atrial fibrillation or flutter and junctional rhythms (Fig. 4–14). Prominent a-waves reflect an obstruction of right heart outflow, as in pulmonary hypertension or pulmonary stenosis. With tricuspid regurgitation, the c- and v-waves are replaced by large regurgitant v-waves. The CVP measurement also allows evaluation of right heart function and compliance. Large v-waves may become prominent with a decrease in right ventricular compliance, as in ischemia, volume overload, or amyloidosis.[40]

MIXED VENOUS SATURATION MONITORING

Pulmonary artery catheters allow mixed venous oxygen saturation (SvO_2), by both blood sampling and continuous oximetry. Fiberoptic technology, specifically reflectance oximetry, allows a computer to continually analyze the reflected light and provide an SvO_2 calculation. This measurement reflects the adequacy of cardiac performance to meet metabolic demands. The use of SvO_2 to determine the adequacy of cardiac output is analogous to measuring the arterial partial pressure of carbon dioxide to evaluate minute ventilation.[20] Therefore the continuous measurement of SvO_2 has been used to assess the adequacy of oxygen supply and demand balance.[41]

An understanding of oxygen delivery, demand, and consumption is necessary to comprehend the utility of SvO_2 as a reflection of oxygen balance. The mixed venous oxygen saturation is dependent on: 1) arterial oxygen saturation; 2) metabolic consumption of oxy-

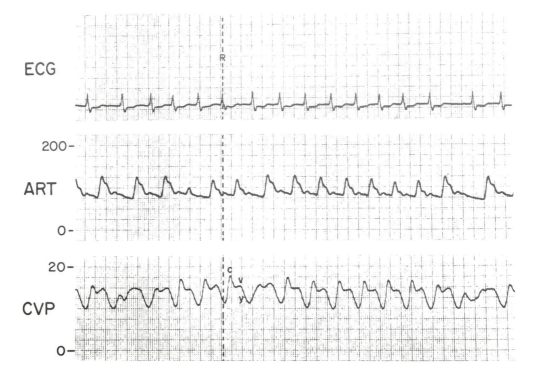

FIGURE 4–14. Traces of patients with atrial fibrillation. On the left is an example of the loss of the a-wave. The trace on the right demonstrates f, or flutter, waves. (From Marks JB: Central venous pressure monitoring: clinical insights beyond the numbers. J Cardiothorac Vasc Surg 5:163, 1991. With permission.)

TABLE 4–3. FACTORS AFFECTING MIXED VENOUS SATURATION

Arterial oxygen saturation
Metabolic consumption of oxygen
Cardiac output
Arterial hemoglobin concentration

gen; 3) cardiac output; and 4) arterial hemoglobin concentration (Table 4–3). Oxygen delivery equals the arterial oxygen content (dependent primarily on the hemoglobin saturation and concentration) times the cardiac output. The global cellular metabolic requirement for oxygen is a reflection of oxygen demand. The total oxygen consumption (VO_2)—the amount of oxygen utilized by the various tissue beds—is calculated as the difference between arterial oxygen content and the mixed venous content. The relation of these factors is given by rearranging the Fick equation:

$$SvO_2 = SaO_2 - VO_2/(CO * Hgb * 1.36)$$

The multiple variables involved in the SvO_2 determination makes this assessment of cardiac performance difficult. In contrast, if other variables (arterial oxygen content and oxygen consumption) are constant, the SvO_2 will reflect cardiac output. Care must be taken in situations where there is an increase in SvO_2, as the increase may not be related to a more favorable supply and demand balance (Table 4–4). Sepsis with abnormal cellular utilization and shunting of blood by tissue beds may result in an elevated SvO_2. Arteriovenous fistulas, cirrhosis, left-to-right shunts, cyanide toxicity, hypothermia, and inadvertent PAC wedging may cause an increase in the mixed venous saturation.[26,33]

For the oxymetric tip to adequately sample blood it must be free within the lumen of the pulmonary artery. Reflection of the infrared signal from the blood vessel wall may cause an error in the calculation. Other artifacts such as motion and positive airway pressure therapy interfere with accurate measurement.

THERMODILUTION CARDIAC OUTPUT

Incorporating a thermistor into PAC has allowed rapid and accurate determination of cardiac output. It allows the clinician to evaluate the heart's function as a pump. Although other methods exist (e.g., Doppler and Fick calculation), cardiac output is most commonly measured by thermodilution. A thermal decay curve is obtained by injecting a known volume of cold or room temperature crystalloid as an indicator and measuring the change in temperature distally. A cardiac output computer can then integrate the area under the curve and calculate the cardiac output. The Stewart-Hamilton equation describes the thermodilution principle:

$$Q = \frac{V(T_B - T_I)(K_1)(K_2)}{T_B(t)dt}$$

where Q = cardiac output; V = volume injected; T_B = blood temperature; T_I = injectate temperature; K_1 and K_2 = computational constants; $T_B(t)dt$ = change in blood temperature as a function of time. A cardiac output computer integrates the temperature change and produces a cardiac output curve. The area under the curve is inversely proportional to the cardiac output.

To minimize error during the cardiac output determination, several technical aspects must be considered. Accurate filling of injectate syringes to match the volume programmed into the computer helps eliminate volume as a source of error.[42] The temperature of the injectate and blood must also be closely recorded. Most of the current thermodilution PAC and computers automatically measure and update the blood and injectate temperature. The computation constant also takes into consideration the injectate temperature. The temperature of the injectate may be altered by warming it in the operator's hand, catheter, or

TABLE 4–4. METABOLIC EFFECTS ON MIXED VENOUS SATURATION

Increased SvO_2
  Increased CO
  Sepsis
  Cyanide toxicity
  Lactic acidosis
  Left-to-right shunts
  Hypothermia
  Cirrhosis
  PAC wedging

Decreased SvO_2
  Decreased cardiac output
  Shivering
  Fever
  AV shunting

TABLE 4–5. SOURCES OF ERROR IN THERMODILUTION CARDIAC OUTPUT

Inaccurate volume of injectate
Variable injectate temperature
Rapid fluid infusion
Poor injectate mixing
Changes in vital signs
Slow injection of injectate
Small variation in temperature from blood to injectate
Blood temperature changes
Inaccurate computation constants
Respiratory variations
Excessive warming of the injectate
Thermistor insulated by vessel lumen
Respiratory variations

syringe. Although cold injectate offers the advantage of a greater signal-to-noise ratio, which is especially helpful during hypothermia, it has been reported to produce arrhythmias.[42] Care must be taken when entering the computation constant into the computer. This constant takes into account the injectate lumen capacity, volume of injectate, temperature of injectate, and pulmonary artery catheter characteristics. Changes in hematocrit and use of either saline or dextrose water for the injectate cause negligible changes in the constants.[43] The variations between computation constants may be reflected in the differences between computers.[44]

Poor mixing of the injectate, changes in heart rate and blood pressure, and abnormal ventilatory patterns may also cause irregular cardiac output curves (Table 4–5). Inadequate mixing of the injectate with venous blood may result from intracardiac shunts, tricuspid regurgitation, or arrhythmias. By ensuring rapid injection (<4 seconds), inadequate mixing can be minimized. Because of the dynamics of intrathoracic pressure during ventilation, injecting the thermal indicator at the same time during each respiratory cycle and averaging a series of injections can minimize these effects.[45,46]

The thermistor needs to be able to freely sense the change in temperature. If the thermistor is "insulated" by the vessel wall, an irregular curve may result. If the injectate port is within the sheath introducer, retrograde injection into the sidearm is possible, which may yield spuriously high outputs owing to the output calculation being based on a larger injectate volume.[9]

The use of cardiac output as an indication of heart function is limited without assessing other clinical parameters (e.g., urine output) or indices of perfusion (mixed venous saturation). A given cardiac output may be luxuriant, adequate, or suboptimal depending on the metabolic needs and arterial oxygen content.[20]

References

1. Cushing HW: On routine determinations of arterial tensions in the operating room and clinic. Boston Med Surg J *148*:250, 1903.
2. Davis RF: Clinical comparison of automated auscultatory and oscillometric and catheter-transducer measurements of arterial pressure. J Clin Monit *1*:114, 1985.
3. Bruner JMR, Krenis LJ, Kunsman JM, et al: Comparison of direct and indirect methods of blood pressure monitoring. Med Instrum *15*:182, 1981.
4. Gorback MS: Considerations in the interpretation of systemic pressure monitoring. *In* Lumb PD, Bryan-Brown CW (eds): Complications in Critical Care Medicine. Chicago, Year Book, 1988.
5. Yong PG, Geddes LA: The effect of cuff pressure deflation rate on accuracy in indirect measurement of blood pressure with the auscultatory method. J Clin Monit *3*:155, 1987.
6. Cohn JN: Blood pressure measurement in shock. JAMA *199*:118, 1967.
7. Geddes LA: Cardiovascular Devices and Their Application. John Wiley & Sons, New York, 1984.
8. Ramsey M: Blood pressure monitoring: automated oscillometric devices. J Clin Monit *7*:161, 1991.
9. Stoller JK, Herbst TJ, Hurford W, et al: Spuriously high output from injecting thermal indicator through an ensheathed port. Crit Care Med *14*:1064, 1986.
10. Yelderman M, Ream AK: Indirect measurement of mean blood pressure in anesthetized patients. Anesthesiology *59*:349, 1979.
11. Borow KM, Newburger JW: Noninvasive estimate of central aortic pressure using the oscillometric method for analyzing systemic artery pulsatile blood flow: comparative study of indirect systolic, diastolic, and mean brachial artery pressure with simultaneous direct ascending aortic pressure measurements. Am Heart J *103*:879, 1982.
12. Celoria G, Dawson JA, Teres D: Compartment syndrome in a patient monitored with an automated blood pressure cuff. J Clin Monit *3*:139, 1987.
13. Bedford RF: Invasive blood pressure monitoring. *In* Blitt CD (ed): Monitoring in Anesthesia and Critical Care Medicine, 2nd ed. New York, Churchill Livingstone, 1990, p. 93.
14. Prys-Roberts C: Invasive monitoring of the circulation. *In* Saidman LJ, Smith NT (eds): Monitoring in Anesthesia, 2nd ed. Boston, Butterworth, Publishing, 1984, p. 79.
15. Tremper KK, Barker SJ: Fundamental principles of monitoring instrumentation. *In* Miller RD (ed), Anesthesia, 3rd ed. New York, Churchill Livingstone, 1990, p. 957.
16. Geddes LA: The Direct and Indirect Measurement of Blood Pressure. Chicago, Year Book, 1970.

17. Gardner RM: Direct blood pressure measurement—dynamic response requirements. Anesthesiology *54*: 227, 1981.
18. Wilkins RG: Radial artery cannulation and ischemic damage: a review. Anaesthesia *40*:896, 1985.
19. Bedford RF, Wollman H: Complications of percutaneous radial artery cannulation: an objective prospective study in man. Anesthesiology *38*:228, 1973.
20. Vender JS: Invasive cardiac monitoring. *In* Vender JS (ed): Intensive Care Monitoring. Philadelphia, Saunders, 1988, p. 468.
21. Civetta JM, Gabel JC: Flow-directed pulmonary artery catheterization: indications and modification of technique. Ann Surg *176*:753, 1972.
22. Forrester JS, Diamond GA, McHugh TJ, et al: Filling pressures in the right and left sides of the heart in acute myocardial infarction. N Engl J Med *285*:190, 1971.
23. Samii K, Conseiller C, Viars P: Central venous pressure and pulmonary wedge pressure. Arch Surg *111*: 1122, 1976.
24. Tuman KJ, Carroll GC, Ivankovich AD: Pitfalls in interpretation of pulmonary artery catheter data. J Cardiothorac Anesth *3*:625, 1989.
25. Schmitt EA, Brantigan CO: Common artifacts of pulmonary artery wedge pressure: recognition and interpretation. J Clin Monit *2*:44, 1986.
26. Shapiro BA, et al: Circulation and perfusion. *In* Clinical Application of Respiratory Care, 4th ed. St. Louis, Mosby, 1991, p. 209.
27. O'Quin R, Marini JJ: Pulmonary artery occlusion pressure: clinical physiology, measurement, and interpretation. Am Rev Respir Dis *128*:319, 1983.
28. West JB, Dollery CT, Naimark A: Distribution of the blood flow in the isolated lung: relation to the vascular and alveolar pressures. J Appl Physiol *19*:713, 1964.
29. Lappas D, Lell WA, Gabel JC: Measurement of left-atrial pressure in surgical patients—pulmonary capillary wedge and pulmonary artery diastolic pressures compared to left-atrial pressure. Anesthesiology *38*: 394, 1973.
30. Kronberg GM, Quan SF, Schlobohm RM, et al: Anatomic locations of the tips of pulmonary artery catheters in supine patients. Anesthesiology *51*:467, 1979.
31. Amin DA, Shah PK, Swan HJC: The Swan-Ganz catheter: indications for insertion. J Crit Illness *1*:54, 1986.
32. Berryhill RE, Benumof JL: PEEP-induced discrepancy between pulmonary arterial wedge pressure and left atrial pressure: the influence of controlled vs. spontaneous ventilation and compliant vs. noncompliant lungs. Anesthesiology *46*:383, 1979.
33. Otto CW: Central venous pressure monitoring. *In* Blitt CD (ed): Monitoring in Anesthesia and Critical Care Medicine, 2nd ed. New York, Churchill Livingstone, 1990, p. 169.
34. Bouchard RJ, Gault JH, Ross J: Evaluation of pulmonary arterial end-diastolic pressure as an estimate of left ventricular end-diastolic pressure in patients with normal and abnormal left ventricular performance. Circulation *44*:1072, 1971.
35. Gabrial S: The difference between the pulmonary artery diastolic pressure and the pulmonary wedge pressure in chronic lung disease. Acta Med Scand *190*: 555, 1971.
36. Barash PG, Nardi D, Hammond G, et al: Catheter-induced pulmonary artery perforation: mechanisms, management, and modifications. J Thorac Cardiovasc Surg *82*:5, 1981.
37. Berman AL, Green LO, Grossman W: Right ventricular diastolic pressure in coronary artery disease. Am J Cardiol *44*:1263, 1979.
38. Lopez-Sendon J, Coma-Canella I, Gamely C: Sensitivity and specificity of hemodynamic criteria in the diagnosis of right ventricular infarction. Circulation *64*:515, 1981.
39. Starkey SW: Beyond the wedge: clinical physiology and the Swan-Ganz catheter. Am J Med *83*:111, 1987.
40. Marks JB: Central venous pressure monitoring: clinical insights beyond the numbers. J Cardiothorac Vasc Surg *5*:163, 1991.
41. Kandel G, Aberman A: Mixed venous oxygen saturation, it's role in the assessment of the critically ill patient. Arch Intern Med *143*:1400, 1983.
42. Riedinger MS, Shellock FG: Technical aspects of the thermodilution method for measuring cardiac output. Heart Lung *13*:215, 1984.
43. Barash PG, Hines R: Pulmonary artery catheters. *In* Blitt CD (ed): Monitoring in Anesthesia and Critical Care Medicine, 2nd ed. New York, Churchill Livingstone, 1990, p. 210.
44. Matthew EB, Vender JS: Comparison of thermodilution cardiac output measured by different computers. Crit Care Med *15*:989, 1987.
45. Armengol J, Man GCW, Balsys AJ, et al: Effects of respiratory cycle on cardiac output measurements: reproducibility of data enhanced by timing of the thermodilution injections in dogs. Crit Care Med *9*:852, 1981.
46. Snyder JV, Powner DJ: Effects of mechanical ventilation on the measurement of cardiac output by thermodilution. Crit Care Med *10*:677, 1982.
47. Stoller JK, Herbst TJ, Hurford W, et al: Spuriously high output from injecting thermal indicator through an ensheathed port. Crit Care Med *14*:1064, 1986.

RESPIRATORY COMPLICATIONS

CHRISTINA M. CHOMKA LEYA
and LEONARD C. BANDALA

Anesthesia and surgery are associated with respiratory changes that start with administration of the premedication and can last for days postoperatively. It is not surprising that the primary cause of life-threatening morbidity in the post anesthesia care unit (PACU) is of respiratory origin. In a review of PACU mishaps leading to malpractice claims against anesthesiologists, the respiratory system was responsible for more than 50 per cent of the critical incidents.[1] Although respiratory critical events occurred less frequently in the PACU than in the operating room, serious outcomes, either death or brain damage, were greater.

Is there any way that we can predict which patients are at greater risk for developing postoperative respiratory complications so such events can be prevented? Are certain surgical procedures or anesthetic techniques responsible for a greater proportion of postoperative respiratory problems?

DRUG EFFECTS

INHALATIONAL ANESTHETICS

All inhalational anesthetics decrease ventilation in a dose-related manner; and a decrease in tidal volume is associated with a simultaneous increase in breathing frequency.[2,3] When a patient is allowed to breath spontaneously while anesthetized, the measurement of tidal volume can be used to reflect anesthetic depth. An elevation in $PaCO_2$ is a consequence of this ventilatory depression, with some agents (i.e., enflurane) being more depressant than others. Not only is the patient's resting $PaCO_2$ elevated, the inhalational anesthetics diminish the responsiveness of ventilation to exogenous CO_2.

The hypoxic ventilatory response, like the

CO_2 response, is impaired in a dose-related manner by inhalational anesthetics.[4] However, in most circumstances a much smaller concentration of anesthetic is required to depress the ventilatory response to hypoxia. Residual anesthetics present in the PACU thus impair the patient's ability to respond appropriately to hypoxemia.

Anesthetics have also been shown to depress the ventilatory response to an external load (i.e., resistance to inspiration).[5] Patients with thoracic or abdominal pressure or binding may be unable to maintain adequate spontaneous ventilation even if only partially anesthetized. Individuals with underlying pulmonary pathology may be the most susceptible to hypercarbia secondary to residual anesthesia while breathing spontaneously.

Not only do anesthetics affect the ventilatory response; oxygenation is also impaired. Reduction of functional residual capacity, progressive pulmonary atelectasis, altered mucociliary function, and impairment of hypoxic pulmonary vasoconstriction[6] have been documented in the presence of inhalational anesthetics.

NARCOTICS

The respiratory depressant effects of narcotics are well known. Not only is the resting $PaCO_2$ elevated, hypoxic ventilatory drive is also decreased by narcotics.[7] Similar to the inhalational anesthetics, the ventilatory response to an external load is blunted,[8] and mucociliary motion is decreased. However, hypoxic pulmonary vasoconstriction is maintained.

Almost all of the opiates can cause delayed or recurring respiratory depression.[9,10] Prominent secondary peaks and fluctuations in plasma opioid levels have been reported during the elimination phase. A potential explanation for this phenomenon is peripheral sequestration and reuptake from the gastrointestinal tract and lungs as well as the peripheral muscles.

MUSCLE RELAXANTS

Studies of neuromuscular function following recovery of the train-of-four ratio to 0.7 or more (four nerve stimuli at an amplitude of 2 Hz each are given every 0.5 second, and the ratio of the evoked muscle response of the fourth to the first nerve stimulation is determined) or maximum negative inspiratory pressures of at least -25 cm H_2O suggest that these parameters may be inadequate to predict the maintenance of a functionally intact airway.[11] The muscles responsible for airway protection may be nonfunctional in the presence of residual muscle relaxants even when ventilation is thought to be adequate. The maneuver recommended to assess adequacy of reversal of neuromuscular blocking agents is a sustained head lift. The ability to sustain a head lift for 5 seconds has been shown to be associated with sufficient muscle strength to prevent airway obstruction and aspiration.

The effects of muscle relaxants are potentiated by inhalational anesthetics, most antiarrhythmic agents, and many antibacterial agents.[12] In fact, the only antibiotics devoid of neuromuscular effects appear to be penicillin G and the cephalosporins. Electrolyte imbalances (K^+, Mg^{2+}, Ca^{2+}), hypothermia, and underlying myopathies can depress neuromuscular function. Respiratory acidosis has also been shown to inhibit the reversal of neuromuscular blockade. Altered hepatic and renal function can affect metabolism and excretion of the muscle relaxants. The adequacy of the reversal of neuromuscular blockade should be carefully assessed in all patients.

PHYSICAL ASSESSMENT

With the advent of routine use of pulse oximetry in many PACUs, the diagnosis of arterial hypoxemia has been significantly facilitated. The interobserver variability in diagnosing cyanosis has been previously documented, and significant reductions in arterial saturation may occur before cyanosis becomes clinically apparent. We are frequently called to evaluate desaturations when clinically there are no apparent signs of respiratory distress. To deal effectively with this new technology, we must rely on our skills as clinicians to evaluate the significance of these numeric abnormalities.

INSPECTION

An initial impression is obtained by observing the patient's level of consciousness, general body habitus, and vital signs. If the patient demonstrates signs of acute distress, the remainder of the examination must be expedited in order to localize the problem quickly, and supportive care must be provided before the etiology of the distress can be defined. When the patient's condition is more stable, a thorough examination can then be performed.

Evaluation of the patient's level of consciousness is a simple but important assessment. The approach to a partially anesthetized, possibly disoriented patient is different than when dealing with a conscious patient in distress, who can answer questions and follow commands.

Airway Obstruction

Pharyngeal obstruction due to a relaxed tongue in a semiconscious patient is a familiar scenario during the immediate postoperative period and can be easily remedied. Partial airway obstruction is characterized by loud or noisy inspiration. Snoring, gurgling, and stridor are normally present in partial airway obstruction. If left untreated, airway obstruction can lead to hypoxia and hypercarbia. Total airway obstruction, a life-threatening emergency, is characterized by absence of airflow, flaring nostrils, exaggerated respiratory effort, use of accessory muscles, and patient agitation.

Both head tilt and forward displacement of the mandible can relieve upper airway soft tissue obstruction[13] (Fig. 5–1). If patency of the airway cannot be maintained by these maneuvers, a nasal or oral airway should be inserted, or the patient may be laterally positioned. Semicomatose or arousable patients usually tolerate a nasopharyngeal airway better than an oropharyngeal airway, as it is stabilized by the nasal passage and lies on the posterior pharyngeal wall rather than anteriorly. Placement of an oral airway may stimulate gagging, vomiting, and occasionally laryngospasm. Epistaxis is an immediate concern with nasopharyngeal airways.

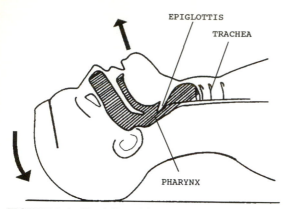

FIGURE 5–1. Head tilt and forward displacement of the mandible can be performed to relieve soft tissue obstruction of the upper airway.

If the above maneuvers fail to relieve the airway obstruction, a laryngeal or subglottic process should be entertained, and the patient will require intubation. Intubation in the PACU should proceed in a similar, controlled fashion, as when it is performed in the operating room. The patient should be preoxygenated if ventilation can be manually assisted. If complete airway obstruction is present, immediate oral intubation should be attempted. Muscle relaxants may be used to facilitate this process. If attempts at intubation are unsuccessful and the airway remains obstructed, an emergency cricothyroidotomy should be performed. A midline vertical incision through the cricothyroid membrane allows entrance into the larynx below the vocal cords. Any type of tube may be inserted to maintain pa-

tency (Fig. 5–2). Commercially available cricothyroidotomy sets (e.g., NuTrake, Melker Catheter) may facilitate tube placement.

If patients require a less emergent intubation, they can be sedated and paralyzed in a manner similar to what would be done in the operating room. However, in a spontaneously breathing patient with altered postoperative oropharyngeal or neck anatomy (i.e., diffuse edema, expanding hematoma, surgical resection), intubation utilizing muscle relaxants should not be attempted unless one is fairly certain the airway can be secured. A fiberoptic brochoscope can be utilized to facilitate the intubation and to define the etiology of the airway obstruction.

In an institution where the overall rate of postoperative reintubation was only 0.17 per cent, the risk of postoperative airway compromise was significantly greater in patients having undergone diagnostic laryngoscopy or panendoscopy, being 1.2 and 3.0 per cent, respectively.[14] These patients should be closely monitored for the development of airway compromise.

Patterns of Ventilation

Visual examination of the chest is useful for assessing the thoracic configuration and the pattern and effort of breathing. The rate, depth, and rhythm of breathing are controlled by the brainstem. Increases in CO_2 or metabolic rate, hypoxemia, or acidemia can stimulate the depth and rate of breathing. Increases in metabolic rate can occur with fever, shivering, heart failure, pulmonary edema, or early

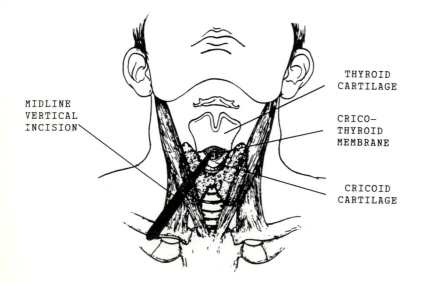

FIGURE 5–2. Cricothyroidotomy procedure. A midline vertical incision is made through the cricothyroid membrane followed by tube placement to maintain patency.

hypoglycemia. Kussmaul's breathing, a rapid, deep ventilatory pattern, is frequently seen with metabolic acidosis, particularly diabetic ketoacidosis.

A rapid, shallow ventilatory pattern is commonly associated with a restrictive lung process and is most frequently encountered in the PACU secondary to pleuritic chest pain and diaphragmatic dysfunction following upper abdominal or thoracic surgery. Persistence of this ventilatory pattern may lead to inefficient gas exchange, hypoxemia, and hypercapnia. Use of adequate systemic or epidural analgesics may help relieve the pain and improve pulmonary mechanics.

A slow, irregular respiratory pattern associated with delays in expiration and a decreased, normal, or increased tidal volume is characteristically seen in patients receiving narcotics. If the respiratory rate is slow enough that the minute ventilation is significantly decreased, leading to CO_2 retention or hemodynamic instability, a narcotic antagonist should be given. Careful titration of naloxone, a narcotic antagonist, can usually restore spontaneous ventilation without reversing the analgesia. Because of the short duration of naloxone, if a longer-acting opioid such as morphine is being antagonized, renarcotization may occur. Repeated injections of naloxone (0.5 to 1.0 μg/kg) or a continuous naloxone infusion (1.0 to 3.0 μg/kg/hr) may be required to maintain adequate spontaneous ventilation. If the patient remains intubated postoperatively, consideration should be given to mechanical ventilatory support in the presence of hypoventilation secondary to narcotics.

PALPATION

Palpation is performed to assess chest wall expansion, tactile fremitus, and the skin and subcutaneous tissues for subcutaneous emphysema. Asymmetric movement of the hemithoraces is seen with unilateral disease processes. Decreased lung expansion can occur secondary to consolidation, atelectasis, collapse, mainstem bronchus intubation, or air or fluid in the pleural space. Patients who develop a tension pneumothorax can develop contralateral tracheal deviation as well. The presence of tracheal deviation can facilitate the diagnosis of other underlying pneumonic processes (Table 5–1). (Treatment of pneumothorax is discussed subsequently.

TABLE 5–1. PNEUMONIC PROCESSES ASSOCIATED WITH TRACHEAL DEVIATION

Trachea Deviates Toward Normal Lung	Trachea Deviates Away from Normal Lung
Pleural effusion	Atelectasis
Tension pneumothorax	Pneumonectomy
Unilateral emphysema	

During the assessment of tactile fremitus, the patient repeats "ninety-nine" while the examiner palpates the thorax. The intensity of the tactile fremitus increases in conditions that increase the density of the lung, e.g., consolidation or atelectasis. If the consolidated lung is sequestered from a patent bronchus, the tactile fremitus is decreased or absent. When a pleural effusion or a pneumothorax is present, tactile fremitus is also significantly decreased. Obese or extremely muscular patients often have reduced tactile fremitus bilaterally, as do patients with emphysema.

PERCUSSION

Percussion, by itself, is rarely useful for making a diagnosis in the PACU. The normal chest is resonant throughout. A suspected consolidation, effusion, or lung collapse can be confirmed when dull or flat percussion is present. Increased resonance is associated with hyperinflated lungs or a pneumothorax.

AUSCULTATION

After initial inspection of the patient, auscultation is the most useful clinical tool. The characteristics of breath sounds include pitch, loudness, distinctive qualities, and the inspiratory/expiratory ratio. Additional sounds are crackles or rales, rhonchi, wheezing, and pleural rubs.

Rales are often produced by the movement of secretions or fluid in the airways as air passes through. Dependent crackles often occur late during inspiration and result from the opening of peripheral airways that may have closed during shallow breathing. Several deep inspiratory maneuvers may clear these abnormal sounds. If crackles persist, the diagnosis of atelectasis, pneumonia, or pulmonary edema should be entertained.

TABLE 5–2. DIFFERENTIAL DIAGNOSIS OF PERIOPERATIVE WHEEZING[a]

Upper airway obstruction
   Laryngeal edema or hemorrhage
   Laryngeal spasm
   Foreign body
   Vocal cord paralysis
   Infection
Lower airway
   Asthma: intrinsic, extrinsic, drug-induced
   Bronchitis
   Chronic obstructive pulmonary disease
   Anaphylaxis
   Aspiration: chemical bronchitis
   Foreign body
   Carcinoid syndrome
Vascular problems
   Cardiac asthma
   Pulmonary embolism
   Vasculitis: allergic
Other problems
   Factitious asthma

[a] Wheezing not present on preoperative examination.

Wheezing results from the vibration of the wall of a narrowed or compressed airway as air passes through at a high velocity. The airway diameter may be reduced by bronchospasm, mucosal edema, extrinsic compression, or a foreign body. The greater the luminal narrowing, the higher the pitch. Wheezes are the hallmark of airway obstruction, the characteristic feature of chronic bronchitis, bronchial asthma, or emphysema.

Wheezing is a nonspecific manifestation of airway obstruction. Virtually any process that involves the tracheobronchial tree can produce wheezing. During the immediate postoperative period one must determine whether the wheezing is secondary to an exacerbation of underlying asthma or is a manifestation of the airway response to an acute process. Bronchoconstriction may be centrally mediated as in asthma or other allergic reactions, or it may be a local response to airway irritation. Table 5–2 lists possible etiologies of wheezing originating during the perioperative period.

The airway obstruction may be completely reversible in asthmatics but only partially reversible in bronchitics. Cigarette smokers and those with chronic bronchitis have irritable airways that are more reactive to stimulation. A combination of wheezing and crackles may indicate bronchopneumonia, bronchiectasis, or severe airway obstruction. Unilateral wheezing suggests discrete bronchial narrowing resulting from a mucous plug, foreign body, or tumor and thus may be present with inspiration as well as exhalation. Noxious stimuli such as secretions, blood, or vomitus in the airway and artificial airways themselves may precipitate bronchospasm. Acute pulmonary embolism must be considered in an adult with new onset of wheezing and signs and symptoms of right heart failure or lower extremity thrombosis.

The intensity of wheezing is related to flow. Loud wheezing indicates that air movement is occurring, whereas soft wheezing may signal fatigue and respiratory deterioration, rather than an improvement in the patient's condition. Repeated auscultatory examinations coordinated with other clinical signs are required to assess response to therapy.

The basic approach to the wheezing patients involves administration of supplemental oxygen to correct hypoxemia, bronchodilators to reduce airway resistance and improve gas exchange, and ventilatory assistance if the patient manifests deterioration in ventilatory status despite appropriate pharmacologic intervention. The chest roentgenogram is essential for the evaluation of wheezing in nonasthmatic patients. Findings may involve the parenchyma, airways, or mediastinum.

If a patient has aspirated in the supine position, alveolar infiltrates are present in the superior segments of the lower lobes, posterior segments of the upper lobes, or both. The diagnosis of acute congestive heart failure can be made even in the presence of a normal-sized heart when alveolar pulmonary edema is present, typically in the distribution of a butterfly pattern. When pulmonary embolism is suspected, the chest roentgenogram is usually normal.

A radiopaque foreign body can be easily visualized on a chest film. Even if the foreign body cannot be visualized, atelectasis or lung collapse may be present distal to a suspected foreign body. Partial airway obstruction by a foreign body can produce ipsilateral hyperlucent lung syndrome secondary to air trapping during positive-pressure ventilation. In 85 per cent of cases, a chest roentgenogram contributes to the diagnosis of a bronchial foreign body.

The mediastinum and the pulmonary parenchyma should be closely examined for evidence of mediastinal or pleural air resulting from barotrauma.

β-Adrenergic agonists are the mainstay of

pharmacologic therapy for acute broncho-spasm. The choice of adrenergic agonist depends on the desired effect. The catecholamines (epinephrine, isoproterenol, isoetharine) achieve peak bronchodilation within 5 minutes, but their effects dissipate by 1 to 2 hours. In addition to their relatively short duration of action, the catecholamines are relatively β_2 nonselective. The noncatecholamines (metaproterenol, terbutaline, albuterol) are somewhat slower in onset and usually attain near-maximal bronchodilation within 10 to 15 minutes. In addition to being longer-acting, the noncatecholamines are more β_2 selective. Tremor and cardiac side effects such as tachycardia and palpitations increase proportionally to the amount of drug given.

Inhaled β-adrenergic agonists are indicated for the short-term relief of bronchoconstriction and are the treatment of choice for acute exacerbations of asthma.[15] The inhaled route should be the first form of therapy used to relieve airway obstruction.[16] Administration by inhalation delivers the drug directly to the airways, so only small amounts of the medication are required to achieve the therapeutic actions (Table 5–3). In the past, severe episodes of asthma were treated with β-agonists administered subcutaneously because it was thought that severe bronchoconstriction would interfere with delivery of the inhaled medication. Current studies, to the contrary, suggest that in severe disease aerosolized therapy is more effective.[17]

Theophylline is a less effective bronchodila-tor than the β-agonists and is not effective as an inhalant; thus it must be given intravenously as aminophylline. A 5.6 mg/kg loading dose of aminophylline is administered to the patient over a 20- to 30-minute period, after which the patient is maintained on a continuous infusion ranging from 0.2 to 0.9 mg/kg/hr. Potential aminophylline side effects include nervousness, nausea, vomiting, and headache, with cardiac arrhythmias and seizures occurring at high plasma concentrations. Aminophylline should not be considered the first drug of choice for treating acute wheezing.

Inhaled anticholinergic drugs, e.g., atropine sulfate or ipratropium bromide, are rarely used for acute treatment of bronchospasm, as their peak bronchodilator activity may not be reached for 30 to 60 minutes. Moreover, they are considered to be only medium-potency bronchodilators.

HYPOXEMIA

The existence of postoperative hypoxemia appears to be the norm rather than the exception in patients undergoing even the most minor procedures under general anesthesia.[18] It has become routine practice to administer supplemental oxygen (35 to 40 per cent inspired oxygen by face mask or nasal cannula) to all patients in the PACU until they have "recovered" from the effects of general anesthesia and are ready to be discharged.

Supplemental oxygen administration should also be considered for all patients being transported from the operating room to the PACU following general anesthesia. Utilizing pulse oximetry, arterial desaturation below 90 per cent has been documented in a significant number of previously healthy patients (22 to 35 per cent) breathing room air during postoperative transport and on arrival in the PACU.[19–22] Administration of supplemental oxygen at a flow rate of only 2 liters per minute through a nasal cannula has been shown to prevent this desaturation.

The most common mechanisms for postoperative hypoxemia are 1) alveolar hypoventilation, 2) ventilation/perfusion mismatch (shunt effect), 3) right-to-left intrapulmonary shunt (true shunt), and 4) a low inspired concentration of oxygen.[23]

Fortunately, the incidence of the administration of a hypoxic gas mixture is rare, but diffusion hypoxia can occur with the discontinuation of a nitrous oxide anesthetic. The

TABLE 5–3. β_2 SELECTIVE AGONISTS (INHALED)

Drug	Effect
Isoetharine (Bronkosol)	Minor β_1 effects at therapeutic doses but can cause tachycardia at higher doses. Rapid onset. Effects last 1.5–3.0 hours.
Metaproterenol (Alupent, metaprel)	Similar to isoetharine but longer duration of action—up to 5 hours. Onset 5–30 minutes.
Terbutaline (Brethaire)	Greater β_2 effects than metaproterenol. Onset 5–30 minutes. Effects last 4–6 hours.
Albuterol (Proventil, ventolin)	Pure β-drug with the least β_1 effects of currently available inhalers. Onset <15 minutes. Effects last 4–6 hours.

dilution of alveolar gases by the outpouring of nitrous oxide from the circulation can lead to a hypoxic alveolar gas mixture. Additionally, depression of respiration secondary to dilution of alveolar CO_2 may occur.[24] Diffusion hypoxemia can be prevented by administration of 100 per cent oxygen during the period of greatest elimination of nitrous oxide, the first 5 to 10 minutes after discontinuation of anesthesia.

A depressed ventilatory drive secondary to the effects of residual anesthesia superimposed on the resumption of spontaneous ventilation following controlled intraoperative hyperventilation may result in hypoventilation during the immediate postoperative period. Alveolar oxygen tension is reduced as a direct result of hypoventilation, as can be seen from the ideal alveolar gas equation

$$PaO_2 = [P_B - PH_2O]F_{IO_2} - PaCO_2/0.8$$

where the respiratory quotient = 0.8. Hypoxemia is further exacerbated when ventilation/perfusion abnormalities are present or cardiac output is reduced.[25]

Postoperative hypoxemia is most commonly secondary to true shunting and shunt effect. *True shunting* occurs when mixed venous blood enters the left side of the heart without respiring with alveolar gas, whereas *shunt effect* refers to blood that respires but attains less than ideal oxygen tensions. Shunt effect mechanisms are referred to as *ventilation/perfusion mismatch* and may result from a poorly ventilated alveolus or an excessive rate of blood flow through the alveolar capillaries. Hypoxemia resulting from true shunting is refractory to correction with supplemental oxygen administration (<10 mm Hg increase in PaO_2 associated with 0.2 increase in F_{IO_2}), whereas hypoxemia resulting from ventilation/perfusion mismatch improves dramatically with only small increases in oxygen.

Atelectasis is the most common cause of true shunting that occurs during the postoperative period. The forms and causes of acute atelectasis include the following.

1. *Compression atelectasis*—resulting from direct compression of the lung parenchyma during surgery by retractors, packing, or surgical manipulation or by space-occupying lesions of the chest including pneumothorax, hemothorax, and pleural fluid.
2. *Absorption atelectasis*—resulting from total obstruction of bronchi or bronchioles with absorption of distal alveolar gas, which most frequently occurs with a main-

TABLE 5–4. COMMON CAUSES OF PERMEABILITY DEFECTS (ARDS)[a]

Anaphylaxis

Aspiration

Disseminated intravascular coagulation

Fat or air emboli

Massive blood transfusion

Oxygen toxicity (altered endothelial function breathing 100% F_{IO_2} >24 hours, with progression to ARDS after 60 hours on 100% F_{IO_2}

Prolonged cardiopulmonary bypass

Sepsis

Shock

Thoracic trauma

[a] Adult Respiratory Distress Syndrome.

stem intubation, inspissated secretions, or a foreign body.
3. *Microatelectasis*—random collapse of alveoli resulting from constant-volume ventilation of increased surface tension (adult respiratory distress syndrome, or ARDS). Common perioperative causes of ARDS are listed in Table 5–4.

Capillary shunting can also occur as a result of alveolar fluid. Potential perioperative causes include pooled secretions, cardiogenic/noncardiogenic pulmonary edema, or pneumonia.

Patients undergoing upper abdominal surgery are at greatest risk for developing atelectasis.[26,27] Postoperative changes in lung function after upper abdominal surgery are similar to those seen in patients with muscle weakness or diaphragmatic paralysis. A reduction in diaphragmatic function has in fact been demonstrated immediately postoperatively.[28] Attempts have been made to determine the contribution of postoperative pain to diaphragmatic dysfunction; however, neither epidural analgesia nor intercostal nerve blockade has significantly improved overall pulmonary function. The reduced function of the diaphragm during the immediate postoperative period may be responsible for the reduced vital capacity, atelectasis, and resultant hypoxemia following abdominal surgery. The incidence of postoperative atelectasis after lower abdominal or peripheral surgery is significantly less than that after upper abdominal surgery. Nonsurgical risk factors associated with an increased incidence of postoperative atelectasis include underlying pulmonary pathology, obesity,[29,30] smoking,[31] age,[32] and duration of anesthesia.

The simplest means of treating postoperative atelectasis is to encourage patients to sustain their inspiratory effort for as long as possible. Such a sustained maximal inspiration can produce transpulmonary pressure gradients in excess of 40 cm H_2O for 5 to 15 seconds, with resultant tidal volumes up to 40 ml/kg.[33] If the patient is unable to generate a vital capacity of at least 10 to 15 ml/kg, intermittent positive-pressure breathing or continuous positive airway pressure delivered at intervals by face mask may be required to treat the atelectasis.[34]

ASPIRATION

Although most commonly intraoperative problems, emesis, regurgitation, and aspiration can also occur postoperatively. Alternatively, the event may have occurred in the operating room but may not have been recognized until the patient begins to have difficulties in the PACU. Olsson et al. reported the incidence of aspiration to be approximately 1 in 2100 anesthetics.[35]

Patients at risk for aspiration include any patient in whom the airway reflexes are obtunded, e.g., those who are emerging from general anesthesia, are excessively sedated, or have neurologic abnormalities (i.e., coma, stupor, and increased intracranial pressure). Patients with increased intragastric contents from either recent ingestion or prolonged gastric emptying times (i.e., patients with ileus, diabetes, pain, or anxiety or the pregnant patient) pose a significant concern for potential aspiration of gastric contents. Increased intraabdominal pressure from the gravid uterus, an abdominal mass, obesity, tight abdominal dressings, or the presence of hiatal hernia create conditions that favor overcoming the lower esophageal sphincter pressure, the normal barrier to regurgitation and vomiting.[36]

The morbidity and mortality due to aspiration are significantly related to the quantity and character of the material that enters the airways and lungs. Aspiration of gastric material has received the most attention in the literature for two reasons. First, it is indeed the most common substance aspirated by patients under or after anesthesia; and, second, it carries a significant possibility for morbidity and mortality. The key factors determining the extent and severity of damage to the pulmonary parenchyma are the pH and the volume of the gastric material aspirated. Significant pulmonary damage has been seen with volumes of 0.4 ml/kg if the pH is less than 2.5. Even lesser volumes at a lower pH can be associated with a significant mortality rate.

The character of the material aspirated is also important. The presence of large particles may lead to complete airway obstruction and asphyxia, as can aspiration of a large amount of material with smaller particles that can obstruct peripheral areas of the lung. Asphyxia can also occur as a result of aspiration of a large amount of clear liquid. Aspiration of feculent material carries a particularly ominous prognosis, often leading to fulminant pneumonia, sepsis, and death.[37]

In addition to gastric contents, other substances that may present potential problems for aspiration are blood and pus. Blood, although not nearly as irritating to the airway as gastric fluid, can present a serious hazard to the airway, as when, for example, a large, obstructing blood clot is drawn into the airway on extubation leading to asphyxiation.[38] A massive amount of bleeding in the airway may compromise gas exchange in a significant portion of the lung and may furthermore lead to clot formation in distal airways, making air movement difficult or impossible. Pus aspirated into the lung can result in abscess formation, pneumonia, and sepsis.

Because therapy for aspiration is mainly supportive once it has occurred, prevention is the primary concern during the perioperative period. Prevention begins with pharmacologic treatment. Clear, nonparticulate antacids, H_2 blocking agents to decrease the volume and acidity of the gastric juice, and metoclopramide to increase lower esophageal tone, speed gastric emptying, and decrease the incidence of postoperative nausea and vomiting should be given to high risk patients preoperatively.[39] Prior to the patient awakening from anesthesia, it is desirable to aspirate the stomach of as much material as possible. Even if solid material remains, the rapidity of regurgitation or vomiting is slower, thereby allowing one to position the patient's head and evacuate the pharynx one more time. Unfortunately, as far as recovery from anesthesia is concerned, these therapies only lessen, but do not eliminate, the risk for significant aspiration of gastric contents. Unintubated patients are at the same risk for aspiration at the conclusion of surgery as they were at the start, and this risk continues in the PACU until the patient is fully awake and able to protect the airway from soilage.

With modern induction agents, a smooth, rapid descent to surgical levels of anesthesia is possible, and the classic Guedel stages of anesthetic depth are not seen. Emergence from anesthesia, however, is a much slower process, and it is possible to see a stage corresponding to that of Guedel's stages II–III in which increased salivation, retching, and vomiting occur. In some cases, the latter may occur when a patient is brought, perhaps inappropriately, to the PACU still essentially anesthetized. Even in the presence of a properly positioned endotracheal tube with an appropriately inflated cuff in place, regurgitated material may be drawn into the trachea around the cuff during abrupt inspiratory efforts, as often occurs when a patient coughs.

Residual anesthetics are present during every patient's recovery from general anesthesia. Although the patient may have "woken up" from the anesthetic in the operating room, once the stimulus of the operating room has subsided the patient may again lapse into an obtunded state. During the transition from the operating room to the PACU, the patient must be continually observed and should be placed in a lateral position during transport if possible. A patient who has been recently extubated may not recover the glottic protective mechanism for several hours after extubation. As previously mentioned, a patient may recover sufficient motor function after a nondepolarizing muscle relaxant but may still lack sufficient coordination of the glottic and pharyngeal musculature to protect the airway from aspiration.

Within the PACU care must be taken to avoid "reanesthetizing" the patient with opiates in an attempt to have a totally comfortable and quiet patient. Excessive amounts of opiates may lead to obtundation of the airway reflexes as well as to some potential for airway obstruction, causing increased diaphragmatic activity, which can lead to opening of the cardioesophageal sphincter and allow regurgitation to occur. The opiates also stimulate the chemoreceptors in the brain, causing nausea and emesis.

Once aspiration has occurred, the physician and nursing responsibilities lie primarily with supportive care, as the damage is immediate in most cases. The diagnosis of aspiration is difficult to establish definitively, especially if it was "silent" or unnoticed. The initial physical presentation of a patient who has aspirated is often an unexplained tachypnea and tachycardia. Auscultation of the lung fields might reveal rales and rhonchi. If significant airway edema is already present, wheezing may be noted. A chest roentgenogram taken soon after the event may fail to reveal the full extent of the damage. Usually the film reveals a diffuse or regional infiltrative process that may progress to consolidation and loss of lung volume as the process matures.

The severity of the immediate injury may be reflected in the degree of hypoxemia demonstrated on arterial blood gas analysis. Arterial PCO_2 is usually decreased, and the pH is increased as a result of hyperventilation by the patient attempting to correct the hypoxemia. Decreased pH might be seen in a situation where the aspiration and hence the hypoxemia that results is so severe as to cause tissue hypoxia and increased lactic acid production. Elevated $PaCO_2$ may indicate a severely obtunded and respiratory depressed patient or is an ominous sign of significant inability to exchange gas—as would occur with major degrees of airway obstruction.[40]

As was mentioned earlier, the extent of damage is related to the character and amount of the aspirated material. A large volume of clear liquid, regardless of the pH, can lead to asphyxiation and is treated by immediately suctioning the oropharynx, trachea, and bronchi while providing supplemental oxygen and indicated ventilatory support. Nonacidic or mildly acidic fluid (pH > 2.5) causes reflex bronchospasm and loss of surfactant. This situation leads to atelectasis and an increase in physiologic shunting within the lungs. Minimal histologic changes are seen within the lung parenchyma itself.

In contrast, liquid aspirate with a pH of less than 2.5 leads to almost immediate focal atelectasis. Progressive damage to the pulmonary parenchyma occurs over the next several hours. Initially, there is breakdown of the alveolar capillary membrane, intraalveolar hemorrhage, capillary congestion, and interstitial edema. These processes lead to the development of alveolar edema, loss of surfactant, and atelectasis. Hypoxemia is a common finding. Later, fluid losses into the lungs are significant, leading to a decrease in lung compliance and a resultant increase in the work of breathing. Additionally, the significant loss of fluid into the lungs leads to hypovolemia and hypotension if the fluid is not aggressively replaced. Pulmonary artery pressure is also often increased as a result of significant hypoxic pulmonary vasoconstriction. Therapy at this point consists in maintaining the airway, oxygen, ventilation, and removal of as much foreign material as possible by blind suctioning of the trachea.

Controversy exists concerning the use of positive airway pressure during the early stages. Some advocate spontaneous ventilation with sufficient oxygen to achieve adequate oxygenation, whereas others favor the aggressive application of continuous positive airway pressure (CPAP) or positive end-expiratory pressure (PEEP) early in the management of these patients, as the process is likely to progress over several hours. The latter group believe that early application of CPAP or PEEP serves to support alveoli that have lost surfactant and are therefore at risk of collapsing. The levels of CPAP or PEEP needed are titrated to allow the FIO_2 to be decreased below 0.5 while maintaining adequate PaO_2 so long as the patient is able to maintain hemodynamic stability.

Early application of positive airway pressure may not require intubation if the patient is awake and able to protect the airway. The application of up to 10 to 15 cm H_2O pressure of CPAP can be achieved with a properly fitted mask. The higher levels of support may be tolerated for only a limited time by the patient, however, as the tight fit of the mask may become uncomfortable and the patient is likely to experience significant gastric distension due to swallowed air. In addition, if the patient's level of consciousness deteriorates, mask CPAP is contraindicated because the tight mask ensures that any emesis that occurs would remain in the pharynx and likely be aspirated as well, worsening the aspiration pneumonitis. Therefore if the patient is unable to tolerate mask CPAP or requires higher levels of airway pressure or mechanical ventilation (or both), an endotracheal tube must be inserted.

Occasionally the loss of intravascular volume into the lungs results in hemodynamic instability, especially in the presence of high levels of airway pressure therapy. Measurement of central blood volume and preferably of left-sided cardiac filling pressures is desirable and necessary. The pulmonary artery catheter additionally allows one to optimize cardiac function using inotropic agents such as dopamine (3 to 10 $\mu g/kg/min$) and to adjust the airway pressure therapy for maximal oxygen delivery and minimal intrapulmonary shunt ($\dot{Q}sp/\dot{Q}t$).

Rigid bronchoscopy after a clear liquid aspiration serves little purpose. If the volume is massive, blind suction of the endotracheal tube achieves the same result as when done through a bronchoscope. With smaller aspirations, the material is dispersed throughout the lung within 20 seconds of the event, and the reactive process that ensues quickly raises the pH of the fluid. Therefore it is unlikely that significant amounts of material can be recovered, and the course is not altered. The technique of fiberoptic bronchoscopy, however, is rather simple and should therefore be performed if significant aspiration of gastric material has occurred. It allows one not only to assess whether any particulate matter has been aspirated but to remove retained secretions that could cause significant atelectasis. Irrigation with small volumes (5 to 10 ml) of sterile saline can then be injected and suctioned via the bronchoscope to clear as much material from the airway as possible, and it may obviate the need for an additional general anesthetic for rigid bronchoscopy.

The administration of steroids remains controversial. Although there is no doubt that an inflammatory response is one of the early findings histologically after acid aspiration, there is no evidence that the course is favorably altered by the administration of steroids. To the contrary, steroids are known to impair the reparative processes and therefore may prolong the course.

The routine use of antibiotics in aspiration pneumonitis is to be discouraged. Antibiotic prophylaxis alters the normal flora and tends to encourage suprainfection with resistant and pathogenic organisms. If clinical signs of pulmonary infection are present, however, or if the aspirated material was obviously infected (i.e., feculent gastric contents or pus), antibiotics must be started immediately because the latter problem is associated with a high mortality rate.

When a patient has aspirated solid material, immediate attention must be directed to clearing the upper airway and assessing the ability of the patient to ventilate spontaneously or with assistance. Large particles may completely occlude the airway and require emergent laryngoscopy or bronchoscopy in an attempt to establish an airway below the level of the obstruction. Once the airway has been established and the patient has been adequately oxygenated and ventilated, flexible or rigid bronchoscopy may be necessary for the removal of any remaining contamination of the lower airway. Food particles that remain in the airway can cause an intense, prolonged inflammatory process and should be removed as soon as the patient has been stabilized from the initial event.

Blood is another potential substance that can be aspirated in the PACU. Patients who have had surgery of the head and neck are at particular risk. Tonsillectomy patients, for example, can swallow significant amounts of blood, which might then be regurgitated and aspirated; alternatively, the blood can be directly aspirated if the patient is overly sedated. Although significant hypoxemia due to markedly increased intrapulmonary shunting occurs with this type of aspiration, little if any inflammatory reaction occurs; and if the patient survives the initial insult, recovery is likely.

PNEUMOTHORAX

Barotrauma is most often seen as a result of pulmonary parenchymal injury due to chest trauma and rib fractures. Less common causes are injuries to large airways and rupture of emphysematous bullae, the latter of which may be responsible for so-called spontaneous pneumothoraces.[41,42] Any time needles are inserted near the lung, there exists the potential for parenchymal injury and the development of a pneumothorax. Supraclavicular, interscalene, and intercostal nerve blocks carry the potential for such lung injury. The most common iatrogenic cause of lung injury and pneumothorax is insertion of central venous catheters.[43]

Although the event causing the injury may have occurred prior to or in the operating room, the pneumothorax may not be discovered until the patient is in the PACU. Diagnosis of a pneumothorax requires an index of suspicion and must be differentiated from other causes of diminished breath sounds and hypoxemia. A small amount of extraparenchymal gas (i.e., 10 per cent of the hemithoracic volume) may be entirely asymptomatic and only be discovered as an incidental finding on a postoperative chest roentgenogram. The awake patient may complain of chest pain that radiates to the neck. Often the patient complains of shortness of breath or is noted to be tachypneic on physical examination.

The loss of lung volume due to the extraparenchymal air leads to compression or collapse of the lung tissue on the affected side. It causes atelectasis and an increase in the intrapulmonary shunting of blood through the lungs, leading to the development of the arterial hypoxemia. Cyanosis, although described, is not an invariable finding, as it requires a level of reduced hemoglobin of more than 5 gm/dl and is a rather subjective assessment. Peripheral pulse oximetry, on the other hand, might reveal a significant desaturation.

Palpation of the chest may reveal subcutaneous emphysema, which can be felt to "crinkle" under the fingers. Often this abnormality is an early sign and, if present unilaterally, may indicate the likely side of the pathology. Percussion of the chest usually reveals hyperresonance in the presence of a pneumothorax as opposed to dullness when atelectasis or fluid is present in the thoracic cavity, and it assists in the differentiation of this process from that seen with a mainstem intubation.

Auscultation of the chest reveals diminished or absent breath sounds over the affected side, and wheezing may be heard as a result of the atelectasis and airway compression. If the amount of pressure due to the extraparenchymal air is great, a shift of the mediastinal structures (i.e., the heart and trachea) away from the affected side is noted. Examination of chest expansion may reveal an asymmetric pattern, which is usually more apparent during the slow and deep breaths of mechanical ventilation, where it is noted that expansion of the affected side lags behind that of the unaffected side. An upright, expiratory chest roentgenogram usually demonstrates the degree of lung collapse better than the usual end-inspiratory film.[44]

Treatment of pneumothorax (Fig. 5–3) depends on the severity of the volume loss in the hemithorax and if the patient is receiving positive pressure mechanical ventilation or shows signs of hemodynamic instability. In the spontaneously breathing patient with up to a 20 per cent pneumothorax who is hemodynamically stable and adequately oxygenated, treatment consists in obtaining serial chest roentgenograms to follow the resolution of the pneumothorax and oxygen. If the pneumothorax is estimated to occupy more than 20 per cent of the hemithorax or a pneumothorax of any size is present in a patient receiving positive pressure ventilation, decompression with a chest tube is necessary.

Positive pressure ventilation in the presence of any size pneumothorax presents a risk for the development of a tension pneumothorax in which the shift of the mediastinal structures

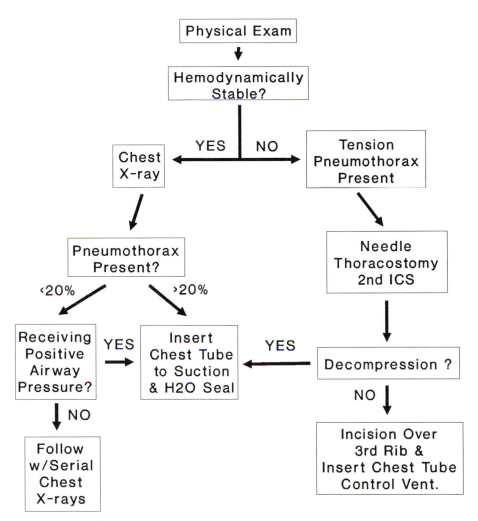

FIGURE 5–3. Diagnosis and treatment protocol for pneumothorax.

away from the affected side is so great that venous return to the right heart is compromised and cardiovascular collapse occurs. This condition is life-threatening and requires immediate attention. There is no justification for delaying definitive therapy for a chest film confirmation of the clinical impression that the patient has a tension pneumothorax. A 14 gauge angiocath should be inserted in the second intercostal space along the midclavicular line of the affected side (Fig. 5–4). The needle is inserted on top of the third rib until bone is contacted and is then walked superiorly off the rib into the intercostal space and subsequently into the thoracic cavity. This technique avoids the risk of accidental injury to the neurovascular bundle, which is located in the groove on the underside of the inferior border of each rib. Usually this maneuver

results in a rush of air being released, and often it is effective in temporarily releasing the tension in the chest and improving the patient's hemodynamic picture.

Occasionally the needle thoracostomy is insufficient to release enough pressure within the chest or to maintain the initially improved state. In this situation, a tube thoracostomy (chest tube) should be inserted in this same location. The skin is incised over the third rib, and a hemostat or large clamp is then inserted onto the rib and walked superiorly into the interspace, where entry to the thoracic cavity can be gained. The clamp is then opened widely to increase the size of the hole into the chest. If a chest tube is not immediately available, an endotracheal tube can be inserted through this incision to continue to vent the thorax. Because this maneuver creates a di-

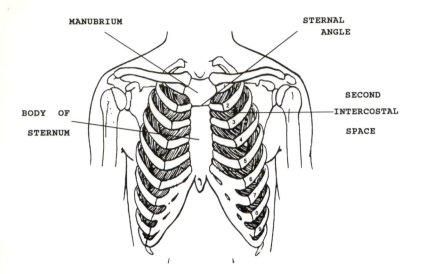

FIGURE 5–4. Emergency treatment of a tension pneumothorax. A 14 gauge angiocath is inserted in the second intercostal space along the midclavicular line of the affected side, just superior to the third rib. If inadequate decompression occurs with this technique, a chest tube may be inserted in this same location.

rect communication between the thorax and the atmosphere, controlled ventilation is required. If the patient is sufficiently stable after the initial release of pressure with the needle thoracostomy, a definitive chest tube with water seal apparatus, which can be connected to suction at 10 to 25 cm H_2O negative pressure, should be placed. For the comfort of the patient, these tubes are usually inserted under local anesthesia along the anterior axillary line in the fifth or sixth intercostal space.

PULMONARY EEDEMA

Pulmonary edema during the acute postoperative period can be a perplexing problem (Fig. 5–5). The causes are numerous, and the

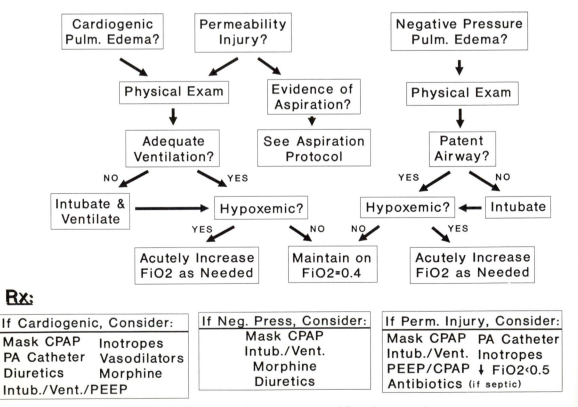

FIGURE 5–5. Diagnosis and treatment protocol for pulmonary edema.

edema may appear suddenly and without warning. Early signs and symptoms may be confusing and lead to the incorrect diagnosis until a more fulminant picture develops. Cooperman and Price, in a survey of 40 postoperative cases of pulmonary edema, found its overall incidence to be 1 in 4500 surgical procedures performed.[45] They noted that none of the 40 cases examined occurred after spinal anesthesia. Most of these cases first became apparent only after the patient was in the PACU. Seventy-five per cent of the cases developed within 1 hour after completion of the anesthetic.

Causes of pulmonary edema during the postoperative period can be grouped into three broad categories: 1) elevated pulmonary capillary hydrostatic pressure; 2) increased pulmonary capillary permeability (ARDS); and 3) sustained reductions in interstitial hydrostatic pressure in the lungs. Tables 5–4 and 5–5 list the common causes leading to the development of pulmonary edema for the first two categories. The third category, which has also been called negative pressure pulmonary edema, is typically seen in patients who develop acute airway obstruction and make vigorous ventilatory efforts against this obstruction[46,47] (Table 5–6). Some data seem to indicate that this latter entity is perhaps causally related to elevation of the capillary hydrostatic pressure and therefore should be classified with the first group described above. Also considered under this third category is reexpansion pulmonary edema, which occurs when a lung that has been collapsed for several hours is suddenly reexpanded.

Multiple factors are present at the conclusion of a general anesthetic that favor abrupt increases in the transmural capillary hydrostatic pressure. Cessation of positive pressure ventilation and the return to spontaneous ventilation are associated with an acute increase in venous return and therefore right heart output. If the left heart is unable to handle this

TABLE 5–5. CAUSES OF ELEVATED PULMONARY CAPILLARY HYDROSTATIC PRESSURE

Excessive volume expansion
Cardiac ischemia
Cardiac valvular disease
Airway obstruction

TABLE 5–6. CAUSES OF NEGATIVE PRESSURE PULMONARY EDEMA

Laryngospasm
Foreign body aspiration
Rapid reexpansion of atelectatic lung
Goiter
Epiglottitis/croup

increased volume, the capillary pressure in the lungs increases. In addition, on awakening the patient begins to experience pain again, causing an increase in the adrenergic tone and leading to systemic hypertension. Associated with the increase in afterload to the heart is a rise in left ventricular end-diastolic pressure, which is reflected in a rise in the pulmonary capillary pressure. These factors, as well as the development of cardiac ischemia or acutely worsened mitral valvular incompetence, may exacerbate the increase in capillary hydrostatic pressure.

Similarly, neurogenic pulmonary edema is thought to occur as a result of a massive and sudden sympathetic discharge due to neurologic injury. This adrenergic outflow suddenly increases the intrapulmonary blood volume, causing increased capillary hydrostatic pressure. Later, permeability edema may also be seen, so it appears that this entity has more than one cause.

Postobstructive or negative pressure pulmonary edema is frequently seen after laryngospasm in children and adults. When laryngospasm develops, in addition to the subatmospheric pressure generated by the diaphragm working against an obstruction, the patient is likely to become hypoxemic. The hypoxic pulmonary vasoconstriction that ensues is thought to play a role in the development of the subsequent edema.[48] Also, with the development of the negative pressure within the alveoli, the right ventricular blood volume and right ventricular ejection fraction decrease, and the left ventricular afterload increases. The left ventricular ejection fraction decreases, which favors a rise in the left atrial and pulmonary blood volumes resulting in edema formation. The development of the pulmonary edema may be delayed for up to 2.0 to 2.5 hours after the inciting event.

The most common presentation of pulmonary edema is that of hypoxemia, as noted by pulse oximetry or blood gas analysis. Tachypnea with a decreased tidal volume and paradoxical or uncoordinated ventilatory pattern sometimes is confused with that seen in a patient who has not had adequate reversal of the neuromuscular blockade. Further administration of anticholinesterase agents, however, fails to improve this situation. Auscultation of the chest may also be confusing during the early stages of pulmonary edema. The incipient edema may cause wheezes to be heard, resulting in the administration of bronchodilators in the mistaken belief that the patient is experiencing an allergic reaction or an acute asthmatic episode.

Tachycardia may also be noted; and if misdiagnosed as a reflex response to hypovolemia, the patient may be given inappropriate fluid challenges that could worsen the problem. Laboratory evaluation of these patients reveals arterial hypoxemia, and a chest film demonstrates diffuse infiltrates.

Treatment of the patient who has hypoxemia related to pulmonary edema consists in maintaining an unobstructed airway and oxygen therapy to correct the hypoxemia. The application of positive airway pressure in the form of low levels (<10 cm H_2O) of CPAP or PEEP may further improve the hypoxemia as well as reduce the patient's work of breathing by restoring the functional residual capacity. If the patient is awake and can tolerate mask CPAP, intubation may be avoided, which is especially desirable in patients who develop the negative pressure type of pulmonary edema, as resolution of their pulmonary problem begins as soon as the obstruction is relieved.

Morphine sulfate can be titrated to alleviate anxiety and vasodilate the venous capacitance vessels. Diuretic therapy, although not necessary for the postobstructive pulmonary edema cases, is probably helpful because intravenous furosemide also acts to dilate the capacitance vessels even before it begins functioning as a diuretic. In both the permeability and the cardiogenic pulmonary edema groups, the underlying cause should be treated.

Patients with cardiogenic pulmonary edema may require placement of central venous access and insertion of a pulmonary artery catheter to monitor intravascular volume status and vasodilator and inotropic therapies, as well as to allow optimal adjustment of the positive airway pressure. Those patients who develop ARDS likely need significant levels of oxygen, PEEP, and ventilatory support for some time in the intensive care unit if they are to survive this insult.

HYPERCARBIA

Postoperative hypercarbia may result from decreased CO_2 elimination, increased production, or a combination of the two. Hypercarbia can be easily diagnosed if the patient remains intubated and the expired gases are being analyzed by capnography. It is more common, however, for the patient to arrive extubated in the PACU. If this is the case and hypercarbia is suspected, the diagnosis can be made only by arterial blood gas sampling and analysis or application of a transcutaneous CO_2 monitor.

Patients with significant obstructive pulmonary disease may be chronic CO_2 retainers. In these patients arterial blood gas analysis reveals an elevated CO_2 tension with normal acid-base status. These patients' ventilatory drive can be easily depressed with small, analgesic doses of narcotics; therefore caution must be used when titrating postoperative analgesics.[49] If an arterial blood gas is obtained in a patient with no apparent underlying pulmonary disease and the $PaCO_2$ is elevated with a normal acid-base measurement, a metabolic alkalosis secondary to electrolyte imbalance should be suspected.

The most common cause of postoperative hypercarbia is hypoventilation secondary to residual anesthesia and narcotic premedication. A single intramuscular injection of morphine may produce respiratory depression up to 4 to 5 hours after administration. The respiratory depression is discernible even when the narcotic blood levels are too low to disturb consciousness. On the other hand, sedating concentrations of the inhalational anesthetics usually cause minimal, if any, carbon dioxide retention.

If the etiology of the hypercarbia is neuromuscular weakness due to inadequate muscle relaxant reversal, the patient usually manifests paradoxical breathing, assuming he or she can maintain a patent airway. With paradoxical breathing, the patient alternates inspiratory work between the diaphragm and the external intercostal muscles, allowing each muscle group to rest intermittently.[50] The diaphragm remains passive when the external intercostals are contracting, so the abdominal wall appears to be sucked in. Careful assessment of muscle strength, either head lift or hand grasp, is indicated for the awake patient, and direct nerve stimulation can be utilized in the anesthetized patient to assess the need for further anticholinesterase drugs to reverse the muscle relaxants.

Patients with restrictive pulmonary function owing to thoracic or upper abdominal procedures, obesity, or underlying pulmonary dysfunction have limited ventilatory reserves and may begin manifesting ventilatory fatigue with paradoxical breathing in the PACU. In these patients additional anticholinesterase drugs are not indicated, and the only treatment for the paradoxical breathing is rest, achieved by mechanical ventilatory support.

With conditions causing increased deadspace, inadequate elimination of CO_2 may be occurring despite maintenance of a normal minute ventilation (6 to 8 L/min in an average-sized adult). Deadspace-producing processes in the spontaneously breathing patient include low cardiac output states, pulmonary embolism, chronic obstructive pulmonary disease, and interstitial lung disease including ARDS. In the intubated patient, mechanical ventilation leads to an increase in physiologic deadspace, and the application of additional tubing through which the patient must both inhale and exhale causes an increase in anatomic deadspace.

PULMONARY EMBOLISM

Although frequently associated with hypoxemia, pulmonary embolism is initially a deadspace-producing process, resulting in hypercarbia if the patient's minute ventilation does not increase. Focal areas of edema and atelectasis often develop in the region of the occluded pulmonary artery, and loss of alveolar surfactant may further promote alveolar collapse and fluid accumulation, resulting in hypoxemia.

Most pulmonary emboli come from deep veins in the legs. Factors predisposing to venous thrombosis include prolonged bed rest, congestive heart failure, limited mobility, deep venous varicosities, and hypercoagulable states. When dealing with these patients, we must be alert to their increased risk for having a pulmonary embolism.

The signs and symptoms of pulmonary embolism—tachypnea, pleuritic chest pain, and hemoptysis—are nonspecific during the postoperative period. The mainstay for the diagnosis is a high degree of clinical suspicion in a patient with predisposing factors complaining of breathlessness.

Proving that pulmonary embolization has occurred is often difficult. Neither a chest roentgenogram nor arterial blood gas assays can prove that embolization has occurred. The most frequent electrocardiographic manifestation of pulmonary embolism is nonspecific ST-T changes. Only with massive pulmonary infarcts is the pattern of right ventricular strain present.

The results of the Prospective Investigation of Pulmonary Embolism Diagnosis (PIOPED) investigators reveal that the pulmonary angiogram is the only reliable test for confirming a pulmonary embolism. Although a high-probability ventilation/perfusion scan was usually associated with a pulmonary embolism, only a few of the patients with a pulmonary embolism had a high-probability scan.[51]

Standard therapy for uncomplicated pulmonary embolism is anticoagulation with heparin followed by warfarin (Coumadin) for several months. Because anticoagulation may be contraindicated in the postoperative patient, an umbrella or other mechanical interruption of the inferior vena cava may be necessary. In addition, the patient should be maintained on supplemental oxygen. Oxygen flows should be adjusted to provide for the patient's increased minute ventilation.

Hypercarbia may also result from an increased production of CO_2. Hypermetabolic states such as fever, malignant hyperthermia, and thyrotoxicosis may become apparent in the PACU. Butyrophenones (i.e., droperidol) and phenothiazines can precipitate neuroleptic malignant syndrome, another hypermetabolic condition. Therapy should be directed at correcting the underlying cause; however, one should be prepared to provide ventilatory assistance if it is apparent that the patient is becoming fatigued from the increased workload.

Inadvertent hypothermia is not an uncommon phenomenon during major surgical procedures, and the shivering that occurs during the rewarming period can cause an increase in CO_2 production (up to 500 per cent above basal levels). A variety of drugs have been used in an attempt to control postoperative shivering. Meperidine, in a dose ranging from 25 to 50 mg IV, appears to be the most effective agent for suppressing visible shivering and reducing the increased CO_2 production.[52]

SUMMARY

Postoperative pulmonary complications are the most frequent causes of death and morbidity in the PACU. Pulse oximetry can detect hypoxemia that occurs in the PACU earlier than traditional methods of monitoring. By detecting early arterial desaturation, appropriate assessment and corrective measures can be undertaken, avoiding the progression to more profound hypoxia and potentially catastrophic sequelae.

References

1. Caplan RA, Posner KL, Ward RJ, Cheney FW: Adverse respiratory events in anesthesia: A closed claims analysis. Anesthesiology 72:828–833, 1990.
2. Hickey RF, Fourcade HE, Eger EI II, et al: The effects of ether, halothane, and Forane on apneic threshold in man. Anesthesiology 35:32–37, 1971.
3. Caverley RK, Smith NT, Jones CW, et al: Ventilatory and cardiovascular effects of enflurane anesthesia during spontaneous ventilation in man. Anesth Analg 57:610, 1979.
4. Knill RL, Gelb AW: Ventilatory responses to hypoxia and hypercapnia during halothane sedation and anesthesia in man. Anesthesiology 49:244–251, 1978.
5. Nunn JF, Esi-Ashi TI: The respiratory effects of resistance to breathing in anesthetized man. Anesthesiology 27:716–728, 1966.
6. Mathers J, Benumof JL, Wahrenbrock EA: General anesthetics and regional hypoxic pulmonary vasoconstriction. Anesthesiology 46:111–114, 1977.
7. Weil JV, McCullough RE, Kline JS, Sodal IE: Diminished ventilatory response to hypoxia and hypercapnia after morphine in normal man. N Engl J Med 292:1103–1106, 1975.
8. Rigg JR, Rondi P: Changes in rib cage and diaphragm contribution to ventilation after morphine. Anesthesiology 55:507–514, 1981.
9. Vejlsted H, Hansen M, Jacobsen E: Postoperative ventilatory response to carbon dioxide following neurolept anaesthesia. Acta Anaesth Scand 21:529–533, 1977.
10. Becker LD, Paulson BA, Miller RD, et al: Biphasic respiratory depression after fentanyl-droperidol or fentanyl alone used to supplement nitrous oxide anesthesia. Anesthesiology 44:291–296, 1976.
11. Pavlin EG, Holle RH, Schoene RB: Recovery of airway protection compared with ventilation in humans after paralysis with curare. Anesthesiology 70:381–385, 1989.
12. Burkett L, Bikhazi GB, Thomas KC, et al: Mutual potentiation of the neuromuscular effects of antibiotics and relaxants. Anesth Analg 58:107–115, 1979.
13. Morikawa S, Safar P, DeCarlo J: Influence on the head-jaw position upon upper airway patency. Anesthesiology 22:265–270, 1961.
14. Hill RS, Koltai PJ, Parnes SM: Airway complications from laryngoscopy and panendoscopy. Ann Otol Rhinol Laryngol 96:691–694, 1987.
15. Barnes PJ: A new approach to the treatment of asthma. N Engl J Med 321:1517–1527, 1989.
16. Kingston HG, Hirshman CA: Perioperative management of the patient with asthma. Anesth Analg 63:844–855, 1984.
17. Fanta CH, Rossing TH, McFadden EJ: Treatment of acute asthma: is combination therapy with sympathomimetics and methylxanthines indicated? Am J Med 80:5–10, 1986.
18. Nunn JF: Hypoxaemia after general anesthesia. Lancet 2:631–632, 1962.
19. Smith DC, Crul JF: early postoperative hypoxia during transport. Br J Anaesth 61:625–627, 1988.
20. Pullerits J, Burrows FA, Roy WL: Arterial desaturation in healthy children during transfer to the recovery room. Can J Anaesth 34:470–473, 1987.
21. McKenzie AJ: Perioperative hypoxaemia detected by intermittent pulse oximetry. Anaesth Intens Care 17:412–417, 1989.
22. Smith DC, Canning JJ, Crul JF: Pulse oximetry in the recovery room. Anaesthesia 44:345:348, 1989.
23. Marshall BE, Wyche MQ: Hypoxemia during and after anesthesia. Anesthesiology 37:178–209, 1972.
24. Fink BR: Diffusion anoxia. Anesthesiology 16:511–519, 1955.
25. Philbin DM, Sullivan SF, Bowman FO, et al: Postoperative hypoxemia: contribution of the cardiac output. Anesthesiology 32:136–142, 1970.
26. Bartlett RH, Brennan ML, Gazzaniga AB, Hanson EL: Studies on the pathogenesis and prevention of postoperative pulmonary complications. Surg Gynecol Obstet 137:925–933, 1973.
27. Wightman JAK: A prospective survey of the incidence of postoperative pulmonary complications. Br J Surg 55:85–91, 1968.
28. Ford GT, Whitelaw WA, Rosenal TW, et al: Diaphragm function after upper abdominal surgery in humans. Am Rev Respir Dis 127:431–436, 1983.
29. Vaughan RW, Engelhardt RC, Wise L: Postoperative hypoxemia in obese patients. Ann Surg 180:877–882, 1974.
30. Strandberg A, Tokics L, Brismar B, et al: Constitutional factors promoting development of atelectasis during anaesthesia. Acta Anaesthesiol Scand 31:21–24, 1987.
31. Holtz B, Bake B, Sixt R: Prediction of postoperative hypoxemia in smokers and non-smokers. Acta Anaesth Scand 23:411–418, 1979.
32. Kitamura H, Sawa T, Ikezono E: Postoperative hypoxemia: the contribution of age to the maldistribution of ventilation. Anesthesiology 36:244–252, 1972.
33. Bartlett RH, Hanson EL, Moore RD: Physiology of yawning and its application to postoperative care. Surg Forum 22:220, 1970.
34. Stock MC, Downs JB, Gauer PK, et al: Prevention of postoperative pulmonary complications with CPAP, incentive spirometry, and conservative therapy. Chest 87:151–157, 1985.
35. Olsson GL, Hallen B, Hanbraeus-Janzon K: Aspiration during anaesthesia: a computer-aided study of 185,358 anesthetics. Acta Anaesthesiol Scand 30:84, 1986.
36. McCormick PW: Immediate care after aspiration of vomit. Anaesthesia 30:658–665, 1975.
37. Bartlett JG, Gorbach SL: The triple threat of aspiration pneumonia. Chest 68:560–566, 1975.
38. Culver GA, Makel HP, Beecher HK: Frequency of aspiration of gastric contents by the lungs during anesthesia and surgery. Ann Surg 133:289–292, 1951.
39. Bond VK, Stoelting RK, Gupta CD: Pulmonary aspiration syndrome after inhalation of gastric fluid containing antacids. Anesthesiology 51:452–453, 1979.
40. Cullen DJ: Recovery room complications. AORN 26:746–763, 1977.
41. Ramachandran M, Dulay VC, Lobo ZA, Kuriyan JB: Bilateral pneumothorax with pneumomediastinum under anesthesia in a healthy female. Can Anaesth Soc J 29:391–394, 1982.

42. Monty CP: Pneumothorax following induction of anesthesia. JAMA *210*:2398, 1969.

43. Cullen DJ, Caldera DL: The incidence of ventilator-induced pulmonary barotrauma in critically ill patients. Anesthesiology *50*:185–190, 1979.

44. Calodney L, Aldrete JA: Pneumothorax: a complication of modern life. South Med J *65*:948–953, 1972.

45. Cooperman LH, Price HL: Pulmonary edema in the operative and postoperative period: a review of 40 cases. Ann Surg *172*:883–891, 1970.

46. Warner LO, Beach TP, Martino JD: Negative pressure pulmonary oedema secondary to airway obstruction in an intubated infant. Can J Anaesth *35*:507–510, 1988.

47. Herrick IA, Mahendran B, Penny FJ: Postobstructive pulmonary edema following anesthesia. J Clin Anesth *2*:116–120, 1990.

48. Arnaud D, Blache JL, Courtinat C, et al: Oedeme pulmonaire apres laryngospasme: a case of post-laryngoscopy pulmonary oedema. Ann Fr Anesth Reanim *6*:42–44, 1987.

49. Beard K, Jick H, Walker AM: Adverse respiratory events occurring in the recovery room after general anesthesia. Anesthesiology *64*:269–272, 1986.

50. Macklem PT: Respiratory muscles: the vital pump. Chest *78*:753–758, 1980.

51. PIOPED Investigators: Value of the ventilation/perfusion scan in acute pulmonary embolism. JAMA *263*:2753–2759, 1990.

52. Macintyre PE, Pavlin EG, Dwersteg JF: Effect of meperidine on oxygen consumption, carbon dioxide production, and respiratory gas exchange in postanesthesia shivering. Anesth Analg *66*:751–755, 1987.

6 POSTOPERATIVE ACID-BASE DISORDERS: Recognition and Management

DAVID M. ROTHENBERG

Perioperative disturbances in acid-base status may be secondary to or a cause of major organ dysfunction. Interpretation of such disorders has been greatly aided by experimental and clinical knowledge acquired during the 1980s. Unfortunately, this knowledge has been accompanied by the development of complex terminology and the use of occasionally redundant and impractical tests. As a result, many physicians consider this field of knowledge difficult to comprehend. Therefore it is the purpose of this chapter to provide a basic understanding of acid-base physiology and to offer a simple, practical approach to managing patients in the perioperative setting who manifest acid-base disorders. This chapter is divided into sections relating to the recognition and treatment of simple respiratory and metabolic acid-base disorders during the perioperative period, as well as a discussion on the acid-base changes during cardiopulmonary resuscitation.

NORMAL ACID-BASE PHYSIOLOGY

Acidity of body fluids is measured primarily in terms of hydrogen ion concentration ($[H^+]$) and is commonly expressed as hydrogen ion activity, or pH. The relation of $[H^+]$ to pH is straightforward and is depicted in Figure 6–1. For any given rise in $[H^+]$ a corresponding fall in pH occurs, whereas any decline in $[H^+]$ is matched by a rise in pH. Hydrogen ions are abundant in the body and readily react with or dissociate from carbon, oxygen, nitrogen, and sulfur. Molecules that accept or donate hydrogen ions are called *buffers* and act to stabilize

though not totally correct alterations in pH. Buffering is often defined by the equation

$$[HA] \rightleftharpoons [A^-] + [H^+]$$

where [HA] is a weak acid and $[A^-]$ is the base. When excess hydrogen ions are present in solution (or in the bloodstream), the reaction is driven in the direction of weak acid [HA] formation, thereby binding hydrogen ions and preventing their physiochemical activity. In the setting of a low $[H^+]$, the reaction moves in favor of hydrogen ion donation, thereby buffering an otherwise more basic solution. The extent to which a body buffer is able to stabilize pH depends on its ability to dissociate, which in turn is determined by its *dissociation constant* (*pK*). The closer the pK is to the normal pH of 7.40, the better is the buffering capacity of that particular acid-base group. Of the biologic fluids that function as buffers, the most important and prevalent system is the carbonic acid–bicarbonate pair. The relation of pH to this buffering system is conveyed by the *Henderson-Hasselbach equation*.

$$pH = pK + \log \frac{[HCO_3^-]}{[H_2CO_3]}$$
$$= 6.1 + \log \frac{[HCO_3^-]}{0.03 \, PaCO_2}$$

The importance of the carbonic acid–bicarbonate buffer pair, despite the marked disparity between its pK and normal pH, is related to the role of the kidney and lung in maintaining an $[HCO_3^-]/[H_2CO_3]$ ratio of approximately $20:1$. Other nonbicarbonate buffers that aid in maintaining normal pH include plasma proteins such as albumin and hemoglobin, mono- and dibasic phosphates, and am-

94

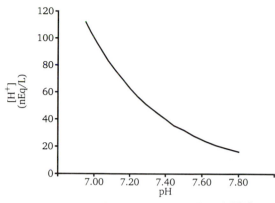

FIGURE 6–1. Relation between pH and $[H^+]$.

monium. Bone also serves as a major buffer source especially for patients with chronic metabolic acidoses, as is seen in those with renal failure. All buffer systems are in equilibrium with the carbonic acid–bicarbonate pair and therefore may alter pH only by changes in either $[H_2CO_3^-]$ (as measured by dissolved $PaCO_2$) or $[HCO_3^-]$. This concept is termed the *isohydric principle*.[1]

Applying the Henderson-Hasselbach equation to a clinical situation is an arduous and clumsy task. A more practical and simpler approach emphasizing the interrelation of $[H^+]$, $PaCO_2$, and $[HCO_3^-]$ uses the *Henderson equation*.[1,2]

$$[H^+] = 24 \frac{PaCO_2}{[HCO_3^-]}$$

Henderson's equation is useful not only for a rapid calculation of $[H^+]$, $PaCO_2$, or $[HCO_3^-]$ once any two of the parameters are known but also for assessing the accuracy and internal consistency of the data presented. It is clear from this equation that the *normal pH is 7.40*, the *normal $PaCO_2$ is 40 mm Hg*, and the *normal $[HCO_3^-]$ is 24 mEq/L*. To interpret acid-base disorders properly, it is important to accept these values as normal. Although ranges in pH of 7.35 to 74.5 may be clinically acceptable, for the sake of acid-base interpretation a pH of 7.39 is acidemic and a pH of 7.41 is alkalemic. (The terms *acidemia* and *alkalemia* apply to blood pH, whereas *alkalosis* and *acidosis* relate to tissue pH and clinical processes.) Extrapolating $[H^+]$ to pH may be done easily from Figure 6–1. Note that between pH 7.2 and 7.5 a pH change of 0.01 units exists for approximately every 1 mEq/L change in $[H^+]$.

The development of a clinical acid-base disorder is determined by changes in the plasma $[HCO_3^-]$, the so-called metabolic or renal component, or by changes in the $PaCO_2$, the so-called respiratory component. A primary metabolic acidosis is caused by a fall in serum bicarbonate; likewise, a metabolic alkalosis occurs with a rise in serum bicarbonate. Primary respiratory acidosis and alkalosis occur with a rise or fall in $PaCO_2$, respectively. The alteration in blood pH is therefore always determined by the $PaCO_2/[HCO_3^-]$ ratio. Maintaining a near-normal pH depends on appropriate *compensatory mechanisms:* A primary metabolic process induces a compensatory respiratory change; a primary respiratory process induces a compensatory metabolic change. Thus a primary metabolic acidosis initiates a compensatory decrease in $PaCO_2$, whereas a primary metabolic alkalosis initiates a compensatory increase in $PaCO_2$. A compensatory increase or decrease in $[HCO_3^-]$ is seen for primary respiratory acidosis and respiratory alkalosis (Table 6–1). Compensation always moves the dependent (secondary) variable in the *same direction* as the independent (primary) variable in order to maintain the $PaCO_2/[HCO_3^-]$ ratio constant. Therefore an easy "rule of thumb" for determining appropriate compensation is to note that the "arrows" always point in the same direction as is seen in Table 6–1. When interpreting an acid-base disturbance, if the "arrows" are opposite a *mixed acid-base disorder* must exist (i.e., two disorders occurring simultaneously). It is important to note that it is physiologically impossible to "overcompensate" to a normal pH of 7.40. The term "overcompensation" is incorrectly used for what is more accurately termed a mixed disorder. The appropriateness of the compensatory response is the essence of acid-base determination and is discussed in each of the primary acid-base disorder sections.

TABLE 6–1. APPROPRIATE COMPENSATORY CHANGES FOR PRIMARY ACID-BASE DISORDERS

Primary Disorder	Status	Compensation
Respiratory acidosis	↑ $PaCO_2$	↑ $[HCO_3^-]$
Respiratory alkalosis	↓ $PaCO_2$	↓ $[HCO_3^-]$
Metabolic acidosis	↓ $[HCO_3^-]$	↓ $PaCO_2$
Metabolic alkalosis	↑ $[HCO_3^-]$	↑ $PaCO_2$

ACUTE RESPIRATORY ACIDOSIS

The acid-base disorder that most commonly occurs in the postoperative setting is acute respiratory acidosis. Initiated by processes that increase $PaCO_2$ and associated with a decrease in pH, respiratory acidosis is almost always secondary to an impairment in effective alveolar ventilation ($\dot{V}_E$). Rarely is an increase in CO_2 production ($\dot{V}CO_2$) the sole cause of a respiratory acidosis. However, in the setting of an impaired or fixed minute ventilation, acute respiratory acidosis due to a marked increase in CO_2 production may occur. (An example of this phenomenon may be seen during malignant hyperthermia in an anesthetized patient undergoing mechanical ventilation at a fixed-minute ventilation.[3]) The magnitude of pH change during acute respiratory acidosis therefore depends on both CO_2 production and CO_2 elimination and can be defined by the equation[4]

$$PaCO_2 = (K) \frac{\dot{V}CO_2}{\dot{V}_E}$$

Note that when $\dot{V}CO_2$ is constant, any change in $PaCO_2$ is indirectly proportional to $\dot{V}_E$. A doubling of $\dot{V}_E$ causes the $PaCO_2$ to fall by one half. During the acute phase of a respiratory acidosis, nonbicarbonate buffering and renal adaptive mechanisms also play an important role in mitigating the decline in pH. The stimulus to increase $\dot{V}_E$ in response to an increase in $\dot{V}CO_2$ is primarily mediated by changes in the $[H^+]$ in the cerebrospinal fluid (CSF) that bathes the chemoreceptor neurons of the central nervous system (CNS) located in the medulla.[5] CSF is essentially devoid of all nonbicarbonate buffers. Therefore owing to the capacity by which CO_2 diffuses across the blood-brain barrier, an acute rise in $PaCO_2$ produces a marked rise in CSF $[H^+]$. A slower rise in CSF $[HCO_3^-]$ from transfer of either cerebral or blood $[HCO_3^-]$ eventually corrects CSF pH toward normal. The responsiveness of the CNS appears to be mediated by the change in medullary CO_2 and, in turn, by the change in medullary $[H^+]$.[5] The location of the neural elements responsive to this change appear to be located along a diffusion path between the blood and CSF. Indeed the neurologic changes seen with acute hypercarbia are likely related to these changes in the medullary $[H^+]$.

Following an acute rise in $PaCO_2$, a small increase in plasma bicarbonate is seen usually within 5 to 10 minutes and is primarily the result of the titration of intracellular nonbicarbonate buffers. These buffers, when combined with hydrogen ions generated from the dissociation of carbonic acid, also generate bicarbonate. A large proportion of this nonbicarbonate buffering is due to the "chloride shift,"[1] whereby extracellular chloride enters red blood cells in exchange for bicarbonate. Renal reabsorption of bicarbonate plays a less important role during the acute phases of respiratory acidosis, though it most certainly aids in maintaining the level of buffer-generated bicarbonate.

A primary acute respiratory acidosis is usually not associated with a plasma bicarbonate concentration of more than 32 mEq/L. A higher value almost certainly implies the association of secondary metabolic alkalosis. The appropriate rise in plasma bicarbonate for an acute respiratory acidosis may be defined by the equation[6]

$$\Delta [HCO_3^-] = \frac{\Delta PaCO_2}{10} \pm 3$$

Simply stated, an acute rise in $PaCO_2$ from 40 mm Hg to 70 mm Hg should be associated with a concomitant rise in plasma bicarbonate of 3 to 6 mEq/L or from a plasma bicarbonate of 24 mEq/L to 27 to 30 mEq/L.

CLINICAL MANIFESTATIONS

The clinical manifestations of acute respiratory acidosis depend not only on the absolute magnitude of the $PaCO_2$ but also on the rate of $PaCO_2$ rise and the degree of associated hypoxemia. As previously mentioned, the CNS is sensitive to an acute rise in $PaCO_2$, with neurologic manifestations ranging from anxiety and confusion to frank psychosis. At extreme levels of $PaCO_2$, a state of carbon dioxide narcosis with stupor and coma may develop.[7] A carbon dioxide level of more than 245 mm Hg may achieve a general anesthetic effect equivalent to 1 minimum alveolar concentration (MAC). Other neurologic signs and symptoms include tremors, myoclonus, and asterixis. Hypercarbia causes cerebral vasodilation that, when severe, may lead to increased intracranial pressure with associated headaches and papilledema.[8] These changes are common with the acute and chronic stages of respiratory acidosis. Cardiovascular manifestations are also common in the setting of acute respiratory acidosis.[9] The increase in heart rate and blood pressure, as well as the frequent occurrence of supraventricular and ventricular dysrhythmias, are thought to be secondary to the direct hypercarbic stimulation of the sympathetic nervous system. At the same time, an acute rise in $PaCO_2$ may cause direct peripheral vasodilation; however, the blood pressure is usually maintained or elevated owing to the increase in cardiac output from sympathetic nervous system stimulation despite the patient appearing warm and flushed.[10]

Clinically significant acute respiratory acidosis is almost always associated with some degree of hypoxemia due to either pure alveolar hypoventilation with a lowered inspired oxygen or concomitant lung pathology and impaired oxygen exchange. It is therefore important to note that many of the signs and symptoms associated with acute respiratory acidosis may be attenuated or exacerbated by an increase or a decrease in the PaO_2, respectively.

ETIOLOGIES

Disorders that may cause acute respiratory acidosis are listed in Table 6–2. This list emphasizes those etiologies that most commonly present in an early postoperative setting. Detected by sonorous and paradoxical respiration, upper airway obstruction is one of the more common causes of acute respiratory acidosis in a post anesthesia care unit (PACU). Mechanical obstruction may occur by posterior pharyngeal displacement of the tongue following anesthesia or by an improperly fitted oral airway. Aspiration of vomitus or blood may cause upper airway obstruction and may lead to acute lung injury with associated hypercarbia and hypoxemia. The presence of stridor suggests acute laryngospasm as a cause of upper airway obstruction and, if severe, may create a negative transpulmonary pressure gradient and induce pulmonary edema.[11,12] Severe postoperative bronchospasm may occur in asthmatics undergoing either general or regional anesthesia and may be related to direct airway irritation, histamine release, mucous plugging, or excessive vagal tone as seen with high epidural or spinal anesthesia. Severe bronchospasm may markedly elevate intrathoracic pressure, impairing cardiac output; and when it is coupled with an increased work of breathing it may lead to tissue hypoxia and a metabolic acidosis secondary to lactate accumulation.[13]

Direct depression of the medullary respira-

TABLE 6–2. ETIOLOGIES OF POSTOPERATIVE ACUTE RESPIRATORY ACIDOSIS

Upper airway obstruction
  Posterior tongue displacement
  Foreign body
  Obstructed endotracheal tube
  Laryngospasm
  Aspiration

Lower airway obstruction
  Severe bronchospasm
  Obstructive sleep apnea

Respiratory center depression
  General anesthesia
  Sedative or narcotic overdose
  Intracranial surgery

Neuromuscular disorders
  Prolonged depolarizing blockade (e.g., pseudocholinesterase deficiency, phase II block in association with succinylcholine)
  Prolonged nondepolarizing blockade (e.g., excess drug, hypothermia, aminoglycosides)
  Cervical cordotomy
  Myasthenia gravis crisis

Restrictive lung disorders
  Hemothorax
  Pneumothorax
  Flail chest
  Acute lung injury

Miscellaneous disorders
  Malignant hyperthermia
  Circulatory arrest
  Maladjusted ventilator
  Shivering

tory center by anesthetic agents often causes an acute respiratory acidosis, with most patients having some degree of alveolar hypoventilation with an impaired CO_2 response curve due to the effect of general anesthesia.[14] Direct cerebral injury may also lead to acute respiratory acidosis; its influence on effective alveolar ventilation depends on the degree of injury. Severe cerebral ischemia, infarct, or hemorrhage may cause central hypoventilation, whereas milder involvement may stimulate ventilation, leading to respiratory alkalosis.

Of the neuromuscular disorders that compromise ventilation, prolonged neuromuscular blockade is the most common. Failure to adequately reverse a nondepolarizing muscle relaxant leads to respiratory muscle weakness and acute respiratory acidosis. "Recurarization'' may also occur in the PACU owing to hypothermia, concomitant use of aminoglycosides, or the respiratory acidosis itself.[15] Patients with pseudocholinesterase deficiencies have prolonged neuromuscular blockade due to the depolarizing muscle relaxant succinylcholine and may require short-term mechanical ventilation in the PACU until this drug can be eliminated. Transection of the cervical spinal cord above the level of the phrenic nerve distribution leads to impaired diaphragmatic strength and respiratory muscle fatigue. Complete respiratory paralysis may be seen with spinal cord trauma above the level of the third cervical vertebra. Finally, myasthenia gravis may be exacerbated during the perioperative period owing to the stress of surgery, general anesthesia, the inappropriate use of long-acting nondepolarizing neuromuscular-blocking agents or drugs with neuromuscular blocking properties such as aminoglycosides.[16]

Many pulmonary disorders may directly restrict ventilation and lead to acute respiratory acidosis. Such disorders include large pleural effusions, tension pneumothoraces, marked obesity, and tense ascites. Pulmonary edema and pulmonary emboli, if severe, also cause CO_2 retention, though profound hypoxemia is generally the rule.

An acute respiratory acidosis due to excessive CO_2 production in the presence of ineffective alveolar ventilation may be seen during malignant hyperthermia, as noted above, as well as in the setting of excessive shivering. Finally, an acute respiratory acidosis occurs when improper adjustments of minute ventilation are made in patients requiring mechanical assistance.

THERAPY

Early recognition and prompt alleviation of acute respiratory acidosis is essential to minimize the CNS and cardiovascular sequelae associated with severe hypercapnia and hypoxemia. During the postoperative period it may require simple maneuvers, e.g., a jaw thrust or airway insertion, to relieve an upper airway obstruction, or full mechanical ventilation with insertion of an endotracheal tube for patients with more severe disorders such as prolonged neuromuscular blockade.

A number of pharmacologic agents are also important not only for minimizing but also reversing acute respiratory acidosis. Table 6–3 lists these particular drugs. The opioid antagonist naloxone is primarily employed for treat-

TABLE 6–3. PHARMACOLOGIC THERAPY OF ACUTE RESPIRATORY ACIDOSIS

Naloxone
Doxapram
Anticholinesterase inhibitors
Aminophylline
Flumazenil
Bronchodilators
Corticosteroids
Diuretics

ing narcotic overdosage. Incremental dosing of naloxone seems prudent, as rapid reversal has been reported to precipitate acute pulmonary edema. This phenomenon is thought to be secondary to a massive catecholamine surge inducing a hydrostatic-mediated pulmonary edema and seems to be unique to the anesthesia recovery period.[17] Use of high-dose naloxone in other settings (e.g., spinal cord trauma) has not been associated with this complication.[18] Doxapram hydrochloride is a central respiratory stimulant that, unlike naloxone, does not reverse the analgesic effects of narcotics. Because of its relatively short clinical effect, however, patients should be monitored closely for signs of recurrent hypoventilation.[19] Anticholinesterase inhibitors reverse residual neuromuscular blockade and are useful for the treatment of myasthenic crises, which may require the systemic use of the anticholinesterase inhibitor pyridostigmine. Aminophylline and physostigmine have been used successfully in the past to treat respiratory depression due to benzodiazepines.[20,21] However, the direct acting benzodiazepine antagonist flumazenil will likely replace these agents for treating this cause of respiratory acidosis.[22,23] Other drugs, such as inhalational bronchodilators and systemic corticosteroids, aid in treating severe bronchospasm, and diuretics such as furosemide help to alleviate severe pulmonary edema. Finally, in regard to alkali loading in patients with a pure, acute respiratory acidosis, it is considered contraindicated to administer sodium bicarbonate for three main reasons: 1) Little if any change in acid-base equilibrium may be expected to occur when a normally functioning kidney excretes most of the bicarbonate fraction.[1] 2) In patients with impaired minute ventilation or impaired pulmonary perfusion, the amount of dissolved CO_2 (260 to 280 mm Hg) in an ampul of sodium bicarbonate may significantly worsen both the venous and arterial acidosis.[24] 3) In patients with compromised cardiac and renal function, sodium bicarbonate administration may precipitate pulmonary edema, thereby worsening the respiratory acidosis and causing hypoxemia. The appropriate use of alkali therapy is discussed in more detail in the section on metabolic acidosis.

ACUTE RESPIRATORY ALKALOSIS

Acute respiratory alkalosis also occurs commonly during the postoperative period and is diagnosed by an arterial pH of more than 7.40 in the presence of $PaCO_2$ of less than 40 mm Hg. The terms "alveolar hyperventilation," "primary hypocarbia," and "hypocapnia" are all synonymous with respiratory alkalosis. The secondary hypocapnia that occurs as a compensatory response to a metabolic acidosis is not considered to be part of the definition of acute respiratory alkalosis. The regulation of alveolar ventilation is governed by chemoreceptors located in the brainstem and in the carotid arteries and aortic arch. The chemoreceptors in the medulla are most sensitive to changes in hydrogen ion concentration (as noted in the previous section on acute respiratory acidosis), whereas those in the carotid arteries and aortic arch are most sensitive to changes in oxygen delivery. Cortical input also plays a role for voluntary control of respiration. Finally, pathophysiologic changes in the lung stimulate pulmonary chemoreceptors as well as "J" or stretch receptors and lead to hyperventilation. In response to the alkalemia induced by alveolar hyperventilation, secondary physiologic responses attempt to mitigate the degree of pH change. Buffering takes place acutely in the extracellular space with blood buffers such as hemoglobin and proteins releasing hydrogen ion. Tissue buffering also occurs, with intracellular phosphates and other proteins playing a major role. Generation of the organic acid lactate in response to an acute respiratory alkalosis appears to play a minor role in buffering this disorder. Steady-state equilibrium is achieved by the kidneys' ability to excrete bicarbonate and, more importantly, by the decrease in titratable acid excretion. The degree of renal compensation for acute respiratory alkalosis is defined by the equation[6]

$$\frac{\Delta\ PaCO_2}{10} \times (1 - 3) = \Delta\ [HCO_3^-]$$

For example, the patient with an arterial pH of 7.50 and a $PaCO_2$ of 27 mm Hg should have a plasma bicarbonate level in the range of 20 to 23 mEq/L.

CLINICAL MANIFESTATIONS

Acute respiratory alkalosis induces changes in the CNS characterized by confusion and dizziness, although generalized seizures may occur. These changes relate to the hypocapnic effect on cerebral blood flow. Cerebrovascular resistance increases with the reduction in $PaCO_2$, with marked impairment in cerebral blood flow at $PaCO_2$ levels below 25 mm Hg.[25] In addition, an associated fall in cerebral venous oxygen tension may lead to cerebral hypoxia, which may be the primary cause of seizures seen with acute respiratory alkalosis.[26] Acute respiratory alkalosis is also associated with paresthesias in the extremities, chest pain, and circumoral numbness.

The cardiovascular changes of acute respiratory alkalosis are controversial, as experimental data differ when comparing the anesthetized hyperventilated patient to the awake hyperventilating patient. The effects most commonly described are tachycardia and a decline in stroke volume with minimal overall change in cardiac output or peripheral resistance.[27] Cardiac dysrhythmias are common at extremes of pH (>7.60) and are often refractory to standard forms of treatment.[28]

Metabolic abnormalities are also common during acute respiratory alkalosis. Intracellular shifts of sodium and potassium occur in response to the buffering effect of the hydrogen ion as it shifts to the extracellular space. Serum phosphate concentration is diminished owing to intracellular alkalosis activating the process of phosphorylation, thus depleting phosphate stores.[29] This effect does not seem to be pronounced during metabolic alkalosis, appearing to be related solely to the intracellular hypocapnia. Finally, protein binding of calcium is increased during respiratory alkalosis and may cause or contribute to neurologic changes, although a fall in ionized calcium is unlikely to be the sole cause of seizures associated with acute respiratory alkalosis.

ETIOLOGIES

Table 6–4 lists the most common postoperative causes of acute respiratory alkalosis. The most common cause, diminished oxygen de-

TABLE 6–4. ETIOLOGIES OF POSTOPERATIVE ACUTE RESPIRATORY ALKALOSIS

Decreased oxygen delivery
 Decreased oxygen content (anemia, hypoxemia)
 Decreased cardiac output

Central nervous system stimulation
 Voluntary stimulation
 Anxiety
 Pain
 Fever
 Stroke syndromes
 Infection (encephalitis, meningitis)
 Trauma
 Tumor
 Drugs (naloxone, doxapram, methylxanthines, salicylates)
 Gram-negative sepsis

Pulmonary disease
 Asthma
 Pulmonary edema
 Pulmonary embolism
 Pneumonia
 Interstitial pneumonitis

Excessive mechanical ventilation

livery, is mediated by the peripheral chemoreceptors in the carotid arteries and aortic arch, which override medullary chemoreceptors that sense the alkaline pH. A slight decline in PaO_2 does not appear to be sufficient to stimulate ventilation, whereas a fall in PaO_2 to less than 65 mm Hg yields clinically apparent hyperventilation. Similar peripheral chemoreceptor stimulation occurs in patients with hypotension or severe anemia (or both), with the patients hyperventilating even in the presence of a normal PaO_2.

Many mechanisms account for CNS-mediated hyperventilation. Stimulation at the cortical level is seen with voluntary or psychogenic hyperventilation, these patients often presenting with the symptoms of substernal chest tightness that is difficult to differentiate from the symptoms of angina or pulmonary embolism. Primary neurologic diseases produce different patterns of hyperventilation. Central hyperventilation may occur secondary to lesions in the pontine-midbrain region, whereas Cheynes-Stokes respiration may be seen with more diffuse cortical lesions. It is important to point out that with severe neurologic involvement respiratory depression may be the rule, with the primary acid-base disorder being an

acute respiratory acidosis. Drugs such as naloxone and doxapram cause a CNS-mediated increase in minute ventilation, whereas other agents such as aspirin directly stimulate the medullary chemoreceptors, also leading to a marked increase in respiratory rate. This change may occur with a dose of 12 gm or more over a 24-hour period and may produce a significant fall in $PaCO_2$.[30] Though salicylism is rarely encountered during the postoperative period, its diagnosis should be considered in any patient presenting with an acute respiratory alkalosis in association with an elevated anion gap, signifying a metabolic acidosis. (It is due to aspirin's ability to uncouple oxidative phosphorylation, causing lactic acidosis; to its effect on glucose metabolism, yielding keto-acidosis; and to the direct contribution of its salicylic acid component.[31] Gram-negative sepsis is associated with acute respiratory alkalosis and often precedes the metabolic acidosis that occurs during septic shock.[32] Whether a central stimulating effect of gram-negative endotoxin is the cause of this phenomenon is yet unknown. Hyperventilation in association with gram-positive bacteremia has also been described.[32]

Many primary pulmonary diseases such as pneumonia, asthma, pulmonary edema, or pulmonary embolism are associated with acute respiratory alkalosis due to chemoreceptor stimulation and associated hypoxemia. Finally, maladjustment of the mechanical ventilator settings of tidal volume and rate cause an iatrogenic respiratory alkalosis. This practice may be therapeutic in the patient with elevated intracranial pressure in whom a mechanically induced hypocapnia of 25 to 30 mm Hg causes an increase in cerebrovascular resistance. The increase in resistance reduces cerebral blood flow, thereby lowering intracranial pressure.[33]

THERAPY

The degree of alkalemia has been shown to correlate with high mortality in intensive care units when the $PaCO_2$ is less than 15 mm Hg[34]; therefore marked alkalemia needs to be treated aggressively. Unlike acute respiratory acidosis, however, there is no pharmacologic armamentarium to treat acute respiratory alkalosis. Therapy therefore is directed solely to the underlying cause. Severe anxiety can be treated by the patient rebreathing from a paper bag or by using anxiolytic agents such as benzodiazepines. Analgesic therapy for the patient in pain, oxygen therapy for the hypoxemic patient, and readjustment of the mechanical overventilation are obvious forms of treating these particular causes of acute respiratory alkalosis.

METABOLIC ALKALOSIS

A metabolic alkalosis exists when plasma bicarbonate is above 24 mEq/L with an arterial pH greater than 7.40. When this form of alkalosis develops, it is primarily due to loss of titratable acid from either the gastrointestinal tract or the kidney, or from the net addition of exogenous bicarbonate. The extrarenal buffering of metabolic alkalosis occurs primarily via the extracellular release of hydrogen ion from plasma proteins, as well as by intracellular sodium–hydrogen and potassium–hydrogen exchange. Respiratory compensation occurs as the result of inhibition of the medullary chemoreceptors, leading to alveolar hypoventilation. The degree of compensation is based on the following equation[6]:

$$\Delta\,[HCO_3^-] \times (0.8) = \Delta\,PaCO_2$$

Therefore a patient with a plasma bicarbonate of 40 mEq/L would be expected to hypoventilate to a $PaCO_2$ of approximately 52 to 53 mm Hg. Because alveolar hypoventilation may be associated with low inspired oxygen concentrations, the maximum pulmonary compensatory response to severe metabolic alkalosis is limited by hypoxemia. Oxygen delivery may be further impaired owing to the shift in the oxyhemoglobin dissociation curve to the left (Bohr effect), thus diminishing oxygen availability at the tissue level.

Metabolic alkaloses can be classified as either chloride-responsive or chloride-resistant and are discussed in more detail below. For most patients, however, postoperative metabolic alkalosis is ordinarily either chloride-responsive or due to an acute alkali load. Therefore chloride-resistant metabolic alkalosis such as that seen in patients with hyperaldosteronism is not discussed in this text.

CLINICAL MANIFESTATIONS

As with acute respiratory alkalosis, CNS changes occur with severe metabolic alkalosis. Confusion, lethargy, and stupor have been attributed to the severity of the pH rise. Re-

fractory cardiac dysrhythmias, as mentioned in the previous section, also may occur. Metabolic changes associated with metabolic alkalosis include low ionized calcium due to increased protein binding at alkalemic pH levels, as well as hypokalemia due to renal losses of potassium when hypovolemia stimulates the release of aldosterone in patients with chloride-responsive metabolic alkalosis. This subject is discussed in more detail in the section on gastric losses as a cause of metabolic alkalosis.

ETIOLOGIES

The causes of metabolic alkalosis that are of concern during the postoperative period are listed in Table 6–5. Acute and sustained alkali loading may overcome the ability of the kidneys to excrete a bicarbonate load and, especially in the patient with volume contraction, may lead to severe metabolic alkalosis. Gastric losses as seen with vomiting or continuous nasogastric suction lead not only to a direct loss of hydrogen and chloride ions but also to losses of sodium and water. The major consequences of these losses is the stimulation and release of aldosterone, which then promotes a sodium–potassium and sodium–hydrogen exchange, causing not only hypokalemia but a perpetuation of the metabolic alkalosis. With chloride relatively unavailable as a major anion for reabsorption with the cation sodium, bicarbonate is reabsorbed despite the presence of a systemic alkalemia, leading to a perpetuation and worsening of this disorder. To correct hypokalemic, metabolic alkalosis secondary to gastric fluid losses, it is imperative to administer chloride in order to restore intravascular volume and "turn off" the release of aldosterone.[1,6]

Patients who use diuretics on a chronic basis for the treatment of edematous states or hypertension may develop hypokalemic metabolic alkalosis due to the enhanced hydrogen

TABLE 6–5. ETIOLOGIES OF POSTOPERATIVE METABOLIC ALKALOSIS

Acute alkali administration
Gastric fluid losses
Postdiuretic therapy
Posthypercapnic states
Massive transfusions

and potassium excretion caused by both thiazide and loop diuretics.[35]

Posthypercapnic metabolic alkalosis occurs when patients with chronic respiratory acidosis are acutely hyperventilated. In these patients plasma bicarbonate levels are chronically high owing to renal compensation for the respiratory acidosis. Sudden hyperventilation may cause an acute and often severe alkalemia due to the delay in renal excretion of bicarbonate.[36] Finally, massive transfusion therapy may cause a mild metabolic alkalosis owing to conversion of the citrate moiety in preserved blood to bicarbonate.[37]

THERAPY

The major goal of therapy for patients with metabolic alkalosis is to minimize the rise in pH, treating levels of pH 7.55 or more so as to prevent the cardiovascular and neurologic sequelae. Prevention of metabolic alkalosis may be accomplished by minimizing excessive use of exogenous alkali or diuretics. Employing histamine-2 blocking agents, e.g., ranitidine or cimetidine, may be beneficial in reducing gastric hydrogen ion secretion, thereby minimizing acid loss in patients undergoing nasogastric suction.[38] The major treatment modality for patients with chloride-responsive metabolic alkalosis is the infusion of sodium chloride. Normal saline offers more chloride per liter than does Ringer's lactate (154 mEq/L versus 104 to 109 mEq/L) and is therefore the agent of choice in the nonedematous, hypovolemic patient.[1,6] Ringer's lactate also may be contraindicated owing to the conversion of lactate to bicarbonate. For patients with edema (e.g., congestive heart failure, cirrhosis, nephrosis), chloride is best administered as potassium chloride so as to avoid the potential for further volume overloading with normal saline. With severe metabolic alkalosis, dilute hydrochloric acid may be used by infusing 1 to 2 liters of 0.10 to 0.15 N hydrochloride acid slowly through a central intravenous catheter, titrating the therapy to lower the pH to less than 7.60.[39] Acetazolamide is also a useful agent, especially in patients with posthypercapnic or edematous metabolic alkalosis. By causing carbonic anhydrase inhibition, acetazolamide creates bicarbonate diuresis, thereby lowering systemic pH.[40,41] Replacement of renal potassium losses should be anticipated and treated accordingly.

METABOLIC ACIDOSIS

Metabolic acidosis is a primary disorder characterized by a reduction in the plasma bicarbonate level, which results in a lowering of the pH. A metabolic acidosis occurs when there is either a net addition of acid or a net loss of bicarbonate from the extracellular compartment. Rapid dilution of the extracellular space by bicarbonate-free solutions such as isotonic saline also lower plasma bicarbonate and yield a metabolic acidosis. The fall in plasma bicarbonate is initially buffered by intracellular proteins, phosphates, and hemoglobin, and bone acts as a major buffer source during periods of severe or chronic acid loads as seen in patients with chronic renal failure. Respiratory compensation occurs as a consequence of the acidic pH stimulating the medullary chemoreceptors. This alveolar hyperventilation often takes 12 to 24 hours to reach a maximal effect. The degree of hyperventilation depends on the degree of metabolic acidosis. As previously mentioned, it is physiologically impossible for respiratory compensation to restore the pH to the preexisting normal level. The relation of respiratory compensation to the fall in plasma bicarbonate is defined by the equation[6]

$$PaCO_2 = \Delta\,[HCO_3^-] \times 1.2$$

Therefore a patient with a pH of 7.30 and a serum bicarbonate level of 16 mEq/L would be expected to hyperventilate to a $PaCO_2$ of 30 to 31 mm Hg. If such a patient were noted to have a $PaCO_2$ of 38 mm Hg, a secondary respiratory alkalosis would be present. The astute clinician would recognize this mixed acid-base disturbance as a sign of potential respiratory muscle fatigue and institute early ventilatory support for the respiratory acidosis, rather than attempting to treat the metabolic acidosis with the infusion of sodium bicarbonate.

A metabolic acidosis may be characterized based on the net gain of acid or the net loss of bicarbonate by utilizing the anion gap.[42] The *anion gap* is based on the physiologic concept of electroneutrality. Simply stated, the cations in the extracellular space precisely balance the anions. The major extracellular fluid cation is sodium (potassium primarily resides in the intracellular fluid space). Unmeasured cations (i.e., those not routinely measured, such as sulfates and phosphates) constitute the remainder of the positively charged ions. The major anions include chloride and bicarbonate as well as the unmeasured anions. Therefore unmeasured cations plus sodium should equal unmeasured anions plus chloride and bicarbonate. The anion gap formula is obtained by rearranging this equation to read:

Unmeasured anions − unmeasured cations
$$= Na^+ - (Cl^- + HCO_3^-)$$

The difference between unmeasured cations and unmeasured anions represents the anion gap. Any process that elevates the unmeasured anions thereby increases the anion gap. The relation between the anion gap and metabolic acidosis is based on the fact that additional unmeasured anions are organic acids. Therefore an anion gap metabolic acidosis signifies the net addition of acid, and a nonanion gap metabolic acidosis signifies the net loss of bicarbonate. Table 6–6 lists the etiologies of metabolic acidosis based on the anion gap calculation, with each disorder being discussed in more detail below.

Finally, the use of the standard bicarbonate or base-excess calculation bears mention in regard to the interpretation of all acid-base disorders, but in particular metabolic acidosis.[43] The basic purpose of these measurements is to eliminate the respiratory component from the analysis of acid-base equilibrium, thereby allowing for the simplified evaluation of the metabolic disorder. These calculations attempt to provide a shortcut approach to acid-base analyses but unfortunately often yield misleading information, especially in regard to the interpretation of mixed or chronic acid-base disorders. A negative base excess is thought to imply the presence of a metabolic acidosis; however, when the pH is more than 7.40, it is clear that a primary respiratory alkalosis exists. Treating a negative base excess with sodium bicarbon-

TABLE 6–6. ETIOLOGIES OF POSTOPERATIVE METABOLIC ACIDOSIS

Nonanion Gap (Net Loss of Bicarbonate)	Anion Gap (Net Addition of Acid)
Diarrhea	Lactic acidosis
Pancreatic drainage	Ketoacidosis (diabetes, (starvation, alcoholism)
Biliary drainage	Uremia
Urinary diversion (obstructed ileal loop conduit)	
Dilutional acidosis	

ate in a patient with an already alkaline pH is inappropriate. Therefore the base-excess or standard bicarbonate calculations offer no additional value when the pH, $PaCO_2$, $[HCO_3^-]$, and anion gap measurements are provided.[44]

CLINICAL MANIFESTATIONS

The clinical features of a metabolic acidosis are often secondary to the underlying disorder. However, direct effects on specific organ systems do occur, related primarily to the change in pH. Pulmonary manifestations include rapid and deep respiration, so-called Kussmaul's respiration, and are most apparent when the pH is less than 7.20. An increase in pulmonary vascular resistance may also occur, thus contributing to the severity of pulmonary hypertension or right ventricular failure (or both). The degree of myocardial dysfunction associated with metabolic acidosis also depends on the level of the pH. When pH values are less than 7.20, the myocardial contractility is greatly diminished.[45] At less severe changes in pH, cardiac output may not be greatly affected, as metabolic acidosis stimulates the release of catecholamines, thereby providing an endogenous inotropic support during the period of acidosis. Clinical and experimental studies also show that a metabolic acidosis lowers the ventricular fibrillatory threshold, predisposing to life-threatening dysrhythmias.[46,47] A decrease in vascular resistance also occurs with a metabolic acidosis, although it may be counterbalanced by the endogenous release of catecholamines.[45] Metabolic acidosis causes a shift in the oxyhemoglobin dissociation curve to the right, thereby promoting the release of oxygen at the tissue level. Chronic metabolic acidosis causes a decrease in red blood cell 2,3-diphosphoglyceric acid, thereby shifting the oxyhemoglobin dissociation curve back to the left,[45] conceivably adding to tissue hypoxia in certain hypoperfusion states. Gastrointestinal function is also thought to be diminished during periods of metabolic acidosis as manifested by delayed gastric emptying.

ETIOLOGIES

Table 6–6 lists the common causes of postoperative metabolic acidosis. An increased anion gap metabolic acidosis is seen with lactic acidosis and is due to either an increase in oxygen demand or a reduction in oxygen supply (or both). Examples of increased oxygen demand include severe seizure disorders, shivering, and malignant hyperthermia. Reduced oxygen supply occurs during reduced tissue perfusion such as with prolonged hypotension or circulatory arrest, or during periods of reduced oxygen content such as severe anemia or hypoxemia. Whenever the production of lactic acid exceeds its metabolism, the plasma bicarbonate level falls and a metabolic acidosis develops. Patients with liver dysfunction fail to metabolize lactic acid adequately, predisposing to pronounced metabolic acidosis under periods of increased lactic acid production. Ketoacidosis resulting from either an absolute or a relative insulin deficiency may occur in patients with diabetes mellitus, particularly during periods of perioperative stress. Ketoacidosis should also be expected in patients with prolonged starvation and in alcohol-intoxicated patients who require emergency surgery. Acute or chronic renal failure leads to accumulation of organic acids and an anion gap metabolic acidosis, with acidosis occurring secondary to the diminished excretion of a daily acid load rather than from an increase in acid production. Diarrhea is the most common cause of a nonanion gap metabolic acidosis and is due to the marked intestinal losses of bicarbonate in the diarrheal fluid.[1,6] Likewise, bicarbonate concentration in biliary and pancreatic secretions is high; therefore during drainage procedures or with external fistulas, a nonanion gap metabolic acidosis may occur.[1,6] Obstructed urinary diversions such as ileo-loop conduits expose bowel mucosa to urine for long periods, causing a chloride–bicarbonate exchange. This exchange results in intestinal losses of bicarbonate, which precipitates a nonanion gap metabolic acidosis.[48] Finally, rapid expansion of the extracellular fluid space with isotonic saline solutions that do not contain bicarbonate reduces plasma bicarbonate levels and causes a hyperchloremic or nonanion gap metabolic acidosis.[49] This effect is more likely to occur in children than in adults. Intravenous solutions such as 5 per cent dextrose in water, 0.9 per cent sodium chloride, or Ringer's lactate have low pH values (4.0, 5.0, 6.5, respectively); however, because these solutions are not buffered and have negligible free hydrogen ion available, they do not directly cause or worsen a metabolic acidosis.[50]

THERAPY

Treatment of the underlying disorder is paramount to correction of a metabolic acidosis. To properly assess this acid-base disturbance, the presence or absence of an anion gap should be determined, and a differential diagnosis based on this calculation should be established.

Therapy for a nonanion gap metabolic acidosis consists in replacing intravascular volume losses with a low chloride, bicarbonate-containing solution. Gastrointestinal losses of bicarbonate due to severe diarrhea or pancreatic or biliary drainage may be accomplished by adding sodium bicarbonate to 0.45 per cent saline (two ampuls of sodium bicarbonate when added to 1 liter of 0.45 per cent saline create a solution with a high bicarbonate, low chloride content and a sodium content similar to that of 0.9 per cent saline). A dilutional nonanion gap metabolic acidosis may be treated by utilizing hypotonic saline solutions when the patient is normovolemic or with a similar bicarbonate-containing solution as mentioned above when the patient is hypovolemic.

Although the treatment of certain anion gap metabolic acidoses is well established (e.g., insulin and intravenous fluids for diabetic ketoacidosis or dialysis for severe renal failure), the adjunctive therapy for other organic acidoses appears to be more controversial. This controversy centers primarily around the administration of sodium bicarbonate for the treatment of lactic acidosis. Based on experimental models, recommendations have been made to limit the use of sodium bicarbonate as a buffering agent for lactic acidosis, citing its minimal effect on correcting systemic pH and its potential for exacerbating the acidemia.[51] The American Heart Association has gone so far as to remove sodium bicarbonate from their treatment algorithms, recommending its use instead only when all other therapeutic modalities have failed.[52] Nonetheless, proponents of bicarbonate therapy for lactic acidosis continue to recommend its use based on the paucity of relevant clinical data.[53]

Arguments against the use of sodium bicarbonate include the following.

1. Due to sodium bicarbonate's high sodium content and high osmolality (2000 mOsm/L), excessive administration may cause severe hypernatremia and hyperosmolality, and therapy may predispose patients to

seizures or other neurologic sequelae.[6,52] Pulmonary and cerebral edema may also be precipitated by excessive administration primarily in patients with poor myocardial, renal, or cerebral function.[1,6]

2. A severe alkalemia may occur owing to excessive bicarbonate administration in the setting of excessive mechanical ventilation. It may lead to a pH high enough to precipitate dysrhythmias or generalized convulsions.[1,6]

3. Sodium bicarbonate administration may result in an increase in $\dot{V}CO_2$ not only because of the titration of bicarbonate by nonbicarbonate buffers to CO_2 but also because of the release of the dissolved fraction of CO_2 in an ampul of sodium bicarbonate (260 to 280 mm Hg). This situation may worsen the pH by adding a respiratory component to the systemic acidosis. A decrease in arterial pH occurs when $\dot{V}_E$ is impaired, and a venous acidosis may ensue when an impairment to pulmonary blood flow fails to deliver CO_2 to the lungs for elimination. This scenario is best exemplified during cardiopulmonary arrest, as is discussed further below.[24,54,55]

4. Lactic acid production may increase owing to the effect of bicarbonate in regard to enhancing the transformation of glucose and amino acids to lactic acid, thereby worsening the metabolic acidosis.[55]

5. Experimental studies fail to show improved survival when bicarbonate is used to treat lactic acidosis.[51]

Arguments for the continued use of $NaHCO_3$ include the following.

1. Careful titration of sodium bicarbonate prevents severe hyperosmolality and pulmonary edema.[1,6,53]

2. Titrating sodium bicarbonate to achieve a serum level of 12 to 15 mEq/L should avoid the complication of severe alkalemia. Based on Henderson's equation, an increase in plasma bicarbonate from 6 mEq/L to 12 mEq/L in a patient with a $PaCO_2$ of 20 mm Hg and pH 7.10 increases the pH to 7.30 despite a potential rise in the $PaCO_2$ to 25 to 27 mm Hg. An appropriate dose of sodium bicarbonate is best determined by calculating the desired increment of change in plasma bicarbonate, multiplying this change by the patient's weight in kilograms and by the volume of distribution of plasma bicarbonate. The volume of distribution depends on the pH, with a pH of 7.00 yielding a volume of distribution of bicarbonate at 80 per cent of total body weight,

whereas at a pH of 7.20 to 7.40 the volume of distribution ranges from approximately 50 to 40 per cent, respectively. Therefore at a pH of 7.10, a 70 kg patient requires approximately 210 mEq of bicarbonate to raise the plasma bicarbonate from 6 mEq/L to 12 mEq/L.

$$70 \text{ kg} \times 0.50 \text{ L/kg} \times 6 \text{ mEq/L} = 210 \text{ mEq}$$

This replacement should be done slowly, with half the dose given over 8 to 12 hours and the remainder over the next 12 to 24 hours.[1,6,53]

3. The increase in $\dot{V}CO_2$ that occurs during sodium bicarbonate administration is of little consequence in a patient who is able to maintain $\dot{V}_E$. However, when $\dot{V}_E$ is impaired or pulmonary blood flow is diminished, this issue may pose more of a problem when severe hypoperfusion or cardiopulmonary arrest is present.[24,52] In such states, CO_2 elimination is impaired not only at the pulmonary level but also at the tissue level. That small proportion of pulmonary blood flow that does deliver CO_2 to the lungs may be effectively eliminated provided ventilation is effective. $PaCO_2$ may therefore be normal. However, at the tissue level continued lactic acidosis and tissue hypercarbia may yield a "paradoxical" or mixed venous acidosis that persists until adequate pulmonary blood flow can improve delivery of CO_2 to the lungs. This mixed venous acidosis represents a tissue or intracellular acidosis that is considered to be the cause of myocardial depression in the setting of electromechanical dissociation. Intravenous infusions of sodium bicarbonate in the setting of poor pulmonary blood flow may therefore worsen the mixed venous acidosis by providing an additional CO_2 load.

4. Provided $\dot{V}_E$ is maintained, the lactic acid that may be generated with the use of sodium bicarbonate does not appear to be of major consequence.[53]

5. Finally, though few experimental studies suggest improved survival when treating lactic acidosis with bicarbonate, there are fewer clinical studies that support this contention.[53,55] At a pH less than 7.20, myocardial performance of a normal heart is usually not impaired owing to an increase in sympathetic stimulation. However, at a pH less than 7.10, severe hemodynamic compromises may occur; and therefore the careful titration of bicarbonate may improve cardiovascular responsiveness while other measures are instituted to correct the cause of the acidosis.[45,53]

On balance, it appears that bicarbonate is an effective buffer, provided the generated or released CO_2 can be eliminated from the tissues. Ensuring proper ventilation is a priority, and maintaining pulmonary blood flow is essential when using bicarbonate to support the patient who has severe lactic acidosis.

Other nonbicarbonate buffers have been utilized with some success for treating lactic acidosis. THAM (tromethamine, tris buffer) is a potent amine buffer that combines with carbonic acid and increases the amount of available bicarbonate.[56] Dichloroacetate reduces lactic acid by stimulating the enzyme pyruvate dehydrogenase, thereby catalyzing the oxidation of lactate to pyruvate.[57,58] Finally, Carbicarb, a combination of sodium carbonate and bicarbonate, is able to generate bicarbonate without elevating levels of $PaCO_2$.[59] All of these drugs offer the advantage of avoiding volume overload, hyperosmolality, and CO_2 loading; however, compelling clinical data to support the use of these new agents are not yet available.

GUIDELINES FOR ASSESSING AN ACID-BASE DISORDER

Successful interpretation of acid-base data requires a systematic approach to each disorder. In so doing, simple and complex abnormalities are detected, differential diagnoses established, and early and appropriate therapeutic intervention initiated. The following steps are offered as guidelines and apply to the clinical evaluation of all acid-base disorders.

1. Perform arterial or venous blood gas analyses (or both) in the proper clinical setting (e.g., apnea, agitation, profound hypotension). Most blood gas laboratories measure pH and $PaCO_2$ directly and calculate bicarbonate based on the Henderson or Henderson-Hasselbach equation; therefore if time permits, simultaneous plasma bicarbonate determination may be more accurate when checking for appropriate compensatory changes.

2. *Assess the pH.* Although pH levels between 7.35 and 7.45 may be considered "normal," for the interpretation of an acid-base disorder a pH of more than 7.40 is considered alkalemic and a pH less than 7.40 is considered acidemic.

3. Determine if the primary disorder is metabolic or respiratory. If the pH is 7.30, the patient has at least a metabolic or respiratory acidosis. If the bicarbonate level is less than 24 mEq/L, the primary disorder is a metabolic acidosis. If the $PaCO_2$ is more than 40 mm Hg, the primary disorder is a respiratory acidosis. (If the bicarbonate is less than 24 mEq/L and the $PaCO_2$ is more than 40 mm Hg, obviously metabolic and respiratory acidosis exists.)

4. Determine the magnitude of compensation based on one of the following "rules of thumb."

Disorder	Appropriate Compensation
Acute respiratory acidosis (pH < 7.40, $PaCO_2$ > 40 mm Hg)	$\frac{\Delta PaCO_2}{10} \pm 3 = \Delta [HCO_3^-]$
Acute respiratory alkalosis (pH > 7.40, $PaCO_2$ < 40 mm Hg)	$\frac{\Delta PaCO_2}{10} \times (1 - 3) = \Delta [HCO_3^-]$
Metabolic alkalosis (pH < 7.40, $[HCO_3^-]$ > 24 mEq/L)	$\Delta [HCO_3^-] \times (0.8) = \Delta PaCO_2$
Metabolic acidosis (pH < 7.40, $[HCO_3^-]$ < 24 mEq/L)	$\Delta [HCO_3^-] \times (1.2) = \Delta PaCO_2$

5. If compensation is not appropriate, determine the secondary problem. For example, a postoperative patient recovering from general anesthesia for major abdominal surgery has a pH of 7.20, a bicarbonate concentration of 18 mEq/L, and a $PaCO_2$ of 38 mm Hg in the PACU. This patient has an obvious acidosis; and because his bicarbonate concentration is less than 24 mEq/L, there must be a metabolic acidosis. However, the appropriate degree of hyperventilation for this degree of metabolic acidosis should be 6×1.2, or a fall in $PaCO_2$ of 7 mm Hg to a $PaCO_2$ of 33 mm Hg. Therefore this patient has an inappropriate respiratory response and appears to be hypoventilating relative to the severity of the metabolic acidosis. In other words, the patient has a primary metabolic acidosis *and* a secondary respiratory acidosis (even though the $PaCO_2$ is less than 40 mm Hg).

6. Check for the presence or absence of an anion gap.

7. Establish a differential diagnosis based on the acid-base disorder.

8. Initiate treatment when appropriate.

References

1. Cohen JJ, Kassirer JP: Acid Base. Boston, Little, Brown, 1982.
2. Kassirer JP, Bleich HL: Rapid estimation of plasma carbon dioxide from pH and total carbon dioxide content. N Engl J Med 272:1067, 1965.
3. Gronert GA, Theye RA: Halothane-induced porcine malignant hyperthermia: metabolic and hemodynamic changes. Anesthesiology 44:36, 1976.
4. West JB: Respiratory Physiology—the Essentials. Baltimore, Williams & Wilkins, 1985, pp. 15–17.
5. Pappenheimer JR, Fencl V, Heisey SR, Held D: Role of cerebral fluids in control of respiration as studied in unanesthetized goats. Am J Physiol 208:436, 1965.
6. Schrier RW: Renal and Electrolyte Disorders. Boston, Little, Brown, 1986.
7. Eisele JH, Eger EI II, Muallem M: Narcotic properties of carbon dioxide in the dog. Anesthesiology 28:856, 1967.
8. Dulfano MJ, Ishikawa S: Hypercapnia: mental changes and extrapulmonary complications: an expanded concept of the "CO₂ intoxication" syndrome. Ann Intern Med 63:829, 1965.
9. Price HL: Effects of carbon dioxide on the cardiovascular system. Anesthesiology 21:652, 1960.
10. Monroe RG, French G, Whittenberger JL: Effects of hypocapnia and hypercapnia on myocardial contractility. Am J Physiol 199:1121, 1960.
11. Jackson FN, Rowland V, Corssen G: Laryngospasm-induced pulmonary edema. Chest 78:819, 1980.
12. Weissman C, Damask MC, Yang J: Noncardiogenic pulmonary edema following laryngeal obstruction. Anesthesiology 60:163, 1984.
13. Appel D, Rubenstein, Schrager K, Williams MH: Lactic acidosis in severe asthma. Am J Med 75:580, 1983.
14. Larson CP, Eger EI II, Muallem M, et al: The effects of diethyl ether and methoxyflurane on ventilation. Anesthesiology 30:174, 1969.
15. Miller RD, Roderick L: The influence of acid-base changes on neostigmine antagonism of pancuronium neuromuscular blockade. Br J Anaesth 50:317, 1978.
16. Eisenkraft JB, Sawhney RK, Papatestas AE: Vecuronium in the myasthenic patient. Anaesthesia 40:848, 1985.
17. Flacke JW, Flacke WE, Williams GD: Acute pulmonary edema following naloxone reversal of high-dose morphine anesthesia. Anesthesiology 47:376, 1977.
18. Bracken MB, Shepard MJ, Collins WF, et al: A randomized controlled trial of methylprednisolone or naloxone in the treatment of acute spinal cord injury: results of the second national acute spinal cord injury study. N Engl J Med 322:1405, 1990.
19. Moser KM, Luchsinger PC, Adamson JS, et al: Respiratory stimulation with intravenous doxapram in respiratory failure. N Engl J Med 288:427, 1973.
20. Wangler MA, Kilpatrick DS: Aminophylline is an antagonist of lorazepam. Anesth Analg 64:834, 1985.
21. Spaulding BC, Choi SD, Gross JB, et al: The effect of physostigmine on diazepam-induced ventilatory depression: a double-blind study. Anesthesiology 61:551, 1984.
22. Haefely W: Pharmacology of benzodiazepine antagonists. Pharmacopsychiatry 18:163, 1985.
23. Ghoneim MM, Dembo JB, Block RI: Time course of antagonism of sedative and amnesic effects of diazepam by flumazenil. Anesthesiology 70:899, 1989.
24. Weil MH, Rackow EC, Trevino R, et al: Difference in acid-base state between venous and arterial blood during cardiopulmonary resuscitation. N Engl J Med 315:153, 1986.
25. Wasserman AJ, Patterson JL: The cerebral vascular response to reduction in arterial carbon dioxide tension. J Clin Invest 40:1297, 1961.
26. Gotoh F, Meyer JS, Takagi Y: Cerebral effects of hyperventilation in man. Arch Neurol 12:410, 1965.
27. Rowe GG, Castillo CA, Crumpton CW: Effects of hyperventilation on systemic and coronary hemodynamics. Am Heart J 63:67, 1962.
28. Ayres SM, Grace WJ: Inappropriate ventilation and hypoxemia as causes of cardiac arrhythmias. Am J Med 46:495, 1969.
29. Mostellar ME, Tuttle EP Jr: Effects of alkalosis on plasma concentration and urinary excretion of inorganic phosphate in man. J Clin Invest 43:138, 1964.
30. Singer RB: The acid-base disturbance in salicylate intoxication. Medicine (Baltimore) 33:1, 1954.
31. Hill JB: Salicylate intoxication. N Engl J Med 288:1110, 1973.
32. Winslow EJ, Loeb HS, Rahimtoola SH, et al: Hemodynamic studies and results of therapy in 50 patients with bacteremic shock. Am J Med 54:421, 1973.
33. Ropper AH: Raised intracranial pressure in neurologic disease. Semin Neurol 4:397, 1984.
34. Mazzara JT, Ayres SM, Grace WJ: Extreme hypocapnia with critically ill patients. Am J Med 56:450, 1974.
35. Bosch JP, Goldstein MH, Levitt MF, et al: Effect of chronic furosemide administration on hydrogen and sodium excretion in the dog. Am J Physiol 232:F397, 1977.
36. Schwartz WB, Hays RM, Polak A, et al: Effects of chronic hypercapnia on electrolyte and acid-base equilibrium. I. Adaptation. J Clin Invest 40:1223, 1961.
37. Litwin MS, Smith LL, Moore FD: Metabolic alkalosis following massive transfusion. Surgery 45:805, 1959.
38. Barton CH, Vaziri ND, Ness RL, et al: Cimetidene in the management of metabolic alkalosis induced by nasogastric drainage. Arch Surg 114:70, 1979.
39. Williams DB, Lyons JH Jr: Treatment of severe metabolic alkalosis with intravenous infusion of hydrochloric acid. Surg Gynecol Obstet 150:315, 1980.
40. Miller PD, Berns AS: Acute metabolic alkalosis perpetuating hypercarbia: a role for acetazolamide in chronic obstructive pulmonary disease. JAMA 238:2400, 1977.
41. Khan MI: Treatment of refractory congestive heart failure and normokalemic hypochloremic metabolic alkalosis with acetazolamide and spironolactone. Can Med Assoc J 123:883, 1980.
42. Oh MS, Carroll HJ: Current concepts: the anion gap. N Engl J Med 297:814, 1977.
43. Astrup P, Jorgensen K, Siggaard-Anderson O, Engel K: Acid base metabolism: new approach. Lancet 1:1035, 1960.

44. Schwartz WB, Relman AS: A critique of the parameters used in the evaluation of acid-base disorders: "whole-blood buffer base" and "standard bicarbonate" compared with blood pH and plasma bicarbonate concentration. N Engl J Med 268:1382, 1963.

45. Mitchell JH, Wildenthal K, Johnson RL Jr: The effects of acid-base disturbances on cardiovascular and pulmonary function. Kidney Int 1:375, 1972.

46. Gerst PH, Fleming WH, Malm JR: Increased susceptibility of the heart to ventricular fibrillation during metabolic acidosis. Circ Res 19:63, 1966.

47. Kerber RE, Pandian NE, Hoyt R, et al: Effect of ischemia, hypertrophy, hypoxia, acidosis and alkalosis on canine defibrillation. Am J Physiol 244:H825, 1983.

48. McConnell JB, Murison J, Stewart WK: The role of the cation in the pathogenesis of hyperchloraemic acidosis in ureterosigmoid anastamosis. Clin Sci 57:305, 1979.

49. Garella S, Chang BS, Kahn SI: Dilutional acidosis and contraction alkalosis: review of a concept. Kidney Int 8:279, 1975.

50. Lebowitz MH, Masuda JY, Beckerman JH: The pH and acidity of intravenous infusion solutions. JAMA 215:1937, 1971.

51. Stacpoole PW: Lactic acidosis: the case against bicarbonate therapy. Ann Intern Med 105:276, 1986 (editorial).

52. Standards and guidelines for cardiopulmonary resuscitation (CPR) and emergency cardiac care (ECC). JAMA 255:2905, 1986.

53. Narins RG, Cohen JJ: Bicarbonate therapy for organic acidosis: the case for its continued use. Ann Intern Med 106:615, 1987.

54. Adrogue HJ, Rashad N, Gorin AB, et al: Assessing acid-base status in circulatory failure: differences between arterial and central venous blood. N Engl J Med 320:1312, 1989.

55. Hindman BJ: Sodium bicarbonate in the treatment of subtypes of acute lactic acidosis: physiologic considerations. Anesthesiology 72:1064, 1990.

56. Rothe KF, Diedler J: Comparison of intra- and extracellular buffering of clinically used buffer substances: tris and bicarbonate. Acta Anaesthesiol Scand 26:194, 1982.

57. Stacpoole PW, Harman EM, Curry SH, et al: Treatment of lactic acidosis with dichloroacetate. N Engl J Med 309:390, 1983.

58. Stacpoole PW, Lorenz AC, Thomas RG, Harman EM: Dichloroacetate in the treatment of lactic acidosis. Ann Intern Med 108:58, 1988.

59. Sun JH, Filley GF, Hard K, et al: Carbicarb: an effective substitute for NaHCO$_3$ for the treatment of acidosis. Surgery 102:835, 1987.

RESPIRATORY CARE: Oxygenation, Bronchial Hygiene, and Mechanical Ventilation

7

WILLIAM T. PERUZZI and JEFFERY S. VENDER

DISORDERS OF OXYGENATION

Hypoxemia can be defined as a relative deficiency of oxygen tension in the arterial blood. Hypoxia exists when there are inadequate cellular oxygen tensions. Distinguishing the terms is important because either one may exist without the other. For example, it is not uncommon for a patient with chronic or acute lung disease to have an arterial oxygen tension (PaO_2) of 65 mm Hg. This value clearly represents hypoxemia; however, in the absence of dyspnea, acidosis, and cardiac arrhythmias, there is no evidence of tissue oxygen deprivation; thus the patient is *not* hypoxic. Conversely, a patient with a PaO_2 of more than 90 mm Hg, normal hemoglobin concentration, cardiac index of 1.5, hypotension, and metabolic acidosis is demonstrating hypoxia resulting from decreased oxygen delivery (cardiac output × arterial oxygen content) and poor tissue perfusion; the patient, however, is *not* hypoxemic.

There are basically only two mechanisms by which arterial hypoxemia can result from pulmonary processes: 1) *shunt effect* (decreased alveolar oxygen tensions); and 2) *true shunting* (blood passing from the right side of the heart to the left side of the heart without undergoing alveolar gas exchange). Shunt effect is characterized by decreased alveolar oxygen tension (PaO_2) due to uneven distribution of alveolar ventilation with respect to alveolar perfusion. This ventilation–perfusion (V/Q) mismatch can result from retained bronchial secretions, bronchospasm, obstructive endobronchial lesions, chronic obstructive pulmonary disease, mild pulmonary edema, or other pulmonary pathology. The hallmark of hypoxemia due to shunt effect is that it is responsive to oxygen therapy. To determine oxygen responsiveness an appropriate oxygen challenge[1] must be given. If, at sea level, the fraction of inspired oxygen (FIO_2) is increased by 0.2 (i.e., from 0.21 to 0.40, or from 0.3 to 0.5) the PaO_2 of all ventilated alveoli should increase by 90 to 100 mm Hg. Subsequently, the PaO_2 increases by significantly more than 10 mm Hg if less than 15 per cent true shunt is present; however, it increases by significantly less than 10 mm Hg if more than 30 per cent true shunt exists. This principle aids in differentiating true shunt pathology from shunt effect.

True shunt can result from several pathologic conditions: intracardiac shunt; alveolar collapse as occurs with acute lung injury; pulmonary consolidation associated with lung infections; segmental or lobar lung collapse due to retained secretions or other lung pathology; pulmonary arteriovenous malformations as sometimes seen with severe liver disease; and large vascular lung tumors. Oxygen therapy is of limited benefit with significantly increased true shunt. The reason for this is that, regardless of the FIO_2 or PaO_2, oxygen transfer cannot occur when blood does not come into contact with functional alveolar units. Therefore true shunt pathology is refractory to oxygen therapy. There is little or no available therapy for several types of pathology resulting in true shunt, whereas antibiotics or surgical intervention may help other types of true shunt that produce disease. The type of lung pathology most responsive to therapy is that involving diffuse or focal lung collapse. Segmental or lobar lung collapse can often be reversed with appropriate bronchial hygiene or removal of the source of obstruction. Diffuse alveolar collapse often results from destabilization of the alveolar architecture due to disruption of the surfactant layer and alveolar epithelial damage associated with acute lung injury (ALI).[2,3] This type of pathology is responsive to positive end-expiratory pressure (PEEP).[4] PEEP levels of 5 to 10 cm H_2O increase alveolar size and redistribute interstitial lung water from the interstitial regions between the alveolar epithelium and pulmonary capillary endothelium to the more areolar peribronchial and hilar regions of the lung.[5,6] PEEP levels of 15 cm H_2O and more no longer increase alveolar size; rather, these levels of PEEP ''recruit'' nonfunctional collapsed alveoli to expanded and functional alveolar units.[7,8]

OXYGEN THERAPY

When dealing with lung pathology amenable to oxygen therapy, the indications for such therapy and the available methods of oxygen administration must be considered. The physiologic responses to hypoxemia and hypoxia must be appreciated in order to understand the indications for oxygen therapy. First, there is an increase in minute ventilation, which increases alveolar ventilation and the work of breathing. Second, there is an increase in cardiac output, which maintains oxygen delivery in the face of decreased oxygen content and increases the stress placed on the cardiovascular system. Therefore the goals of oxygen therapy are to improve oxygen content and subsequently decrease the work of breathing and myocardial stress.

Arterial oxygen content (CaO_2) is determined by the concentration of hemoglobin (Hb) in the blood, the percentage of the Hb that is saturated with oxygen (SaO_2), and the amount of oxygen dissolved in the plasma.

$$CaO_2 = [Hb]\cdot[\%SaO_2]\cdot[1.34] + [PaO_2]\cdot[0.003]$$

It should be obvious that the primary determinant of oxygen content is the hemoglobin concentration (grams per deciliter) and the degree of hemoglobin saturation (expressed as a decimal). At atmospheric pressure the amount of oxygen dissolved in the plasma ($[PaO_2]\cdot[0.003]$) is usually negligible.

OXYGEN DELIVERY SYSTEMS

There are three basic types of gas delivery systems: rebreathing systems, nonrebreathing systems, and partial rebreathing systems. *Rebreathing systems* collect exhaled gases into a reservoir on the expiratory limb of the system, which contains a carbon dioxide absorber. This system permits reentry of expiratory gases into the inspiratory gas flow without rebreathing of carbon dioxide. The system has been used primarily for the delivery of anesthetic gases to conserve expensive volatile anesthetics.

Most oxygen delivery systems are *nonrebreathing systems* in that all expiratory gases are vented in such a fashion that exhaled carbon dioxide is not rebreathed during subsequent breaths. It is often accomplished with one-way valves to prevent mixing of inspired and expired gases.

A *partial rebreathing system* is one in which the initial portion of the expired gases, consisting mainly of gas from the anatomic deadspace, is expired into a reservoir while the latter portions of the expiratory gases are vented to the atmosphere through one-way valves. The expiratory gases from the anatomic deadspace contain little carbon dioxide and therefore can be rebreathed without significant consequences. The reservoir also receives fresh inspiratory gas flow; thus the patient breathes both expiratory gas, containing little carbon dioxide, and fresh inspiratory gas—hence the term partial rebreathing system.

Nonrebreathing systems are further divided into high flow (fixed performance) and low flow (variable performance) systems. A *high flow system* means that the inspiratory gas flow rate delivered by the system is sufficient to meet the peak inspiratory flow demands of the patient. Thus all inspiratory gas is supplied by the oxygen delivery system, and the FIO_2 is both known and stable. To accomplish this goal the inspiratory gas flows must be three to four times the measured minute ventilation.[9,10] High flow oxygen delivery systems are indicated whenever there is a need for a consistent and predictable FIO_2, especially in patients with unstable ventilatory patterns.

Conversely, a *low flow system* delivers a fixed amount of oxygen to the patient, and entrainment of room air is necessary to meet the patient's peak inspiratory flow rates. In this circumstance the FIO_2 is variable and unpredictable if the patient has an abnormal or changing pattern of ventilation. If the patient has a stable, normal pattern of ventilation, however, low flow oxygen delivery systems can deliver a predictable and consistent FIO_2 (Table 7–1).

TABLE 7–1. LOW FLOW OXYGEN DELIVERY DEVICES, FLOW RATES, AND FiO₂

Oxygen Flow Rates (L)	FiO₂
Nasal cannula	
1	0.24
2	0.28
3	0.32
4	0.36
5	0.40
6	0.44
Simple face mask	
5–6	0.40
6–7	0.50
7–8	0.60
Partial rebreathing mask	
6	0.60
7	0.70
8	0.80
9	0.80+
10	0.80+
Nonrebreathing mask	
10	0.80+
15	0.90+

Predicted FiO₂ values for low flow systems assume a normal and stable pattern of ventilation.

TABLE 7–2. VARIABILITY IN FiO₂ WITH LOW FLOW O₂ DELIVERY SYSTEMS AND VARIABLE PATTERNS OF VENTILATION

Parameter	$V_t = 500$ cc	$V_t = 250$ cc
Anatomic reservoir	50 cc O_2	50 cc O_2
Inspiratory phase (1 second)	100 cc O_2	100 cc O_2
Entrained room air	350 cc	100 cc
Oxygen from entrained room air (21% oxygen)	70 cc O_2	20 cc O_2
Total volume O_2/V_t	220/500 cc	170/250 cc
FiO₂	0.44	0.68

Low flow oxygen devices are the most commonly employed oxygen delivery systems because of their simplicity, ease of use, familiarity, economics, and patient acceptance. In most clinical situations these systems are acceptable and even preferable.

Low Flow Systems

Nasal Cannula. The nasal cannula is the most frequently used oxygen delivery device because of its simplicity, ease of use, and comfort. To be effective the nasal passages must be patent to allow filling of the anatomic reservoir; however, the patient does not need to breathe through the nose. Oxygen is entrained from the anatomic reservoir even in the presence of mouth breathing. If the oxygen flow rate exceeds 4 L/min, the gases should be humidified to prevent drying of the nasal mucosa.[11] Flows of more than 6 L/min do not significantly increase FiO₂ more than 0.44 and are often poorly tolerated by the patient.

Simple Face Mask. A simple face mask consists of a mask with two side ports. The mask provides an additional 100 to 200 cc oxygen reservoir and a higher FiO₂ than does a nasal cannula. There are open side ports in the sides of the mask to allow entrainment of room air and venting of exhaled gases. A minimum flow of 5 L/min is necessary to prevent carbon dioxide accumulation and rebreathing. Flow rates of more than 8 L/min do not increase the FiO₂ significantly more than 0.6.

Partial Rebreathing Mask. A partial rebreathing mask is similar in construction to the simple face mask, but it also incorporates a 600- to 1000-ml reservoir bag into which

It must be understood that use of a low-flow oxygen delivery system does not imply delivery of low oxygen concentrations. For example, it is possible to calculate the FiO₂ for a low flow system, e.g., a nasal cannula, if certain assumptions are made: 1) the anatomic reservoir (nose, naropharynx, and oropharynx) comprises approximately one third of the anatomic deadspace (total ~150 cc) and so is approximately 50 cc; 2) oxygen is being delivered at a rate of 6 L/min (100 ml/s) via the nasal cannula; 3) the patient's respiratory rate of 20 breaths/min results in a 1 second inspiratory phase and a 2 second expiratory phase; 4) there is negligible gas flow during the terminal 0.5 second of the expiratory phase, thereby allowing the anatomic reservoir to fill completely with oxygen. Using the above assumptions the FiO₂ can be calculated for variable tidal volumes (V_t) as outlined in Table 7–2.

This variability in FiO₂ at 6 L/min oxygen flow clearly demonstrates the effects of a variable ventilatory pattern on FiO₂. In general, the larger the V_t or the faster the respiratory rate, the lower the FiO₂; and the smaller the V_t or lower the respiratory rate, the higher the FiO₂. With a stable, unchanging ventilatory pattern and oxygen flow rate, low flow systems can deliver a relatively consistent FiO₂.

fresh gas flows. The first one third of the patient's exhaled gas fills the reservoir bag. Because this gas is primarily from anatomic deadspace, it contains little carbon dioxide. With the next breath, the patient inhales a mixture of the exhaled gas and fresh gas. If the fresh gas flows are 8 L/min or more and the reservoir bag remains inflated throughout the entire respiratory cycle, adequate carbon dioxide evacuation and the highest possible FIO_2 should occur. The rebreathing capacity of this system allows some degree of oxygen conservation, which may be useful during transportation with portable oxygen supplies.

Nonrebreathing Mask. A nonrebreathing mask is similar to a partial rebreathing mask but with the addition of three unidirectional valves. Two of the valves are located on opposite sides of the mask. They permit venting of exhaled gas and prevent entrainment of room air. The remaining unidirectional valve is located between the mask and the reservoir bag and prevents exhaled gases from entering the fresh gas reservoir. As with the partial rebreathing mask, the reservoir bag should be inflated throughout the entire ventilatory cycle to ensure adequate carbon dioxide clearance from the system and the highest possible FIO_2.

To avoid air entrainment around the mask and diluton of the delivered FIO_2, masks should fit snugly on the face but should avoid excessive pressure. If the mask is fitted properly, the reservoir bag should respond to the patient's inspiratory efforts. Unfortunately, if fresh gas flows and the volume of the reservoir bag are insufficient to meet inspiratory demands, the patient could be compromised. Therefore, masks may be fitted with a spring-loaded tension valve that opens and allows entrainment of room air as needed to meet inspiratory demands. If such a valve is not present, another option is to remove one of the unidirectional valves that prevent room air entrainment. If the total ventilatory needs of the patient are met by the nonrebreathing system, it functions as a high flow system. If room air entrainment occurs, a low flow system is operating.

Tracheostomy Collars. Tracheostomy collars are used primarily to deliver humidity to patients with artificial airways. Oxygen may be delivered with these devices; but, similar to other low flow systems, the FIO_2 is unpredictable, inconsistent, and depends on the ventilatory pattern.

High Flow Systems

Venturi Mask. The Venturi mask entrains air using the Bernoulli principle and constant pressure-jet mixing.[12] This physical phenomenon is based on a rapid velocity of gas (e.g., oxygen) moving through a restricted orifice, which produces viscous shearing forces, in turn creating a subatmospheric pressure gradient downstream relative to the surrounding gases. This pressure gradient causes room air to be entrained until the pressures are equalized. In this manner, flows high enough to meet peak inspiratory demands of the patient can be generated. As the desired FIO_2 increases, the air/oxygen entrainment ratio decreases with a net reduction in total gas flow. Therefore the probability of the patient's needs exceeding the total flow capabilities of the device increases with higher FIO_2 settings. Occlusion of or impingement on the exhalation ports of the mask can cause backpressure and alter gas flow ("Venturi stall"). In addition, the oxygen injector port can become clogged, especially with water droplets. Therefore aerosol devices should not be used with these devices; if humidity is necessary, a vapor-type humidity adaptor collar can be used.

There are two basic types of Venturi system: 1) a fixed FIO_2 model that requires specific color-coded inspiratory attachments with labeled jets that produce a known FIO_2 with a given flow; and 2) a variable-FIO_2 model, which has a graded adjustments of the air entrainment port that can be set to allow variation in delivered FIO_2.

Aerosol Mask and T-Piece. An FIO_2 of more than 0.40 with a high flow system is best provided with a large volume nebulizer and wide bore tubing. Aerosol masks, in conjunction with air entrainment nebulizers or air/oxygen blenders, can deliver a consistent and predictable FIO_2 regardless of the patient's ventilatory pattern. A T-piece is used in place of an aerosol mask for patients with an endotracheal or tracheostomy tube.

An air entrainment nebulizer can deliver an FIO_2 of 0.35 to 1.00, produce an aerosol, and generate flow rates of 14 to 16 L/mn. As with Venturi masks, a higher FIO_2 results in less room air entrainment and lower flow rates. Should a greater total flow be required, two nebulizers can feed a single mask and increase the total flow.

Air/oxygen blenders can deliver a consistent FIO_2 in the range of 0.21 to 1.00 with flows up to 100 L/min. These devices are usually used in conjunction with humidifiers.

Humidification

The administration of dry oxygen lowers the water content of the inspired air. The use of an artificial airway bypasses the nasopharynx and oropharynx, where a significant amount of warming and humidification of inspired gases takes place. As a result, oxygen administration and the use of artificial airways increase the demand on the lung to humidify the inspired gases, ultimately leading to drying of the tracheal and bronchial mucosa, decreased mucociliary clearance, and inspissated secretions. To prevent these complications, a humidifier or nebulizer should be used to increase the water content of the inspired gases.

A humidifier increases the water vapor in a gas, which can be accomplished in several ways: passing gas over heated water (heated passover humidifier); fractionating gas into tiny bubbles as gas passes through water (bubble humidifiers); allowing gas to pass through a chamber that contains a heated, water-saturated wick (heated wick humidifier); or vaporizing water and selectively allowing the vapor to mix with the inspired gases (vapor phase humidifier).

A nebulizer increases the water content of the inspired gas by generating aerosols (small droplets of particulate water) of uniform size that become incorporated into the delivered gas stream and then evaporate into the inspired gas as it is warmed in the respiratory tract. There are two basic types of nebulizer. Pneumatic nebulizers operate from a pressurized gas source and are either jet or hydronomic. Electrical nebulizers are powered by an electrical source and are referred to as "ultrasonic." There are several varieties of the above nebulizers that are more dependent on design differences than on the power source.

COMPLICATIONS OF OXYGEN THERAPY

Absorption Atelectasis

Absorption atelectasis occurs when high alveolar oxygen concentrations cause alveolar collapse. Nitrogen, already at equilibrium, remains within the alveoli and "splints" alveoli open. When a high FIO_2 is administered, nitrogen is "washed out" of the alveoli and the alveoli are filled primarily with oxygen. In areas of the lung with reduced V/Q ratios, oxygen is absorbed into the blood faster than ventilation can replace it. The affected alveoli then become progressively smaller until they reach the critical volume at which surface tension forces cause alveolar collapse. This phenomenon is precipitated primarily by the administration of an FIO_2 of more than 0.5.[13]

Oxygen Toxicity

High inspired oxygen concentrations can be injurious to the lungs. The mechanism of oxygen toxicity is related to a significantly higher production rate of oxygen free radicals such as superoxide anions (O_2^-), hydroxyl radicals (OH^-), hydrogen peroxide (H_2O_2), and singlet oxygen (O'). These radicals affect cell function by inactivating sulfhydryl enzymes, interfering with DNA synthesis, and disrupting the integrity of cell membranes. During periods of lung tissue hyperoxia the normal oxygen radical scavenging mechanisms are overwhelmed and toxicity results.[14]

The FIO_2 at which oxygen toxicity becomes important is controversial and variable depending on animal species, degree of underlying lung injury, ambient barometric pressure, and duration of exposure. In general, it is best to avoid exposure of an FIO_2 of more than 0.5 for more than 24 hours.

BRONCHIAL HYGIENE

Bronchial hygiene is useful and effective when the patient is carefully evaluated, the goals of therapy are clearly defined, and the appropriate modalities are applied. Prophylactic bronchial hygiene therapy is administered to patients who are essentially free of acute pulmonary pathology with the intention of preventing inadequate bronchial hygiene. Therapeutic bronchial hygiene therapy is aimed at the reversal of preexisting inadequate bronchial hygiene, specifically the mobilization of retained secretions and the reinflation of atelectatic lung regions.

INCENTIVE SPIROMETRY

The incentive spirometer is an effective and inexpensive prophylactic bronchial hygiene tool. This device provides a visual goal or "incentive" for the patient to achieve and sustain a maximal inspiratory effort. When performed on an hourly basis, this modality provides optimal lung inflation, distribution of ventilation, and an improved cough. Thus atelectasis and the retention of bronchial secretions are prevented. Incentive spirometry can also be helpful in the diagnosis of acute pulmonary pathology in that a sudden decrease in the ability of a patient to perform at a previously established level may herald the onset of severe atelectasis, pneumonia, or other pulmonary pathology. For incentive spirometry to be effective the patient must be cooperative, motivated, and well instructed in the technique (by the respiratory therapist, nurse, or physician); a vital capacity of more than 14 ml/kg or an inspiratory capacity of more than 12 ml/kg should be obtainable; and the patient should not be tachypneic or on a high FIO_2.

SUCTIONING

Removal of bronchial secretions via suction is a commonly employed bronchial hygiene technique. Performed appropriately, this procedure is safe and effective. Performed without appropriate caution, it can result in significant complications or death.

Airway suctioning can be accomplished safely in patients with artificial airways (endotracheal or tracheostomy tubes) in place. In this circumstance, the patient should be ventilated with a manual resuscitation bag providing a high FIO_2 ("preoxygenation"). This practice minimizes the hypoxemia induced by removing the patient from an oxygen source and the application of suction to the airways. A sterile suction catheter should then be placed into the airway and advanced, without application of a vacuum, beyond the tip of the artificial airway until it can no longer be easily advanced. The catheter should then be withdrawn slightly before suction is applied. Suctioning is accomplished by intermittent application of a vacuum and gradual withdrawal of the catheter in a rotating fashion. The duration of the entire procedure should not exceed 20 seconds. After completion of suctioning the patient should be manually ventilated with an oxygen-enriched atmosphere to ensure adequate lung reexpansion and oxygenation. The patient should be monitored for signs of distress, bronchospasm, hemodynamic instability, or arrhythmias throughout the entire procedure.

Suctioning of the tracheobronchial tree without an artificial airway in place (i.e., naso-tracheal suctioning) carries several risks. Because the patient cannot be manually ventilated and "preoxygenated" prior to the procedure, hypoxemia and hemodynamically significant arrhythmias can occur.[15,16] In addition, passing the suction catheter through the vocal cords can result in laryngospasm or vocal cord injury with subsequent airway obstruction. Because of these concerns, suctioning the tracheobronchial tree in the absence of an artificial airway cannot be recommended.

Tracheobronchial tree suctioning should be undertaken only in the presence of appropriate indications. The primary indication is the presence of bronchial secretions that can be identified visually or on auscultation. Rising airway pressures in mechanically ventilated patients may also indicate the presence of retained bronchial secretions. Mucosal irritation, trauma, and bleeding can be precipitated by frequent and aggressive suctioning in the absence of bronchial secretions. "Routine" suctioning of the airway should be discouraged except in neonates where small airway diameters can be acutely obstructed by a small accumulation of secretions.

HUMIDIFICATION

Air inspired through the nose is warmed and nearly 90 per cent humidified by the time it passes through the pharynx. This humidification process is bypassed in patients with artificial airways in place. If adequate humidification of inspired gases is not provided prior to gas entry into the trachea, the deficit of humidity is provided by moisture from the mucous blanket of the tracheobronchial tree. This action results in drying of the tracheobronchial tree, ciliary dysfunction, impairment of mucous transport, inflammation and necrosis of the ciliated pulmonary epithelium, retention of dried secretions, atelectasis, bacterial infiltration of the pulmonary mucosa, and pneumonia. Inspired gases must always be humidified for patients with artificial airways in place.

AEROSOL THERAPY

An aerosol is a suspension of fine particles of a liquid in a gas. Aerosols have three basic applications in respiratory care: 1) as an aid to bronchial hygiene; 2) for humidifying inspiratory gases; and 3) for delivering medications.

When dealing with medical aerosols for inhalation, the particle size is important. Particle size should be 3 μm or less in order for gravitational effects to be sufficiently small to permit deposition in the pulmonary tree.

When used as an aid to bronchial hygiene, water is one of the most important physically active agents. Aerosol therapy can be useful for the hydration of dried, retained secretions and the restoration and maintenance of the mucous blanket. In conjunction with appropriate cough mechanisms and other bronchial hygiene techniques, aerosol therapy permits mobilization of retained secretions. Care must be taken, however, because aerosols used for these purposes can result in clinical deterioration due to either increased airway resistance (bronchospasm) or swelling and expansion of dried secretions, with worsening hypoxemia. These detrimental effects can be ameliorated by the administration of a bronchodilator, techniques to mobilize the expanding secretions, or both.

The delivery of medications for the reversal and prevention of bronchoconstriction is an important application of aerosol therapy. Table 7–3 lists the names, dosages, mechanisms of action, and so on for the most commonly used aerosolized pharmacologic agents.

CHEST PHYSICAL THERAPY

Chest physical therapy (CPT) techniques can be classified into those that promote bronchial hygiene, improve breathing efficiency, or promote physical reconditioning. The CPT techniques considered here are those concerned with bronchial hygiene.

Postural drainage is a technique that utilizes different body positions to facilitate gravitational drainage of mucus from various lung segments. Diseases amenable to postural drainage therapy include cystic fibrosis, bronchiectasis, chronic obstructive pulmonary disease, acute atelectasis, and lung abscess. In hospitalized patients the basilar lung regions often benefit from postural drainage because most hospital bed positions do not permit adequate drainage of these segments. When dealing with postural drainage of unilateral lung disease, it is best to follow it with drainage of the contralateral lung because cross-contamination of the nondiseased lung is always a possibility. It is important to avoid inappropriate positioning during postural drainage. Patients with increased intracranial pressure or congestive heart failure may not tolerate head-down positioning to facilitate drainage of the basilar lung segments. Also, it is important to avoid direct pressure on sites of injury, surgery, or burns.

Chest percussion and vibration are techniques used to loosen and mobilize secretions adherent to bronchial walls.[17] When used in conjunction with appropriate postural drainage and coughing techniques, they can facilitate bronchial hygiene efforts significantly. Chest percussion is performed by rhythmic "clapping" with cupped hands over the lung areas in question. This action generates a mechanical energy wave that is transmitted through the chest wall to the lung tissue and loosens adherent mucus. Chest vibration is accomplished by placing the hands on the chest wall and generating a rapid vibratory motion in the arms, from the shoulders, and gently compressing the chest wall in the direction that the ribs normally move during exhalation.[18] It is most effective when performed during exhalation. Relative contraindications to these techniques include fractured ribs, "fragile bones" (i.e., osteoporosis), coagulopathies, and undrained empyema.

INTERMITTENT POSITIVE PRESSURE BREATHING

Intermittent positive pressure breathing (IPPB) is the application of inspiratory positive pressure to the airway in order to provide a significantly larger tidal volume, with a physiologically advantageous inspiratory to expiratory pattern, than the patient can produce spontaneously. It should not be confused with positive pressure ventilation delivered with a mechanical ventilator that is intended to provide ventilatory support. IPPB is useful for disease states in which the patient's depth of breathing is limited. Because it is expensive, this mode of therapy is indicated only when the patient's vital capacity (VC) is less than 15 cc/kg; the IPPB treatment should augment it by at least 100 per cent.

MECHANICAL VENTILATORY SUPPORT

The need for mechanical ventilatory support arises when the patient's cardiopulmonary reserves are overwhelmed or compro-

TABLE 7-3. AEROSOLIZED BRONCHODILATORS AND ANTIASTHMATIC DRUGS

Drug	Method	Dosages[a]	Frequency	Duration of Action (hr)	Effects	Mechanism
Sympathomimetics						
Isoetharine hydrochloride 1% (Bronkosol)	Nebulized MDI[b]	0.25–0.50 ml in 4.0 cc 2 puffs (10 mg/puff)	q2–4h	1.5–3.0	Bronchodilation, tachycardia	β_2-Agonist increase in cAMP
Metaproterenol sulfate 5% (Alupent)	Nebulized MDI	0.3 ml in 4.0 cc 2 puffs (0.65 mg/puff)	q4–6h or qid	≤5	Bronchodilation	β_2-Agonist increase in cAMP
Albuterol (Ventolin, Proventil)	MDI Nebulized	2 puffs (90 μg/puff) 2.5–5.0 mg in 4 cc	q4–6h or qid	≤6	Bronchodilation	β_2-Agonist increase in cAMP
Racemic epinephrine 2.25%	Nebulized	0.5 ml in 3.5 cc	q1h, prn	<1	Mucosal decongestion	Weak β_2 and mild α mucosal vasoconstrictor
Isoproterenol (.5%)	Nebulized	0.25–0.50 mg in 3.5 ml	q2–4h	1.5–2.0	Bronchodilation, tachycardia, vasodilation, flushing	Prototype β-agonist; significant β_1 side effects
Anticholinergic drugs						
Ipratroprium bromide (Atrovent)	MDI	2 puffs (18 μg/puff)	q4h or qid	3–4	Bronchodilation	Cholinergic blocker increasing β stimulation
Antiallergy agents						
Cromolyn sodium 1% (Intel)	Nebulized MDI	20 mg in 2–4 cc 2 puffs (1 mg/puff)	q6h or qid	6	Stabilization of mast cell membranes	Suppression of mast cell response to Ag-Ab reactions; used prophylactically.
Beclomethasone acetonide (Vanceril, Beclovent)	MDI	2 puffs (42 μg/puff)	q6h or qid	6	Antiinflammatory	Antiinflammatory; inhibit leukocyte migration; potentiate effects of β-agonists
Dexamethasone sodium phosphate (Decadron)	Nebulized	0.25 ml (1 mg) in 2.5 cc	q6h	6	Antiinflammatory	Antiinflammatory; inhibit leukocyte migration; potentiate effects of β-agonists

Ag-Ab = antigen-antibody.
[a] Dosages may vary. References to specific drug inserts are recommended.
[b] MDI = metered dose inhaler.

mised by a pathologic situation. In these circumstances either the ventilatory mechanism is rendered ineffectual, or the work of breathing becomes detrimental to the patient's physiologic homeostasis and respiratory muscle fatigue develops. In either event, mechanical ventilatory support permits the clinician to support the patient while the underlying pathologic process is being reversed. Although an artificial airway (endotracheal tube or tracheostomy tube) is required whenever mechanical ventilation is to be undertaken, it must be noted that the indications for artificial airways and for mechanical ventilatory support are not the same.

INDICATIONS

Artificial Airways

An artificial airway (endotracheal tube or tracheostomy) is indicated in the presence of four basic clinical situations: 1) upper airway obstruction; 2) loss or impairment of airway protective reflexes; 3) the inability to maintain clearance of bronchial secretions; and 4) the need for mechanical ventilatory support. Some include hypoxemia/hypoxia as an indication for an artificial airway, but there are many ways to establish adequate oxygenation without intubation or tracheostomy. Additionally, the presence of an artificial airway does not mandate the need for mechanical ventilatory support.

Mechanical Ventilation

There are four basic clinical indications for mechanical ventilatory support: 1) apnea; 2) acute ventilatory failure; 3) impending ventilatory failure; and 4) hyperventilation for intracranial pressure (ICP) control. *Apnea* can occur in a variety of clinical situations. It is often related to prescribed or illicit drug administration, e.g., narcotics or neuromuscular blocking agents. It can also occur with certain types of central nervous system (CNS) injury or profound cardiovascular instability. *Acute ventilatory failure* is a diagnosis based on arterial blood gas analysis demonstrating an acute rise in $PaCO_2$ and an acute fall in pH.[19] This circumstance indicates that, for whatever reason, the patient is incapable of spontaneously maintaining normal carbon dioxide homeostasis. If the situation is not corrected or the patient is not appropriately supported, the pro-

cess can be expected to progress eventually to death. *Impending ventilatory failure* is a clinical diagnosis made independent of arterial blood gas analysis. In this circumstance the clinician is making the assessment that the patient's clinical presentation is consistent with significantly increased work of breathing (WOB)—exceeding the patient's cardiopulmonary reserves and detrimental to the physiologic homeostasis. If left unabated, this condition eventually progresses to respiratory muscle fatigue and acute ventilatory failure. Clinical signs of detrimental WOB include tachypnea, dyspnea, intercostal retractions, use of accessory muscles of ventilation, tachycardia, hypertension, and diaphoresis.

Hyperventilation for ICP control is included here because, although many patients with CNS injuries hyperventilate spontaneously, mechanical ventilation is the only way to ensure consistent maintenance of a desired $PaCO_2$.

PRINCIPLES OF MECHANICAL VENTILATORY SUPPORT

Ventilator Commitment

First, establish the airway and manually support the ventilation with a manual resuscitation bag. Manual ventilation allows the clinician to gradually take over ventilation and vary the pattern in conjunction with patient efforts. During the early stages of mechanical ventilation, this method permits a smooth transition to positive pressure ventilation (PPV).

Second, establish hemodynamic stability. It is not uncommon for patients to demonstrate cardiovascular instability during this process. Often delays in establishing the airway, stress of intubation, sedative drugs, and inappropriate support are blamed for this occurrence. However, such instability often occurs in the absence of any of the above mentioned factors and is due to 1) a decrease in catecholamine levels with subsequent vasodilatation and decreased cardiac output related to the relief of respiratory distress; 2) decreased venous return related to PPV; or 3) a combination thereof.

Third, if not already in place, establish appropriate monitors and support, e.g., intravenous and intraarterial catheters, electrocardiographic monitor.

Fourth, establish the ventilatory pattern by

manually supporting the patient until he or she relaxes and adopts the slow, deep pattern of PPV. If patients do not tolerate the anticipated ventilatory pattern, appropriate sedation should be applied until they are comfortable, stable, and in synchrony with ventilatory support. Finally, connect the patient to the ventilator for maintenance of PPV.

Full Ventilatory Support

When initiating mechanical ventilatory support during an acute episode of ventilatory failure, it is imperative that the patient be adequately supported. In this context the concept of full ventilatory support is important. Full ventilatory support means that the ventilator provides all of the work that is required to maintain carbon dioxide excretion, which can be accomplished with ventilator rates of 8 to 10 breaths/min and tidal volumes of 12 to 15 cc/kg. In patients who are stable hemodynamically, this technique usually results in a $PaCO_2$ of less than 45 mm Hg. Patients with significantly decreased cardiac output may demonstrate high deadspace ventilation (high ventilation/perfusion ratios), and the $PaCO_2$ may be higher.

Partial Ventilatory Support

Spontaneous ventilation carries some benefits (e.g., improved V/Q matching, improved venous return) that are negated by mechanical ventilatory support. After the acute deterioration when patients are more stable and rested, and therapy has been in place, they may be able to tolerate a portion of the WOB but not all of it. In this circumstance it is possible to allow the ventilator to perform WOB that is detrimental to the patient's cardiopulmonary homeostasis while allowing the patient to perform the amount of work that produces beneficial effects. This concept has been termed partial ventilatory support and is usually accomplished with the same tidal volumes as outlined for full ventilatory support but with slower rates ($\leq$6 breaths/min).

Eucapnic Ventilation

Eucapnic ventilation is maintenance of the $PaCO_2$ within a normal range, usually defined as 35 to 45 mm Hg. However, when providing mechanical ventilatory support, one must take into consideration what is normal for the individual patient. Thus patients who normally maintain a $PaCO_2$ of 60 to 70 mm Hg should be mechanically ventilated within that same range.

Modes of Mechanical Ventilation

Volume Preset Modes

Control mode ventilation is one of the earliest forms of mechanical ventilation. This mode delivers a preset tidal volume (V_t) at predetermined time intervals. With this mode, spontaneous ventilatory efforts cannot take place. *Assist mode ventilation* is a volume preset mode; however, rather than breaths occurring at preset time intervals, the patient's inspiratory efforts determine the ventilatory frequency. *Assist-control mode* is a volume preset mode that permits the patient's spontaneous ventilatory efforts to determine the frequency of ventilation provided the spontaneous respiratory rate exceeds a certain preset minimum rate. *Intermittent mandatory ventilation* is a mode of mechanical ventilation that delivers a preset V_t at preset time intervals, but a continuous gas flow is provided to the patient so spontaneous ventilation can occur between breaths in an unrestricted fashion. *Synchronized intermittent mandatory ventilation* is a ventilatory mode that utilizes a demand valve system to synchronize the delivery of a mechanical breath with the spontaneous ventilatory efforts of the patient. The mechanical breaths are delivered within preset time intervals, and the patient's spontaneous ventilatory efforts are unassisted between these synchronized breaths.

Volume-Variable Modes

Pressure support ventilation is a mode of ventilation in which the patient's spontaneous efforts determine the ventilatory rate. Upon initiation of each breath the ventilator generates a preset inspiratory circuit pressure by rapidly adjusting inspiratory flow rates as necessary. The V_t varies depending on lung compliance, the strength of the patient's inspiratory efforts, and the degree of other restrictive or obstructive pulmonary pathology. *Pressure control ventilation* is a volume-variable mode in which inspiration is initiated and discontinued at preset time intervals. The breath is delivered by generation of a preset inspiratory circuit pressure in a fashion similar to that of pressure support ventilation. *Airway pressure release ventilation,* a volume-variable mode of mechanical ventilation, initiates and terminates the inspiratory cycle at predetermined time intervals. Pressure is maintained by administration of a continuous gas flow through threshold resistor devices that generate various levels of airway pressure. The patient can breathe spontaneously throughout the mechanical ventilatory cycle.

The volume-variable modes of mechanical ventilation do not necessarily deliver constant tidal volumes; therefore minute ventilation may vary significantly at times. Hence these modes have been reserved primarily for use in the stabilized patient during maintenance mechanical ventilation or during withdrawal of mechanical ventilatory support, or "weaning." When a patient requires a consistent and reliable minute ventilation, it is probably best to choose a volume-preset mode.

References

1. Shapiro BA, Kacmarek RM, Cane RD, et al: Limitations of oxygen therapy. *In* Shapiro BA, Kacmarek RM, Cane RD, et al. (eds): Clinical Application of Respiratory Care, 4th ed. Chicago, Year Book, 1991, pp. 135–150.
2. Soliday NH, Shapiro BA, Grancey DR: Adult respiratory distress syndrome. Chest *69*:207, 1976.
3. Lamay M, Fallat RJ, Koeniger E, et al: Pathologic features and mechanisms of hypoxemia in adult respiratory distress syndrome. Am Rev Respir Dis *114*:267, 1976.
4. Shapiro BA, Cane RD, Harrison RA: Positive end-expiratory pressure in acute lung injury. Chest *83*:558, 1983.
5. Shapiro BA, Cane RD: Metabolic malfunction of the lung: noncardiogenic edema and adult respiratory distress syndrome. Surg Annu *13*:271, 1981.
6. Miller WC, Rice DL, Unger KM, et al: Effect of PEEP on lung water content in experimental noncardiogenic pulmonary edema. Crit Care Med *9*:7, 1981.
7. Daly BDT, Edmonds CH, Norman JC: In vivo alveolar morphometric with positive end expiratory pressure. Surg Forum *24*:217, 1973.
8. Shapiro BA, Cane RD, Harrison RA: Positive end expiratory pressure therapy in adults with special reference to acute lung injury: a review of the literature and suggested clinical correlations. Crit Care Med *12*:127, 1984.
9. Schacter EN, Littner MR, Luddy P, et al: Monitoring of oxygen delivery systems in clinical practice. Crit Care Med *8*:405, 1980.
10. Shapiro BA, Kacmarek RM, Cane RD, et al: Oxygen therapy. *In* Clinical Application of Respiratory Care, 4th ed. Chicago, Year Book, 1991, pp. 123–134.
11. American College of Chest Physicians–Heart, Lung and Blood Institute: National Conference of Oxygen Therapy. Chest *85*:234–247, 1984.
12. Scacci R: Air entrainment masks: jet mixing is how they work; the Bernoulli and Venturi principles are how they don't. Respir Care *24*:928–931, 1979.
13. Shapiro BA, Kacmarek RA, Cane RD et al: Limitations of oxygen therapy. *In* Shapiro BA, Kacmarek RA, Cane RD, et al. (eds): Clinical Application of Respiratory Care, 4th ed. Chicago, Year Book, 1991, pp. 135–150.
14. Deneke SM, Fanberg BL: Normobaric oxygen toxicity of the lung. N Engl J Med *303*:76–86, 1980.
15. Shim C, Fine N, Fernandes R, William MH: Cardiac arrhythmias resulting from tracheal suctioning. Ann Intern Med *71*:1149, 1969.
16. Sloan HE: Vagus nerve in cardiac arrest. Surg Gynecol Obstet *91*:257, 1950.
17. Radford R: Rational basis for percussion—augmented mucociliary clearance. Respir Care *27*:556, 1982.
18. Shapiro BA, Kacmarek RM, Cane RD, et al: Applying and evaluating bronchial hygiene therapy. *In* Shapiro BA, Kacmarek RA, Cane RD, et al. (eds): Clinical Application of Respiratory Care, 4th ed. Chicago, Year Book, 1991, pp. 85–108.
19. Shapiro BA, Harrison RA, Cane RD, Templin R: Respiratory acid-base balance. *In* Shapiro BA, Harrison RA, Cane RD, Templin R (eds): Clinical Application of Blood Gases, 4th ed., Chicago, Year Book, 1989, pp. 38–56.

8 POSTOPERATIVE CONSIDERATIONS AFTER MAJOR VASCULAR SURGERY

JANE D. LOWDON and IRA J. ISAACSON

Postoperative care of the patient who has undergone major vascular surgery can be a challenging and complex task. Patients with peripheral vascular disease classically present to the anesthesiologist with diseases of multiple organ systems. This preexisting compromised state is then further stressed by a surgical procedure that may result in more extensive pathophysiologic derangements. This chapter examines the potential postoperative consequences of three major vascular procedures.

CAROTID ENDARTERECTOMY

After surgery for extracranial carotid occlusive disease, the patient requires the same careful monitoring and attention provided in the operating suite. Labile arterial blood pressures are a characteristic and potentially devastating event after carotid surgery. Altered baroreceptor function is the most likely explanation for the fluctuations in arterial pressure.[1] Baroreceptors are found in the walls of the large arteries in the neck and thorax but are concentrated in the aortic arch and the carotid sinuses, located just superior to the bifurcation of the internal and external carotid arteries.[2] Hering's nerve carries impulses from the carotid sinuses to the glossopharyngeal nerve and then to the medulla. The carotid baroreceptors modulate and buffer arterial blood pressure rapidly in response to changes in posture and Valsalva maneuvers. The number of impulses from the carotid sinus nerves vary directly with the arterial blood pressure. Nerve impulses travel to the brainstem, where they inhibit the vasoconstrictor center of the medulla and stimulate the vagal center with the net results being peripheral vasodilation, decreased heart rate, and decreased inotropy. In contrast, low arterial pressure results in fewer impulses reaching the brainstem, less inhibition of the vasoconstrictor center, and an increase in arterial pressure.[2]

Reflex hypotension after carotid endarterectomy occurs commonly, with a reported incidence of 13.3 per cent[3] to 45 per cent.[4] It may be explained as a misinterpretation of arterial pressure by the carotid sinuses. Prior to surgery the carotid sinuses function at a certain set point that is elevated in most patients with chronic arterial hypertension. It is these hypertensive patients who most frequently experience reflex hypotension after carotid endarterectomy.[1] Reflex hypotension may appear after surgical dissection of the carotid artery with removal of the atheromatous plaques that had previously dampened the arterial pressures to which the carotid sinuses were exposed. The patient's preoperative arterial pressure is now interpreted as hypertension by the carotid sinuses, thus triggering reflex hypotension and bradycardia until (Table 8–1) the carotid sinus mechanism can reset.[1,5] The hypotension may be exacerbated by preexisting hypovolemia[5] and does not usually manifest until 60 minutes after surgery, although its onset may be delayed as long as 5 hours after surgery.[6]

Treatment of reflex hypotension includes infusion of a vasopressor such as phenylephrine to maintain the systolic blood pressure higher than 100 mm Hg in normotensives or within approximately 30 per cent of preoperative values in hypertensive patients. Additionally, if a bradycardia of less than 50 beats per minute

TABLE 8–1. POSTCAROTID ENDARTERECTOMY

Reflex hypotension and bradycardia: Postcarotid Endarterectomy

Incidence 13–45%

Onset 1–5 hours after surgery

Symptoms: nausea, emesis, complaints of confusion

Signs
  Decrease in systolic blood pressure (SBP) to <100 mm Hg in normotensive patient or decrease in SBP by 30% in hypertensive patient
  Confusion, agitation, or disorientation
  Focal signs of CVA
Treatment
  Vasopressor: phenylephrine infusion
  Anticholinergic: glycopyrrolate 0.2 mg IV or atropine 0.4 mg IV
  Maintain oxygenation
Differential diagnosis
  Hypovolemia
  Myocardial ischemia

TABLE 8–2. HYPERTENSION POSTCAROTID ENDARTERECTOMY

Incidence up to 66%

Occurs most frequently after the second CEA and in patients with preexisting hypertension

Symptoms: usually none; occasionally headache

Signs: >30% increase in SBP over baseline change in mental status

Treatment: vasodilators
  Nitroglycerin infusion 0.25–1.00 μg/kg/min
  Labetalol by bolus and/or infusion
  Sodium nitroprusside 0.5–2.0 μg/kg/min
Differential diagnosis
  Pain
  Myocardial ischemia

accompanies the hypotension, treatment with an anticholinergic such as atropine or glycopyrrolate is suggested. Other causes of hypotension that must be considered include sensitivity to vasodilators (e.g., preoperative antihypertensives or anesthetics) and myocardial ischemia. The consequences of hypotension can be devastating and include cerebral hypoperfusion,[7] an increased possibility of thrombosis at the endarterectomy site,[8] and myocardial hypoperfusion.

Postendarterectomy hypertension (Table 8–2) has been reported with an incidence of up to 66 per cent.[9] Its occurrence is closely associated with the severity and control of preoperative hypertension.[3,10,11] Neurologic complications are reported more frequently in patients with postoperative hypertension.[3,6,10] Other sequelae of uncontrolled hypertension include damage to the surgical anastomosis, hematoma formation,[12] and myocardial dysfunction.[9,12]

The mechanism of postoperative hypertension remains illusive. The most popular theory involves baroreceptor dysfunction, which may occur when carotid sinus nerves are subject to trauma or neural blockade.[1] If fewer impulses reach the medulla, the reflex response is vasoconstriction.[1] Another theory suggests a correlation between postoperative hypertension and increased renin production by the brain.[13] Additionally, pain must be considered an etiology of hypertension and treated with appropriate analgesia.

The treatment for postoperative hypertension may include infusion of a peripheral vasodilator such as nitroglycerin or sodium nitroprusside with the goal being maintenance of systolic blood pressure within 30 per cent of preoperative values. Use of the combined α- and β-blocking agent labetalol by bolus and infusion is another therapeutic option for controlling hypertension, particularly if it is accompanied by an elevated heart rate.

A national survey of carotid endarterectomy found a 3.4 per cent operative mortality (within 30 days of surgery) and a 9.8 per cent risk of major operative complications.[14] Coronary atherosclerotic heart disease occurs frequently in patients with extracranial cerebrovascular disease. In patients undergoing carotid endarterectomy, Hertzer and Lees reported a 65 per cent incidence of coronary artery disease based on the history of electrocardiograms and found coronary artery disease to be the most common cause of postoperative mortality.[15] Riles and coworkers reported myocardial infarction (MI) as the second leading cause of morbidity and mortality after carotid endarterectomy (2.3 per cent) of patients sustained an MI within 72 hours of surgery).[16] The mortality rates are much higher in patients with angina pectoris (18.2 per cent) than in those with no cardiac symptoms (1.5 per cent).[17]

Although each patient is regarded as being at risk for myocardial ischemia, the high risk patients must be identified preoperatively and closely monitored. All preoperative medications for angina should be continued during the perioperative period or appropriate substitutions made. Hemodynamic monitoring in the operative suite should also be used during the postoperative period. A continuous electrocardiogram must be observed for arrhythmias as well as ST segment and T wave changes. If the intraoperative monitors include a pulmonary artery catheter, the clinician must be prepared to treat abnormalities in pulmonary artery pressures that may signal impending myocardial ischemia. If myocardial ischemia is detected, prompt treatment is mandatory. Adequate oxygenation must always be maintained, as hypoxemia is poorly tolerated in this population of patients. Hemodynamic variables must be carefully considered with attention to coronary perfusion (adequate diastolic arterial pressure and the absence of high pulmonary artery filling pressures), heart rate (avoidance of tachycardia to maintain diastolic perfusion of the myocardium), and normovolemia. If myocardial ischemia occurs and arterial pressure is adequate, a nitroglycerin infusion may improve myocardial oxygen balance. If coronary spasm is suspected, a calcium channel blocker such as nifedipine (10 mg sublingually) may improve myocardial perfusion.

Neurologic deficits (Table 8–3) are an unfortunate but sometimes unavoidable conse-

quence of carotid endarterectomy. The reported incidence of neurologic complications are variable and range from 1.7 per cent[18] to 21 per cent[19] with large, multicenter evaluations of data reporting an approximately 6 per cent risk of stroke or death due to neurologic complications.[20,21] Patients with a contralateral occlusive lesion or multiple cerebral arterial lesions present an especially high risk for perioperative neurologic deficit or a cerebral infarction.[22] The degree of impairment ranges from subtle changes detectable only by psychological testing to profound deficits such as aphasia or hemiplegia.[12] Etiologies of neurologic deficits include intraoperative embolization,[7,23–26] ipsilateral cerebral hyperperfusion following relief of a high grade stenosis,[26,27] postoperative hypotension[7] or hypertension,[3,10] intraoperative ischemia secondary to poor collateral flow during cross-clamp,[25] and intracerebral hemorrhage.[25,28–31] The identification of carotid thrombosis[24,32] is critical, as reexploration within 12 hours of surgery may reverse some of the neurologic deficit.[12,33]

The acute postoperative patient should undergo frequent neurologic assessment. Within the limits of adequate analgesia, the patient must remain free of excess sedation. If a neurologic complication occurs, the neurologic examination, hemodynamic variables, adequacy of oxygenation, and ventilation must be assessed in detail.

The extent of the neurologic deficit and the presumed etiology determine the course of action. Although the topic is controversial, some investigators advocate observation and supportive care of patients with minor, focal deficits.[34] Digital subtraction angiography or conventional cerebral angiography should be considered for those patients with moderately severe or progressive deficits.[25] Immediate surgical intervention is the treatment for distal intimal dissection and for carotid artery occlusion.[8,25] Therapy for a distal arterial embolus ranges from ongoing evaluation and antiplatelet therapy to complete anticoagulation.[25]

Isolated nerve injuries can occur after carotid endarterectomy and include damage to the hypoglossal, recurrent laryngeal, superior laryngeal, glossopharyngeal, facial (marginal mandibular branch),[35] and greater auricular nerves and the cervical sympathetic trunk (Table 8–4).[36] In a prospective study by Hertzer and coworkers, cranial nerve injuries were reported as having an incidence of 15.8 per cent (240 surgeries), with five patients sustaining

TABLE 8–3. NEUROLOGIC DEFICITS POSTCAROTID ENDARTERECTOMY

Incidence 1.7–21.0%

Etiology
  Intraoperative embolization
  Intraoperative ischemia (poor collateral flow)
  Postoperative hypotension or hypertension
  Cerebral hyperperfusion
  Intracerebral hemorrhage
  Carotid thrombosis
  Cranial nerve injuries
Symptoms: dysphagia, dysarthria, dyspnea, headache, change in mental status
Signs: hoarseness, stridor, airway obstruction; focal neurogic signs
Treatment
  Maintain airway and oxygenation
  Maintain blood pressure within preoperative limits
  Anticoagulation when appropriate
  Cerebral angiography for moderately severe or progressive deficits
  Surgical intervention when appropriate

TABLE 8–4. CRANIAL NERVE INJURIES AFTER CEA

Nerve	Symptom
Hypoglossal	Tongue deviated to affected side
Recurrent laryngeal	Vocal cord paresis
Glossopharyngeal	Discordinate tongue movements
Facial nerve	Drooping of lower lip
Greater auricular	Anesthesia of ear lobe and cheek
Cervical sympathetics	Horner syndrome

injury to two or more nerves.[37] Patients were described as minimally affected, with most injuries resolving in 1 to 12 months.[37] Dysfunction of the marginal mandibular nerve causes drooping of the corner of the mouth.[37] Injury to the recurrent laryngeal nerve results in paralysis of the ipsilateral vocal cord, which comes to rest in the median or paramedian position. Bilateral recurrent nerve injury, albeit rare, may result in airway obstruction.[38] Unilateral paralysis of cranial nerve XII causes glossal deviation toward the affected site or discoordinate movements of the tongue during speech and mastication.[37] If the injuries are multiple, bilateral, or severe, however, the airway may be jeopardized and require prolonged intubation or tracheostomy.[39] The importance of cranial nerve dysfunction is magnified when staged carotid endarterectomies are planned, as subsequent bilateral injury to the recurrent laryngeal or hypoglossal nerves can cause life-threatening airway obstruction.[40]

The development of a hematoma (Table 8–5) at the endarterectomy site is an uncommon (reported incidence 1 to 4 per cent) yet potentially devastating complication of the procedure.[41] Factors associated with the development of a significant wound hematoma include hypertension and perioperative treat-

TABLE 8–5. HEMORRHAGE: POST CEA

Incidence up to 4%

Associated with hypertension and antiplatelet drugs

Symptoms: pain, hoarseness, dyspnea

Signs: expanding neck mass, respiratory distress

Treatment
  Maintain oxygenation (consider helium-oxygen blend), airway
  Evacuate clot under local anesthesia

ment with antiplatelet drugs, e.g., aspirin and dipyridamole.[41,42] The size of the hematoma and the patient's respiratory status must be monitored closely. Should respiratory distress develop, sutures and clot should be removed immediately under local anesthesia.[42,43] Difficulty with tracheal reintubation in patients with a large hematoma may range from challenging in optimal circumstances to frankly impossible. The trachea may be deviated, and oropharyngeal edema may preclude identification of normal anatomy.[42–44]

Fiberoptic laryngoscopy may offer an alternative to conventional laryngoscopy, and the use of a small endotracheal tube is advised.[43,44] Ultimately, cricothyroidotomy or tracheostomy may become necessary but must be undertaken with caution and with recognition of the grossly distorted anatomy.[42] Although not a substitute for a secured airway, a helium-oxygen mixture with decreased resistance to gas flow[45] may facilitate oxygenation through a stenotic orifice and allow time for definitive surgical intervention.[43] Helium-oxygen mixtures limit the inspired oxygen concentration and must be used with great caution in patients with marginal oxygenation. Continuous pulse oximetry is mandatory when helium-oxygen blends are employed.

Unique physiologic impairments are observed in the patient who has undergone the second of two carotid endarterectomy procedures. Bilateral carotid endarterectomy may result in a significantly impaired ventilatory response to hypoxia and chronic elevation of PCO_2 (5.8 mm Hg mean increase in resting PCO_2).[46] These ventilatory changes result from damage to both the carotid bodies and their nerves or to their blood supplies. Any drugs that depress ventilation (including opioids, barbiturates, and anesthetics) must be used with caution in these individuals, as relatively small doses profoundly affect ventilatory drive.[46] Patients with bilateral carotid body denervation have lost their peripheral chemoreceptors and with them the ability to compensate for drug-induced central respiratory depression.[46,47] It is recommended that bilateral carotid endarterectomy not be performed as one operative procedure because of the exponentially increased risk of complications, such as airway obstruction and neurologic or myocardial morbidity. The recommended time lapse between procedures in the patient needing bilateral carotid endarterectomy (Table 8–6) remains controversial, al-

TABLE 8–6. UNIQUE PROBLEMS AFTER BILATERAL CEA

Impaired ventilatory response to hypoxia
Chronic elevation of PCO_2
Extreme sensitivity to sedative drugs

though 3 to 6 weeks between procedures is not uncommon.

AORTIC RECONSTRUCTIVE SURGERY

Patients undergoing abdominal aortic reconstructive surgery (Table 8–7) present an array of complex problems for the surgeon, anesthesiologist, and critical care team. Although the etiologies of aortic disease are varied, including degenerative, inflammatory, traumatic, and congenital processes,[48] each patient who undergoes aortic reconstructive surgery sustains significant physiologic trespass by the nature of the procedure. Numerous studies of outcome have documented a mortality rate of 2 to 5 per cent after elective aortic surgery[49–54] and mortality ranging from 23 per cent[53] to 55.8 per cent[50] after repair of a ruptured abdominal aortic aneurysm.[50–53,55–57] As with the patients undergoing carotid endarterectomy, coexisting disease of multiple organ systems is the rule and not the exception in this group of patients.[58,59]

Because preexisting cardiac disease is prevalent in this population of patients and predictive of serious sequelae, the preoperative identification of the high risk patient may alert the clinician and allow early, definitive intervention of postoperative problems. In a large series of patients, Hertzer and colleagues found severe, correctable coronary artery disease (CAD) by coronary angiography in 31 per cent of patients with abdominal aortic aneurysms.[60] Of patients with a positive cardiac history and an abnormal electrocardiogram,

TABLE 8–7. AORTIC RECONSTRUCTIVE SURGERY

Associated medical problems
    Coronary artery disease
    Hypertension
    Renal dysfunction
    Chronic obstructive pulmonary disease
    Diabetes mellitus

the incidence of perioperative myocardial infarction and operative mortality during aortic reconstructive surgery was approximately 9 per cent compared to a 1 to 3 per cent incidence of such an outcome in patients without evidence of CAD.[61,62] In a statistical analysis of outcome, Yeager and coworkers identified a history of myocardial infarction to be the primary predictor of death or myocardial infarction during the first month after aortic surgery.[63] Congestive heart failure has been identified as the other major risk factor for postoperative morbidity and mortality (Table 8–8) following aortic reconstructive surgery.[63,64]

In contrast to elective aortic reconstruction, the mortality associated with myocardial infarction or congestive heart failure in patients with ruptured aneurysms is reported to be as high as 100 per cent.[55]

During the acute postoperative period, all patients who have undergone aortic reconstructive surgery are considered to be at risk for myocardial ischemia, and careful monitoring for such events is indicated. Most myocardial reinfarctions take place on the third postoperative day and can occur without angina pectoris. The mortality following reinfarction is as high as 50 to 70 per cent.[65] Therefore attention to hemodynamic monitors and other indicators of myocardial dysfunction must not be discontinued prematurely.

Chronic arterial hypertension is a major health problem found in 40 to 60 per cent of vascular surgery patients.[58] After surgery, it remains important to keep arterial pressure within reasonable limits to maintain cerebral, coronary, and renal perfusion and to avoid

TABLE 8–8. POSTOPERATIVE COMPLICATIONS

Mortality:
    Elective surgery 2–5%
    Ruptured aneurysm 23–56%
Perioperative myocardial infarction: up to 9% in patients with coronary artery disease
Gastrointestinal complications: ranging from ileus to bowel infarction
Lower extremity ischemia
Spinal cord ischemia
Cerebrovascular accident
Hypothermia
Bleeding
Respiratory compromise

jeopardizing the integrity of the vascular anastomosis. The etiology of postoperative perturbations in arterial pressure includes the omission of routine antihypertensive medications, residual anesthetic, vasoactive drugs, and profound hyper- or hypovolemia. The goal of therapy is maintenance of systolic arterial pressure within 20 to 30 per cent of preoperative resting values. Treatment modalities include the use of direct vasodilators (nitroglycerin, nitroprusside, or hydralazine), sympathetic receptor blocking agents (α- or β-blockers, or both), diuretics, and, if appropriate, liberal analgesics for pain.

Renal dysfunction may occur after aortic reconstructive surgery and may be associated with intraoperative or postoperative renal hypoperfusion, nephrotoxic agents (dyes, antibiotics), anesthetic agents,[66] renal microembolization,[67] aneurysmal or occlusive disease involving the renal arteries,[54] or preoperative renal dysfunction.[62] Intraoperative oliguria does not, however, necessarily predict postoperative renal dysfunction.[68] Early mortality after repair of unruptured abdominal aortic aneurysm has been considered to be of primary renal origin in 10 per cent of cases,[53] and nearly 26 per cent of patients with ruptured abdominal aortic aneurysms developed renal failure with a 66 per cent mortality rate.[55] Of the patients who developed renal failure, most (59 per cent) had nonliguric renal failure. The remainder (41 per cent) manifested oliguria or anuria, with most requiring at least temporary dialysis.[62] Monitoring urine output and renal function is therefore important postoperatively. The differential diagnosis of decreased urine output (Table 8–9) must include not only parenchymal causes of acute renal failure but also hypoperfusion secondary to decreased cardiac output, hypovolemia, hypotension,

and anatomic dysfunction at the anastomosis of the renal arteries. Tests of renal function that may aid in diagnosis include plasma and urine electrolytes and creatinine for evaluation of renal failure indices.

Therapeutic interventions are based on etiology, with the goal being maintenance of urine output at 0.5 to 1.0 ml/kg/hr. Hypovolemia is the simplest cause of oliguria to treat with administration of the appropriate fluid (crystalloid, colloid, or blood products). Loop diuretics are useful for treating volume overload or for converting oliguric to nonoliguric acute renal failure. Dopamine by infusion in low doses (1–3 μg/kg/min) may improve renal blood flow and thus urine output. Renovascular problems may be diagnosed by nuclear or Doppler techniques and may require surgical intervention to restore adequate renal blood flow.

Gastrointestinal (GI) complications after aortic reconstructive surgery include ischemic intestine, ileus, peptic ulceration, undiagnosed GI bleeding, and aortoenteric fistulas.[69] Acute GI sequelae are reported to occur with an incidence as high as 6.7 per cent, with intestinal ischemia noted most frequently.[69] The mortality associated with severe intestinal ischemia (Table 8–10) ranges from 67 per cent[70] to 100 per cent.[55,69]

The clinical syndrome of colonic ischemia varies with the degree of injury. Colonic mucosal injury usually manifests as diarrhea and is often self-limiting. Colonic mucosal and muscularis injury results in bloody diarrhea occasionally accompanied by fever. Infarction of the colon appears early during the postoperative period and may be characterized by fever,[71] diarrhea, hypotension, abdominal pain, and metabolic acidosis.

The treatment of bowel ischemia is straight-

TABLE 8–9. DIFFERENTIAL DIAGNOSIS OF DECREASED URINE OUTPUT

Renal Causes	Other Causes	Treatment
Preoperative renal dysfunction	Decreased cardiac output	Assess hemodynamic and volume status
Intraoperative ischemia	Hypovolemia	Consider loop diuretic if patient is hypervolemic
Nephrotoxic agents: dyes, antibiotics	Hypotension	Dopamine infusion: 2.0–2.5 μg/kg/min
Microembolization	Anatomic dysfunction of renal artery anastomosis	Serial urine/plasma electrolytes and creatinine
Renovascular disease: aneurysmal or occlusive		Hemodialysis for renal failure

TABLE 8–10. INTESTINAL ISCHEMIA

Signs	Diagnosis	Treatment
Diarrhea	Plain roentgenogram of the abdomen	Surgical resection of gangrenous bowel
Nausea and vomiting	Sigmoidoscopy	
Fever	Colonoscopy	
Abdominal pain	Barium enema	
Hypotension and shock		
Metabolic acidosis		

forward: early surgical intervention to resect the gangrenous bowel.[72,73] Careful intraoperative surgical attention to the patency of the inferior mesenteric artery reduces the likelihood of this devastating complication.

Lower extremity ischemia is a complication of aortic reconstruction (reported incidence is 0.57 per cent[74] to 10.3 per cent[74]) and is associated with an increase in morbidity and mortality.[74] The etiologies of leg ischemia include intraoperative thrombosis,[74] embolism of atheromatous debris, inadequate heparinization, prolonged cross-clamp time, hypercoagulability, and technical problems such as a faulty anastomosis or a kinked or twisted prothesis.[75] Monitoring of distal pulses by palpation of Doppler studies at regular and frequent intervals is essential during the postoperative period. If limb ischemia is noted postoperatively, angiographic studies may help to determine the appropriate intervention.[75]

Spinal cord ischemia during surgery on the abdominal aorta may evolve into severe, devastating neurologic deficits. Such events occur uncommonly with an incidence of 0.25 per cent after unruptured aneurysms and 2.5 per cent after ruptured aneurysms.[76] The extraspinal blood supply in the thoracic region arises from radicular arteries, which branch off intercostal arteries predominantly on the left side (80 per cent). Six to eight radicular arteries supply the anterior spinal artery trunk, and 10 to 23 supply the posterior spinal artery trunks.[77] The largest radicular artery is the arteria radicularis magna, also known as the artery of Adamkiewiz.[78] This artery usually exits the aorta with the ninth, tenth, eleventh, or twelfth thoracic nerve roots but may exit as low as the first or second lumbar nerve roots (in 10 per cent of patients) or as high as the fifth, sixth, seventh, or eighth thoracic nerve roots (in 15 per cent of patients).[78] The anterior spinal artery is formed from fusion of

two radicular arteries arising from the vertebral arteries[79] and supplies all the gray matter except the posterior horns and all the white matter except the posterior columns.[80] The two posterior spinal arteries[79] arise directly from the vertebral arteries[78] and supply the gray matter of the posterior horns and the white matter of the posterior columns.[80]

Perfusion of the spinal cord may be compromised by arterial hypotension, inadequate flow after aortic cross-clamping,[78] or thrombosis or embolism.[76] The neurologic deficits range from paresis without sensory loss to a complete sensory loss with flaccid paralysis.[81] The extent of the paralysis may progress over days owing to thrombosis of posterior spinal arteries, and regression is seen in only a few cases.[81] The classic anterior spinal artery syndrome involves paraplegia, rectal and urinary incontinence, and loss of pain and temperature sensation with sparing of vibration and proprioception.[78]

Cerebrovascular accident, a complication of aortic reconstructive surgery, has a reported incidence of less than 1 per cent.[53,62] However, if this complication occurs in a patient with a ruptured abdominal aortic aneurysm, the mortality is reported to be as high as 100 per cent.[55] Thus in the context of potential neurologic sequelae, careful and frequent neurologic examinations take on the utmost importance during the early postoperative period.

Hypothermia is a problem seen frequently after abdominal surgery and complicates postoperative management.[82] Although anesthesia attenuates some responses, postoperative hypothermia elicits a large sympathetic outpouring with a concomitant rise in heart rate, stroke volume, arterial blood pressure, cardiac output, and oxygen consumption[83] (see Chapter 13). In fact, shivering may cause up to a fivefold increase in oxygen consumption.[84]

Such increased demands on a myocardium with diminished reserve are obviously undesirable. Furthermore, conduction problems and dysrhythmias can occur more commonly with hypothermia. The electrocardiographic changes include sinus bradycardia, prolonged P-R interval, widened QRS, prolonged Q-T interval, and the characteristic ST segment change known as the J, or Osborne, wave.[83]

Organ perfusion changes with hypothermia and includes a significant decrease in flow to skeletal muscle, a smaller decrease in flow to the kidneys, and an even smaller decrease in splanchnic flow. Perfusion of the heart and brain is minimally compromised.[85,86] Hypothermia increases blood viscosity by hemoconcentration due to plasma loss,[87,88] a direct effect of temperature on plasma,[87] and a low flow state induced by hypothermia.[87] Hypothermia can also result in erythrocyte aggregation and rouleaux formation. All the above factors may adversely affect regional blood flow, especially the microcirculation.

Hypothermia can also significantly impair blood coagulation. Platelet function decreases with hypothermia, and platelets disappear from the systemic circulation, being sequestration in the portal system, especially in the liver.[83] Upon rewarming, however, platelet function returns to normal.[89] The effect of hypothermia on clotting factors and their effectiveness is variable and incompletely described.[83]

Management of hypothermic patients involves protecting them from their own potentially maladaptive physiologic responses. Any increase in myocardial oxygen demand must be scrupulously avoided. If the patient's temperature postoperatively is less than 35°C, conservative management involves maintenance of the well anesthetized state; that is, the patient's oxygenation and ventilation are supported while neuromuscular blockade is maintained. During the period of postoperative rewarming, the clinician must not forget to ensure adequate amnesia (with benzodiazepines) and to block sympathetic responses to surgical pain or to the endotracheal tube (with opioids or adrenergic receptor antagonists).

DESCENDING THORACOABDOMINAL ANEURYSMS

The descending thoracoabdominal aorta encompasses more extensive pathophysiologic processes than abdominal aortic aneurysms, with an accompanying increase in surgical risk. Crawford and colleagues reported an early mortality rate (within 30 days of surgery) of 8.9 per cent.[90] The cause of death was attributed to cardiac origin in most cases (44 per cent), followed by renal (37 per cent), pulmonary (33 per cent), and infectious (19 per cent) etiologies.[90] Preoperative risk factors associated with death during the early postoperative period included advanced age (>70 years), chronic obstructive pulmonary disease, renal artery occlusive disease, coronary artery disease, renal insufficiency, and a prolonged aortic cross-clamp time (>60 minutes).[90]

Postoperative neurologic deficits are an important issue for this group of patients. The mechanisms of spinal cord ischemia are the same as those during abdominal aortic reconstruction. The incidence of postoperative motor deficit with thoracoabdominal aneurysms was reported as 11 per cent in one large series of patients but can be as high as 40 per cent with extensive, dissected aneurysms.[90] Predicting such as outcome is difficult because the intraoperative use of somatosensory evoked potentials did not change the incidence of postoperative paralysis or paraparesis.[91] Air emboli are another source of postoperative neurologic deficits. Air bubbles can travel cephalad after unclamping a superior anastomosis of the aortic graft.[92,93] In one study cerebrovascular accident accounted for a small but significant number (9 per cent) of early (within 30 days) postoperative deaths after surgery.[90]

Respiratory dysfunction can be catastrophic after both abdominal and thoracic aortic reconstructive surgery, especially in the older patient population with limited organ reserve. Given the high incidence of chronic obstructive pulmonary disease (25 to 50 per cent),[58] patients undergoing aortic reconstruction experience many pulmonary complications common to surgical patients (see Chapter 5). There is a syndrome unique to patients who sustain transient peripheral tissue ischemia (e.g., secondary to the cross-clamp). Klausner and colleagues have described a clinical course of respiratory failure with pulmonary hypertension, hypoxemia, and noncardiogenic pulmonary edema after reperfusion of the lower extremities. The explanation of this phenomenon involves the release of arachidonic acid metabolites (thromboxane and leukotriene B_4) and sequestration in the lung of neutrophils that had accumulated distal to the surgical cross-clamp.[94] Changes in lung permeability then results from the neutrophils, collection of oxygen free radicals, and thromboxane. Because this type of respiratory dysfunction is usually transient, treatment includes supportive care, maintenance of oxygenation, and positive pressure ventilation if necessary.[94]

CONCLUSION

Patients who undergo major vascular surgery have significant disease, usually in multiple organ systems. Postoperative care offers a number of challenging problems for real or potential disaster. The approach to these patients requires vigilance and careful attention to each and every detail.

References

1. Bove EL, Fry WJ, Gross WS, Stanley JC: Hypotension and hypertension as consequences of baroreceptor dysfunction following carotid endarterectomy. Surgery 85:633–637, 1979.
2. Guyton AC: Textbook of Medical Physiology. Philadelphia, Saunders, 1981, pp. 246–258.
3. Asiddao CB, Donegan JH, Whitesell RC, Kalbfleisch JH: Factors associated with perioperative complications during carotid endarterectomy. Anesth Analg 61:631–637, 1982.
4. Angell-James JE, Lumley JSP: The effects of carotid endarterectomy on the mechanical properties of the carotid sinus and carotid sinus nerve activity in atherosclerotic patients. Br J Surg 61:805–810, 1984.
5. Tarlov E, Schmider H, Scott RM, et al: Reflex hypotension following carotid endarterectomy: mechanism and management. J Neurosurg 39:323–327, 1973.
6. Skydell JL, Machleder HI, Baker JD et al: Incidence and mechanism of post-carotid endarterectomy hypertension. Arch Surg 122:1153–1155, 1987.
7. Owens ML, Wilson SE: Prevention of neurologic complications of carotid endarterectomy. Arch Surg 117:551–554, 1982.
8. Simma W, Hesse H, Gilhofer G, et al: Management of immediate occlusion after carotid-reconstruction. J Cardiovasc Surg 28:176–179, 1987.
9. Davies MJ, Cronin KD: Post carotid endarterectomy hypertension. Anaesth Intensive Care 8:190–194, 1980.
10. Towne JB, Bernhard VM: The relationship of postoperative hypertension to complications following carotid endarterectomy. Surgery 88:575–580, 1980.
11. Corson JD, Chang BB, Leopold PW, et al: Perioperative hypertension in patients undergoing carotid endarterectomy: shorter duration under regional block anesthesia. Circulation 74 (suppl):I1–I4, 1986.
12. Marschall KE, Turndorf H: Anesthesia for carotid endarterectomy. In Cottrell JE, Turndorf H, eds. Anesthesia and Neurosurgery. St. Louis, Mosby, 1986, pp. 444–452.
13. Smith BL: Hypertension following carotid endarterectomy: the role of cerebral renin production. J Vasc Surg 1:623–627, 1984.
14. Winslow CM, Solomon DH, Chassin MR, et al: The

appropriateness of carotid endarterectomy. N Engl J Med 318:721–727, 1988.
15. Hertzer NR, Lees CD: Fatal myocardial infarction following carotid endarterectomy. Ann Surg 194:212–218, 1981.
16. Riles TS, Kopelman I, Imparato AM: Myocardial infarction following carotid endarterectomy: a review of 683 operations. Surgery 85:249–252, 1979.
17. Ennix CL, Lawrie GM, Morris GC, et al: Improved results of carotid endarterectomy in patients with symptomatic coronary disease: an analysis of 1,546 consecutive carotid operations. Stroke 10:122–125, 1979.
18. Connolly JE, Kwaan JHM, Stemmer EA: Improved results with carotid endarterectomy. Ann Surg 186(3):334–340, 1977.
19. DeWeese JA, Rob CG, Satran R, et al: Results of carotid endarterectomies for transient ischemic attacks-five years later. Ann Surg 178:258–263, 1973.
20. Fode NC, Sundt TM, Robertson JT, et al: Multicenter retrospective review of the results and complications of carotid endarterectomy in 1981. Stroke 17:370–376, 1986.
21. Toronto Cerebrovascular Study Group: Risks of carotid endarterectomy. Stroke 17:848–852, 1986.
22. Skillman JJ: Neurological complications of cardiovascular surgery: I. Procedures involving the carotid arteries and abdominal aorta. Int Anesthesiol Clin 24:135–157, 1986.
23. Piepgras DG, Sundt TM, Marsh WR, et al: Recurrent carotid stenosis. Ann Surg 203:205–213, 1986.
24. Hafner CD: Minimizing the risks of carotid endarterectomy. J Vasc Surg 1:392–397, 1984.
25. Sutherland GR, Barr HWK: Postoperative complications following carotid endarterectomy and their management. Int Anesthesiol Clin 22:165–173, 1984.
26. Sundt TM, Sharborough FW, Pipgras DG, et al: Correlation of cerebral blood flow and electroencephalographic changes during carotid endarterectomy. Mayo Clin Proc 56:533–543, 1981.
27. Sundt TF: The ischemic tolerance of neural tissue and the need for monitoring and selective shunting during carotid endarterectomy. Stroke 14:93–97, 1983.
28. Pomposelli FB, Lamparello PJ, Riles TS, et al: Intracranial hemorrhage after carotid endarterectomy. J Vasc Surg 7:248–255, 1988.
29. Hafner DH, Smith RB, King OW, et al: Massive intracerebral hemorrhage following carotid endarterectomy. Arch Surg 122:305–307, 1987.
30. Piepgras DG, Morgan MK, Sundt TM, et al: Intracerebral hemorrhage after carotid endarterectomy. J Neurosurg 68:532–536, 1988.
31. Solomon RA, Loftus CM, Quest DO, Correll JW: Incidence and etiology of intracerebral hemorrhage following carotid endarterectomy. J Neurosurg 64:29–34, 1986.
32. Oller DW, Welch H: Complications of carotid endarterectomy. Am Surg 52:479–484, 1986.
33. Treiman RL, Cossman DV, Cohen JL, et al: Management of postoperative stroke after carotid endarterectomy. Am J Surg 142:236–238, 1981.
34. Rosenthal D, Zeichner WD, Lamis PA, Stanton PE: Neurologic deficit after carotid endarterectomy: pathogenesis and management. Surgery 94:776–780, 1983.
35. Schmidt D, Zuschneid W, Kaiser M: Cranial nerve injuries during carotid arterial reconstruction. J Neurol 230:131–135, 1983.
36. Forssell C, Takolander R, Bergqvist D, et al: Cranial

nerve injuries associated with carotid endarterectomy. Acta Chir Scand *151*:595–598, 1985.

37. Hertzer NR, Feldman BJ, Beven EG, Tucker HM: A prospective study of the incidence of injury to the cranial nerves during carotid endarterectomy. Surg Gynecol Obstet *151*:781–784, 1980.
38. Knight FW, Yeager RM, Morris DM: Cranial nerve injuries during carotid endarterectomy. Am J Surg *154*:529–532, 1987.
39. Matsumoto GH, Cossman D, Callow AD: Hazards and safeguards during carotid endarterectomy. Am J Surg *133*:458–462, 1977.
40. Dehn TCB, Taylor GW: Cranial and cervical nerve damage associated with carotid endarterectomy. Br J Surg *70*:365–368, 1983.
41. Gomez ER, Kunkel JM, Jarstfer BS, Collins GJ: Wound hematomas after carotid endarterectomy. Am Surg *51*:111–113, 1985.
42. Kunkel JM, Gomez ER, Spebar MJ et al: Wound hematomas after carotid endarterectomy. Am J Surg *148*:844–847, 1984.
43. O'Sullivan JC, Wells DG, Wells GR: Difficult airway management with neck swelling after carotid endarterectomy. Anaesth Intensive Care *14*:460–464, 1986.
44. Bukht D, Langford RM: Airway obstruction after surgery in the neck (Letter). Anaesthesia *38*:389–90, 1983.
45. Lu TS, Ohmura A, Wong KC, Hodges MR: Helium-oxygen in treatment of upper airway obstruction. Anesthesiology *45*:678–680, 1976.
46. Wade JG, Larson CP, Hickey RF et al: Effect of carotid endarterectomy on carotid chemoreceptor and baroreceptor function in man. N Engl J Med *282*:823–829, 1970.
47. Lee JK, Hanowell S, Kim YD, Macnamara TE: Morphine-induced respiratory depression following bilateral carotid endarterectomy. Anesth Analg *60*:64–65, 1981.
48. Rutherford RB: Arterial aneurysms—overview. *In* Rutherford RB, ed. Vascular Surgery. Philadelphia, WB Saunders, 1984, pp. 745–754.
49. Lausten GS, Engell HC: Postoperative complications in abdominal vascular surgery. Acta Chir Scand *150*:457–461, 1984.
50. Campbell WB, Collin J, Morris PJ: The mortality of abdominal aortic aneurysm. Ann R Coll Surg Eng *68*:275–278, 1986.
51. Hicks GL, Eastland MW, DeWeese JA, et al: Survival improvement following aortic aneurysm resection. Ann Surg *181*:863–869, 1975.
52. Ruberti U, Scorza R, Biasi GM, Odero A: Nineteen year experience on the treatment of aneurysms of the abdominal aorta: A survey of 832 consecutive cases. J Cardiovasc Surg *26*:547–553, 1985.
53. Crawford ES, Saleh SA, Babb JW III, et al: Infrarenal abdominal aortic aneurysm: Factors influencing survival after operation performed over a 25-year period. Ann Surg *193*:699–709, 1981.
54. Crawford ES: Symposium: Prevention of complications of abdominal aortic reconstruction. Surgery *93*:91–96, 1983.
55. Fielding JWL, Black J, Ashton F, Slaney G: Ruptured aortic aneurysms: postoperative complications and their aetiology. Br J Surg *71*:487–491, 1984.
56. Crew JR, Bashour TT, Ellertson D, et al: Ruptured abdominal aortic aneurysms: experience with 70 cases. Clin Cardiol *8*:433–436, 1985.
57. Jenkins AM, Ruckley CV, Nolan B: Ruptured abdominal aortic aneurysm. Br J Surg *73*:395–398, 1986.

58. Clark NJ, Stanley TH: Anesthesia for vascular surgery. *In* Miller RD, ed. Anesthesia. New York, Churchill Livingstone, 1986, pp. 1519–1562.
59. Whittemore AD, Clowes AW, Hechtman HB, Mannick JA: Reduced operative mortality associated with maintenance of optimal cardiac performance. Ann Surg *192*:414–421, 1980.
60. Hertzer NR, Beven EG, Young JR, et al: Coronary artery disease in peripheral vascular patients. Ann Surg *199*:223–233, 1984.
61. Hertzer NR: Myocardial ischemia. Surgery *93*:97–101, 1983.
62. Diehl JT, Cali RF, Hertzer NR, Beven EG: Complications of abdominal aortic reconstruction. Ann Surg *197*:49–56, 1983.
63. Yeager RA, Wiegel RM, Murphy ES, et al: Application of clinically valid cardiac risk factors to aortic aneurysm surgery. Arch Surg *121*:278–281, 1986.
64. Bjerkelund CE, Smith-Erichsen N, Solheim K: Abdominal aortic reconstruction. Acta Chir Scand *152*:111–115, 1986.
65. Rao TLK, Jacobs KH, El-Etr AA: Reinfarction following anesthesia in patients with myocardial infarction. Anesthesiology *59*:499–505, 1983.
66. Bush HL: Renal failure following abdominal aortic reconstruction. Surgery *93*:107–109, 1983.
67. Iliopoulos JI,k Zdon MJ, Crawford BG et al: Renal microembolization syndrome. Am J Surg *146*:779–783, 1983.
68. Alpert RA, Roizen MJ, Hamilton WK et al: Intraoperative urinary output does not predict postoperative renal function in patients undergoing abdominal aortic revascularization. Surgery *95*:707–711, 1984.
69. Crowson M, Fielding JWL, Black J, et al: Acute gastrointestinal complications of infrarenal aortic aneurysm repair. Br J Surg *71*:825–828, 1984.
70. Fiddian-Green RG, Amelin PM, Herrmann JB, et al: Prediction of the development of sigmoid ischemia on the day of aortic operations. Arch Surg *121*:654–660, 1986.
71. Johnson WC, Nabseth DC: Visceral infarction following aortic surgery. Ann Surg *180*:312–318, 1974.
72. Miller RE, Knox WG: Colon ischemia following infrarenal aortic surgery. Ann Surg *163*:639–642, 1966.
73. Lannerstad O, Bergentz S, Bergqvist D, Takolander R: Ischemic intestinal complications after aortic reconstructive surgery. Acta Chir Scand *151*:599–602, 1985.
74. Imparato AM: Abdominal aortic surgery: prevention of lower limb ischemia. Surgery *93*:112–116, 1983.
75. Strom JA, Bernhard VM, Towne JB: Acute limb ischemia following aortic reconstruction. Arch Surg *119*:470–473, 1984.
76. Szilagyi DE, Hageman JH, Smith RF, Elliott JP: Spinal cord damage in surgery of the abdominal aorta. Surgery *83*:38–56, 1978.
77. Connolly JE: Prevention of paraplegia secondary to operations on the aorta. J Cardiovasc Surg *27*:410–417, 1986.
78. Costello TG, Fisher A: Neurological complications following aortic surgery. Anaesthesia *38*:230–236, 1983.
79. Gray H: Anatomy of the human body. In Clemente CD, ed. Philadelphia, Lea and Febiger, 1985, pp. 964–969.
80. Picone AL, Green RM, Ricotta JR, et al: Spinal cord ischemia following operations on the abdominal aorta. J Vasc Surg *3*:94–103, 1986.

81. Nielsen BP: Ischaemic injury to the spinal cord as a complication to abdominal aortic surgery. Acta Chir Scand *151*:433–435, 1985.

82. Shanks CA: Control of heat balance during arterial surgery. Anaesth Intensive Care *3*:118–121, 1975.

83. Rupp SM, Severinghaus JW: Hypothermia. *In* Miller RD, ed. Anesthesia. 2nd ed. New York, Churchill Livingstone, 1986, pp. 1995–2022.

84. Bay J, Nunn JF, Prys-Roberts C: Factors influencing arterial Po_2 during recovery from anaesthesia. Br J Anaesth *40*:398–406, 1968.

85. Zarins CK, Skinner DB: Circulation in profound hypothermia. J Surg Res *14*:97–104, 1973.

86. Delin NA, Kjartansson KB, Pollock L, Schenk WG: Redistribution of regional blood flow in hypothermia. J Thorac Cardiovasc Surg *49*:511–516, 1965.

87. Chen RYZ, Chien S: Hemodynamic functions and blood viscosity in surface hypothermia. Am J Physiol *235*:H136–H143, 1978.

88. Nose H: Transvascular fluid shift and redistribution of blood in hypothermia. Jpn J Physiol *32*:831–842, 1982.

89. Thomas R, Hessel EA, Harker LA, et al: Platelet function during and after deep surface hypothermia. J Surg Res *31*:314–318, 1981.

90. Crawford ES, Crawford JL, Safi HJ, et al: Thoracoabdominal aortic aneurysms: preoperative and intraoperative factors determining immediate and long-term results of operations in 605 patients. J Vasc Surg *3*:389–404, 1986.

91. Crawford ES, Mizrahi EM, Hess KR, et al: The impact of distal aortic perfusion and somatosensory evoked potential monitoring on prevention of paraplegia after aortic aneurysm operation. J Thorac Cardiovasc Surg *95*:357–367, 1988.

92. Crawford ES, Snyder DM: Thoracoabdominal aortic aneurysm. *In* Rutherford RB, ed. Vascular Surgery. Philadelphia, WB Saunders, 1984, pp. 772–785.

93. Najafi H, Javid H, Hunter J, et al: Descending aortic aneurysmectomy without adjuncts to avoid ischemia. Ann Thorac Surg *30*:326–335, 1980.

94. Klausner JM, Patterson IS, Mannick JA, et al: Reperfusion pulmonary edema. JAMA *261*:1030–1035, 1989.

HEMORRHAGIC PROBLEMS DURING THE IMMEDIATE POSTOPERATIVE PERIOD

9

BRUCE D. SPIESS

The incidence of major hemorrhage is low considering the total number of surgeries performed annually. Approximately 4 million red blood cell transfusions are given in the United States annually,[1] and most of them are utilized during the perioperative period. Anesthesiologists, surgeons, critical care physicians, and nurses affect the utilization of blood products by their decision-making. The impact of the human immunodeficiency virus (AIDS) crisis has been seen in transfusion medicine.[2] An understanding of the issues—risks and benefits of transfusion, hemorrhage and anemia in patients with normal physiology or disease—is essential for the rational application of transfusion therapy. This chapter discusses the physiology of anemia, the risks of transfusion, blood component therapy, coagulopathies, and monitoring as they relate to the surgical patient during the immediate postoperative period.

PATIENTS AT RISK

Patients who have undergone procedures that incur abnormal bleeding intraoperatively may well continue to hemorrhage during the postoperative period. Any, except the most minor, procedure may produce unexpected blood loss. A partial list of procedures that put the patient at risk includes liver transplantations or hepatic resections, major abdominal resections, radical prostatectomy, transurethral resection of the prostate, cardiopulmonary bypass, aortic aneurysm repair, orthopedic joint replacemnts, long bone fractures, major spinal surgery, and multiple trauma. It is impossible to discuss what would

be normal blood loss for each of these categories, but, for example, the expected blood loss for total hip arthroplasty has been reported to be between 500 and 1000 ml.[3,4] That blood loss, however, does not cease at closure of the wound; some degree of oozing blood loss is present for 12 to 24 hours after the operation.

In many cases the presence of abnormal bleeding is readily evident when one inspects drains, dressings, or wound sites. Tissue drains are not always effective. They may either be remote from a source of bleeding or have tissue or clot blocking them. These indicators of hemorrhage may therefore prove unreliable, and so other signs of hemorrhage must be utilized.

A high index of suspicion is helpful if physiologic changes are encountered. The site of surgery itself is important when deciding what types of change signal bleeding. In enclosed spaces, e.g., the cranial vault, small collections of blood may change the levels of consciousness or cause seizures. In a less constrained space, e.g., the abdomen, large quantities of blood can accumulate without outward signs, especially in postoperative patients who may have abdominal distension due to surgery or dressings and whose pain sensations are blunted by narcotics.

Quantities of blood loss that could be hazardous vary from one surgical site to another. In the cranial vault, for example, quantities of 100 ml may be enough to cause damage. Patients who have undergone tonsillectomy may be at risk from even small amounts of hemorrhage if that blood causes laryngospasm or is aspirated into the trachea. Postoperative tonsillectomy bleeding is discussed in Chapter 18. Hypovolemia may present with certain classic

131

signs in the young, healthy patient. In contrast, patients who are elderly, those with cardiovascular disease, or those who take β-blockers may exhibit few of those signs.

The decision to reoperate a patient because of bleeding must take into account the site of surgery. A 400 or 500 ml blood loss after total hip arthroplasty may be expected, whereas in cardiopulmonary bypass patients that amount of bleeding may be the upper limit of what would be tolerated during a given 8 hour period.

PHYSIOLOGY OF ANEMIA

Oxygen transport to the tissues is the most important biologic function of hemoglobin and erythrocytes. Sufficient amounts of hemoglobin and cardiac output must be present to supply tissue demands. The transfer of oxygen from blood cells to tissue mitochondria has been well understood for more than 60 years.[5,6] However, controversies exist concerning the lower limits of oxygen supply, hemoglobin, or cardiac output in certain disease states.[7] If practitioners are to transfuse blood, a procedure that carries risks, they must understand the controversies regarding anemia. The decision of whether to reexplore for bleeding after any surgical procedure must be based on experience, expectations for a given patient, and knowledge of the evolution of that bleeding.

Maintenance of intravascular circulating volume is of the greatest importance when hemorrhage occurs.[8] The changes that occur with volume loss are different from those seen with euvolemic anemia alone. Volume loss, if moderately severe (20 to 30 per cent), leads to hypotension and shock. The end result of shock is tissue hypoxia due to inadequate oxygen delivery. If circulating volume is maintained, profound levels of anemia can be tolerated in animals or humans without cardiovascular disease. Hematocrit levels as low as 7 per cent in experimental dogs have been survived.[9] Acute human surgical hemodilution to a hemoglobin level of 1.2 gm/dl has been survived without transfusion or use of a hyperbaric chamber (personal observation). Therefore the absolute lower limits of hemoglobin and hematocrit in patients with normal compensatory mechanisms are unclear.

As red blood cell (RBC) mass is lost, the first physiologic change to be encountered is an increase in cardiac output. That increase is a compensatory reaction to a decrease in the systemic vascular resistance.[10–12] The formed elements of the blood—RBCs, white blood cells (WBCs), and proteins provide the greatest contribution to blood viscosity.[13,14] With dilution their concentration decreases, and tissue blood flow increases in direct proportion to the changes in viscosity and vascular resistance up to certain limits.[15,16] This fact may be qualified in some manner in tissues where autoregulation controls blood flow, most notable of which are the circulations to the brain, heart, and kidneys.[17–20] At markedly low hematocrit levels (10 to 12 per cent) coronary vasodilation may be at its maximum and blood flow does not increase further. Further reduction of the hematocrit may cause a debt in oxygen supply and demand. As the hemoglobin concentration is decreased and cardiac output is increased, there is little increase in the myocardial oxygen demand until hematocrit levels below 10 per cent are reached.[7,21] Cardiac output is increased by stroke volume changes (i.e., vascular resistance); and if preload is maintained (euvolemia), effective emptying of the left ventricle occurs.[7] Preload may be slightly increased as the hematocrit is decreased from 40 per cent to 20 per cent. This increase may be due to changes in venous flow characteristics. Such hemodynamic changes do not cause an increase in heart rate, and myocardial oxygen demand is stable or only slightly increased.[7] For anemia to cause tachycardia at hemoglobin levels below 7 gm/dl, hypovolemia or other concomitant problems such as infection and acidosis must be present. If tachycardia is encountered in a bleeding patient, hypovolemia must be suspected. Of course, the differential diagnosis of tachycardia during the postoperative period is extensive.

The results of the changes of anemia are that tissue oxygen delivery is probably "best" at a hematocrit of about 33 to 35 per cent—not at 40 per cent or more. In contrast, as the hematocrit rises there is an increase in blood viscosity and therefore an increase in the vascular resistance and myocardial work. Tissue oxygen delivery actually decreases and can reach low levels equal to those seen with moderate to severe anemia. Polycythemia is responsible for hyperviscosity and early thrombosis, so it definitely should be avoided. From our knowledge of anemia there is no exact number or rule ascribed to the hemoglobin or hematocrit at which transfusion should occur.

In patients with coronary artery disease

there is evidence of tolerance for mild to moderate anemia (to 17 per cent hematocrit).[22] Hematocrit levels up to 30 per cent have been shown to cause no change in thallium scans in patients with known coronary lesions. In several patients hemodilution has actually improved the thallium scan.[23] In patients with peripheral vascular ischemia, hemodilution is a useful treatment. Sudden anemia, especially if seen in conjunction with hypovolemia, can, however, cause myocardial ischemia and angina.[24] A hematocrit of 30 per cent is considered safe for most individuals with coronary artery disease, and some clinicians would transfuse the patient if that percentage dropped. However, in postoperative cardiopulmonary bypass patients the hematocrit is routinely allowed to be 20 to 25 per cent. Such levels are well tolerated during and immediately after bypass; and although surgery is corrective, coronary disease still exists. One study showed a significant amount of myocardial ischemia during the early postbypass period, although a cause-and-effect relation between hematocrit and ischemia has not been demonstrated.[25] The question of the level at which to transfuse these patients remains controversial.

TRIGGER FOR TRANSFUSION

Historically, RBC products have been transfused when either a hemoglobin level of 10 gm/dl has been reached or a 20 per cent blood loss has been encountered. This practice was based on a statement by John Lundy during the 1940s stating that patients should have at least 8 to10 gm of hemoglobin per deciliter before elective surgery.[26] That statement was reprinted in almost every anesthesia and surgery text from the 1950s until the present AIDS crisis. Prior to the 1940s hemoglobin levels were maintained at a high enough level that the examiner could detect cyanosis by observing the mucosa or nail beds. This criterion required a hemoglobin level of at least 5 to 7 gm/dl.

From 1984 through 1988 the National Institutes of Health held a series of three consensus development conferences to suggest guidelines for component transfusion.[27] Each conference had a panel of experts who heard testimony and scientific presentations on the indications and risks of transfusion. They then developed acceptable guidelines as a national policy on blood transfusion.

Although the trigger for transfusion has now decreased to an individualized number for each patient based on the disease state and the anticipated medial problems, compliance with this policy is not universal. Education has had major effects on transfusion practice, but it requires ongoing reinforcement.

The use of autologous blood products has grown rapidly since the early 1980s.[28] This practice eliminates the risk of viral disease transmission and therefore appeals to most patients. It remains a greatly underutilized resource, however.[30] Three major methods involving autologous blood may be utilized: preoperative donation, euvolemic hemodilution, and cell salvage. All three subtypes require advanced planning.

Preoperative donation requires the patient for elective surgery to come to a collection facility at least once prior to surgery. Inconveniences of time off work, travel, and scheduling can create problems for both the patient and the surgeon.

Euvolemic hemodilution involves removal of the RBC mass at the time of surgery and replacement with either colloid or crystalloid to maintain intravascular volume. The theory is that once the patient has a lower hematocrit any blood lost thereafter is of lower hematocrit; hence the patient will benefit from a conservation of RBC mass. Although controversial, there does seem to be some benefit to this technique at least in cases of moderate blood loss.[31] Once again, however, anticipation and planning are necessary. Units collected in the operating room or elsewhere should be labeled appropriately with the patient's name and hospital number. The usual paperwork from a blood bank does not accompany these units, and anyone caring for the patient during the perioperative period should take extra care when checking the accuracy of the identifiers on the blood pack. The shelf-life of these products is about 6 hours without refrigeration to 4°C. Concern about bacterial growth precludes their routine usage after that time.[32] One advantage of warm storage is that these units maintain normal platelet activity.

Cell salvage can be accomplished intraoperatively and into the postoperative period as well. Blood collected by automated cell washing devices is the type utilized most commonly intraoperatively. It is contraindicated in cases where infection is present and remains controversial where cancer cells may be encountered.[33–36] The product produced is packed RBCs with a hematocrit of 55 to 60 per cent. The automated cell washers clear plasma and platelets, and therefore there is no clotting function transfused with the product. An advantage of cell savers is that there is also little debris, fibrin degradation products, or fat particles contained within the packed cells. There is even evidence that such cell savers could be used for cesarean sections as they can clear blood of the amniotic fluid.[38] The shelf life of these products is similar to that of cells obtained by euvolemic hemodilution, and the same problem exists regarding adequate labeling. Cell viability after transfusion is similar to that of homologous transfusions.[39]

These systems all use some type of anticoagulant, either heparin or citrate, so there is some concern about contamination of the final product with anticoagulant. If the blood is washed properly and the manufacturer's recommendations are followed, however, the amount of anticoagulant present in the final product is insignificant.[40] If large amounts of cell-saver blood are utilized, the coagulopathies that develop are most likely due to effects of dilutional thrombocytopenia or the loss of factor V due to continuous loss of plasma. Routine coverage of the cell-saver blood with dosages of protamine is unnecessary and may cause further coagulopathy by depressing platelet count and function transiently. Free hemoglobin levels may be elevated after transfusion of cell-salvaged blood, and appropriate precautions regarding renal function are necessary. This problem appears to be reduced by larger volumes of saline washing.[41]

Intraoperative and postoperative blood collection for reinfusion utilizing a number of devices that filter rather than wash blood are now available. Their use for orthopedic surgery and after cardiopulmonary bypass has become widespread.[42–45] The blood product produced by such filtering devices is safe for intravascular reinfusion and can make rather significant contributions to RBC requirements for transfusion. As a product it is different from what is obtained from the cell-saver devices. Because the blood so collected has already clotted and undergone lysis, it is depleted of consumable factors and contains high levels of D-dimer and other fibrin degradation products.[46,47] Platelets are present, although they function poorly because they have already been utilized for clot formation. Transfusion of either shed mediastinal blood or wound blood does not itself cause further coagulopathies in moderate amounts. If can, however, increase the levels of circulating fibrin degradation products and therefore give a laboratory picture that could be confused with disseminated intravascular coagulation.

All three strategies should be maximized to reduce the dependence on homologous blood supplies. The practitioner during the postoperative period may have little input into the preoperative planning and therefore have little control over the utilization of these products. The postanesthesia care unit (PACU) personnel should transfuse autologous units whenever they are available before using homologous units. *The indications for transfusion, however, should be the same.* Patient's who need blood should receive it, but those who can be treated without it should avoid transfusion. Often there is a belief that because patients have donated their own blood they should get it back after surgery. This practice is controversial and perhaps unsafe. Autologous blood carries the same risk for clerical error as does routine homologous blood. Those units of blood obtained by intraoperative salvage, euvolemic hemodilution, or postoperative salvage may even have a higher risk of human error, although the question has not been studied. Bacterial infection of a given unit can occur with either homologous or autologous units. The incidence of clerical error has not changed in 50 years, however, it is considerably less than the incidence of AIDS transmission in blood.[48] Therefore there is no adequate rationale for transfusing unneeded autologous units. Autologous blood is more expensive than homologous blood. Transfusion of autologous units that would not have been indicated except that "the patient paid for it" is difficult to defend if mishap occurs and the blood was not truly indicated.

RISKS OF TRANSFUSION

Understanding the risks of blood transfusion is the heart of rational patient care in terms of blood utilization. The effects of anemia have already been discussed. Essentially, it is difficult to demonstrate that there is benefit derived from individual transfusions or even that relief of anemia by itself produces a better outcome. Certain exceptions can be made in terms of immunosuppression with solid organ transplantation.[49] The only advantage to routine transfusion to achieve a relatively normal hematocrit is that subjectively some patients do "feel better." The myth that relief of anemia creates better wound healing has been disproved.[50] Indeed, mild anemia appears to speed the production of fibroblasts. When one knows these facts, a discussion of the risks of transfusion becomes more important.

Transfusion of homologous blood is still not without risk, although a number of studies have shown it to be the safest it has ever been.[51] The most common reaction is a WBC-mediated allergic-type reaction heralded by the signs of histamine release or a febrile reaction.[52] Unfortunately, the early signs of a major transfusion reaction may also be those of histamine or an allergic reaction. Patients who are emerging from an anesthetic may not complain of many of the side effects of histamine release. Therefore these reactions may not be easy to discern.

Human error is responsible for transfusion reactions in conjunction with approximately one of every 2600 to 6000 U transfused.[53,54] Such reactions do not trigger major cell lysis or cause extensive organ damage. Fatal hemolytic transfusion reactions occur with 1/40,000 to 1/100,000 U transfused. Most of these events (71 per cent) are due to ABO or Rh incompatibility problems that must have occurred because of human error.[55] Mislabeling of samples, laboratory errors, or confusion when checking blood products prior to administration is always the cause of such catastrophes, and they are therefore preventable. The incidence of these events has not changed in 50 years, and it appears that further education of personnel does not substantially change those numbers. Perhaps the future world of computerized data management will create a foolproof system wherein the human factor is removed from the loop of identification. For the postoperative patient the key is a high index of suspicion if any untoward events occur temporally related to the transfusion of blood products. The first line of therapy should always be to stop any possibly offending transfusion and then proceed with further workup and treatment. For patients requiring large amounts of blood products or rapidly transfused products, the identification of 1 U as a source of transfusion reaction may be difficult or impossible. However, every effort should be made to identify an offending unit by returning it to the blood bank for workup.

The risk of disease transmission is of the greatest concern to both the public and health care professionals. Hepatitis B and C (previously non A, non B) are the greatest risks. The incidence of transfusion of active virus has been reported to be somewhere between 1 per 100 to 1 per 200 units transfused. Since the development of new hepatitis C screening for blood, those numbers have decreased. At least one report from Italy noted that the incidence of posttransfusion hepatitis has decreased by almost 50 per cent. However, they also noted an approximately 3 per cent incidence of posttransfusion hepatitis—down from 6 to 10 per cent, and they commented on the degree of safety associated with transfusions today. Their data reflect a definite improvement, but no practitioner should be lulled into thinking that the risks have vanished. AIDS remains the most feared complication of blood transfusion. The incidence of AIDS transmission has been cited to be approximately one case per 50,000 U transfused.[56] These numbers may be tending toward the one case per 1 million units at the present time. The use of hepatitis C testing and a number of clerical and voluntary disqualification methods for donors has helped to make the blood supply safe.[51]

Other viruses may also be transmitted in blood transfusions: Epstein-Barr, cytomegalovirus, and HTLV-I and HTLV-II. Malaria and other parasitic diseases may also be transmitted. Bacterial contamination of stored blood can occur, and a number of cases of *Yersinia enterocolitica* and other pathogen-infected units have been reported.[57–59] If septic blood products are transfused, a picture of septic shock could arise that may be difficult to distinguish from other transfusion reactions.

Red blood cell transfusions are associated with a number of abnormalities depending on how the blood was stored and for how long. Blood stored under refrigeration contains 70 per cent viable RBCs at 42 days of age.[60] Restoration of RBC mass therefore requires 1.5 times normal volume to achieve normal viable erythrocyte function. The cellular debris transfused may be considerable. The utilization of micropore filters (40 μm or less) has been controversial, and to date no absolute indication for filtering below 100 μm exists. Hyperkalemia initially followed by hypocalcemia, hypokalemia, acidosis, and shifts in the oxyhemoglobin dissociation curve are other complications of transfusion.

COAGULATION FUNCTION

The most commonly encountered coagulopathy after all types of surgery is dilutional thrombocytopenia.[61-63] Blood loss with subsequent volume replacement using crystalloids or colloids can, if in large enough doses, significantly decrease the platelet count. Mild and even moderate blood losses may not cause significant thrombocytopenia, as the spleen may release large quantities of platelets into the circulation.[64] There is no magic number below which all patients should receive platelet transfusions. Platelet counts below 20,000/cu mm may contribute to spontaneous hemorrhage, and levels between 50,000 and 100,000/cu mm are generally accepted as adequate for elective surgery. Postoperatively, platelet function, vascular integrity, and the degree of coagulation stimulus may be more important than just platelet number.

Platelet function can be altered by many medications, including aspirin, β-blockers, and calcium channel blockers.[65-69] Aspirin, widely studied, should be discontinued 5 to 7 days prior to elective surgery if normal platelet activity is desirable. A number of other nonsteroidal antiinflammatory agents are being introduced, some of which are now available in intravenous forms; all of them have prostaglandin-inhibiting capability. The effect of these agents on postoperative platelet function and ultimately bleeding has not yet been extensively studied.

The protein coagulation cascade has been reviewed extensively by many others. Both arms of the cascade are activated during surgery and continue to be so into the postoperative period. This effect is both local (at the sight of tissue injury) and systemic. Hypofibrinogenemia may occur owing to dilution, and thrombocytopenia occurs. For normal coagulation, a fibrinogen concentration of at least 150 mg/dl must be present. That level is nearly 100 per cent of the normal concentration and is in contrast to the requirements for other proteins. All other protein procoagulants must present in concentrations of only 20 to 30 per cent of normal or less for adequate coagulation function. Factor V may be decreased because of consumption during an active coagulation process. In the event a massive stimulus for coagulation has occurred, all proteins of the coagulation cascade may decrease in concentration. Disseminated intravascular coagulation (DIC) does occur pe-

rioperatively and may be associated with sepsis, shock, neurosurgery, fat embolism due to orthopedic surgery or trauma, amniotic fluid embolism, dissecting thoracic aneurysm, and massive hemorrhage.[70,71] DIC may be encountered in gradations from mild and compensated to life-threatening. Capillary deposition of coagulation factors and platelets can lead to tissue ischemia and eventual patient demise. Although clot lysis does occur with DIC, it need not always to be present. Fibrinogen and factor V assays, as well as platelet counts, are useful for following the consumptive process and its treatment. Fibrin breakdown products, particularly the D-dimer fragment, may be present with DIC but are not diagnostic.

There is a tendency for any normal patient undergoing surgery to become relatively hypercoagulable as the length of surgery progresses, and this state continues into the postoperative period.[72] Release of tissue thromboplastin and fibrinopeptides can cause generalized stimulation of the coagulation function. Pain and the effects of stress hormones can increase the blood levels of both platelets and fibrinogen.[72-74] Postoperative hypercoagulability may be the result of these changes. Deep venous thrombosis and pulmonary embolism are the feared complications. Patients who are immobilized or who have undergone certain operations, e.g., hip replacement, appear to be at the greatest risk for embolic complications. A number of techniques are being utilized to decrease these risks. Low dose heparin, pneumatic extremity compression devices, and elastic stocking are all being utilized. A number of studies have explored this problem, and no single technique affords complete protection or is universally applicable. Combinations of techniques may also be possible, but some level of embolism still occurs. The use of certain anesthetic and postoperative pain management techniques may decrease hypercoagulability and possibly perioperative thrombotic complications, but this area requires further study.[75] Epidural anesthesia may decrease intraoperative blood loss, decrease stress hormone release, and, if continued into the postoperative period, decrease complications and hypercoagulability. The use of platelet-inhibiting infusions and perhaps in the future short-acting platelet inhibitors may be useful.

Coagulation monitoring during the postoperative period has largely focused on a number of screening tests. The prothrombin time (PT), partial thromboplastin time (PTT), and thrombin time (TT) act as initial gross tests of serum protein cascade function. The extrinsic system is monitored with the PT, the intrinsic system with the PTT, and the final common pathway with the TT. As screening tests they are useful; and if patients have oozing hemorrhage postoperatively these tests should be undertaken. At times, however, the results are misleading. These tests cannot predict the patients who will bleed perioperatively.[76,77] Isolated abnormalities in one or another test do not always signal the need to treat with a blood product (fresh frozen plasma). False-positive tests can occur; and even when all three tests are normal, the platelet number or function abnormalities may overwhelm normal protein function. In vivo the protein cascade must interact with the phospholipid of activated platelets; therefore in vitro serum tests, though useful, do not provide a complete picture of coagulation.

Platelet number can be easily assessed by the platelet count. Platelet function abnormalities are common—perhaps most common after cardiopulmonary bypass. Tests for platelet function have in the past been clinically inadequate. The bleeding time is a gross test for platelet function abnormalities if platelet number is adequate and tissue elastic function, nutrition, and capillary action are normal. The test requires a trained technician so its results are reproducible, and during the evenings and weekends such personnel may not be readily available. Moreover, a review of the literature regarding the bleeding time has shown that it has little predictive value for postoperative bleeding.[78] Other complex tests for platelet function do exist but are time-consuming, are expensive, and may yield little clinically useful information.

Two whole blood tests of clot strength are useful. Thromboelastography (TEG) and Sonoclot were utilized initially for liver transplantations but now are also employed for cardiac and other surgery.[75–77,79,80] Both tests assess the interaction of the coagulation cascade and platelet activity from the time of initiation of clotting through clot growth, retraction, and eventual lysis. They provide a gross overview of clot dynamics but do not provide an in-depth analysis of abnormalities. A key to tracing shapes and abnormal parameters for the TEG has been published and suggests the diagnosis of some coagulopathies. The TEG has

been shown to be predictive of postcardiopulmonary bypass hemorrhage. The application of this technology to all open-heart surgical procedures at our institution has allowed discrimination of surgical versus coagulopathic bleeding postoperatively. Unless hemodynamically compromised, patients have their TEGs normalized before being returned to the operating rooms for reexploration of the mediastinum.

Coagulopathies after cardiopulmonary bypass have been extensively investigated, but this chapter cannot adequately cover the complex nature of those changes. In summary, however, conventional thoughts have always been that a combination of dilutional thrombocytopenia and platelet function abnormalities are the most common causes of bleeding. Studies have shown that continuous stimulation for fibrinolysis occurs during bypass, and that it can be a major contributor to the platelet abnormalities already noted.[81–83] Hemorrhage after bypass can be caused by these problems as well as inadequate reversal of the anticoagulant heparin or even partial reheparinization due to differential hepatic metabolism and redistribution of protamine. Monitoring the activated clotting time intraoperatively and early during the postoperative period identifies situations wherein heparin continues to be present. The future may bring a number of advances in coagulation during and after cardiopulmonary bypass. For example, the use of heparin-bound bypass circuits and the administration of aprotinin appear exciting.

Treatment of coagulopathies depends on proper identification of the abnormality. The length of time it takes to get test results during the early postoperative period has often been such that treatment must be instituted based on clinical judgment. It is now found, though, that the TEG, platelet count, and fibrinogen level can provide data within 30 to 40 minutes that covers almost all coagulopathies. Treatment with platelets, fresh frozen plasma cryoprecipitate, and even ε-aminocapric acid (EACA) simultaneously, as a "shotgun" approach, reveals a misunderstanding of the coagulopathies, exposes a patient to unnecessary infectious risk, and may be harmful by causing a hypercoagulable state. Patients rarely expire from coagulopathic bleeding. Desperate unguided therapy is therefore rarely appropriate.

The available options for coagulopathy

treatment are limited. D-8-Arginine vasopressin (DDAVP) has been shown to be useful for the treatment of von Willebrand's disease and has been tested for cardiac surgery.[84,85] Only one study supports its use in that situation, and a number of repeat studies have shown no advantage to the use of DDAVP in terms of decreasing postoperative hemorrhage. EACA and tranexamic acid stop plasminogen activation and, if given prophylactically, decrease hemorrhage after bypass.[86,87] They may also be used in cases of primary fibrinolysis, but one must be careful to distinguish that condition from secondary lysis due to DIC.

Platelet concentrates (plasma with a high concentration of platelets) can be transfused. Each unit contains 50 to 70 ml of plasma and 5.5×10^{10} platelets. A single unit of platelets should raise the normal patient's platelet count approximately 10,000/ml. Therefore multiple platelet units are usually required, and they are most often from multiple donors, thereby increasing the risk of disease transmission as the population of donors is increased per transfusion. Fresh frozen plasma is the most overutilized and inappropriately transfused blood product, although it does carry all of the plasma proteins necessary for coagulation in the normal concentrations seen in plasma. If a patient has a large enough deficit to require fresh frozen plasma administration, the volume required to raise the patient's plasma protein concentration may be large. The 2-U transfusion does nothing to change either the fibrinogen concentration or other procoagulant activities and therefore is an unnecessary transfusion in most cases. Cryoprecipitate contains a higher concentration of fibrinogen (250 mg/dl) and factor VIII than is seen in fresh frozen plasma. Normal volumes per unit are 10 to 15 ml; therefore if fibrinogen or factor VIII is deficient, some advantage can be gained without giving the large volumes of fresh frozen plasma. Like platelet transfusions, multiple units are often required to correct abnormalities; therefore often 10 or more donor exposures may occur for each treatment. Other individual factor concentrates are available and are also most often prepared from multiple donors.

In summary the judicious use of coagulation blood products during the postoperative period dictates a knowledge of their composition and especially of the coagulopathy to be treated. The fact most often overlooked, especially with postoperative bypass patients, is

that time and rewarming of the patient frequently correct coagulopathies. Hasty treatment may be misconstrued to have helped when these factors were indeed responsible for the cessation of hemorrhage.

SUMMARY

The use of blood products, hemorrhage, and coagulopathies are topics that are timely during the early 1990s. Postoperative care givers routinely encounter bleeding. The decisions of when to transfuse and what products to utilize in the face of coagulopathies are now governed by different criteria from those utilized even during the 1980s. Practitioners must pay attention to each individual decision to transfuse, as it will affect the individual patient and the public health of the nation.

References

1. Spiess BD (ed): Hemorrhagic disorders. Anesthesiol Clin North Am 8:441–692, 1990.
2. Stehling L: Trends in transfusion therapy in hemorrhagic disorders. Anesthesiol Clin North Am 8:519, 1990.
3. Donadoui R, Baele G, Devolder J, et al: Coagulation and fibrinolytic parameters in patients undergoing total hip replacement: influence of anaesthesia technique. Acta Anaesthesiol Scand 33:588–592, 1984.
4. Thompson GE, Miller RD, Stevens WC, et al: Hypotensive anesthesia for total hip arthroplasty: a study of blood loss and organ function (brain, heart, liver and kidney). Anesthesiology 48:91–96, 1978.
5. Krogh A: The number and distribution of capillaries in muscles with calculations of the oxygen pressure head necessary for supplying the tissue. J Physiol (Lond) 52:409, 1919.
6. Krogh A: The supply of oxygen to the tissues and the regulation of capillary circulation. J Physiol (Lond) 52:459, 1919.
7. Tuman KJ: Tissue oxygen delivery: the physiology of anemia. Anesthesiol Clin North Am 8:451, 1990.
8. Messmer K: Hemodilution. Surg Clin North Am 55:659, 1975.
9. Messmer K, Lewis DH, Sunder-Plassmann L, et al: Acute normovolemic hemodilution. Eur Surg Res 4:55, 1972.
10. Cain SM: Oxygen delivery and uptake in dogs during anemic and hypoxic hypoxia. J Appl Physiol 42:228, 1977.
11. Dedichen H, Race D, Scheck WG Jr: Hemodilution and concomitant hyperbaric oxygenation. J Thorac Cardiovasc Surg 53:341, 1967.
12. Fouler NO, Holmes JC: Blood viscosity and cardiac output in acute experimental anemia. J Apply Physiol 39:453, 1975.
13. Farhaeus R, Lindquist T: The viscosity of blood in narrow capillary tubes. Am J Physiol 96:562, 1931.

14. Chien S, Usami S, Taylor HB, et al: Effects of hematocrit and plasma proteins on human blood rheology at low shear rates. J Appl Physiol 21:81, 1966.
15. Mirhashemi S, Messmer K, Intaglietta M: Tissue perfusion improvement during normovolemic hemodilution exhibited by a hydraulic model of cardiovasculature. Microvasc Res 29:240, 1985.
16. Messmer K, Kessler M, Frumme A, et al: Microvascular hemodynamics during normovolemic hemodilution: rheological changes during normovolemic hemodilution. Arzneimittelforschung 25:1670, 1975.
17. Biro GP: Comparison of acute cardiovascular effects and oxygen supply following hemodilution with dextran, strove-free hemoglobin solution and fluorocarbon suspension. Cardiovasc Res 16:194, 1982.
18. Crystal GJ, Salem MR: Myocardial oxygen consumption and segmental shortening during isovolemic hemodilution above and in combination with adenosine-induced controlled hypotension. Anesth Analg 67:339, 1988.
19. Von Restroff W, Hofling B, Holtz J, et al: Effect of increased blood fluidity through hemodilution on coronary circulation at rest and during exercise in dogs. Pflugers Arch 357:15, 1975.
20. Brazier J, Cooper N, Maloney JV Jr, et al: The adequacy of myocardial oxygen delivery in acute normovolemic anemia. Surgery 75:508, 1974.
21. Cain SM, Chapler CK: O$_2$ extraction of hindlimb versus whole dog during anemic hypoxia. J Appl Physiol 45:966, 1978.
22. Most AS, Ruocco NA, Gerwitz H: Effect of reduction in blood viscosity on maximal myocardial oxygen delivery distal to a moderate coronary stenosis. Circulation 74:1085, 1986.
23. Laxenaire MC, Aug F, Voisin C, et al: Effects of hemodilution on ventricular function in coronary heart disease patients. Ann Fr Anesth Reanim 5:218, 1986.
24. Ansari A: The angina that signaled more than heart disease. Geriatrics 42:87, 1987.
25. Smith RC, Leung JM, Mangano DT, et al: Postoperative myocardial ischemia in patients undergoing coronary artery bypass graft surgery. Anesthesiology 74:464–473, 1991.
26. Adams RC, Lundy JS: Anesthesia in cases of poor surgical risk: some suggestions for decreasing the risk. Surg Gynecol Obstet 71:1011, 1941.
27. Ellison N, Silberstein LE: A commentary on three consensus development conferences on transfusion medicine. Anesthesiol Clin North Am 8:609, 1990.
28. Stehling L: Perioperative Autologous Transfusion. Arlington, VA, American Association of Blood Banks, 1991.
29. Maffei LM, Thurer RL: Autologous Blood Transfusion: Current Issues. Arlington, VA, American Association of Blood Banks, 1988.
30. Toy P: Autologous transfusion. Anesthesiol Clin North Am 8:533, 1990.
31. Kafer ER, Collins ML: Acute intraoperative hemodilution and perioperative blood salvage. Anesthesiol Clin North Am 8:543, 1990.
32. Ezzedine H, Baele P, Robert A: Bacteriologic quality of intraoperative autotransfusion. Surgery 109:259, 1991.
33. Bondreaux JP, Bornside GH, Cohn I Jr: Emergency autotransfusion: partial cleansing of bacteria-laden blood by cell washing. J Trauma 23:31, 1983.
34. Dale RF, Kipling RM, Smith MF, et al: Separation of malignant cells during autotransfusion. Br J Surg 75:581, 1988.
35. Klimberg I, Serois R, Waysman Z, et al: Intraoperative autotransfusion in urologic oncology. Arch Surg 121:1326, 1986.
36. Klimberg I: Autotransfusion and blood conservation in urologic oncology. Semin Surg Oncol 5:286, 1989.
37. Orr MD: Autotransfusion: intraoperative scavenging. Int Anesthesiol Clin 20:97, 1982.
38. Keeling MM, Gray LA, Brink MA, et al: Intraoperative autotransfusion: experience in 725 consecutive cases. Ann Surg 197:536, 1983.
39. Ray JM, Flynn JC, Bierman AH: Erythrocyte survival following intraoperative autotransfusion in spinal surgery: an in vivo comparative study and 5 year update. Spine 11:879, 1986.
40. Breyer RH, Engleman RM, Rouson JA, et al: Blood conservation for myocardial revascularization. J Thorac Cardiovasc Surg 93:512, 1987.
41. Henn A, Hoffmann R, Muller HAG: Haptoglobin determination in the serum of patients following intraoperative autotransfusion using the Haemonetics Cell Saver III: studies on the loading of patients with free hemoglobin in retransfused erythrocyte concentrate. Anaesthesist 37:741, 1988.
42. Schoff HV, Haver JM, Bell WR, et al: Autotransfusion of shed mediastinal blood after cardiac surgery. J Thorac Cardiovasc Surg 75:632, 1978.
43. Thurer RL, Lytle BW, Cosgrove DM, Loop FD: Autotransfusion following cardiac operations: a randomized, prospective study. Ann Thorac Surg 27:500, 1979.
44. Napoli VM, Symbas PJ, Vroon DH, Symbas PN: Autotransfusion from experimental hemothorax: levels of coagulation factors. J Trauma 27:296, 1987.
45. Lepore V, Radegrau K: Autotransfusion of mediastinal blood in cardiac surgery. Scand J Thorac Cardiovasc Surg 27:47, 1989.
46. Griffith LD, Billman GF, Daily PO, Lane TA: Apparent coagulopathy caused by infusion of shed mediastinal blood and its prevention by washing of the infusate. Ann Thorac Surg 47:400, 1989.
47. Marcovity MJ, Smith RC, Brown M, et al: Hematosis markers in cardiac surgery patients following postoperative autotransfusion. Anesth Analg 67:S140, 1988.
48. Wenz B, Burus ER: Improvement in safety using a new blood unit and patient identification system as part of safe transfusion practice. Transfusion 31:401, 1991.
49. Opelz G, Sengar DPS, Mickey MR, et al: Effect of blood transfusions in subsequent kidney translants. Transplant Proc 5:253, 1973.
50. Heughan C, Crislig G, Hunt TK: The effect of anemia on wound healing. Ann Surg 179:163, 1974.
51. Sirchia G, Giovanetti AM, Parravicini A, et al: Prospective evaluation of posttransfusion hepatitis. Transfusion 31:299, 1991.
52. De Rie MA, van der Plas-van Dalen CM, Engelfriet CP, et al: The serology of febrile transfusion reactions. Vox Sang 49:126, 1985.
53. Sazama K: Reports of 355 transfusion-associated deaths: 1976 through 1985. Transfusion 30:583, 1990.
54. Binder LS, Ginsberg V, Harnel MH: A six year study of incompatible blood transfusions. Surg Gynecol Obstet 108:19, 1959.
55. Edinger SE: A closer look at fatal transfusion reactions. Med Lab Observ 17:41, 1985.

56. Warner MA, Faust RJ: Risks of transfusion. Anesthesiol Clin North Am 8:501, 1990.
57. Collins PS, Salander JM, Youkey B, et al: Fatal sepsis from blood contaminated with Yersinia enterocolitica. Milit Med 150:684, 1985.
58. Galloway SJ, Jones PD: Transfusion acquired Yersinia enterocolitica. Aust NZ J Med 16:248, 1986.
59. Wright DC, Selss IF, Vinton KJ, et al: Fatal Yersinia enterocolitica sepsis after blood transfusion. Arch Pathol Lab Med 109:1040, 1985.
60. Beutler E: Preservation of liquid red cells. In Rossi E, Simon TL, Moss GS (eds): Principles of Transfusion Medicine. Baltimore, Williams & Wilkins, 1991, pp. 47–56.
61. Miller RD, Robbins TO, Toug MJ, et al: Coagulation defects associated with massive blood transfusions. Ann Surg 174:794, 1971.
62. Addonizio VP, Colman RW: Platelets and extracorporeal circulation. Biomaterials 3:9, 1982.
63. Mammen E, Koets M, Washington B, et al: The hemostasis mechanism after open heart surgery. J Thorac Cardiovasc Surg 70:298, 1975.
64. Weinfeld A, Branehog I, Kutl J: Platelets in the myeloproliferative syndrome. Thromb Haematol 38:1085, 1977.
65. Kiyomoto A, Saski Y, Odawara A, et al: Inhibition of platelet aggregation by diltiazem: comparison with verapamil, nifedipine and inhibitory potencies of diltiazem metabolites. Circ Res 52(suppl 1):115, 1983.
66. Lichtenthal PR, Rossi EC, Louis G, et al: Dose related prolongation of the bleeding time by intravenous nitroglycerin. Anesthesiology 64:30, 1985.
67. Mehta J, Mehta P: Comparative effects of nitroprusside and nitroglycerin on platelet aggregation in patients with heart failure. J Cardiovasc Pharmacol 2:25, 1980.
68. Mills CDB: The mechanism of action of antiplatelet drugs. In Colman RW, Hirsh J, Marder VJ, et al (eds): Hemostasis and Thrombosis. Philadelphia, Lippincott, 1982, pp. 1058–1067.
69. Chesebro JH, Steele PM, Fuster V: Platelet-inhibitor therapy in cardiovascular disease: effective defense against thromboembolism. Postgrad Med 78:48, 1985.
70. Brozovic M: Disseminated intravascular coagulation. In Bloom AL, Thomas DP (eds): Haemostasis and Thrombosis. New York, Churchill Livingstone, 1981, pp. 415–421.
71. Muller-Berghaus G: Pathophysiology of generalized intravascular coagulation. Semin Thromb Hemost 3:209, 1977.
72. Tuman K, Spiess BD, McCarthy R, et al: Effects of progressive blood loss on coagulation as measured by thromboelastography. Anesth Analg 66:856, 1987.
73. Caprini JA, Zuckerman L, Cohen E, et al: The identification of accelerated coagulability. Thromb Res 9:167, 1976.
74. Amundsen MA, Spittel JA, Thompson JH, et al: Hypercoagulability associated with malignant disease and with postoperative state: evidence for elevated levels of antihemophilic globulin. Ann Intern Med 58:608, 1963.
75. Tuman KJ, McCarthy RJ, Spiess BD, Ivankovich AD: Epidural anesthesia and analgesia decreases postoperative hypercoagulability. Anesth Analg 70:S414, 1990.
76. Tuman KJ, Spiess BD, McCarthy RJ, et al: Comparison of visoelastic measures of coagulation after cardiopulmonary bypass. Anesth Analg 69:69, 1989.
77. Spiess BD, Tuman KJ, McCarthy RJ, et al: Thromboelastography as an indicator of post cardiopulmonary bypass coagulopathies. J Clin Monit 3:25, 1987.
78. Channing Rodgers RP, Levin J: A critical reappraisal of the bleeding time. Semin Thromb Hemostas 16:1, 1990.
79. Kang YG, Martin D, Marquez J, et al: Intraoperative changes in blood coagulation and thromboelastographic monitoring in liver transplantation. Anesth Analg 64:888, 1985.
80. Saleen A, Blifeld C, Salsh SA, et al: Visoelastic measurement of clot formation: a new test of platelet function. Ann Clin Lab Sci 13:115, 1983.
81. Mammen E, Kocts MH, Washington B, et al: Hemostasis changes during cardiopulmonary bypass surgery. Semin Thromb Hemost 11:281, 1985.
82. Tanaka K, Takao M, Yada I, et al: Alterations in coagulation and fibrinolysis associated with cardiopulmonary bypass during open heart surgery. J Cardiothorac Anesth 3:181, 1989.
83. Bagge L, Lilieuberg G, Nystrom SO, et al: Coagulation fibrinolysis and bleeding after open heart surgery. Scand J Thorac Cardiovasc Surg 20:151, 1986.
84. Reich DL, Hammerschlag BC, Rand JH, et al: Desmopressin acetate is a mild vasodilator that does not reduce blood loss in uncomplicated cardiac surgical procedures. J Cardiothorac Vasc Anesth 2:142, 1991.
85. Salzman EW, Weinstein MJ, Weintraub RM, et al: Treatment with desmopressin acetate to reduce blood loss after cardiac surgery: a double-blind randomized trial. N Engl J Med 314:1402, 1986.
86. Vander Salm TJ, Ansell JE, O'Kike ON, et al: The role of epsilon-aminocaproic acid in reducing bleeding after cardiac operation: a double-blind randomized study. J Thorac Cardiovasc Surg 96:538, 1988.
87. Horrow J, Hlavacek J, Strong MD, et al: Prophylactic transexamic acid decreases bleeding after cardiac operations. J Thorac Cardiovasc Surg 99:70, 1990.

ACUTE PERIOPERATIVE RENAL DYSFUNCTION 10

LOREN A. BAUMAN and DONALD S. PROUGH

Acute renal failure (ARF) is the sudden reduction of renal function, with or without decreased urine flow, severe enough to result in retention of nitrogenous waste products. The cause of renal failure is multifactorial; hypotension, dehydration, aminoglycoside therapy, and pigmenturia play principal roles.[1,2]

Elevations of blood urea nitrogen and creatinine occur in approximately 5 per cent of all general hospital admissions and in up to 20 per cent of intensive care unit (ICU) patients. In traumatized patients, the risk of ARF increases as the severity (and number) of injuries increase. Ten to fifty per cent of ICU patients suffering from respiratory failure, sepsis, or hepatic failure develop ARF; and most of those affected succumb. Although the incidence of acute perioperative ARF has declined since the 1970s, the mortality rate remains at 50 to 90 per cent.[3] Despite highly sophisticated supportive care, including dialysis, the mortality rate has remained similar for 30 years.

This review focuses on two areas. The first section discusses the mechanisms of renal injury seen in perioperative patients, the clinical settings in which renal injury occurs, and treatment approaches that may minimize injury. The second section summarizes the available types of renal replacement therapy including hemodialysis, hemofiltration, peritoneal dialysis, and continuous hemofiltration.

CLINICAL ASPECTS OF ACUTE RENAL DYSFUNCTION

PATHOGENESIS

Oliguria (urinary output <0.5 ml·kg^{-1}·hr^{-1}) precedes ARF in approximately one half of patients and is conventionally divided into three functional categories: prerenal, renal, and postrenal.[4] Because both prerenal and postrenal oliguria can progress to renal parenchymal disease, rapid treatment may restore urinary flow and prevent the development of ARF.

Prerenal Oliguria

Prerenal oliguria, the most common form of postoperative oliguria, frequently results from decreased renal blood flow (RBF). In response to circulatory compromise, the endocrine mediators renin, angiotensin II, aldosterone, and antidiuretic hormone (ADH) reduce urinary output to conserve water and sodium. Renal vascular disease (renal artery stenosis or renal vein thrombosis) may also compromise RBF.

Renal blood flow, approximately 20 per cent of cardiac output, is regulated by alterations of afferent and efferent arteriolar resistance. The renin-angiotensin and prostaglandin systems, the principal regulators of afferent and efferent resistance, autoregulate renal perfusion over a range of mean arterial pressures of 80 to 160 mm Hg.[5] The distribution of intrarenal blood flow, normally 90 per cent cortical, 8 per cent medullary, and 2 per cent papillary, appears to be regulated by the afferent arteriole, where a large pressure drop has been measured. Autoregulation can be overridden by sympathetic vasoconstriction or by circulating catecholamines, which decrease both cortical perfusion and the glomerular filtration rate (GFR) by increasing afferent arteriolar resistance.[6] Maximal sympathetic stimulation diverts nearly one additional liter of blood per minute from the kidneys to the systemic circulation. Initially, despite decreased RBF, the GFR is well maintained by efferent arteriolar vasoconstriction, thereby elevating the filtration fraction.

Renal underperfusion stimulates conservation of water and sodium. Moderate hypovolemia reduces the stimulation of atrial stretch receptors, thereby initiating ADH release and increasing reabsorption of water in the collecting ducts. Frank hypotension stimulates the vagally innervated aortic arch and carotid sinus baroreceptors, leading to further ADH secretion. Maximum ADH stimulation increases urine osmolality to nearly 1200 mOsm·L^{-1}, although acutely stressed patients may not achieve maximal urinary concentration. To excrete the normal dietary solute load of 400 to 600 mOsm·day^{-1}, the kidneys must excrete urine at a rate of 300 to 500 ml·day^{-1}; stress-induced loss of concentrating ability necessitates greater urinary output to maintain solute balance. Additional solute generated by hypercatabolism, as occurs in burned or septic patients, may require even greater urinary flow.[7]

The renin-angiotensin system powerfully regulates sodium excretion, RBF and GFR. Renin is released from the juxtaglomerular apparatus in response to decreased afferent arteriolar pressure,[8] catecholamine secretion, and increasing tubular concentrations of sodium and chloride delivered to the macula densa.[9] Renin releases angiotensin I, which is converted by angiotensin-converting enzyme to angiotensin II, a potent vasoconstrictor. Angiotensin II constricts both afferent and efferent arterioles, thereby reducing GFR, and it releases aldosterone, which leads to increased sodium reabsorption in the distal tubule.[10]

Trauma, including surgical trauma, and anesthesia typically produce renal hemodynamic and endocrine changes that result in a "prerenal" state, i.e., intense conservation of sodium and water. The primary treatment of prerenal obliguria aims to improve renal perfusion. Prompt restoration of RBF may increase urinary flow, diminish hormonal responses to circulatory depression, and prevent ARF.

Postrenal Oliguria

Postrenal (obstructive) oliguria can present as anuria, oliguria, fluctuating oliguria, and polyuria or as nonoliguric renal failure. It occurs because of extrarenal obstruction at the level of the urethra, bladder neck, or ureters or because of intrarenal obstruction caused by tubular deposition of crystals (e.g., uric acid, oxalate) or necrotic tissue debris. The diagnosis of postrenal obstruction requires identification of the site of obstruction. Malfunction of existing urinary catheters must be excluded in postoperative patients. Bladder catheterization, essential in severely traumatized patients, does not preclude unilateral obstruc-

tion, ureteral injury, or intraperitoneal leakage of urine. If the site of obstruction is obscure, abdominal ultrasonography may be diagnostic. Computed tomography, cystoscopy, and retrograde pyelography may be necessary for accurate diagnosis in selected circumstances.

Renal Oliguria

Oliguric ARF implies that renal dysfunction cannot be corrected by improving prerenal or postrenal factors.[11] Multiple perioperative events may produce ARF. The following sections outline those events, the mechanism by which they cause renal injury, and the potential for treatment.

Hemodynamically Mediated ARF. Inadequately replaced intravascular fluid loss during the perioperative period may reduce cardiac output and renal perfusion. Altered renal perfusion, with or without systemic hypotension, leads to a series of compensatory (prerenal) responses that may ultimately cause renal dysfunction. Although hemodynamically mediated ARF often resolves within 4 to 6 weeks, severe metabolic derangements result from accumulated sodium, potassium, water, and protein catabolic products.

The terminology of ARF has evolved considerably over the past half-century, leaving an array of historically interesting, but confusing terms. Acute tubular necrosis, a term first used in 1951 to describe the renal lesion produced by mercury poisoning,[12] is now used commonly to describe ARF produced by renal hypoperfusion. Classically, patchy loss of individual tubular epithelial cells focally denudes portions of the tubular basement membrane.[13] Hypertrophied actin filaments in the basement membranes form diverticular outpouchings that suggest contraction of basement membranes,[14] possibly mediated by angiotensin II or thromboxane. The brush border of tubular cells becomes markedly attenuated; sufficient accumulation of debris in the tubular lumen may obstruct the distal tubules. Dilated tubules, lined by flattened cells, are filled with casts of hyaline granular or pigmented material.[15]

Possible mechanisms of hemodynamically mediated ARF (Fig. 10–1) include the following:

1. Altered renal blood flow. In response to declining renal perfusion pressure, RBF and GFR may decrease to a fraction of baseline values. Redistribution of blood flow from

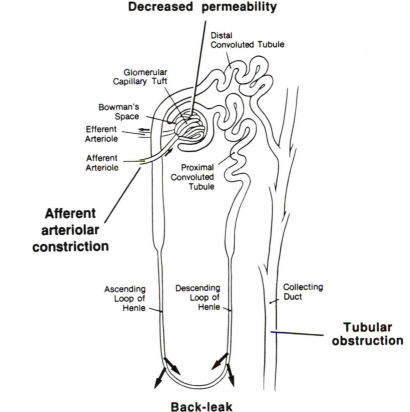

FIGURE 10–1. Mechanisms of hemodynamically mediated ARF. 1) Altered renal blood flow by afferent arteriolar constriction; 2) altered glomerular permeability; 3) tubular obstruction from cellular debris; 4) tubular backleak.

cortical to juxtamedullary nephrons reduces glomerular perfusion in disproportion to the reduction in total RBF.[16]

2. Glomerular abnormalities. The glomeruli in postischemic ARF appear structurally normal, but the filtration fraction declines, perhaps as a consequence of reduced glomerular permeability or afferent arteriolar vasoconstriction.

3. Tubular debris. Obstruction of tubular flow by intratubular debris, produced by ischemic desquamation of brush border microvilli[17] or pigmented casts, can result in back-pressure that opposes glomerular filtration.[18] Although rarely the primary mechanism of ARF (except that caused by pigmenturia or crystallinuria), tubular obstruction may be important for the maintenance of ARF. Mannitol, by maintaining high tubular flow, may prevent ARF by tubular obstruction.[19]

4. Tubular integrity. Disruption of the integrity of tubular epithelium permits "back-leak" of filtrate into the peritubular interstitium and peritubular capillaries. Back-leak, which is aggravated by tubular obstruction from intraluminal debris, may result in retention of nearly 50 per cent of total filtrate, leading to accumulation of waste products and water.[20,21]

Nephrotoxic ARF. AMINOGLYCOSIDE NEPHROTOXICITY. Aminoglycoside antibiotics are associated with nephrotoxicity in 9 to 21 per cent of patients.[22,23] Eisenberg et al. reported that aminoglycoside-related renal dysfunction doubled the duration of hospitalization and significantly increased total hospital charges.[24] Nearly three fourths of ARF secondary to aminoglycosides is nonoliguric,[25] although oliguric ARF may occur.

Aminoglycoside-induced renal injury is characterized by enzymuria, reduced glomerular permeability, vasopressin-resistant concentrating defect, and progressive reduction in GFR.[16] Progressive excretion of enzymes derived from the proximal tubular brush border and from lysosomes reflects proximal tubular injury. Reduced glomerular permeability results from a reduction in the number and density of endothelial fenestrations. Urinary diagnostic tests typically show impaired sodium conservation and reduced concentrating ability. Because the aminoglycosides are cleared exclusively by the kidney, progressive reduction of the GFR produces a steady rise in the "trough" concentration, thereby progressively increasing drug levels and potentiating renal toxicity.

All aminoglycosides are not equally nephrotoxic. Neomycin, which binds most avidly to proximal tubular cells, is sufficiently nephrotoxic that it cannot be given systemically. Most investigators rank gentamicin, tobramycin, and amikacin in order of decreasing nephrotoxicity.[26,27] However, in a prospective, controlled trial, Matzke et al.[25] found an 8 to 10 per cent incidence of gentamicin-induced nephrotoxicity and an 18 per cent incidence associated with tobramycin.

Factors that aggravate aminoglycoside nephrotoxicity include sustained high blood levels, cephalosporin, antibiotics, potent diuretics, advanced age, volume depletion, acidemia, endotoxemia, and a history of recent exposure to aminoglycosides and nonsteroidal antiinflammatory drugs (NSAIDs). Aminoglycoside toxicity can be minimized by limiting risk factors. Although periodic monitoring of serum trough levels reduces toxicity, renal failure may occur despite normal serum levels. Intermittent assessment of urinary concentrating ability and measurement of the tubular enzyme β_2-microglobulin in urine may detect early renal toxicity.[28]

AMPHOTERICIN-INDUCED RENAL INJURY. Amphotericin, a polyene antifungal agent, causes dose-dependent, nonallergic renal insufficiency.[29] The onset of amphotericin-induced renal dysfunction is associated with increased urinary accumulation of crystalline and amorphous material. Hypokalemia and a vasopressin-resistant concentrating defect precede the elevation of creatinine.[30]

Amphotericin-induced nephrotoxicity causes necrosis of the proximal and distal tubular epithelial cells, resulting in tubular atrophy, interstitial edema, and fibrosis.[31] Tubular back-lead of urea probably explains the disproportionately rapid increase in blood urea nitrogen associated with the lesion. RBF, though markedly decreased, is initially compensated by efferent arteriolar constriction and an increased filtration fraction.[32] Experimentally, the intense renal vasoconstriction can be blocked by aminophylline.[33] Minimizing renal injury due to amphotericin can best be accomplished by urinary alkalinization, avoidance of volume depletion, and experimentally by administering amphotericin in a liposome carrier.[34]

CEPHALOSPORIN NEPHROTOXICITY. All cephalosporins have been sporadically associated with two forms of nephrotoxicity. Direct toxicity may produce acute tubular nephrosis, or a hypersensitivity reaction may generate acute interstitial nephritis, accompanied by rash, eosinophiluria, fever, and the presence of cellular casts.[35,36] Cephalosporin-induced ARF appears to be more likely in patients given excessive doses or in those concurrently treated with aminoglycosides[37] or diuretics. Despite widespread use, cephalothin, a semisynthetic, β-lactam antibiotic commonly used to treat gram-positive and gram-negative infections, has rarely been associated with nephrotoxicity.

ANESTHETIC AGENTS AND ARF. Although the renal effects of surgery and trauma are the predominant cause of perioperative renal insufficiency, certain anesthetic agents have also been associated with acute renal dysfunction. Enflurane, for example, is metabolized to F^- but rarely produces renal toxic levels. Because enflurane is highly fat-soluble, enflurane-induced renal dysfunction is more likely in obese patients.[38] If patients with preoperative renal dysfunction undergo prolonged enflurane anesthesia, serum F^- levels may reach 90 to 100 $\mu M \cdot L^{-1}$.[39,40] If renal function is normal, even prolonged enflurane anesthesia is unlikely to generate toxic levels of F^-. Hepatic metabolism of halothane and isoflurane rarely, if ever, produces sufficient F^- to induce ARF.

Contrast-Medium-Induced ARF. The risk of ARF following administration of contrast media is increased by multiple risk factors (Table 10–1), the most significant of which is preexisting renal insufficiency. If the creatinine is less than 1.5 mg/dl, the risk of contrast-induced ARF is 0.6 per cent, increasing to 3 per cent if creatinine is 1.5 to 4.5 mg/dl.[41] Other risk factors include diabetes mellitus, multiple myeloma, dehydration, congestive heart failure, hyperuricemia, liver disease, proteinuria, and vascular disease. Following contrast studies, renal injury produces evidence of azotemia beginning 24 to 48 hours after exposure; creatinine rapidly increases 3 to 5 days after injury, then typically becomes normal within 2 weeks. The newer radiocontrast agents are minimally toxic in the absence of risk factors.[42]

Possible mechanisms of acute renal injury secondary to contrast media include 1) direct cellular toxicity; 2) tubular obstruction; 3) uricosuria (associated with cholecystographic

TABLE 10–1. RISK FACTORS IN THE DEVELOPMENT OF CONTRAST-INDUCED ARF

Definite risk factor
  Preexisting renal insufficiency
Probable risk factors
  Diabetes mellitus
  Multiple myeloma
  Dehydration
  Prior contrast-induced acute renal failure
  Large contrast load
  Congestive heart failure
Possible risk factors
  Advanced age
  Vascular disease
  Proteinuria
  Hyperuricemia
  Hepatic diseases

Reproduced with permission from Coggins CH, Fang LST: Acute renal failure associated with antibiotics, anesthetic agents, and radiographic contrast agents. *In* Brenner BM, Lazarus JM, eds. Acute Renal Failure. New York, Churchill Livingstone, 1988, p. 295.

agents); 4) intrarenal vasoconstriction, mediated by the renin-angiotensin system; and 5) crenation of red blood cells, leading to agglutination and aggregation, local vascular obstruction, and renal tissue hypoxia.

Agents that alter the agglutination of red blood cells (dextran and volume expansion) protect against ARF induced by contrast media. Volume expansion effectively reduces the risk of contrast-induced ARF by minimizing proteinaceous tubular obstruction.[43,44] Mannitol (25 gm) attenuates experimental contrast-induced ARF.[45,46] Minimizing the total dose of contrast medium used also helps to limit injury.

Myoglobin-Induced ARF. Myoglobin, if released in large quantities from injured skeletal muscle, causes ARF (Table 10–2). Several clinical situations associated with myoglobin-induced ARF are 1) the Crush syndrome, in which concomitant hypovolemia occurs owing to hemorrhage and fluid sequestration; 2) strenuous exertion such as with military training, status epilepticus,[47] status asthmaticus,[48]

TABLE 10–2. CAUSES OF MYOGLOBIN-INDUCED ARF

Extensive tissue ischemia
Crush syndrome
Status epilepticus (grand mal)
Severe exertion
Alcohol or drug overdose
Electrolyte imbalance (low phosphate, low potassium)

or prolonged labor[49]; 3) embolic arterial ischemia and rhabdomyolysis; 4) nontraumatic myonecrosis associated with heroin or alcohol abuse, diabetic ketoacidosis, heavy metal poisoning, and several primary muscle diseases; 5) severe hypokalemia, especially if combined with exercise[50]; and 6) hypophosphatemia, especially in alcoholics and severely malnourished patients. Hypophosphatemia limits the regeneration of ATP from ADP.[51] Myoglobinuria is confirmed by orthotolidine-positive (Dipstick) or Hematest-positive urine in the absence of red blood cells on a centrifuged urine sample.

Myoglobin is most toxic when combined with dehydration and reduced tubular flow. Acidic urine (pH < 5.6) converts myoglobin and hemoglobin to highly toxic hematin (ferrihematin).

Myoglobinemia is associated with a precipitous fall in GFR, probably because of swelling of glomerular epithelial and mesangial cells combined with tubular obstruction. Cortical vasoconstriction may result from enhanced sympathetic nervous system tone, activation of the renin-angiotensin system, decreased renal prostaglandin production, or increased ADH release. Precipitation of hematin and urate crystals leads to tubular obstruction.

Because the treatment of pigment-induced ARF is largely unsuccessful, prevention is crucial. Mannitol in doses of 25 to 50 gm prevents the functional anatomic changes seen in experimental pigment-induced ARF. Mannitol induces diuresis and prevents tubular obstruction by decreasing glomerular edema and maintaining tubular flow. In experimental models, furosemide aggravates ARF associated with myoglobinuria. Alkalization of urine with sodium bicarbonate prevents conversion of myoglobin to hematin, decreases tubular obstruction, and reduces associated toxic tubular effects.[52]

ACUTE INTERSTITIAL NEPHRITIS. Acute interstitial nephritis (AIN), often misdiagnosed as acute tubular nephritis because of its presentation, demands a different approach to treatment. AIN is characterized histopathologically by a severe interstitial lymphocytic infiltration. Electron microscopy reveals severe, focal, tubular destruction and disintegration of tubular basement membranes.[15,53] Severe tubular back-leak probably accelerates the onset of uremia. A hypersensitivity mechanism is suggested by the lack of dose dependency, the long latent period between the inciting factor and the onset of renal dysfunction, and the frequent association with skin rash and blood eosinophilia. Fever is common. The urine contains red blood cells, white blood cells, and renal epithelial cells. White blood cell casts are common, and eosinophiluria is diagnostic. Drugs, systemic infection, immunologic diseases, transplant rejection, and pyelonephritis are associated with AIN. Antibiotics, particularly penicillin-related β-lactam antibiotics (methicillin, ampicillin, nafcillin, and oxacillin) produce a nonallergic ARF, usually after at least 10 days of therapy.[54] Other drugs associated with AIN include cimetidine, rifampin, NSAIDs, barbiturates, phenytoin, thiazide diuretics, and furosemide. Both oliguric and nonoliguric forms of AIN have been reported, with the latter constituting 20 to 60 per cent of cases.[55–57]

Both oliguric and nonoliguric AIN may require dialysis, but the prognosis is favorable, providing the offending agent is removed. Although corticosteroids are often used, their clinical efficacy is uncertain.

ATHEROEMBOLIC RENAL DISEASE. Atheromatous material can be dislodged by thoracic or abdominal trauma, cardiac or aortic surgery, or intraaortic catheters. The clinical diagnosis, often difficult, rests on a high index of suspicion and the recognition of peripheral embolization (e.g., ischemic injury to fingers and toes). Livido reticularis, an irregular skin mottling at sites of small vessel occlusion, strongly suggests atheroembolic disease. No specific findings or laboratory values are diagnostic; the only clinical manifestation may be oliguria with increasing hypertension. Biopsy of ischemic areas may be helpful. There is no specific therapy.

Nonoliguric Acute Renal Failure. Nonoliguric acute renal failure (NOARF), rare when first reported during the early 1940s, now represents most[55,58] of the ARF encountered in a general medical-surgical hospital.[59] The increasing incidence has been attributed to widespread use of aminoglycosides, aggressive early use of potent loop diuretics[60] and renal vasodilators, and improved detection through routine serum chemistry panels.

Nephrotoxins, primarily aminoglycosides, cause one fourth of the cases of ARF, most of which are nonoliguric (Table 10–3). Approximately 50 per cent of ARF results from inadequate renal perfusion, often associated with surgical trauma. Improved intraoperative fluid and hemodynamic management appear to favor the development of NOARF rather than oliguric ARF following severe trauma.[61,62] NOARF often follows brief intervals of total

TABLE 10–3. ETIOLOGY OF NONOLIGURIC ARF

Traumatic hypovolemia
Extensive burns
Perioperative renal ischemia
Antibiotics
  Aminoglycosides
  Amphotericin
  Cephalosporins
Radiologic contrast media
Nontraumatic rhabdomyolysis
Hypercalcemia
Hyperuricemia
Cisplatin

renal ischemia.[11] Hypercalcemia and hyperuricemia can also cause NOARF. Ninety per cent of severely burned patients who develop ARF have a nonoliguric or polyuric ARF with a low fractional excretion of sodium. The overall frequency of ARF is 38 per cent in patients sustaining a second or third degree burn that exceeds 30 per cent of surface area.[63] Aminoglycosides, volume depletion, and sepsis commonly contribute to ARF in burned patients.

Converting Oliguric ARF to NOARF. NOARF represents a milder form of the same injury seen with oliguric ARF. Glomerular filtration and tubular function are better maintained with NOARF than with oliguric ARF.[59] In a heterogeneous population of patients with NOARF, complications, duration, and mortality are reduced in comparison to oliguric ARF.[64] Severely traumatized patients with NOARF also demonstrate reduced mortality and morbidity in comparison to oliguric ARF.[62] However, conversion of established, oliguric ARF to NOARF using high doses of loop diuretics and dopamine does not improve the outcome.[65] Renal vasodilators and potent diuretic agents are of limited value in increasing urinary output when administered late in ARF.

LABORATORY EVALUATION OF RENAL FUNCTION

BLOOD AND URINE TESTS

Serum Creatinine

An increase of creatinine (Cr) exceeding 0.5 $mg \cdot dl^{-1}$ suggests ARF, although Cr and Cr clearance determinations may be artificially elevated by non-Cr chromogens and physiologic variability (Table 10–4). Cr also can be

TABLE 10–4. POTENTIAL CONFOUNDING FACTORS IN CREATININE DETERMINATION

Diurnal variation
Proteinuria
Noncreatinine chromagens
   Methyldopa
   Acetoacetate
   Acetone
   α-Ketoglutarate
   Oxaloacetate

TABLE 10–5. URINARY DIAGNOSTIC TESTS FOR ACUTE OLIGURIA

Test	Prerenal	Renal
Urine sodium (mEq·L^{-1})	<20	>40
Urine osmolality (mOsm·L^{-1})	>500	<350
Urine/plasma osmolality	>1.3	<1.1
Urine/plasma urea	>8	<3
Urine/plasma creatinine	>40	<20
Fractional excretion of sodium (%)	<1	>2

falsely elevated by the presence of ketone bodies. Artifactual increases in Cr result in underestimation of Cr. If GFR ceases, Cr clearance increases by 1.0 to 3.0 mg·dl^{-1}·day^{-1}.

Urinary Sodium and Concentrating Ability

Sodium conservation and retained concentrating ability strongly suggest that oliguria results from renal hypoperfusion. With prerenal oliguria, avid sodium reabsorption in the distal tubule usually reduces urinary sodium to 20 mEq·L^{-1} or less. With ARF, impaired sodium conservation results in urinary sodium concentrations that exceed 40 mEq·L^{-1}. However, the specificity and sensitivity of urinary sodium measurements are too poor to permit confident use in acute situations.

Concentrating ability can be assessed by determination of urinary specific gravity or urinary osmolality. Specific gravity, the ratio of the weight of equal volumes of urine and water, is heavily influenced by the weight of any particles in the urine (e.g., protein, blood, or contrast medium) and may not reflect concentrating capability. Urinary osmolality, not influenced by particle weight, can be precisely measured. With prerenal oliguria, urinary osmolality should exceed 400 mOsm·L^{-1} (1.3 × serum); with ARF, the loss of concentrating ability results in isosthenuria (~285 to 300 mOsm·L^{-1}). Unfortunately, with acute oliguria the diagnostic value of urinary osmolality is limited.

Fractional Excretion of Sodium

In an effort to more accurately distinguish prerenal from renal oliguria, investigators have proposed the fractional excretion of sodium (FENa) assay. The FENa is calculated by dividing the urine/plasma sodium ratio by the urine/plasma Cr ratio, then multiplying by 100.[66] Values less than 1 per cent suggest prerenal azotemia (Table 10–5). Despite early enthusiasm about the value of the FENa calculation, its diagnostic and prognostic utility are limited in the acute situation.[67,68] The FENa suggests established parenchymal injury at a time when hemodynamically mediated prerenal factors are still reversible. Moreover, in sodium-avid patients (those with liver failure, nephrotic syndrome, and cirrhosis) the FENa may remain low despite inexorably progressive renal failure.[69]

Urinalysis

Urinalysis in ARF reveals increased hyaline and finely granular casts and increased numbers of tubular epithelial cells. Increased numbers of coarse, granular, pigmented casts are associated with rhabdomyolysis, although they also occur in jaundiced patients without renal injury. Postrenal oliguria secondary to hydronephrosis is characterized by increased urine histiocytes. Crystallinuria, consisting of "coffin-lid" triple phosphate crystals, envelope-like calcium oxalate crystals, or football-shaped uric acid crystals, suggests the cause of tubular obstruction.

ULTRASONOGRAPHY

Renal ultrasonography, a highly sensitive, moderately specific means of detecting urinary tract obstruction, has largely replaced intravenous pyelography for the evaluation of potential obstruction in acutely oliguric patients. This noninvasive, complication-free technique can also identify retroperitoneal hemorrhage or fluid accumulation.

ROENTGENOGRAPHIC EVALUATION

Plain film roentgenography of the abdomen may reveal a calcium-containing stone or an enlarged kidney suggesting postrenal ARF. Intravenous pyelography, because of the risk of aggravating ARF, has been replaced by ultrasonography for evaluating postrenal and many renal causes of oliguria. Retrograde pyelography, which allows more thorough evaluation of the collecting system by dilating the ureters and pelves during injection of contrast medium[70] is occasionally helpful for evaluating perioperative oliguria. Computed tomography can evaluate renal size and the presence of hydronephrosis.

Acute renal failure secondary to emboli, thoracic or aortic aneurysms, dissection, or thrombosis or subsequent to aortic or renal surgery may require renal arteriography.[71] Arteriography also reveals hypoperfusion of interlobar and arcuate arteries in renal transplants undergoing graft rejection.[72,73]

PULMONARY ARTERY CATHETERIZATION

Intravascular volume cannot be effectively assessed in critically ill patients. Occasionally, empiric infusion of fluid into an oliguric patient, especially one who has compromised cardiac function, may precipitate acute pulmonary edema. Although pulmonary artery catheterization provides no specific information about renal status, it provides data that facilitate patient management. When empiric fluid administration seems unduly hazardous, pulmonary artery catheterization permits continued volume expansion while keeping pulmonary artery occlusion pressure below 15 to 18 mm Hg (usually considered the practical upper limit). Hemodynamic monitoring may be particularly helpful in patients with diseases that mandate particular care of fluid management, e.g., cirrhosis or intracranial hypertension.

RENAL BIOPSY

Renal biopsy is rarely employed for the perioperative assessment of acute oliguria. Biopsy is especially helpful when diseases such as acute interstitial nephritis or renal vasculitis figure prominently in the differential diagnosis.

PREVENTION OF ARF

Because of the high mortality associated with postoperative ARF, prevention of renal ischemia and preservation of ischemic renal tissue are essential. Particular attention should be directed to patients with specific risk factors for ARF, including underlying renal disease, hepatic disease, sepsis, cardiac disease, and trauma resulting from cardiac, major vascular, or intraabdominal operations.[7]

The fundamental strategy for the prevention of ARF consists in measures designed to limit the magnitude and duration of renal ischemic insults. In most patients, acute oliguria signals inadequate systemic perfusion. Therefore carefully monitored efforts to improve perfusion should be employed, including volume expansion, inotropic support, and vasodilation, directed when necessary by pulmonary artery catheterization. Adequate preoperative and intraoperative restoration and maintenance of intravascular volume are vital to the prevention of ARF, especially in patients who may have suffered iatrogenic dehydration because of angiography, bowel preparation, or prolonged fasting.[74] Diagnostic data from acutely oliguric patients must be interpreted with caution. Excessive reliance on the interpretation of urinary electrolytes, osmolality, or specialized indices may lead to the delay, interruption, or premature termination of appropriate, timely therapy.

Mannitol, furosemide, and dopamine promote urinary flow and reduce the renal damage produced by experimental renal ischemia. Mannitol improves renal cortical blood flow and may exert a renal cellular protective effect.[75] Mannitol, by maintaining high tubular flow, may decrease the incidence and severity of ARF secondary to contrast media or pigmenturia. Dopamine, a selective renal vasodilator at doses of 1 to 3 $\mu g \cdot kg^{-1} \cdot min^{-1}$, increases renal cortical blood flow with minimal systemic effects. Dopamine induces natriuresis, increases GFR, and improves urinary flow in oliguric renal failure,[76] and it is a useful adjunct to the treatment of oliguria. However, the use of diuretic agents in the absence of adequate volume expansion may transiently increase urinary flow, thereby delaying effective therapy and further depleting intravascular volume.

Clinical use of vasoconstricting inotropic agents, especially norepinephrine, in severely vasodilated, septic patients may improve renal function by increasing renal perfusion pressure.[77,78] Care must be taken, however, that the increase in perfusion pressure is not associated with excessive systemic vasoconstriction.[77,78]

RENAL REPLACEMENT THERAPY

Patients who develop sufficiently severe perioperative renal compromise require short- or long-term renal replacement therapy. In the United States alone, 7500 patients per year develop ARF. In two thirds of those patients ARF is associated with critical medical and surgical illness.[79]

Although maintaining even severely impaired renal function may be superior to dialytic therapy, much of the function of the kidney can be replaced by artificial means. Hemodialysis, peritoneal dialysis, continuous arteriovenous hemofiltration, continuous arteriovenous hemodialysis, and venovenous hemofiltration are capable of removing excess water and sodium and of eliminating waste products. Based on the operational characteristics of each of these techniques, the management of critically ill patients with ARF can be individualized. This section summarizes the principles of renal replacement therapy and reviews the physiologic effects and complications of various forms of therapy. Additional information is available in several reviews and texts.[80–86]

RENAL REPLACEMENT ALTERNATIVES

Two terms essential to understanding renal replacement therapy are ''ultrafiltration'' and ''dialysis.'' *Ultrafiltration* is the movement of serum and solutes through pores in membranes. The primary forces governing filtration are hydrostatic pressure and pore size. When molecules are sufficiently small to pass freely through the pores in the membrane, the filtration then varies directly with the magnitude of hydrostatic pressure.

Dialysis is a generic term that describes diffusive transport of solute down an osmotic gradient across a semipermeable membrane. Accumulated waste solutes such as urea and potassium move from high concentrations in blood into a chemically prescribed dialysate. Substances such as bicarbonate move from higher concentrations in the dialysate into blood.

Hemodialysis

Solute is transported from blood into dialysate across the semipermeable membrane in direct relation to the surface area and permeability of the membrane and to the difference in molecular concentrations on either side of the membrane. Transport of substances across the dialysis membrane is governed by a relation expressed mathematically as

$$J_S = DA(C_B - C_D)$$

where J_S is solute flux; D is the diffusion coefficient of the membrane for the solute; A is the area of membrane; C_B is the concentration of the solute in blood; and C_D is the concentration of the solute in the dialysate. In the hollow-fiber type of dialyzer, 7,000 to 15,000 fibers, having a total length of 1 to 2 miles, provide a membrane area for solute exchange of 0.8 to 2.0 sq meters.[87] Blood and dialysate flow rapidly in opposite directions through the dialyzer (blood inside and dialysate outside the hollow fibers) to achieve maximal solute exchange. Both diffusive and convective transport occur during this countercurrent flow.

The diffusive transport of substances across the dialyzer membrane is different from the convective transport of substances across the renal glomerular membrane. The glomerulus quantitatively filters molecules, independent of size, up to a molecular weight of 7,000 to 10,000 daltons. As molecular weight increases further, glomerular filtration rapidly declines until the upper limit of filtration size (around 100,000 daltons) is attained. In contrast, clearance of solutes by dialysis is inversely proportional to molecular weight across the entire range of 0 to 100,000 daltons. Small molecules, e.g., urea, are cleared readily by dialysis, their clearance being dependent primarily on blood flow through the dialyzer. The largest discrepancies between filtration by the normal kidney and clearance by the dialyzer occur for molecules with molecular weights ranging from 300 to 5000 daltons, the so-called middle molecules.[87]

Hemodialysis efficiently removes small molecules because a large proportion are cleared during each pass through the dialyzer. In contrast, convective removal of undesired solutes by ultrafiltration is relatively slow and inefficient because only the solute present in the filtrate is removed. Although the human kidney also initiates urine formation by filtration, high clearances result from the high rate of filtration. Normal adult kidneys filter approximately 20 per cent of renal plasma flow, or approximately 7 $L \cdot hr^{-1}$. Subsequent reabsorption of salt and water maintains intravascular volume while permitting urinary excretion of undesired wastes. Renal replacement devices that utilize ultrafiltration filter far less volume per hour and lack the ability to modify the filtrate.

Hemodialyzers are also capable of convective transport, the magnitude of which is directly proportional to the transmembrane hydrostatic pressure. To increase transmembrane pressure, arterial pressure can be increased using a blood pump, venous pressure can be increased by partially occluding the venous outflow from the dialyzer, or negative pressure can be generated in the dialysate compartment by application of a vacuum.

Activation of the coagulation cascade by contact with the surface of the dialyzer must be counteracted by systemic or regional anticoagulation during hemodialysis. If regional heparinization is used, heparin is added to the blood in the arterial line and is neutralized with protamine in the venous line before it is returned to the patient, thereby limiting the consequences of systemic heparinization. With either systemic or regional heparinization, careful monitoring of anticoagulation is required.

Hemodialysis requires vascular access sufficient to provide adequate blood flow. Emergent perioperative hemodialysis is frequently performed through a percutaneously inserted Shaldon catheter. Blood is returned through a peripheral vein or, when necessary, through a second Shaldon catheter inserted in the same or a contralateral femoral vein. Double-lumen catheters[88,89] permit simultaneous withdrawal and return through a single percutaneous access site, usually the subclavian vein. Chronic hemodialysis is usually performed through a surgically constructed arteriovenous fistula.

Peritoneal Dialysis

Peritoneal dialysis is an intracorporeal, diffusive method in which the semipermeable membrane consists of the tissue layers that separate peritoneal capillary blood from intraperitoneal dialysate. Peritoneal dialysis utilizes the large capillary network in the peritoneal cavity to provide contact between blood and dialysate. Peritoneal dialysis clears small molecules such as urea more slowly than hemodialysis but clears larger molecules such as inulin more rapidly.[90] The decreased rate at which peritoneal dialysis clears small molecules can be overcome partially by increasing the duration of treatments.

Clearance of solute during peritoneal dialysis depends on the volume and composition of the dialysate, the rate of blood flow in the peritoneal capillaries, the permeability of the tissue between blood and dialysate, the area of the peritoneal membrane, and the circulation of the fluid film in the peritoneal cavity. In adults the volume of dialysate per exchange is usually 2 liters. Higher volumes increase the efficiency of dialysis but may restrict diaphragmatic motion. The composition of the dialysate is modified to increase or decrease blood concentrations of solute. For example, lactate is added to the dialysate as a substrate from which bicarbonate can be synthesized to correct metabolic acidosis. The tonicity of the dialysate may be increased by increasing the dextrose concentration, which then increases the rate of ultrafiltration of water and solute out of the capillary bed. An osmotic pressure gradient across the peritoneal membrane promotes ultrafiltration, as does a hydrostatic gradient across a hemodialysis membrane. If 2 liters of dialysate containing 1.5 per cent dextrose ($347 \ mOsm \cdot L^{-1}$) is infused, that volume increases by 50 to 100 ml within 1 hour and by approximately 130 ml if the dwell time is 4 hours.[87] If the dextrose concentration is increased to 4.25 per cent ($486 \ mOsm \cdot L^{-1}$), 300 to 400 ml of ultrafiltrate is added to the 2 liter dialysate volume within 1 hour and 750 ml by 4 hours.[87] Dextrose concentrations of more than 4.25 per cent are no longer used. Remarkably, peritoneal blood flow remains sufficiently high, even in shock states, to permit peritoneal dialysis.[91] Acute peritoneal dialysis can be employed for correction of severe accumulation of water or solutes.

Peritoneal dialysis is performed through an indwelling peritoneal catheter similar to the model first described by Tenckhoff and Schechter.[92] Short-term peritoneal access may be obtained with a percutaneously inserted catheter,[93] but there is risk of bowel perforation, catheter loss, or both.[94,95]

Continuous Arteriovenous Hemofiltration

Continuous arteriovenous hemofiltration (CAVH) and continuous venovenous hemofiltration (CVVH) are innovative techniques for the purely convective removal of fluid and solute.[96,97] The hydraulic driving pressure produced by systemic arterial pressure or by the addition of a blood pump produces continuous ultrafiltration. The apparatus consists of an arterial or venous withdrawal cannula connected to a filter that empties into a venous return cannula. The rate of ultrafiltration with these devices is described by the equation

$$QF = KA(P_{tm} - P_{onc})$$

where QF is flow of filtrate; K is the filtration characteristic of the membrane; A is membrane area; P_{tm} is the transmembrane hydrostatic pressure gradient; and P_{onc} is the serum oncotic pressure.

The rate of ultrafiltration is directly proportional to the mean arterial pressure and to blood flow through the filter, and it is inversely proportional to the serum oncotic pressure. The addition of a blood pump on the arterial side (mandatory with venovenous techniques) increases the hydrostatic pressure and may increase the formation of ultrafiltrate to as much as 2400 ml·hr^{-1}.[97] The application of negative pressure to the ultrafiltrate line also increases ultrafiltration by increasing the transmembrane pressure.[98] CAVH or CVVH may therefore remove large quantities of protein-free fluid that contains solute in roughly the same concentrations as serum. The serum concentrations of solutes are not changed by the filtration process itself but, rather, by the dilution produced by intravenous infusion of fluid. The net fluid removal during CAVH is prescribed according to the need to remove excess sodium and water versus the need to alter solute concentrations. For instance, CAVH may be used to remove sufficient salt and water to permit full-calorie, high-protein nutritional support of critically ill patients.[99]

Like the human glomerulus, CAVH eliminates solutes in a manner independent of molecular weight up to 10,000 daltons. Middle-weight molecules are cleared more effectively by CAVH than by hemodialysis. However, because there is no subsequent modification of the filtrate, as would occur in the renal tubular system, there may be some loss of physiologically useful substances, e.g., small carrier proteins. Lower clearances are obtained for substances of small molecular weight. Urea clearance equals the filtration rate, which rarely exceeds 35 to 40 ml·min^{-1} and usually is less than 10 ml·min^{-1}. In contrast, hemodialysis may clear urea from 150 ml of plasma in 1 minute.[86]

Continuous arteriovenous hemodialysis (CAVHD) is a modification of CAVH. Here dialysate resembling peritoneal dialysate is passed through the CAVHD device, thereby adding the clearance capabilities of diffusive transport.

The relative indications for and limitations of hemodialysis, peritoneal dialysis, and continuous hemofiltration and continuous arteriovenous hemodialysis are listed in Table 10–6.

PHYSIOLOGIC EFFECTS AND COMPLICATIONS OF RENAL REPLACEMENT THERAPY

In most instances, renal replacement therapy improves the profound physiologic abnormalities induced by renal failure, i.e., fluid overload, pericarditis, electrolyte abnormalities, coagulopathy, and uremic encephalopathy. However, despite major advances, the complications of hemodialysis, peritoneal dialysis, and continuous hemofiltration still represent problems in the management of patients with acute or chronic renal failure.[100,101] The most important physiologic effects and com-

TABLE 10–6. SELECTION OF RENAL REPLACEMENT THERAPY

Therapy	Indications	Limitations
Hemodialysis	Rapid catabolism Severe volume, electrolyte, or acid-base disorders	Hypotension Anticoagulation risk Need for vascular access
Peritoneal dialysis	Lower cost Anticoagulation risk Difficult vascular access Hypotension Infants and small children	Rapid catabolism Diaphragmatic defects Severe volume, electrolyte, or acid-base disorders
CAVH	Hemodynamic instability Inexpensive equipment	Rapid catabolism Severe volume, electrolyte, or acid-base disorders
CAVHD	Hemodynamic instability Inexpensive equipment	Severe volume, electrolyte, or acid-base disorders (Superior to CAVH)

plications of renal replacement therapy involve the central nervous system, cardiovascular system, and respiratory system.

Central Nervous System Effects

The disequilibrium syndrome is an uncommon, potentially severe complication of acute hemodialysis.[102,103] Usually mild, the syndrome may progress to stupor, coma, and seizures. Predisposing factors include a predialysis blood urea nitrogen concentration of more than 150 mg·dl^{-1}, hypernatremia, profound acidemia, and preexisting brain disease. One proposed mechanism of the disequilibrium syndrome is a paradoxical brain acidosis. Rapid hemodialysis increases brain hydrogen ion concentration, even though the serum concentration decreases.[104] Therefore brain tissue osmolality is reduced less rapidly than serum osmolality.[104]

Management of the disequilibrium syndrome is primarily preventive; i.e., urea and sodium concentrations are reduced gradually in high risk patients. Symptomatic treatment includes the administration of mannitol.[102] The disequilibrium syndrome is rarely associated with peritoneal dialysis and does not occur with chronic ambulatory peritoneal dialysis or with CAVH because solute concentrations decrease more slowly during these techniques than during hemodialysis.

Cardiovascular Effects

Symptomatic hypotension complicates 25 per cent of chronic hemodialysis treatments.[105] Critically ill patients are more likely to become hypotensive during hemodialysis. Septic patients are particularly prone to develop hypotension.[106,107]

The cause of hemodialysis-induced hypotension is multifactorial (Table 10–7). Although intravascular volume is reduced, hemodialysis produces more frequent, more severe hypotension than hemofiltration despite comparable volume reduction. Patients undergoing hemodialysis often fail to vasoconstrict in response to reductions in plasma volume and cardiac output. Uremic patients appear to have defective carotid and aortic body reflex arcs.[108,109] Peripheral resistance declines during hemodialysis despite hypotension and a decreased cardiac filling pressures.[110]

The failure of compensatory vasoconstriction may be due to acetate in the dialysate. Acetate, a vasodilator that may interfere with reflex vasoconstriction,[111,112] is metabolized in the liver to bicarbonate, replacing bicarbonate consumed by buffering the hydrogen ions from nonexcreted acids. Dialysate that contains bicarbonate is unstable in solution and must be prepared near the time of dialysis,[114] whereas dialysate containing acetate is stable during extended storage. Removal of fluid and solute by dialysis against a bicarbonate bath may produce less hemodynamic instability than removal of similar quantities of fluid with acetate-containing dialysate.[111,113,114]

Critically ill, septic patients frequently exhibit hemodynamic instability of sufficient severity to preclude effective hemodialysis.[106,107] Cardiac output, left ventricular stroke work index, and mean arterial pressure decrease less in critically ill patients during dialysis if bicarbonate is substituted for acetate.[115] In such patients, dialysis using a bicarbonate-containing bath may improve hemodynamic stability and improve metabolic acidosis more rapidly.[106] During acetate hemodialysis in septic patients, bicarbonate initially moves out of blood into dialysate, causing a temporary worsening of hypobicarbonatemia until acetate, which is simultaneously moving from dialysate into blood, is metabolized in the liver to produce an increase in serum bicarbonate level.[106] This short-term aggravation of metabolic acidosis may be poorly tolerated by critically ill patients as well as by patients who, usually because of liver disease, metabolize acetate slowly.[116] Because acetate is so poorly tolerated, many nephrologists prefer to initiate hemodialysis in critically ill patients by using a bicarbonate-containing dialysate.

Studies suggest that an increase in plasma ionized calcium is the most important factor in the preservation of left ventricular contractility during dialysis.[117] An increase in the calcium concentration of dialysate from 5.5 to 7.5 mg·dl^{-1} produces substantially higher intradialytic blood pressure,[118] although the precise mass transfer of calcium during dialysis is variable.[119]

TABLE 10–7. MECHANISMS OF HYPOTENSION DURING HEMODIALYSIS

Preload reduction
    Sodium and water removal
    Blunted sympathetic reflexes
Afterload reduction
    Acetate-induced arterial dilation
    Temporary decrease in pH
    Blunted sympathetic reflexes
Myocardial depression
    None: myocardial function improved or unchanged

Hemodialysis-induced hypotension also is less severe if plasma volume is reduced slowly. Decreasing the transmembrane pressure in the dialyzer slows the rate of ultrafiltration. Decreasing the osmotic gradient from serum sodium concentration to dialysate sodium concentration decreases the rate of sodium removal. Leg elevation, intravenous fluid administration, and occasionally vasoconstrictors can be used for the short-term management of hypotension. Myers and Moran hypothesized that norepinephrine may be the drug of choice for blood pressure elevation during hemodialysis in patients with ARF owing to the blunted renal response to vasoconstrictors in such patients.[21]

Hypotension occurs less commonly during peritoneal dialysis and CAVH. Hypotension during peritoneal dialysis, usually caused by excessively rapid removal of water and solute, may require substitution of dialysate containing a lower dextrose concentration. CAVH is associated with a low incidence of hypotension.[96] Because transmembrane pressure determines the rate of ultrafiltration, a decrease in systemic blood pressure decreases the rate of ultrafiltration, thereby limiting further rapid fluid removal. However, if a blood pump is included in the arterial circuit, intravascular volume can be depleted rapidly.[97,98] Appropriate intravenous replacement of fluid infusion prevents excessive depletion of intravascular volume. Because CAVH does not interfere with sympathetic reflex responsiveness, even critically ill, septic patients tolerate the modality well.[97]

Respiratory System Effects

Although PaO_2 may increase because of dialysis, especially if cardiogenic pulmonary edema is present, hemodialysis commonly results in hypoxemia. Two mechanisms contribute to hypoxemia during hemodialysis: ventilation-perfusion mismatch and hypoventilation. Some investigators explain hypoxemia on the basis of ventilation-perfusion mismatch secondary to leukocyte-mediated pulmonary dysfunction.[120] However, other data demonstrate that ventilation-perfusion matching and the alveolar-arterial oxygen gradient may remain unchanged despite hypoxemia.[121,122]

Patients may hypoventilate during hemodialysis without becoming hypercarbic, a mechanism first proposed by Aurigemma and colleagues.[123] Sherlock and colleagues[122] attributed the decline in PaO_2 during hemodialy-

sis to loss of carbon dioxide across the dialyzer membrane. They explained the resulting effects[121,122,124,125] in terms of the alveolar gas equation

$$PAO_2 = PiO_2 - \frac{PaCO_2}{RE}$$

where PAO_2 is alveolar oxygen tension; PiO_2 is $FiO_2 \times$ (barometric pressure $- 47$); FiO_2 is the fractional inspired concentration of oxygen; and RE is carbon dioxide excretion by the lung divided by oxygen consumption. During dialysis against acetate, carbon dioxide is both excreted by the lung and lost through the dialyzer membrane. The decline in carbon dioxide excretion by the lung decreases RE, thereby necessarily decreasing PAO_2. If the $P(A-a)O_2$ remains the same, the PaO_2 must fall. If the decrease in PaO_2 exceeds the decrease in PAO_2, ventilation-perfusion mismatch must be increased. Substitution of bicarbonate for acetate in the dialysate limits carbon dioxide loss through the dialyzer.[126]

Hypoxemia during hemodialysis responds to an increase in FiO_2.[126] In rare cases, bicarbonate rather than acetate dialysis is necessary. Occasionally, a less rapid rate of plasma volume reduction may be employed if a decrease in cardiac output is contributing to hypoxemia through production of a lower mixed-venous oxygen content.

During peritoneal dialysis, hypoxemia occurs if upward displacement of the diaphragm is poorly tolerated or if fluid traverses the diaphragm.[127] Hypoxemia seldom occurs during CAVH.

SUMMARY

Minimizing acute renal insults is an important goal of acute perioperative care. Recognition of the perioperative risk factors and surgical/anesthetic perturbations to renal function provides clinicians with an important opportunity to support the kidneys in the perioperative state. When acute renal failure does occur, one should have a basic understanding of the major technical advances in supporting perioperative patients with this disease.

References

1. Hou S, Bushinsky DA, Wish JB, et al: Hospital-acquired renal insufficiency: a prospective study. Am J Med 74:243–248, 1983.
2. Rasmussen HH, Ibels LS: Acute renal failure: multi-

variate analysis of causes and risk factors. Am J Med *73*:211–218, 1982.

3. Beaman M, Turney JH, Rodger RS, et al: Changing pattern of acute renal failure. Q J Med *62*:15–23, 1987.

4. Harrington JT, Cohen JJ: Acute oliguria. N Engl J Med *292*:89–91, 1975.

5. Arendshorst WS, Finn WF, Gottschalk CW: Autoregulation of blood flow in the rat kidney. Am J Physiol *228*:127–133, 1975.

6. Vander AJ: Renal Physiology, 3rd ed. New York, McGraw-Hill, 1985, pp. 70–74.

7. Davis RF: Acute renal failure following traumatic injury or major operation. Int Anesthesiol Clin *25*:117–142, 1987.

8. Vander AJ: Control of renin release. Physiol Rev *47*:359–382, 1967.

9. Thurau K, Schnermann J, Nagel W, et al: Composition of tubular fluid in the macula densa segment as a factor regulating the function of the juxtaglomerular apparatus. Circ Res *21*(suppl II):II-79–II-90, 1967.

10. Vander AJ: Renal Physiology, 3rd ed. New York, McGraw-Hill, 1985, p. 78.

11. Schrier RW: Acute renal failure. JAMA *247*:2518–2522, 1982.

12. Iversen P, Brun C: Aspiration biopsy of the kidney. Am J Med *11*:324–330, 1951.

13. Solez K, Morel-Maroger L, Sraer JD: The morphology of "acute tubular necrosis" in man: analysis of 57 renal biopsies and a comparison with the glycerol model. Medicine (Baltimore) *58*:362–376, 1979.

14. Olsen S: Pathology of acute renal failure. *In* Andreucci VE, ed. Acute Renal Failure. Boston, Martinus Nijhoff, 1984, p. 149.

15. Olsen S, Solez K: Acute renal failure in man: pathogenesis in light of new morphological data. Clin Nephrol *27*:271–277, 1987.

16. Hollenberg NK, Adams DF, Oken DE, et al: Acute renal failure due to nephrotoxins. N Engl J Med *282*:1329–1334, 1970.

17. Donohoe JF, Venkatachalam MA, Bernard DB, Levinsky NG: Tubular leakage and obstruction after renal ischemia: structural-functional correlations. Kidney Int *13*:208–222, 1978.

18. Thurau K: Pathophysiology of the acutely failing kidney. Clin Exp Dialysis Apheresis *7*:9–24, 1983.

19. Oken DE, Arce ML, Wilson DR: Glycerol-induced hemoglobinuric acute renal failure in the rat. I. Micropuncture study of the development of oliguria. J Clin Invest *45*:724–735, 1966.

20. Moran SM, Myers BD: Pathophysiology of protracted acute renal failure in man. J Clin Invest *76*:1440–1448, 1985.

21. Myers BD, Moran SM: Hemodynamically mediated acute renal failure. N Engl J Med *314*:97–105, 1986.

22. Fanning WL, Gump D, Jick H: Gentamicin- and cephalothin-associated rises in blood urea nitrogen. Antimicrob Agents Chemother *10*:80–82, 1976.

23. Hewitt WL: Reflections on the clinical pharmacology of gentamicin. Acta Pathol Microbiol Scand [Suppl 241]*81B*:151–156, 1977.

24. Eisenberg JM, Koffer H, Glick HA, et al: What is the cost of nephrotoxicity associated with aminoglycosides? Ann Intern Med *107*:900–909, 1987.

25. Matzke GR, Lucarotti RL, Shapiro HS: Controlled comparison of gentamicin and tobramycin nephrotoxicity. Am J Nephrol *3*:11–17, 1983.

26. Contrepois A, Brion N, Garaud JJ, et al: Renal dis-

position of gentamicin, dibekacin, tobramycin, netilmicin, and amikacin in humans. Antimicrob Agents Chemother *27*:520–524, 1985.

27. Brier ME, Mayer PR, Brier RA, et al: Relationship between rat renal accumulation of gentamicin, tobramycin, and netilmicin and their nephrotoxicities. Antimicrob Agents Chemother *27*:812–816, 1985.

28. Cabrera J, Arroyo V, Ballesta AM, et al: Aminoglycoside nephrotoxicity in cirrhosis: value of urinary beta 2-microglobulin to discriminate functional renal failure from acute tubular damage. Gastroenterology *82*:97–105, 1982.

29. Coggins CH, Fang LST: Acute renal failure associated with antibiotics, anesthetic agents, and radiographic contrast agents. *In* Brenner BM, Lazarus JM, eds. Acute Renal Failure, 2nd ed. New York, Churchill Livingstone, 1988, pp. 295–352.

30. Barbour GL, Straub KD, O'Neal BL, Leatherman JW: Vasopressin-resistant nephrogenic diabetes insipidus: a result of amphotericin B therapy. Arch Intern Med *139*:86–88, 1979.

31. Holeman CW Jr, Einstein H: The toxic effects of amphotericin in man. Calif Med *99*:90–93, 1963.

32. Butler WT, Hill GJ II, Szwed CF, Knight V: Amphotericin B renal toxicity in the dog. J Pharmacol Exp Ther *143*:47–56, 1964.

33. Gerkens JF, Heidemann HT, Jackson EK, Branch RA: Effect of aminophylline on amphotericin B nephrotoxicity in the dog. J Pharmacol Exp Ther *224*:609–613, 1983.

34. Juliano RL, Lopez-Berestein G, Hopfer R, et al: Selective toxicity and enhanced therapeutic index of liposomal polyene antibiotics in systemic fungal infections. Ann NY Acad Sci *446*:390–402, 1985.

35. Barza M: The nephrotoxicity of cephalosporins: an overview. J Infect Dis *137*:S60–S73, 1978.

36. Benner EJ: Renal damage associated with prolonged administration of ampicillin, cephaloridine and cephalothin. Antimicrob Agents Chemother *9*:417–420, 1969.

37. Foord RD: Cephaloridine, cephalothin and the kidney. J Antimicrob Chemother *1*:119–133, 1975.

38. Miller MS, Gandolfi AJ, Vaughan RW, Bentley JB: Disposition of enflurane in obese patients. J Pharmacol Exp Ther *215*:292–296, 1980.

39. Hartnett MN, Lane W, Bennett WM: Non-oliguric renal failure and enflurane. Ann Intern Med *81*:560, 1974 (letter).

40. Eichhorn JH, Hedley-Whyte J, Steinman TI, et al: Renal failure following enflurane anesthesia. Anesthesiology *45*:557–560, 1976.

41. VanZee BE, Hoy WE, Talley TE, Jaenike JR: Renal injury associated with intravenous pyelography in nondiabetic and diabetic patients. Ann Intern Med *89*:51–54, 1978.

42. Brezis M, Epstein FH: A closer look at radiocontrast-induced nephropathy. N Engl J Med *320*:179–181, 1989.

43. Talner LB: Does hydration prevent contrast material renal injury? AJR *136*:1021–1022, 1981 (editorial).

44. Eisenberg RL, Bank WO, Hedgcock MW: Renal failure after major angiography can be avoided with hydration. AJR *136*:859–861, 1981.

45. Snyder HE, Killen DA, Foster JH: The influence of mannitol in toxic reactions to contrast angiography. Surgery *64*:640–642, 1968.

46. Anto HR, Chou SY, Porush JG, Shapiro WB: Mannitol prevention of acute renal failure (ARF) associ-

ated with infusion intravenous pyelography (IIVP). Clin Res 27:407A, 1979.

47. Singhal PC, Chugh KS, Gulati DR: Myoglobinuria and renal failure after status epilepticus. Neurology 28:200, 1978.

48. Chugh KS, Singhal PC, Khatri GK: Rhabdomyolysis and renal failure following status asthmaticus. Chest 73:879, 1978.

49. Singhal PC, Muthusethupathi MA, Chugh KS: Case report: rhabdomyolysis and postpartum renal failure. Int J Gynaecol Obstet 15:250, 1977.

50. Knochel JP, Schlein EM: On the mechanism of rhabdomyolysis in potassium depletion. J Clin Invest 51:1750–1758, 1972.

51. Farber E: ATP and cell integrity. Fed Proc 32:1534–1539, 1973.

52. Ron D, Taitelman MD, Michaelson MD, et al: Prevention of acute renal failure in traumatic rhabdomyolysis. Arch Intern Med 144:277–280, 1984.

53. Olsen TS, Wassef NF, Olsen HS, Hansen HE: Ultrastructure of the kidney in acute interstitial nephritis. Ultrastruct Pathol 10:1–16, 1986.

54. Van Ypersele de Strihou C: Acute oliguric interstitial nephritis. Kidney Int 16:751–765, 1979.

55. Frankel MC, Weinstein AM, Stenzel KH: Prognostic patterns in acute renal failure: the New York Hospital, 1981–1982. Clin Exp Dialysis Apheresis 7:145–167, 1983.

56. Linton AL, Clark WF, Driedger AA, et al: Acute interstitial nephritis due to drugs: review of the literature with a report of nine cases. Ann Intern Med 93:735–741, 1980.

57. Ditlove J, Weidmann P, Bernstein M, Massry SG: Methicillin nephritis. Medicine (Baltimore) 56:483–491, 1977.

58. Rasmussen HH, Ibels LS: Acute renal failure: multivariate analysis of causes and risk factors. Am J Med 73:211–218, 1982.

59. Anderson RJ, Linas SL, Berns AS, et al: Nonoliguric acute renal failure. N Engl J Med 296:1134–1138, 1977.

60. Myers BD, Hilberman M, Spencer RJ, Jamison RL: Glomerular and tubular function in non-oliguric acute renal failure. Am J Med 72:642–649, 1982.

61. Myers BD, Miller DC, Mehigan JT, et al: Nature of the renal injury following total renal ischemia in man. J Clin Invest 73:329–341, 1984.

62. Shin B, Mackenzie CF, Crowley RA: Changing patterns of posttraumatic acute renal failure. Am Surg 45:182–189, 1979.

63. Planas M, Wachtel T, Frank H, Henderson LW: Characterization of acute renal failure in the burned patient. Arch Intern Med 142:2087–2091, 1982.

64. Levinsky NG, Bernard DB, Johnston PA: Enhancement of recovery of acute renal failure: effects of mannitol and diuretics. In Brenner BM, Stein JH, eds. Acute Renal Failure. Contemporary Issues in Nephrology. Edinburgh, Churchill Livingstone, 1980, pp. 163–179.

65. Brown CB, Ogg CS, Cameron JS: High dose frusemide in acute renal failure: a controlled trial. Clin Nephrol 15:90–96, 1981.

66. Epsinel CH, Gregory AW: Differential diagnosis of acute renal failure. Clin Nephrol 13:73–77, 1980.

67. Oken DE: On the differential diagnosis of acute renal failure. Am J Med 71:916–920, 1981.

68. Pru C, Kjellstrand CM: The FENa test is of no prognostic value in acute renal failure. Nephron 36:20–23, 1984.

69. Diamond JR, Yoburn DC: Nonoliguric acute renal failure associated with a low fractional excretion of sodium. Ann Intern Med 96:597–600, 1982.

70. Rudnick MR, Bastl CP, Elfinbein IB, Narins RG: The differential diagnosis of acute renal failure. In Brenner BM, Lazarus JM, eds. Acute Renal Failure, 2nd ed. New York, Churchill Livingstone, 1988, pp. 209–219.

71. Halpern M: Acute renal artery embolus: a concept of diagnosis and treatment. J Urol 98:552–61, 1967.

72. Foley WD, Bookstein JJ, Tweist M, et al: Arteriography of renal transplants. Radiology 116:271, 1975.

73. Lawson RK, Puileau MA: Renal transplantation and urinary diversion. In Witten DM, Meyers GH, Utz DC, eds. Emmett's Clinical Urography, Vol. 3. Philadelphia, Saunders, 1977, p. 2054.

74. Hesdorffer CS, Milne JF, Meyers AM, et al: The value of Swan-Ganz catheterization and volume loading in preventing renal failure in patients undergoing abdominal aneurysmectomy. Clin Nephrol 28:272–276, 1987.

75. Cronin RE, de Torrente A, Miller PD, et al: Pathogenic mechanisms in early norepinephrine-induced acute renal failure: functional and histological correlates of protection. Kidney Int 14:115–125, 1978.

76. Hollenberg NK, Adams DF, Mendell P, et al: Renal vascular responses to dopamine: haemodynamic and angiographic observations in normal man. Clin Sci Mol Med 45:733–742, 1973.

77. Fukuoka T, Nishimura M, Imanaka H, et al: Effects of norepinephrine on renal function in septic patients with normal elevated serum lactate levels. Crit Care Med 17:1104, 1989.

78. Hesselvik JF, Brodin B: Low dose norepinephrine in patients with septic shock and oliguria: effects on afterload, urine flow, and oxygen transport. Crit Care Med 17:179–80, 1989.

79. Kasiske BL, Kjellstrand CM: Perioperative management of patients with chronic renal failure and postoperative acute renal failure. Urol Clin North Am 10:35–50, 1983.

80. Beck CH Jr: Etiologies of acute renal failure: the dialytic treatment of acute renal failure. In Critical Care: State of the Art, Vol. 5. Fullerton, CA, Society of Critical Care Medicine, 1984, pp. 1–27.

81. Levey AS, Harrington JT: Continuous peritoneal dialysis for chronic renal failure. Medicine (Baltimore) 61:330–339, 1982.

82. Nolph KD: Continuous ambulatory peritoneal dialysis. Am J Nephrol 1:1–10, 1981.

83. Kliger AS: Complications of dialysis: hemodialysis, peritoneal dialysis, CAPD. In Arieff AI, DeFronzo RA, eds. Fluid, Electrolyte, and Acid-Base Disorders, Vol. 2. New York, Churchill Livingstone, 1985, pp. 777–819.

84. Cogan MG, Garovoy MR, eds: Introduction to Dialysis. New York, Churchill Livingstone, 1985.

85. Drukker W, Parsons FM, Maher JF, eds. Replacement of Renal Function by Dialysis: A Textbook of Dialysis, 2nd ed. Boston, Martinus Nijhoff, 1983.

86. Alfred HJ, Cohen AJ: Use of dialytic procedures in the intensive care unit. In Rippe JM, Irwin RS, Alpert JS, et al, eds. Intensive Care Medicine. Boston, Little, Brown, 1985, pp. 562–582.

87. Gotch FA, Keen ML: Dialyzers and delivery systems. In Cogan MG, Garovoy MR, eds. Introduction to Dialysis. New York, Churchill Livingstone, 1985, pp. 1–40.

88. Uldall PR, Joy C, Merchant N: Further experience

with a double-lumen subclavian cannula for hemodialysis. Trans Am Soc Artif Intern Organs 28:71–75, 1982.

89. Lewinstein C, Silberman H, Goren G, et al: Experience with a coaxial dialysis cannula for temporary vascular access. Trans Am Soc Artif Intern Organs 29:357–359, 1983.

90. Maher JF: Characteristics of peritoneal ·transport: physiological and clinical implications. Mineral Electrolyte Metab 5:201–211, 1981.

91. Erbe RW, Greene JA Jr, Weller JM: Peritoneal dialysis during hemorrhagic shock. J Appl Physiol 22:131–135, 1967.

92. Tenckhoff H, Schechter H: A bacteriologically safe peritoneal access device. Trans Am Soc Artif Intern Organs 14:181–187, 1968.

93. Weston RE, Roberts M: Clinical use of stylet-catheter for peritoneal dialysis. Arch Intern Med 115:659–662, 1965.

94. Simkin EP, Wright FK: Perforating injuries of the bowel complicating peritoneal catheter insertion. Lancet 1:64–66, 1968.

95. Cope C, Kramer MS: Laparoscopic retrieval of dialysis catheter. Ann Intern Med 81:121, 1974.

96. Synhaivsky A, Kurtz SB, Wochos DN, et al: Acute renal failure treated by slow continuous ultrafiltration: preliminary report. Mayo Clin Proc 58:729–733, 1983.

97. Lauer A, Saccaggi A, Ronco C, et al: Continuous arteriovenous hemofiltration in the critically ill patient: clinical use and operational characteristics. Ann Intern Med 99:455–460, 1983.

98. Kaplan AA, Longnecker RE, Folkert VW: Continuous arteriovenous hemofiltration: a report of six months' experience. Ann Intern Med 100:358–367, 1984.

99. Bartlett RH, Mault JR, Dechert RE, et al: Continuous arteriovenous hemofiltration: improved survival in surgical acute renal failure? Surgery 100:400–408, 1986.

100. Freeman RB: Treatment of chronic renal failure: an update. N Engl J Med 312:577–579, 1985 (editorial).

101. Twardowski ZJ, Nolph KD: Blood purification in acute renal failure. Ann Intern Med 100:447–449, 1984.

102. Mahoney CA, Arieff AI: Uremic encephalopathies: clinical, biochemical, and experimental features. Am J Kidney Dis 2:324–336, 1982.

103. Arieff AI, Massry SG, Barrientos A, Kleeman CR: Brain water and electrolyte metabolism in uremia: effects of slow and rapid hemodialysis. Kidney Int 4:177–187, 1973.

104. Arieff AI, Guisado R, Massry SG, Lazarowitz VC: Central nervous system pH in uremia and the effects of hemodialysis. J Clin Invest 58:306–311, 1976.

105. Henderson LW: Symptomatic hypotension during hemodialysis. Kidney Int 17:571–576, 1980.

106. Huyghebaert MF, Dhainaut JF, Monsallier JF, Schlemmer B: Bicarbonate hemodialysis of patients with acute renal failure and severe sepsis. Crit Care Med 13:840–843, 1985.

107. Samii K, Rapin M, Le Gall JR, Regnier B: Haemodynamic study of patients with severe sepsis during haemodialysis. Intens Care Med 4:127–131, 1978.

108. Lazarus JM, Hampers CL, Lowrie EG, Merrill JP: Baroreceptor activity in normotensive and hypertensive uremic patients. Circulation 47:1015–1021, 1973.

109. Lilley JJ, Golden J, Stone RA: Adrenergic regulation of blood pressure in chronic renal failure. J Clin Invest 57:1190–1200, 1976.

110. Endou K, Kamijima J, Kakubari Y, Kikawada R: Hemodynamic changes during hemodialysis. Cardiology 63:175–187, 1978.

111. Graefe U, Milutinovich J, Follette WC, et al: Less dialysis-induced morbidity and vascular instability with bicarbonate in dialysate. Ann Intern Med 88:332–336, 1978.

112. Kirkendol PL, Devia CJ, Bower JD, Holbert RD: A comparison of the cardiovascular effects of sodium acetate, sodium bicarbonate and other potential sources of fixed base in hemodialysate solutions. Trans Am Soc Artif Intern Organs 23:399–405, 1977.

113. Raja R, Kramer M, Rosenbaum JL, et al: Prevention of hypotension during iso-osmolar hemodialysis with bicarbonate dialysate. Trans Am Soc Artif Intern Organs 26:375–377, 1980.

114. Fournier G, Man NK: Prevention of hemodialysis-induced hypoxemia by use of bicarbonate-containing dialysate. Kidney Int 17:701–702, 1980 (abstract).

115. Leunissen KM, Hoorntje SJ, Fiers HA, et al: Acetate versus bicarbonate hemodialysis in critically ill patients. Nephron 42:146–151, 1986.

116. Novello A, Kelsch RC, Easterling RE: Acetate intolerance during hemodialysis. Clin Nephrol 5:29–32, 1976.

117. Hung J, Harris PJ, Uren RF, et al: Uremic cardiomyopathy—effect of hemodialysis on left ventricular function in end-stage renal failure. N Engl J Med 302:547–551, 1980.

118. Maynard JC, Cruz C, Kleerekoper M, Levin NW: Blood pressure response to changes in serum ionized calcium during hemodialysis. Ann Intern Med 104:358–361, 1986.

119. Carney SL, Gillies AH: Effect of an optimum dialysis fluid calcium concentration on calcium mass transfer during maintenance hemodialysis. Clin Nephrol 24:28–30, 1985.

120. Craddock PR, Fehr J, Brigham KL, et al: Complement- and leukocyte-mediated pulmonary dysfunction in hemodialysis. N Engl J Med 296:769–774, 1977.

121. Francos GC, Besarab A, Burke JF Jr, et al: Dialysis-induced hypoxemia: membrane independent causes. Am J Kidney Dis 5:191–198, 1985.

122. Sherlock J, Ledwith J, Letteri J: Determinants of oxygenation during hemodialysis and related procedures: a report of data acquired under varying conditions and a review of the literature. Am J Nephrol 4:158–168, 1984.

123. Aurigemma NM, Feldman NT, Gottlieb M, et al: Arterial oxygenation during hemodialysis. N Engl J Med 297:871–873, 1977.

124. Quebbeman EJ, Maierhofer WJ, Piering WF: Mechanisms producing hypoxemia during hemodialysis. Crit Care Med 12:359–363, 1984.

125. Eiser AR, Jayamanne D, Koksong C, et al: Contrasting alterations in oxygen consumption (VO_2) and respiratory quotient (RQ) during acetate (A) and bicarbonate (B) hemodialysis (HD). Kidney Int 19:145, 1981 (abstract).

126. De Backer WA, Verpooten GA, Borgonjon DJ, et al: Hypoxemia during hemodialysis: effects of different membranes and dialysate compositions. Kidney Int 23:738–743, 1983.

127. Edwards SR, Unger AM: Acute hydrothorax—a new complication of peritoneal dialysis. JAMA 199:853–855, 1967.

FLUID AND ELECTROLYTE ABNORMALITIES AND MANAGEMENT

11

KENNETH J. TUMAN

Fluid and electrolyte management is an integral part of the care of the postoperative patient and in some patients may be a critical factor in their care. The physiology of body fluids and electrolytes is affected by many preoperative diseases as well as operative trauma. A thorough understanding of the metabolism of electrolytes in body water is essential to the care of the postoperative patient, and this chapter defines the physiologic principles relating to fluid and electrolyte therapy during the postoperative period.

BODY FLUID COMPARTMENTS: SIZE AND COMPOSITION

A prerequisite to the understanding of fluid and electrolyte management is knowledge of the size and composition of the various body fluid compartments. Water constitutes between 50 and 70 per cent of total body weight. The average normal total body water (TBW) of young adult men is 60 ± 10 per cent of body weight and 50 ± 10 per cent of body weight of young adult women. These compartments are relatively constant in size for the individual patient and are a function of several variables, including lean body weight and age. Because adipose tissue contains little water, lean individuals have a greater ratio of water to total body weight than do obese patients. An extremely obese patient may have 25 to 30 per cent less body water than a lean individual of the same weight. The highest proportion of total body water is found in newborn infants, with a maximum of 75 to 80 per cent.

There are three functional compartments of TBW. The intracellular fluid (ICF) compartment is approximately two thirds of the TBW (between 30 and 40 per cent of the body weight). The extracellular fluid (ECF) compartment represents approximately one third of TBW (approximately 20 per cent of body weight). Approximately one fourth of the ECF exists in the intravascular fluid, or plasma, which represents approximately 5 per cent of body weight. The remaining three fourths of ECF exists in the interstitial or extravascular, extracellular fluid, which constitutes 15 per cent of body weight. Potassium and magnesium are the principal cations in ICF and phosphates, sulfates, and proteins the principle anions. In contrast, sodium is the principal cation and chloride and bicarbonate the principal anions in ECF.

The physical and chemical activity of electrolytes in the various body fluid compartments depends on the number of particles present per unit volume (e.g., millimoles per liter), the number of charges per unit volume (e.g., milliequivalents per liter), and the number of osmotically active particles per unit volume (e.g., milliosmoles per liter).

A *millimole* of a substance is the molecular weight of that substance expressed in milligrams; it may not convey direct information regarding the number of osmotically active particles in solution or the electrical charges they carry. The *milliequivalent* amount of an ion is its atomic weight expressed in milligrams divided by the valence of that ion. For univalent ions, the milliequivalent value is the same as the millimolar value. In the case of divalent ions, e.g., calcium or magnesium, the millimolar value is equal to two milliequivalent values of these ions. The *osmotic pressure* of a solution depends on the actual number of osmotically active particles present in the solution. For example, sodium chloride, which dissociates nearly completely, contributes two milliosmoles for every millimole of compound. Conversely, one millimole of calcium chloride, which dissociates into three

157

particles, contributes three milliosmoles for every millimole of compound.

The total concentration of intracellular ions is larger than that of the extracellular compartment. Although it seems to violate the concept of osmolar equilibrium between the two compartments, it is consistent with the Gibbs-Donnan equilibrium equation because the concentration of ions is expressed in milliequivalents without regard to osmotic activity. In addition, some of the intracellular cations probably exist as undissociated moieties.

The differences in ionic concentration between the ICF and ECF are maintained by the semipermeable cell membrane. Although the total osmotic pressure of both fluid compartments is the same and equals the sum of the partial pressures contributed by each of the solutes in each fluid compartment, the effective osmotic pressure depends on the substances that fail to pass through the semipermeable cellular membranes. Therefore the plasma proteins are the primary determinants of effective osmotic pressure between the plasma and the interstitial fluid compartments (colloid osmotic pressure). The effective osmotic pressure between the ECF and ICF compartments can be contributed to by any substance that does not traverse the cell membranes freely. Therefore ions such as sodium, the principal extracellular cation, contribute a major portion of the osmotic pressure; but substances that fail to penetrate the cell membrane freely, e.g., glucose or mannitol, may increase the effective osmotic pressure. Any condition that alters the effective osmotic pressure in either fluid compartment results in redistribution of water between the compartments, as the cell membrane is completely permeable to water. For example, an increase in effective osmotic pressure in the ECF, which occurs most frequently as a result of increased sodium concentration, would cause a net transfer of water from the ICF to the ECF compartment. This transfer of water would continue until the effective osmotic pressure in the two compartments equalize. Conversely, a decrease in the ECF sodium concentration causes a transfer of water from the ECF to the ICF compartment. Depletion of ECF volume without a change in the concentration of the ions does not result in the transfer of free water from the ICF compartment. Thus, practically, most losses and gains of body fluid are directly from the extracellular compartment.

Acute deprivation and fluid losses during the preoperative period, intraoperative blood and fluid losses, and surgical trauma that results in tissue edema ("third-space loss") all cause stimulation of a number of homeostatic reflexes to maintain intravascular volume. The principal elements in the regulation of intravascular volume result in responses at the renal tubular level, which lead to salt and water retention and restoration of the intravascular fluid compartment. The release of antidiuretic hormone (ADH) is associated with renal water retention, whereas secretion of aldosterone and other corticosteroids result in sodium retention. The release of atrial natriuretic hormone may be inhibited during hypovolemic states because of the lack of distension of the cardiac atria, and this situation results in additional volume retention in the kidney. Finally, vascular responses affecting the glomerular filtration rate for water and sodium are activated in response to changes in intravascular volume.

DISORDERS OF VOLUME AND CONCENTRATION

Disorders of fluid balance may be classified into three general categories: disturbance of volume, concentration, or composition. The first two are discussed in this section. Composition disorders are discussed later in the chapter.

DISTURBANCE OF VOLUME

The most common disturbance of fluid balance seen postoperatively involves volume changes (Fig. 11–1). Acute volume deficit such as that seen during surgical procedures is accompanied by little, if any, change in the ICF volume because the fluid loss is primarily isotonic and fluid is not transferred from the ICF space to refill the depleted ECF compartment so long as the osmolarity of the two compartments remains unchanged.

The ECF deficit most common in the postsurgical patient is the loss of fluid, which is generally isotonic with that of normal ECF. The most common causes for such fluid loss include sequestration of fluid in soft tissue injuries, intraabdominal and retroperitoneal inflammation secondary either to surgical or other trauma, or infection such as acute peri-

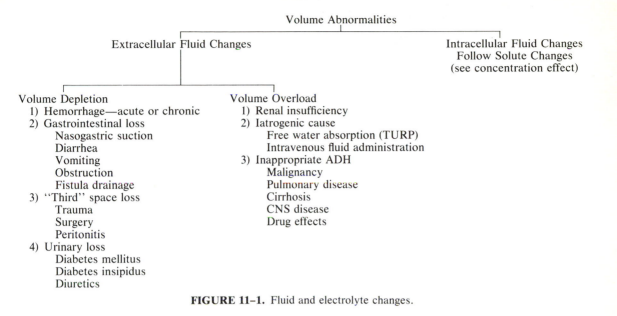

FIGURE 11–1. Fluid and electrolyte changes.

tonitis. The general surgical patient also commonly has losses of ECF volume due to losses of gastrointestinal fluids due to vomiting, nasogastric suction, diarrhea, or drainage from fistulas, in addition to third-space losses intramurally and intraluminally secondary to intestinal obstruction.

When these fluid losses are chronic in nature and have occurred over a prolonged period before surgery and arrival in the recovery area, there may be clinical evidence of this volume deficit. Such evidence includes increases in the serum blood urea nitrogen level, decreased skin turgor, increased thirst, and dry mucous membranes. These signs of tissue desiccation may be absent unless the deficit has existed for at least 18 to 24 hours. However, cardiovascular signs occur much earlier with acute volume deficits.

Varying degrees of altered perfusion result in orthostatic hypotension, tachycardia, collapsed veins, systemic hypotension with low central venous filling pressures, diminished heart sounds, and, in extreme cases, cool extremities and weak peripheral pulses. Oliguria is an early sign of volume deficit; and as dehydration increases, hallucinations, delirium, hyperpnea, stupor, and even coma may ensue. Losses of intravascular volume are compounded in some cases by fever or a warm environment, which increases water loss from the lungs and skin. In unusual cases, intravascular volume loss may be compounded by the inability of the kidney to conserve water be-

cause of inadequate ADH responses (diabetes insipidus), insensitivity to ADH (nephrogenic diabetes insipidus), osmotic diuresis (diabetes mellitus), or inadequate renal tubule function due to intrinsic renal disease. Impaired tubular reabsorption of water may occur in cases of severe potassium depletion and after correction of obstructive uropathy. The use of diuretic therapy (given inappropriately) in the face of an existing volume deficit in order to generate urine output may further compound intravascular volume deficits.

Acute changes in the ECF volume often result in changes in hematocrit levels. When plasma volume is lost because of internal fluid shifts with the development of a third space of sequestered fluid or with external losses of ECF, hemoconcentration occurs and elevated hematocrit levels are often seen. If blood loss is responsible for the loss of intravascular volume, the hematocrit may or may not reflect this blood loss or its replacement with red blood cells because of the time needed for equilibration of a stable final hematocrit level. When preoperative volume deficits have occurred, measurement of body weight compared to the euvolemic state is often useful. If there is an abnormal external fluid loss, the body weight decreases in proportion to the amount of fluid lost so long as the deficit remains. However, when third-space sequestration of fluid occurs, the sequestered fluid remains within the body and there is no loss of weight even though the intravascular fluid compartment is diminished. In fact, a gain in weight results from the necessary replacement of diminished plasma and interstitial fluid volumes of the rest of the body when the deficits are due to the development of a third space of sequestered fluid. These changes in hematocrit and body weight are useful for estimating volume deficits in children so long as one is able to differentiate between external and sequestered fluid losses.

Excesses of ECF that may be seen postoperatively are usually due to renal insufficiency or iatrogenic causes. In such cases the plasma and interstitial fluid volume are generally both increased. When the fluid excess has been present for a prolonged period, subcutaneous edema may be present; and as circulatory overload increases, elevation of central venous filling pressures is noted, as well as distension of central and peripheral veins. Functional murmurs of the heart may be enhanced, and overload of the pulmonary circulation may result in an increase in the intensity of the second heart sound. Although increased cardiac output may be seen with moderate degrees of ECF volume excess, acute congestive heart failure and hydrostatic pulmonary edema may occur with severe ECF volume overload, especially in elderly patients.

DISTURBANCE OF CONCENTRATION

The second major type of disorder of fluid balance consists of changes in the concentration of the osmotically active particles of the ECF space (Fig. 11–2). The best index of osmolarity is the measurement of plasma solute concentrations in the laboratory by determining freezing point depression. Serum osmolarity can be estimated from the formula

$$2(Na^+ mEq/L) + glucose(mg/dl)/18 + BUN(mg/dl)/2.8$$

As seen from this formula, sodium ions generally account for 90 per cent of the osmotically active particles in the ECF and are the primary determinants of its tonicity. If this compartment is depleted of sodium, water passes into the ICF until osmolarity is again equal in the two compartments. Both hyper- and hypoosmolar states may be seen during the postoperative period.

A decreased concentration of sodium in the ECF may result from loss of sodium, dilution by retention of water, or administration of excess amounts of free water. Loss of sodium is seen with adrenal insufficiency, vigorous diuretic therapy, unusual losses of gastrointestinal secretions, and some forms of renal insufficiency. When the deficit of water is replaced with fluids containing inadequate amounts of sodium, hyponatremia results. Patients with cancer, heart disease, liver disease, renal insufficiency, or chronic infection are likely to have an expanded ECF space even before surgical treatment. They are particularly prone to retain water and electrolytes and further expand and dilute the ECF intraoperatively. Water and sodium retention are exaggerated postoperatively in such patients who usually have a poor tolerance for the administration of large volumes of solutions such as Ringer's lactate or 0.9 per cent saline. These patients also tolerate free water (as glucose in water) poorly,

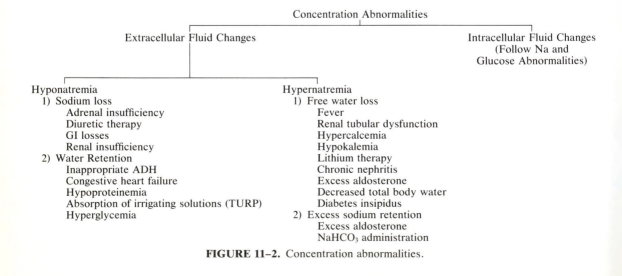

FIGURE 11–2. Concentration abnormalities.

holding onto excessive water intake with further dilution. An expanded ECF space with hyponatremia is the most common pattern of electrolyte abnormality seen in surgical patients and is one of the most difficult to treat once it becomes established.

Inappropriate secretion of ADH may be stimulated by drugs, pulmonary disease, or central nervous system (CNS) disease; and it may be seen in association with malignant tumors. In edematous states such as congestive heart failure, hepatic cirrhosis, nephrotic syndrome, and hypoproteinemia, a decreased circulating blood volume stimulates ADH secretion. Whether ADH is secreted inappropriately or in response to a decreased circulating blood volume, a dilutional syndrome may be produced characterized by hyponatremia with a normal or high total body sodium content.

Acute hyponatremia following intravascular absorption of irrigating solutions is a well described complication of transurethral resection of the prostate (TURP). Intravascular absorption of the irrigating solutions may lead to acute, profound hyponatremia. Moderate hyponatremia may be associated with muscle twitching, hyperactive tendon reflexes progressing to convulsions with loss of reflexes, and even increased intracranial pressure as severe levels of acute hyponatremia occur. The neurologic sequelae of the water intoxication syndrome have been thought in the past to be due to the rapid decrease in serum sodium. However, the exact pathophysiology of the water intoxication syndrome associated with TURP remains somewhat controversial. The key to interpreting the pathophysiology of these neurologic changes depends on differentiating hypotonic hyponatremia from isotonic hyponatremia utilizing the osmolar gap. The osmolar gap is the difference between the measured and the calculated osmolarity. When the measured serum osmolarity exceeds the calculated osmolarity by more than 10 mOsm/kg, an increased osmolar gap exists. This situation implies unmeasured solute must be present in plasma water in significant amounts and therefore may influence the net movement of water across cells. Substances such as glycine, mannitol, and sorbitol (all agents used in irrigating solutions during TURP) are relatively impermeant. Accumulation of these solutes in the plasma therefore influences tonicity and net transcellular water movement. Cerebral cellular swelling or shrinking depends on decreased or increased effective plasma osmolarity. Provided a relatively normal effective osmolarity is maintained, cerebral edema rarely occurs despite low serum sodium levels. Therefore with the use of osmotically active irrigating solutions the concomitant intravascular absorption of osmotically active solute occurs, and marked shifts in brain water are usually attenuated. Acute hyponatremia in this setting may result in cation-induced alterations in glial transmembrane potentials but are unlikely to cause acute cerebral edema.

It must be remembered, however, that the plasma water content is normally about 93 per cent, and that this factor is taken into account in the empiric formula for calculating osmolarity. Should the plasma water content be abnormally low because of an abnormally high level of protein or lipid, the measured plasma sodium appears low when expressed as millimoles per liter, although the concentration in millimoles per kilogram of water, and thus its osmotic effect, is normal. This state has been called *pseudohyponatremia* and is associated with hyperproteinemia and hyperlipidemia. With pseudohyponatremia the calculated value for osmolarity is spuriously low and the osmolar gap is high. This point must be considered when interpreting the significance of the osmolar gap in the setting of acute hyponatremia.

Hyperglycemic hyponatremia occurs whenever hyperglycemia is marked because the osmotic effect of glucose in plasma moves water out of cells into the plasma (in the absence of insulin effect). Plasma sodium decreases approximately 1.6 mEq/L for each increase of 100 mg of plasma glucose per deciliter above normal. This type of hyponatremia is another exception to the rule that hyponatremia means decreased plasma osmolality. The sum of the osmolalities due to glucose and sodium salts does not decrease as hyponatremia progresses.

Differentiation of hypotonic hyponatremia from isotonic hyponatremia is important because it affects the treatment of these patients. Treatment of patients with isotonic hyponatremia utilizing hypertonic saline may lead to a more life-threatening hyperosmolar state, which has been associated with well documented morbidity and mortality. In contrast, if significant fluid absorption occurs without simultaneous absorption of an osmotically active agent, hypotonicity ensues and intracellular cerebral edema occurs. Patients with acute hypotonic hyponatremia are the only patients for whom treatment with hypertonic saline is indicated (see below).

Acute hyponatremia may be associated not only with neurologic but also with cardiovascular signs, including hypertension, which may be related to acute increases of intravascular volume or elevations in intracranial pressure. In addition, cardiac arrhythmias, including ventricular fibrillation, can occur when the serum sodium concentration decreases to below 110 mEq/L. Congestive heart failure may also occur in this setting.

Hyperosmolar concentrations of solutes may occur during the postoperative period and are harmful to patients because shifts of water from the intracellular to the extracellular space cause true intracellular dehydration. Sodium and glucose are the solutes most commonly involved. Although volume changes frequently occur without a change in serum sodium, the converse is unusual. Hypernatremia is almost always accompanied by a loss of body fluid containing more water than sodium. The hypovolemia and hyperosmolarity is often associated with a decrease in body weight, elevation in the blood urea nitrogen/creatinine ratio, dry mucous membranes, tachycardia, oliguria, and hypotension if severe hypovolemia exists. Fever, delirium, hyperpnea, and even coma may result from severe loss of volume and hyperosmolarity. Loss of water without an accompanying loss of electrolytes is not a common occurrence postoperatively but is associated with deficiency or absence of ADH (diabetes insipidus) or resistance of the renal tubules to ADH (nephrogenic diabetes insipidus). Pure water loss due to renal tubular unresponsiveness to ADH can accompany hypercalcemia, hypokalemia, lithium therapy, and chronic nephritic states. Pure water deficits may also occur in elderly or confused patients who do not respond to the sensation of thirst. Elevated serum sodium levels may also reflect a total body excess of sodium. Such excess accumulation of sodium is unusual unless there is altered renal function. Increased reabsorption of sodium by the renal tubules occurs in response to excess aldosterone secretion in the adrenal cortex. This situation may be seen in patients with primary aldosteronism in whom hypernatremia predominates with little evidence of expansion of the interstitial fluid volume. The most common cause of hypernatremia during the postoperative period, however, is not an excess of total body sodium but, rather, a decrease in the total body water content.

Because glucose slowly equilibrates across cell membranes, especially in the absence of insulin, it serves as an osmotically active agent in the ECF. With hyperglycemia, water is lost from cells with an increase in the ECF volume and a consequent dilution of extracellular electrolytes (especially sodium). When glycosuria occurs, the osmotic diuresis results in a loss of total body water and sodium. Contraction of the ECF volume and the continuing hyperosmolarity result in a further shift of water and electrolytes from the intracellular to the extracellular space. Sodium concentrations do not increase if sufficient free water is administered, but the continuing sodium loss depletes body sodium stores. A decrease in circulating blood volume ensues if a prolonged osmotic diuresis occurs; and hypotension, tachycardia, and increased blood urea nitrogen are often found. The presence of clinical evidence of a low blood volume is the best indicator of a sodium deficit, and the serum sodium level is not a reliable index of this setting.

Combined volume and concentration abnormalities, which are common in the postoperative state, occur as a consequence of disease states or inappropriate parenteral fluid therapy. The clinical state associated with combined volume and concentration abnormalities tends to be a composite of the signs and symptoms of the individual abnormalities. For example, when postoperative gastrointestinal fluid losses are replaced with hypotonic sodium solutions, e.g., 5 per cent dextrose with 0.2 per cent saline, one may encounter one of the more common mixed abnormalities that is a combination of an ECF deficit and hyponatremia. Conversely, the excessive administration of water or hypotonic salt solutions to the patient with oliguric renal failure may rapidly produce an ECF excess and hyponatremia. Normal renal function tends to minimize the changes associated with the disease states perturbing normal fluid and electrolyte balance as well as compensate for errors associated with parenteral fluid therapy. However, patients with anuric or oliguric renal failure are particularly prone to develop these mixed volume and osmolar concentration abnormalities. Fluid and electrolyte management in these patients therefore must be precise.

Understanding the basic principles governing the balance of the internal and external exchanges of water and salt is mandatory for developing a plan for fluid and electrolyte therapy of the postoperative patient. Even with maximum concentration of urine solutes, the water produced by oxidative metabolism is inadequate to provide for urinary excretion of the end products of metabolism and to account for the losses of water from the bowel, respiratory tract, and skin.

A normal adult consumes an average of 2000 to 2500 ml of water per day in order to maintain water balance. The water of oxidation adds 200 to 400 ml per day. The daily water losses take place by four routes: 1) urinary output and 2) the water content of stool, both of which are measurable; and by evaporation from 3) the respiratory tract and 4) the skin (insensible losses). An adult deprived of all external access to water must still excrete a minimum of 500 to 600 ml urine per day in order to rid the body of the products of catabolism. The insensible loss of water is increased by hypermetabolism, hyperventilation, and fever.

In addition to the metabolism of water, salt exchange occurs. In normal individuals, salt intake varies between 50 and 90 mEq of sodium per day, and sodium balance is maintained primarily by normal kidneys, which excrete the excess salt. If sodium intake is reduced or extrarenal losses occur, normal renal function allows reduction of sodium excretion to less than 5 mEq per day. Patients with salt-wasting nephropathies, however, may have an obligatory loss exceeding 150 to 200 mEq/L of urine.

In normal individuals, sweat and urine represent hypotonic losses of fluid, with the average sodium loss between 10 and 70 mEq per day in each of these body fluids, respectively. Insensible fluid loss from the lungs, by definition, is pure water. Conversely, most gastrointestinal secretions are isotonic or slightly hypotonic. Thus replacement of gastric, duodenal, ileal, pancreatic, or biliary fluid loss should be performed with an essentially isotonic salt solution.

Knowledge of the normal daily volume of secretions of the gastrointestinal tract is important, as the average values may be used for semiquantitative replacement of gastrointestinal losses. It is estimated that 8,000 to 10,000 ml of gastrointestinal tract secretions are produced in normal adults, of which saliva constitutes 1 to 2 liters, gastric juice about 2500 ml, bile 500 to 750 ml, and pancreatic juice more than 1000 ml per day. In addition, secretion of the upper small bowel contributes between 2000 and 3000 ml. All but 100 to 200 ml is normally reabsorbed by the distal small bowel and the colon. If gastrointestinal tract losses exceed 2000 ml in 24 hours, or when substantial losses continue for more than a few days, it is wise to send an aliquot of the 24 hour drainage for analysis of electrolytes and to determine the pH of a freshly obtained specimen so that replacement can be more precise. It is important to remember that sequestration losses of ECF (third-space losses) that occur operatively or postoperatively also represent isotonic losses of salt in water.

THERAPY FOR VOLUME AND CONCENTRATION DISTURBANCES

Fluid and electrolyte therapy of volume and concentration abnormalities during the postoperative period can generally be considered in three steps. First, one must consider what the baseline maintenance requirements are for water and electrolytes in the absence of oral intake. Next, the presence of abnormal losses must be defined in order to prevent ongoing abnormal fluid and electrolyte deficits resulting from disease, its treatment, or both. Finally, the deficit (or excess) that exists with regard to water, electrolytes, blood volume, and plasma proteins must be assessed. This third step involves deciding what should be done to correct these abnormalities and at what rate reconstitution should be effected.

In addition to these basic guidelines, management of the common fluid disturbances seen during the postoperative period requires an orderly approach with close clinical observation of the patients and frequent reevaluation of their fluid and electrolyte status. In addition, assumptions should not be made regarding the status of fluid balance based on the presence or absence of abnormalities in the concentration of body fluids. For example, an ECF volume deficit or excess may exist concomitantly with a normal, low, or high serum sodium concentration. As noted above, depletion of the ECF compartment without changes in the concentration or composition of that fluid compartment is the most common abnormality seen during the acute postoperative period. The diagnosis of this fluid depletion is generally based entirely on clinical findings, whose presence depends not only on the amount of ECF lost but also the rate of loss and the presence or absence of associated disease states. Preoperative medications, as well as those administered intraoperatively, may alter the clinical presentation of hypovolemia.

For example, patients who are receiving β-adrenergic blockers may not develop tachycardia even with acute losses of intravascular volume. Although exact quantification of the ECF deficit is not possible, it can be estimated on the basis of the severity of clinical signs in most patients.

No specific formulas or single clinical sign should be relied on to determine the adequacy of fluid resuscitation. Because most losses of ECF during the acute postoperative period have occurred acutely, cardiovascular signs predominate, and there are few or no tissue signs reflecting the ECF deficit. Therefore reversal of these signs of volume deficit, e.g., improvement of the systemic blood pressure, correction of a narrowed pulse pressure, slowing of the heart rate, and improvement in the hourly urine volume and a fall in specific gravity (in the absence of an osmotic diuresis), are useful guidelines for gauging fluid replacement. In addition to osmotic diuresis from agents such as mannitol or glucose, other patients may have inappropriately high urine volumes for their intravascular volume status. Patients with chronic renal disease, incipient acute renal damage, and central or nephrogenic diabetes insipidus may also have inappropriately high urine volumes.

Fluid replacement must take into account not only the estimated deficit but also the amount of fluid required for maintenance as well as ongoing losses, most commonly from the site of injury or operative trauma. The magnitude of these losses is usually not appreciated unless one realizes that only a slight increase in the thickness of the peritoneum, bowel wall, and mesentery results in a functional loss of several liters of ECF volume. These "third-space" fluid losses remain a part of the ECF space but are nonfunctional because they are unable to contribute to the intravascular volume. Patients with large amounts of third-space losses may have an enormous total ECF volume, although the functional component (i.e., the intravascular space) may be markedly reduced. Operative trauma frequently involves loss or transfer of significant amounts of blood, plasma, or ECF, which is often underestimated intraoperatively. Operative blood loss as estimated by the operating surgeon is often 20 to 30 per cent less than the isotopically measured blood loss. Several liters of extravascular, extracellular fluid can be lost as third-space fluid in areas of injury and associated only with oliguria and a mild depression of blood pressure,

narrowing of the pulse pressure, and some tachycardia. Because third-space losses are isotonic and operative blood loss involves the loss of isotonic plasma in addition to red blood cell mass, volume replacement of these deficits requires isotonic salt solution.

Several balanced isotonic salt solutions are available, including Ringer's lactate, Plasmalyte, and Normosol-R. Ringer's lactate solution contains sodium 130 mEq/L, potassium 4 mEq/L, calcium 3 mEq/L, chloride 109 mEq/L, and lactate 28 mEq/L. When lactate is metabolized, it yields 28 mEq of bicarbonate per liter. Plasmalyte replacement solution contains sodium 140 mEq/L, potassium 5 mEq/L, magnesium 3 mEq/L, chloride 98 mEq/L, acetate 27 mEq/L, and gluconate 23 mEq/L. Normosol-R replacement solution contains the same sodium, potassium, and magnesium concentrations as Plasmalyte but (per liter) only 90 mEq chloride, 8 mEq acetate, and 50 mEq gluconate.

Acetate and gluconate may each be converted to bicarbonate through a variety of metabolic pathways in the liver. Therefore all of the above-mentioned balanced, isotonic salt solutions have been recommended as replacement-type fluids for loss of ECF, as their use reconstitutes plasma ECF to what closely resembles its normal composition. However, there is no solid evidence favoring use of these solutions over any other isotonic solution, e.g., 0.9 per cent saline, for volume expansion. Indeed these fluids are somewhat contraindicated in patients with hyperkalemia, hypercalcemia, hypermagnesemia, and possibly metabolic alkalosis. In addition, so long as there is reasonable hepatic function and adequate perfusion is restored, lactate, acetate, and gluconate are converted to bicarbonate and should not contribute to the production of lactic acidosis. Some practitioners, however, prefer not to use Ringer's lactate solution in patients who already have lactic acidosis because of concern over worsening a preexisting acid-base problem. In instances where the clinician decides not to use one of the above-mentioned balanced isotonic replacement fluids, 0.9 per cent sodium chloride should be employed with the addition of glucose, potassium, calcium, and sodium bicarbonate as indicated.

For patients with circulatory instability caused by loss of ECF and intravascular volume, the rate of administration of volume replacement with isotonic salt solution depends on the severity of the cardiovascular instability. For patients who are hypotensive, isotonic salt solution should be administered as rapidly as possible in order to replete cardiac preload and improve the perfusion status of the patient. It may involve administering 1000 to 2000 ml of fluid over a 5- to 10-minute period if acute intravascular volume repletion must be performed. More casual administration of fluid may be employed if oliguria and mild tachycardia are the only abnormalities and circulatory insufficiency is not present. However, the volume that may be safely administered is contingent on the patient's cardiac status. Patients with impaired cardiovascular reserves may benefit from measurement of the central venous pressure and the pulmonary artery occlusion pressure to detect limitations in cardiac competence, assess the efficacy of rapid volume replacement, and avoid acute cardiac decompensation and pulmonary edema.

If there is a question of the cardiac competence, a fluid challenge of 100 or 200 ml of fluid may be administered over a period of less than 5 minutes while the central venous pressure (CVP), pulmonary artery occlusion pressure (PAOP), or both are monitored. If a rapidly administered infusion of fluid does not increase the PAOP by at least 3 mm Hg and the ventricle is still on the horizontal portion of its diastolic pressure–volume curve, and, conversely, if it rises by more than 7 mm Hg, the less compliant ascending limb has been reached.

Further volume infusion may not improve stroke volume significantly and so should be undertaken judiciously. Continued volume infusion after the PAOP is made to rise acutely may result in hydrostatic pulmonary edema. The clinician may construct a family of Starling curves only if able to infer that end-diastolic volume has changed in response to a rapid volume infusion by noting a substantial increase in PAOP or CVP. Slow volume infusions may not allow such a relation to be tested because the ventricular diastolic pressure–volume relation may vary abruptly for a variety of reasons and because intravenously administered fluid (even isotonic crystalloid) may rapidly leave the intravascular space. After inferring a change in the end-diastolic volume, the corresponding change in stroke volume allows the clinician to determine if the Frank-Starling relation between stroke volume and PAOP is displaced to the right, as might occur with decreased left ventricular compliance due to an ischemic or hypertro-

phied left ventricle or pericardial disease. Because the usual relation between diastolic pressure and volume is not valid when myocardial compliance changes, the PAOP may not be an accurate monitor of left ventricular performance, and clinical assessment of the patient's response to therapy is essential for optimizing treatment. The effects of volume infusion, vasodilating agents, ventilatory changes, and disease states on left ventricular preload are not entirely predictable when PAOP is measured, although the net effect can usually be surmised from resultant changes in the measured stroke volume.

When acute hemorrhage is the primary cause of intravascular volume depletion, enough red blood cells are lost such that erythrocyte replacement may be required. The decision to transfuse blood is a complex one and involves consideration of the patient's circulatory status, absolute hemoglobin level, underlying disease state, and ability to employ compensatory homeostatic mechanisms in response to acute anemia (see Chapter 9).

In the absence of the need to transfuse blood, acute volume expansion of the intravascular space may be achieved with either isotonic crystalloid or colloid solution. Isotonic crystalloid provides osmotic particles that are distributed evenly throughout the ECF. Because the intravascular space comprises approximately one fourth of the entire ECF, normally only one fourth of the infused crystalloid solution remains within the intravascular space and three fourths is distributed into the interstitial space. This unequal distribution is more exaggerated in the critically ill, in whom as much as 90 to 95 per cent of isotonic crystalloid reaches the interstitial space because of defects in capillary impermeability. Colloids, on the other hand, are acutely confined mainly to the intravascular space and, even in the presence of leaky capillary membranes, require longer to distribute themselves into the interstitial space.

When expansion of the intravascular space involves resuscitation with isotonic crystalloid, for the relatively small amount of fluid that finally circulates in the intravascular space, there is gross overexpansion of the interstitial space. Expansion of the interstitial space is an inevitable sequela of resuscitation with isotonic crystalloid solutions. In addition, when hypotonic solutions are employed for intravascular volume expansion, even less of the original infused volume remains intravascularly. For example, when 5 per cent dextrose in water is employed, 1 of every 12 parts of volume infused remains intravascular, with the remainder distributed in the interstitial and intracellular fluid compartments: Glucose is readily transportable across cell membranes, especially in the presence of circulating insulin. Some data support the concept that patients who require large volumes of fluid for resuscitation may benefit from colloid compared with crystalloid administration, although this point remains controversial. It is clear, however, that if colloid solutions are to be used for fluid resuscitation, their use should be limited to situations that require rapid correction of hypovolemia. The use of colloids versus crystalloids is most controversial in situations that require less aggressive replacement of fluid losses. When large deficits in the interstitial space are present, such as may occur in cases of diabetic ketoacidosis, crystalloid solution should be used for resuscitation because isotonic crystalloid causes greater expansion of the interstitial space than colloid. Colloid solutions should be used only for resuscitation of the intravascular space.

In addition to correcting preexisting deficits that are present during the postoperative period, consideration must be given to maintenance of fluid requirements and accurate assessment and replacement of ongoing losses. During the acute perioperative period, activation of the normal stress responses results in release of ADH. Although normal kidneys are able to conserve sodium efficiently, unless salt is added to maintenance fluids a significant degree of hyponatremia may occur during the postoperative period owing to the retention of free water because of an ADH effect. In addition, elderly patients with inadequate renal function, salt-wasting nephropathies, or inappropriate ADH secretion may have an even more profound inability to retain salt while retaining excessive amounts of free water. Although a normal adult with maximum urinary concentration may be able to excrete obligatory metabolic solutes in a minimum of 500 to 600 ml of water, it is probably unnecessary to stress the kidneys to this degree.

With the above considerations, it is reasonable to administer approximately 800 to 1000 ml of solutions such as 5 per cent dextrose with 0.45 per cent saline to provide maintenance fluid for obligatory urinary excretory function. Use of solutions with less salt often results in postoperative hyponatremia because of excessive free water administration. Conversely, administration of solutions containing more than 0.45 per cent saline, e.g., lactated Ringer's solution or 0.9 per cent saline, often contain more salt than necessary, and so long as renal function is normal the excess sodium is excreted in the urine. Insensible losses are usually replaced with 5 per cent dextrose because insensible losses are generally considered to be nearly salt-free except in special instances, e.g., cystic fibrosis. Use of salt-containing solutions, e.g., 5 per cent dextrose with 0.45 per cent saline, for replacement of insensible loss has no significant clinical effect so long as renal function is normal. Use of such solutions to replace insensible losses may even compensate for any possible inadequate salt replacement of isotonic losses.

In summary, daily maintenance requirements of water and sodium for the normal 70 kg adult range between 2000 and 3000 ml of water and 75 and 150 mEq of sodium to prevent hyponatremia. When lean body mass is markedly different from that in the "typical" 70 kg adult, one may use the following formula to estimate daily maintenance fluid requirements: 100 ml/kg/day for the first 10 kg plus 50 ml/kg/day for the next 10 kg plus 20 ml/kg/day for the remainder of the body weight (which exceeds 20 kg). Alternatively, daily maintenance requirements may be estimated on an hourly basis by providing 1.5 ml fluid/kg/hr. This amount must be adjusted upward or downward depending on the patient's cardiovascular and renal function.

Patients with anuric or oliguric renal failure may require only replacement of insensible (evaporative) water losses from the skin and respiratory tract (500 to 800 ml per day) minus the amount of water produced from endogenous metabolism (300 ml per day). Conversely, patients with nonoliguric ("high output") renal failure may have large obligate salt and water losses and may require as much as 3000 to 5000 ml per day as maintenance fluid to avoid abnormal fluid balance in the presence of impaired renal concentrating ability. In addition, patients with fever develop larger water deficits owing to insensible losses from sweating. The water deficit increases by 100 to 150 ml per day in the average adult for each degree of body temperature exceeding 37°C. Many postsurgical patients have gastrointestinal losses that are usually isotonic or slightly hypotonic, and their losses should be replaced with essentially isotonic salt solutions. Thus all measured and insensible losses must be replaced with fluids of appropriate composition, allowing for any preexisting deficit.

Administration of one half of the estimated deficits during the first 8-hour period of replacement with the remainder being replaced over the ensuing 16 hours is a commonly cited guideline for replacement of estimated deficits. This restriction should not be applied if it will not result in an adequate circulating blood volume, as this state remains the foremost priority during the acute postoperative period. In addition, correction of concentration abnormalities (e.g., hyponatremia or hypernatremia) or of compositional abnormalities of plasma may need to be undertaken at a more rapid rate if imbalances such as severe acute hypokalemia exist.

In all cases, although initial fluid prescriptions may be written according to the basic guidelines noted above, for the patient with complications who has received or lost large amounts of fluid, it is frequently difficult to estimate the exact fluid requirements for the ensuing 12 to 24 hours. In these situations the patient should be checked frequently to determine the adequacy of their response to the fluid therapy until the situation is clarified. Proper replacement of fluids during this relatively short time during the postoperative period facilitates subsequent fluid management and patient care.

The ECF space can occasionally be overexpanded during the postoperative period when isotonic salt solutions (or other intravenous fluid therapy) have been administered in excess of volume losses (external or internal). Patients with normal cardiovascular and renal function are able to tolerate acute plasma overexpansion without serious problems.

Volume-overexpanded patients may have signs of interstitial space edema with edematous facies, especially scleral and eyelid edema, and peripheral edema. Circulatory and pulmonary signs of volume overload may occur (especially in patients with cardiopulmonary disease) and represent the most serious complication of fluid overload. Dyspnea, enlargement of the normal alveolar–arterial oxygen gradient, increases in intrapulmonary venoarterial admixture, overt pulmonary edema, and congestive heart failure may occur in patients with overexpansion of the ECF space. It may not be observed during the immediate postoperative period but may present several hours later when postoperative pain results in increases in blood pressure and vascular resistance, resulting in increases in both preload and afterload with acute cardiac decompensation.

This situation is not uncommon after spinal and epidural anesthesia involving significant degrees of sympathetic blockade, which is treated intraoperatively with aggressive fluid resuscitation and minimal amounts of vasopressor in order to return blood pressure toward normal. After surgery, when sympathetic blockade has dissipated, the above scenario is not uncommon.

It is important to note that overexpansion of the total ECF space may exist with depletion of the functional ECF compartment. Intravascular hypovolemia commonly occurs with interstitial fluid overload in conditions such as cirrhosis, chronic congestive heart failure, nephrotic syndrome, and postresuscitative states and sepsis. Use of CVP and PAOP measurements may be helpful for determining the size of the intravascular fluid compartment but may be misleading for a variety of reasons, primarily because altered ventricular compliance prevents the consistent differentiation of primary pump failure from the normovolemic or hypervolemic state when the PAOP is elevated. However, if central venous filling pressures are low, one can almost always rule out intravascular volume excess.

When fluid excess is present, the use of loop diuretics combined with temporary restriction of fluid input is usually sufficient to effect correction of this problem. In patients with adequate renal function, the use of low dose dopamine (2 to 5 μg/kg/min) to stimulate renal dopaminergic receptors and renal blood flow may help augment the needed diuresis. In patients with inadequate renal function, the use of continuous arteriovenous ultrafiltration (hemofiltration) or dialysis may be required to remove fluid excesses. When excess fluid results in increases of pulmonary extravascular water, supplemental oxygen and positive airway pressure may be needed. If patients are able to breathe spontaneously without excessive work of breathing, either face mask oxygen or continuous positive airway pressure (CPAP) delivered by face mask of endotracheal tube is sufficient. If the work of breathing is excessive despite the latter therapy, standard positive pressure ventilation with positive end-expiratory pressure (PEEP) may be required. Although volume excess is not as common as hypovolemia during the postoperative period, it may contribute to significant perioperative morbidity and even mortality in patients with significant underlying cardiopulmonary disease.

Imbalances in the ECF volume rarely occur

in pure form and are often accompanied by alterations in concentration. Hypernatremia is usually associated with water depletion caused by unreplaced losses and occasionally associated with increased output (e.g., osmotic diuresis, diarrhea). A water deficiency results in a decrease in the volume of all body fluid compartments; and because solute content does not change, hyperosmolarity ensues. Osmole receptors are stimulated, and ADH secretion is increased, with more water being reabsorbed from the distal renal tubule. A rough working estimate of the magnitude of water deficit can be calculated assuming that normal total body water (TBW) is 60 per cent of body weight and that normal plasma sodium (P_{Na} is 140 mEq/L. Actual total body water can be estimated using the following relation:

$$\text{Actual TBW} = \text{normal TBW} \times \text{normal } P_{Na}/\text{actual } P_{Na}$$

Water deficit is the normal total body water minus actual total body water. If intravascular volume is not markedly depleted, intravenous water can be given as either 5 per cent dextrose in water or 0.5 N saline to treat hypertonicity and replace water deficits. Excessive rates of correction of water deficits may result in cerebral edema even if the plasma sodium concentration and osmolality remain above normal. Patients with excessive renal water loss because of central diabetes insipidus may be treated with aqueous vasopressin administered intramuscularly or desmopressin (DDAVP) administered nasally.

Water deficits are frequently associated with hypernatremia, hypertonicity, and clinical signs of hypovolemia (e.g., tachycardia, orthostasis, oliguria). Treatment must begin with restoration of the circulation using isotonic salt solutions or colloid; once cardiovascular parameters and urine volume reflect correction of the intravascular volume deficit, one can change to hypotonic fluids. If the patient has normal renal function, volume repletion allows the urinary sodium concentration to rise, in turn aiding correction of the hypertonicity. As with cases of water deficit without concomitant ECF volume depletion, full correction of hypertonicity in this setting should proceed cautiously to avoid "isotonic water intoxication" and resultant brain swelling.

With the exceptions of hyperglycemia, hyperlipidemia, and severe hyperproteinemia, a reduction in serum sodium concentration most commonly indicates hypotonicity of body fluids. Postoperative hyponatremia is occasion-

ally seen following all types of surgical procedure and in this setting is usually due to hypotonic fluid administration in the presence of nonosmotic secretion of arginine vasopressin. When evaluating a patient with hyponatremia, it is useful to classify the patient into one of three categories (hypovolemic states, edematous states, or neither).

Hypovolemic hyponatremia presents with clinical evidence of ECF volume depletion, the absence of edema or ascites, low central venous filling pressures, and a blood glucose level of less than 250 mg/dl. In the presence of hypovolemia, ADH release is stimulated, and water is retained even at the expense of the occurrence of hypoosmolality. Parasympathetic afferent pathways from the aortic arch, carotid sinus, and possibly the cardiac atria respond to changes in either arterial or atrial pressure, with subsequent changes in parasympathetic tone and ADH release. The two main sources of fluid loss that result in hyponatremic hypovolemia are the gastrointestinal tract (e.g., vomiting, diarrhea) or renal losses secondary either to salt-losing nephropathy or excessive diuretic use. Hyponatremia and ECF volume depletion may also be a sign of adrenal insufficiency. Examination of the urinary sodium concentration is often helpful for narrowing down the diagnostic possibilities. When the fluid and electrolyte loss are from the gastrointestinal tract or when loss occurs into a "third space," the renal excretion of sodium should be minimal (<10 mEq/L), and the urine should be concentrated if renal function is intact. In contrast, overuse of diuretics, salt-losing nephritis, and primary adrenal insufficiency are associated with renal salt-wasting and an inappropriately high urine sodium concentration for the degree of hypovolemia (>20 mEq/L).

Hyponatremia may also be associated with an expanded ECF volume and is classified as *edematous hyponatremia* in this situation. Edematous hyponatremia is associated with the absence of clinical evidence of ECF depletion, the presence of edema or ascites, and elevated central venous filling pressures and blood glucose levels of less than 250 mg/dl. Hyponatremia occurs most frequently in association with edematous states. Although total body sodium and total body water are increased in these states, total body water is increased to a greater extent. The edematous disorders, including cirrhosis, cardiac failure, and nephrotic syndrome, impair renal water excretion and are associated with hyponatremia in the absence of diuretic use. Cardiac failure and hepatic failure result in impaired water excretion because of persistent release of ADH diminished distal fluid delivery to the diluting segment of the nephron. Nephrotic syndrome is associated with impaired renal water excretion, which may be mediated primarily by an increased release of ADH caused by hypovolemia. With all the edematous disorders, renal retention of sodium is high, and urinary excretion of sodium usually is less than 10 mEq/L unless the patient is receiving diuretic agents.

Normovolemic hyponatremia is defined as hyponatremia occurring without evidence of either hypovolemia or edema. These patients generally have excess ADH effect due either to pharmacologic agents or the syndrome of inappropriate ADH secretion (SIADH). The diagnosis of SIADH is made primarily by excluding other causes of hyponatremia. The diseases generally associated with SIADH fall into three categories: malignancies, pulmonary disorder, and CNS disorders. When SIADH is present, the urine is concentrated despite the presence of hyponatremia. The urinary solute concentration is generally increased, and the main defect is the inability to excrete free water.

Normovolemic hyponatremia, a common finding postoperatively, is caused by the administration of relatively hypotonic fluid in the presence of stress-related secretion of ADH. Cautious use of isotonic fluids during the perioperative period helps minimize the development of hyponatremia.

Classification of hyponatremic states into normovolemic, edematous, or hypovolemic states helps to define appropriate therapy. Water and sodium restriction are usually the requirements for treatment of edematous states, and saline administration is best used in patients with hyponatremia and volume depletion. Hypertonic saline is generally not indicated in the presence of volume depletion and could lead to further cellular dehydration, as these patients already have losses of both sodium and water from all body compartments. Administration of isotonic saline usually allows the osmole receptor–ADH system to normalize plasma osmolality once the ECF space has been reconstituted. When water retention occurs in SIADH, it is best treated with the use of water restriction, although diuretic-induced water losses may be necessary depending on the severity of the hyponatremia.

Acute, severe hyponatremia may result in significant morbidity and mortality. Acute hyponatremia associated with water retention and actual hypotonicity can result in generalized cell swelling, including brain swelling. Severe acute postoperative hyponatremia after elective surgery is occasionally associated with fatal or permanently crippling CNS effects. It is not clear whether it is the severity of the hyponatremia or the speed of correction that causes these neuropathologic complications. Rapid treatment of hyponatremia has been associated with central pontine myelinolysis and may be related to a phenomenon known as the osmotic demyelination syndrome. As noted earlier in the chapter, acute hyponatremia should be aggressively treated only when CNS abnormalities occur in the presence of *measured* hypotonicity. Isotonic hyponatremia, as may occur in cases of TURP syndrome, should not be treated with hypertonic saline. If hypertonic (3 per cent) saline solution is required for the treatment of symptomatic hypotonic hyponatremic states, volumes of approximately 100 to 200 ml are required, and they should be administered through a central venous catheter with close monitoring of the cardiovascular response, including measurement of central venous filling pressures (CVP, PAOP), blood pressure, heart rate, and cardiac output. Rapid correction of acute hyponatremia is not without neurologic and cardiovascular risk, and its application is controversial.

Essential hyponatremia, also known as the sick cell syndrome, is one of the few types of hyponatremia that does not result from a defect in water diuresis. Changes in cellular metabolism lead to a primary reduction in cellular osmolality that causes water to shift out of cells, thereby diluting the ECF and initiating hyponatremia. With this process (commonly seen in chronically ill patients, especially those with a malignancy) the osmoreceptor cells in the hypothalamus are reset, and a decreased plasma osmolality is maintained. This type of hyponatremia is usually asymptomatic and does not require treatment.

COMPOSITIONAL ABNORMALITIES

POTASSIUM

Disorders of potassium metabolism (Fig. 11–3) are common during the acute postopera-

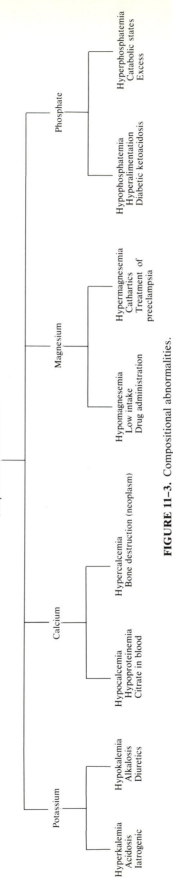

FIGURE 11–3. Compositional abnormalities.

tive period. The greatest proportion (approximately 97 per cent) of total body potassium is within cells, where it exists at a mean concentration of about 150 to 160 mEq/L. Active transport of potassium into cells balances the rate of passive outward diffusion and maintains a steep concentration gradient, so the ECF normally contains only 4 to 5 mEq of potassium per liter. The distribution of potassium between the intracellular and extracellular spaces is greatly influenced by the relative acid-base status of the two compartments. Extracellular acidosis tends to drive potassium out of cells and elevate its plasma concentration, whereas extracellular alkalosis has the opposite effect. Certain drugs such as insulin and β-adrenergic agonists facilitate the cellular uptake of potassium. The ratio of intra- to extracellular potassium concentrations is the major determinant of the membrane potential in muscle and nervous tissue. Because the extracellular potassium concentration is generally low, small alterations in its absolute concentration greatly influence the ratio. The normal intake of potassium is approximately 50 to 100 mEq per day, and urinary potassium excretion is normally regulated to equal this dietary intake. Multiple factors, e.g., aldosterone, level of sodium excretion, and acid-base status, interact to control renal potassium excretion. Aldosterone and alkalosis both stimulate potassium excretion. Renal excretion of potassium is increased when large quantities of sodium are available for excretion. The more sodium available for reabsorption, the more potassium is exchanged for it in the renal tubule, which is probably the basis for increased potassium requirements after massive isotonic fluid volume replacement or in the presence of steroid administration.

Hypokalemia in the postoperative surgical patient may be associated with either decreased total body potassium content or an alteration in the transcellular distribution of potassium. Because of the large transcellular potassium gradient, enormous total body potassium deficits can be present with only a small decrease in the serum potassium concentration. For example, it has been estimated that a chronic reduction in serum potassium concentration of 1 mEq/L can reflect a total body deficit of 600 to 800 mEq of potassium ion. Causes of decreased total body potassium content include gastrointestinal losses (nasogastric suctioning, vomiting, diarrhea) and renal losses, which may be induced by diuretics, hyperglycemia, hyperaldosteronism, or the excessive cortisol activity that sometimes occurs after surgical trauma.

When potassium deficiencies are due primarily to gastrointestinal losses, urinary potassium levels are low (usually <10 mEq/L); however, when potassium depletion occurs because of renal loss of potassium, the urinary potassium levels usually exceed 40 mEq/L. It has been estimated that the average postoperative adult loses approximately 50 mEq of potassium per day for the first two postoperative days because of increases in circulating aldosterone and cortisol (which itself has some mineralocorticoid activity). Altered transcellular distribution of potassium may occur because of respiratory or metabolic alkalosis, and it is estimated that a 0.5 mEq/L fall of potassium concentration occurs for every 0.1 rise in serum pH.

Respiratory alkalosis is a common cause of hypokalemia during the perioperative period. In addition, administration of glucose and the subsequent insulin effect (either endogenous or exogenous) result in a translocation of potassium to the intracellular space. In addition, some patients with familial, periodic paralysis have hypokalemia on the basis of an altered transcellular potassium distribution.

The clinical significance of hypokalemia depends in large part on whether the hypokalemia is acute or chronic and whether it is due to potassium loss or simply to an intracellular shift. Although hypokalemic patients are thought to have an increased potential for arrhythmias during the acute perioperative period, some data exist to suggest that chronic hypokalemia per se is not associated with a high incidence of perioperative arrhythmias. This point is probably true of modest hypokalemia (2.5 to 3.5 mEq/L); however, severe hypokalemia (<2.5 mEq/L) has been associated with the development of dangerous ventricular tachyarrhythmias, even in the absence of heart disease or digitalis therapy. Acute lowering of serum potassium may be more arrhythmogenic than chronic hypokalemia. Although clinical studies have shown consistent alterations in the electrocardiogram with progressive lowering of the serum potassium consisting of a sagging ST segment, a low T wave, and a prominent U wave, the effects of modest, chronic hypokalemia on the occurrence of serious cardiac arrhythmias is less consistent. The lack of correlation between chronic hypokalemia and significant arrhythmias has been demonstrated not only in generally healthy patients but also in those with significant cardiovascular disease (even in the presence of long-term digoxin therapy).

Because potassium administration may precipitate serious morbidity and is a potentially hazardous practice, it should be used cautiously during the perioperative period in patients who have chronic preoperative hypokalemia. When acute hypokalemia exists as a result of potassium loss (but not altered transcellular distribution), more aggressive correction of hypokalemia appears to be indicated. Nonetheless, even in these settings, intravenous potassium solutions should not contain concentrations of more than 40 mEq/L and are most safely infused with a rate-controlling device using ancillary intravenous lines.

Although potassium infusions can be tolerated at rates as high as 0.5 mEq/kg/hr, most guidelines list safe rates of infusion at 15 to 20 mEq/hr. Inadvertent intravenous potassium boluses of as little as 2 to 5 mEq, especially if administered via a central venous catheter, may result in cardiac concentrations of 10 to 12 mEq/L because of incomplete venous mixing and may result in cardiac arrest. Patients who are receiving intravenous potassium therapy at a rate exceeding 20 mEq/h should have electrocardiographic (ECG) monitoring.

Hypokalemia has been associated with skeletal muscle weakness, increased sensitivity to nondepolarizing neuromuscular blocking agents, paralytic ileus, and renal tubular dysfunction with decreased tubular concentrating ability and polyuria. When concomitant magnesium deficiency is present, simultaneous administration of magnesium may be required to increase serum and cellular potassium. When hypokalemia is associated with hypochloremic metabolic alkalosis, correction of serum potassium is difficult unless serum chloride levels are repleted and the metabolic alkalosis corrected.

Hyperkalemia is associated with increased total body potassium or a shift of potassium out of cells. Many cases of increased total body potassium content with resultant hyperkalemia are iatrogenic. These cases occur primarily in patients with renal insufficiency (glomerular filtration rate <15 per cent normal) who are challenged with excessive potassium loads such as rapid intravenous administration of old, banked blood, which may have a plasma potassium content approaching 30 mEq/L. Rapid intravenous administration of potassium penicillin may also result in significant hyperkalemia in patients with renal disease. Other causes of excessive total body

content of potassium include the use of potassium-sparing diuretics, Addison's disease, and the hyporeninemic, hypoaldosterone syndrome.

Altered distribution of body potassium stores occurs in a number of settings. When succinylcholine is used in patients with significant burns, muscle trauma, or spinal cord injuries, the cells of the body can release massive amounts of potassium. When respiratory or metabolic acidosis occurs, a decrease in the pH of 0.1 unit results in an increase in serum potassium of approximately 0.5 mEq/L. Cell lysis may occur secondary to chemotherapy or hemolysis and in the presence of malignant hyperpyrexia. Patients who are severely thrombocytotic may have a spurious hyperkalemia due to the release of potassium from platelets during aggregation in the blood collection tube. The pseudohyperkalemia that occurs when potassium is released from cells during blood sample clotting in states of leukocytosis, thrombocytosis, or hemolysis can be differentiated by the appearance of an abnormally high serum potassium level but a normal plasma (unclotted sample) potassium level. Some forms of familial, periodic paralysis are also associated with hyperkalemia. Finally, patients with diabetes mellitus who have insulin deficiency, as well as patients who are receiving β-adrenergic blocking drugs have impaired uptake of potassium into cells and may develop hyperkalemia in response to small amounts of exogenously administered potassium.

Hyperkalemia impairs cardiac automaticity, conductivity, and contractility. As serum potassium levels progressively rise, prolongation of the PR interval, peaking of the T wave, and ST segment elevation occur. At serum potassium levels higher than 7 mEq/L, ventricular arrhythmias, ventricular fibrillation, and diastolic cardiac standstill are likely. Hyperkalemia depolarizes the postjunctional membrane of skeletal muscle, and severe hyperkalemia is often accompanied by muscle weakness.

Any patient with ECG changes or other evidence of hyperkalemic cardiac toxicity must be treated immediately. The goals of treatment of hyperkalemia are to: 1) protect the cardiac cells from the effects of potassium; 2) shift potassium from the ECF to the ICF; and 3) reduce total body potassium stores. Because life-threatening arrhythmias may occur at any time during therapy, continuous ECG monitoring is required.

Once hyperkalemia has been diagnosed, potassium intake must be stopped immediately. Direct antagonism of the cardiac effects of hyperkalemia can be achieved by administering calcium gluconate or calcium chloride intravenously (5 to 10 ml of a 10 per cent solution) over a 2- to 4-minute period with constant ECG monitoring. A second dose may be given if no apparent response occurs within 5 minutes. Although calcium administration usually has immediate effects they are temporary, and other modalities should be initiated as soon as possible, including shifting potassium intracellularly by the administration of glucose, insulin, and bicarbonate. Treatment with bicarbonate is especially important in patients with metabolic acidosis but is effective even in those patients who have a neutral serum pH. One ampul of 8.4 per cent sodium bicarbonate (50 mEq) is usually given intravenously over a 3- to 5-minute period and repeated in 5 to 10 minutes if ECG abnormalities persist. Sodium bicarbonate solutions contain sufficient sodium that volume overload or hypernatremia (or both) may occur.

If patients are intubated during the postoperative period, active hyperventilation with production of a respiratory alkalosis also helps shift potassium intracellularly. A variety of methods of combining glucose and insulin infusions have been applied in this setting; 5 to 10 units of regular insulin is usually given intravenously at the same time as one ampul of 50 per cent dextrose (25 gm) over a 5-minute period. An alternative method is to administer 500 ml of 10 per cent dextrose with 10 to 15 units of regular insulin.

When hyperglycemia is present, insulin alone may be administered. Serum potassium usually decreases over a 30- to 60-minute period and remains so for a few hours. In addition, administration of glucose and insulin may result in volume expansion or an osmotic diuresis with a loss of intravascular volume. Hypoglycemia is also possible, and serial glucose levels should be measured after this therapy has been instituted.

It is important to remember that the above therapies do not remove potassium from the body but, rather, temporize until other therapies can be instituted. Cation-exchange resins, e.g., sodium polystyrene sulfonate, exchange sodium for potassium in the bowel and can be administered either by mouth (usually 15 to 30 gm in 50 ml of 20 per cent sorbitol) or as a retention enema (50 gm in 200 ml of 20 per cent sorbitol). The sorbitol is added as an osmotic agent, as the resin itself is constipating.

Dialysis with or without hemofiltration is the other method of removing potassium.

CALCIUM

Calcium is essential for nerve and muscle excitability, and the physiologically active form is the ionized fraction, which normally constitutes approximately 45 per cent of the total serum calcium. When serum albumin concentrations are decreased, less calcium is bound to protein; total serum calcium levels decrease, but the ionized portion remains unchanged. Measurement of the total serum calcium concentration during the postoperative period may therefore provide deceiving results, and the serum ionized calcium assay is required.

Causes of reduced ionized calcium concentrations during the postoperative period include respiratory or metabolic alkalosis, hypoparathyroidism following neck surgery, hypo- or hypermagnesemia, hyperphosphatemia, sepsis, pancreatitis, and fat embolism syndrome. Decreases in ionized calcium values may occur during transfusion of large amounts of blood and correlate with elevations in circulating citrate levels and the speed of transfusion. At normothermia, with normal hepatic function, administration of citrated blood generally does not result in decreased ionized calcium unless infusion rates exceed 2 ml/kg/min, or about 1 unit of blood every 5 minutes in an average size adult. The metabolism of citrate is effected by tissue perfusion, acid-base balance, and the activity of the enzyme aconitase, which is present in muscle, kidney, and liver. When the transfusion rate exceeds the rate of citrate metabolism, citrate levels rise and ionized calcium levels fall. When citrate clearance is impaired in hypothermic states or in patients with severe hepatic disease (especially during liver transplantation), even slower rates of administration of lesser amounts of citrated blood can increase plasma citrate to levels that cause clinically significant ionized hypocalcemia with resulting cardiovascular depression.

The clinical manifestations of decreased ionized calcium include hypotension with a narrow pulse pressure, elevated left ventricular end-diastolic and right atrial pressures, and decreased cardiac output. A prolonged Q-T interval may be seen on the ECG, although it is not a consistent finding. Bradycardia and ventricular fibrillation may occur, and there may be failure to respond to drugs that act through calcium-related mechanisms (e.g., digoxin, norepinephrine, and dopamine). Calcium is also important for maintaining peripheral vascular resistance. Patients with hypocalcemia may develop peripheral nerve irritability (Chvostek and Trousseau signs), circumoral paresthesias, confusion, seizures, and even tetany. Laryngospasm has been reported in critically ill patients who become hypocalcemic after neck surgery. Hypocalcemia results in an alteration in the presynaptic release of acetylcholine with resulting weakness and carpopedal spasm.

Acute symptomatic hypocalcemia (Fig. 11–3) is a medical emergency that necessitates therapy with intravenous calcium salts. Prompt administration of either calcium gluconate or calcium chloride (10 ml of a 10 per cent solution) intravenously over a 10-minute period usually results in reversal of the neuronal irritability and the cardiovascular abnormalities. In patients with profound ionized hypocalcemia or those who are anhepatic (e.g., during orthotopic liver transplantation), more rapid administration and larger doses may be required. Determination of serum ionized calcium levels should be delayed for 10 to 15 minutes after administration to allow equilibration in order to guide further therapy.

Administration of calcium to hyperphosphatemic patients may cause calcium salt precipitation. In addition, patients who are hypo- or hypermagnesemic often respond poorly to calcium therapy unless the serum magnesium level is normalized. One should avoid hyperventilation or the excessive use of bicarbonate, as alkalosis further reduces serum ionized calcium levels. In the acute postoperative state, severe hypocalcemia may be responsible for the potentiation of nondepolarizing neuromuscular blockade. Because calcium is a cofactor at several points in the coagulation cascade, coagulation abnormalities could also theoretically accompany extreme reductions in ionized calcium. This situation is rarely seen, as cardiovascular effects occur at levels of ionized hypocalcemia well above those levels required to effect coagulation.

Hypercalcemia occurs must less commonly during the postoperative period. The most common causes of hypercalcemia postoperatively are neoplastic disorders (especially with bone metastases) and hyperparathyroidism. The latter may occur as part of the multiple endocrine neoplasia syndrome, but parathyroid adenomas are more common. These adenomas may be primary or, more commonly, are associated with renal failure. Other etiologies include immobilization, granulomatous diseases such as sarcoidosis, and abuse of thiazide diuretics. Postoperatively, patients with hypercalcemia may present with prolonged obtundation, nausea and vomiting, and slowing of the electroencehpalogram; mild increases in intracranial pressure may also occur. ECG changes include the presence of a shortened Q-T interval, bradycardia, increased P-R interval, atrioventricular block, and widening of the QRS complex. There may be potentiation of digitalis-induced arrhythmias.

The cornerstone of treatment of hypercalcemia during the postoperative period is hydration with 0.9 per cent sodium chloride solution. Circulating blood volume must be assessed and plasma volume deficiencies corrected. Once plasma volume has been normalized or increased above normal, diuresis with loop diuretics such as furosemide or ethacrynic acid facilitates renal loss of calcium. Urinary losses of other electrolytes (especially potassium and magnesium), as well as water losses, must be monitored carefully and replaced to maintain hydration and electrolyte balance. Excessive use of furosemide or ethacrynic acid without water and electrolyte replacement leads to volume depletion, which exacerbates the hypercalcemia. If renal impairment is present, dialysis may be required to remove calcium from the body. Another approach is to transfer calcium into bone stores. Mithromycin inhibits bone resorption and is used for treatment of hypercalcemia in advanced malignancy. In addition, synthetic calcitonin may lower the serum calcium concentration, but this effect is only temporary. Synthetic calcitonin is most effective for severe hypercalcemia due to carcinoma, multiple myeloma, or primary hyperparathyroidism, and its use is considered only if rehydration and salt loading with diuresis are ineffective. When any of the above therapies are used, it is prudent to monitor the ECG to detect adverse effects on cardiac conduction by rapid shifts of ionized calcium levels.

Inorganic phosphate supplementation has been recommended by some investigators as a final therapeutic option for the acute management of hypercalcemia. Intravenous inorganic phosphate therapy should be administered with great caution, if at all, as severe tissue calcification, renal cortical necrosis, and death have been reported after its use.

MAGNESIUM

Hypomagnesemia is probably the most underdiagnosed electrolyte disturbance during the postoperative period; the incidence of hypomagnesemia exceeds 50 per cent of patients admitted to either surgical or medical intensive care units. Hypomagnesemia may occur as a consequence of inadequate magnesium intake, gastrointestinal or renal losses of magnesium, or intracellular shifts of magnesium ion. The administration of drugs such as aminoglycosides, cyclosporin, amphotericin, diuretics, and digoxin have been associated with increased renal magnesium wasting. Patients with poor nutritional status (e.g., cancer patients, those with esophageal disease that requires surgery, and perhaps the elderly) are more likely to develop hypomagnesemia during the postoperative period than the general population. Administration of catecholamines may cause an intracellular shift of magnesium and contribute to hypomagnesemia.

Approximately 50 per cent of total body magnesium exists in the insoluble state in bone, about 5 per cent is present as extracellular cation, and the remaining 45 per cent is intracellular. Approximately one third of plasma magnesium is bound to protein, and two thirds circulates as free cation. Magnesium exerts physiologic effects on the nervous system resembling those of calcium. Low concentrations produce irritability, disorientation, muscle spasm, hyperreflexia, and seizures. Calcium ion exerts an antagonistic action, probably by decreasing acetylcholine release at the myoneural junction, which is increased in the presence of low magnesium levels. Hypomagnesemia may also result in significant cardiovascular problems. Tissue magnesium deficiency is associated with the development of serious ventricular arrhythmias (including torsade de pointes), although total serum magnesium concentration may not be a useful marker of tissue levels (see below). In addition, hypomagnesemia has been associated with an increased frequency of ventricular tachyarrhythmias in the presence of acute myocardial ischemia. Administering magnesium as either a bolus injection or an infusion can reduce the incidence of arrhythmias after acute myocardial infarction. The movement of sodium out of cells and potassium into cells is largely regulated by the magnesium-dependent enzyme Na-K-ATPase. With magnesium deficiency, the function of this pump may be impaired, disrupting normal cellular sodium-potassium balance and interfering with normal potassium homeostasis. Such a situation may lead to inadequate potassium concentrations in cardiac cells, resulting in cardiac irritability.

Several studies have shown a strong association between hypokalemia and hypomagnesemia. The effectiveness of potassium replacement therapy correlates with the presence of adequate tissue magnesium. In the presence of magnesium deficiency, tissue replacement of potassium in hypokalemic patients may be achieved effectively only after administration of magnesium. In addition, ventricular ectopic beats may not be effectively treated with potassium infusion unless tissue magnesium levels are adequate, even if hypokalemia is corrected. Patients on digitalis therapy who are magnesium deficient may also have a lower threshold for digitalis-induced arrhythmias. Although there is a strong association between hypomagnesemia and hypokalemia, a definite cause-and-effect relation has not been demonstrated. It is possible that there are common etiologies for both abnormalities in many instances, e.g., renal potassium or magnesium wasting secondary to diuretic use.

As noted above, tissue magnesium deficiency may not be adequately reflected by the measurement of serum magnesium concentration. Although serum magnesium determinations are the only test of magnesium metabolism currently available for routine clinical use, postoperative patients may be better served by measuring ultrafilterable or cellular (lymphocytic or erythrocytic) magnesium levels. Currently, it is prudent to measure serum magnesium concentrations during the acute postoperative period in patients who have any of the conditions noted to be associated with hypomagnesemia, especially those with unexplained or difficult-to-treat hypokalemia or who have ventricular arrhythmias despite correction of hypokalemia.

Magnesium deficiency may be treated by the parenteral administration of magnesium sulfate or magnesium chloride solutions. Magnesium sulfate is more commonly used, and 1 to 2 gm of magnesium sulfate (8 to 16 mEq Mg^{2+}) may be given intravenously over a 30- to 60-minute period. As much as 1 to 2 mEq magnesium per kilogram may be required over 24 hours in cases of severe depletion. When such large doses are required, heart rate, blood pressure, respirations, and the ECG should be monitored. Because magnesium toxicity may result in hypotension, impaired ventilation, and even cardiac arrest, the patellar deep tendon reflex should be monitored; and if it becomes depressed or disappears, magnesium infusion should be discontinued.

Magnesium sulfate may produce peripheral vasodilation, and this effect has been used therapeutically to treat severe hypertension that is not responsive to other agents. Its use in this setting has been reported in a patient with hypertension secondary to a pheochromocytoma.

Some clinical signs are associated with progressive rises in serum magnesium levels. At levels of 3 to 7 mEq/L patients usually become slightly sedated; at levels of 7 to 10 mEq/L, a decrease in the patellar deep tendon reflex is noted and muscle weakness may be present, although alveolar ventilation is usually normal; at levels of 10 to 16 mEq/L, profound respiratory depression may be seen; and cardiac arrest almost uniformly occurs when serum magnesium levels exceed 16 mEq/L. It is advisable to have calcium chloride solution available during magnesium sulfate infusions to counteract any potential adverse cardiac, respiratory, or neuromuscular effects of rising plasma magnesium levels. Patients who have chronic magnesium deficits but who are asymptomatic during the postoperative period may have replacement of these deficits over several days using the intramuscular route or including magnesium sulfate or magnesium chloride in the maintenance intravenous fluids (usually 4 to 8 mEq per day is required for maintenance). Care should be taken when administering magnesium ion to patients with oliguria or those with renal insufficiency. In these situations, careful monitoring for signs or symptoms of magnesium toxicity must be undertaken, and smaller doses are required.

Hypermagnesemia is less common in postoperative patients and occurs primarily in those with renal failure. It is common when magnesium sulfate is used as a cathartic, and enough magnesium may be absorbed to produce toxicity when renal function is impaired. Manifestations of hypermagnesemia include muscle weakness, hypotension, drowsiness, and hyporeflexia. Progressively increasing levels of serum magnesium may result in prolongation of the Q-T interval, atrioventricular block, and cardiac arrest. Obstetric patients treated for preeclampsia or eclampsia with intravenous magnesium sulfate may develop signs or symptoms of magnesium excess.

When cardiac arrest occurs in this setting, it is usually due to respiratory muscle paralysis. Severe hypermagnesemia is treated with intravenous calcium chloride, which temporarily reverses the symptoms. Because hypermagnesemia is exacerbated by acidosis, treatment also consists in immediate measures to correct any acidosis and replenish any preexisting ECF deficit. Fluid loading with normal saline and administration of diuretics may enhance magnesium elimination through the renal tubules. When renal failure is present, dialysis may be indicated.

PHOSPHATE

Hypophosphatemia (Fig. 11–3) may occur postoperatively in the presence of normal phosphate stores. Conversely, serious depletion of body phosphate stores may coexist with low, normal, or even high concentrations of serum phosphate. Severe hypophosphatemia may result in serious physiologic consequences, especially when acute decreases in serum phosphate levels occur. At very low serum phosphate levels there may be serious hemolytic anemia with increased erythrocyte fragility, impaired oxygen delivery to tissues because of decreases in 2,3-diphosphoglyceric acid in erythrocytes, and a leftward shift of the oxyhemoglobin curve, impairing oxygen unloading. When acute hypophosphatemia occurs and is accompanied by acidosis (e.g., diabetic ketoacidosis), overzealous treatment of the acidosis could unmask the effect of hypophosphatemia and lead to profound tissue hypoxemia. Hypophosphatemic patients may have muscle weakness, especially of the respiratory muscles including the diaphragm, which may impede withdrawal of mechanical ventilatory support. This condition is most crucial in patients who are critically ill and have increased ventilatory requirements with limited ventilatory reserves. Severe hypophosphatemia with serum phosphate levels of less than 1 mg/dl have been associated with cardiac failure. Rapid shifts of inorganic phosphate between body compartments may occur soon after initiation of hyperalimentation, during treatment of diabetic ketoacidosis, during the diuretic phase of acute tubular necrosis, or in the presence of respiratory alkalosis.

Treatment of hypophosphatemia depends on the severity of the associated physiologic abnormalities and whether the phosphate deficiency is chronic or acute. Phosphate may be administered intravenously as a mixture of KH_2PO_4 and K_2HPO_4. If the patient is asymptomatic and hypophosphatemia is of recent onset, a dose of 0.08 mmol/kg is recommended. If the patient is asymptomatic but has had hypophosphatemia for a protracted period of time, the initial dose is doubled to 0.16 mmol/kg. Symptomatic patients should have this dose increased by 25 to 50 per cent; and if the patient is hypercalcemic, the initial dose should be decreased by 25 to 50 per cent to avoid a salting-out effect and the formation of calcium phosphate precipitate.

Prevention of hypophosphatemia during the postoperative period is the best therapy in many clinical settings. For example, most patients receiving hyperalimentation should receive phosphate supplementation to minimize phosphate depletion. In all cases, because neither the body deficit nor its response to therapy can be predicted, close monitoring of serum phosphate levels is necessary, especially in the presence of hypercalcemia or renal insufficiency.

If hypocalcemia coexists, calcium should be supplemented. Adding calcium to solutions containing phosphate or administration through the same intravenous line must be avoided.

Hyperphosphatemia usually occurs with renal insufficiency but may also be seen with hypothyroidism, catabolic states, and excessive administration of phosphate to patients who have limited renal excretory function. Acute increases in phosphate levels often cause a fall in serum calcium, producing signs of hypocalcemia. A reduction in serum bicarbonate usually accompanies increased phosphate anion in order to maintain plasma neutrality.

A major complication is metastatic calcification. Treatment includes phosphate restriction, use of inorganic phosphate-binding antacids, and in severe cases dialysis.

SUMMARY

Abnormalities of body fluid volume, concentration, and composition occur commonly during the acute postoperative period. Many of these abnormalities may be largely avoided by careful attention to the details of patient management and understanding the pathophysiology of the individual patient's condi-

tion. The accurate clinical assessment of the patient's condition is the first and usually the most difficult step in successful management of most fluid and electrolyte disorders during the acute postoperative period. Frequent reassessment of the patient along with a high index of suspicion about certain abnormalities (e.g., hypomagnesemia) are essential. Many diseases and operative trauma have a great impact on the physiology of fluid and electrolytes within the body, but a thorough understanding of the metabolism of salt, water, and electrolytes allows successful management of these common postoperative problems.

Bibliography

General Information

Lindeman RD, Papper S: Therapy of fluid and electrolyte disorders. Ann Intern Med *82*:64–70, 1975.

Schrier RW, ed: Renal and Electrolyte Disorders, 2nd ed. Boston, Little, Brown, 1980.

Shires GT, Canizaro PC: Fluid, electrolyte and nutritional management of the surgical patient. *In* Schwartz SI, ed. Principles of Surgery, 5th ed. New York, McGraw-Hill, 1988, pp. 67–103.

Fluid Volume and Sodium

Arieff AI: Hyponatremia, convulsions, respiratory arrest and permanent brain damage after elective surgery in healthy women. N Engl J Med *314*:1529–1535, 1986.

Chung HM, Kluge R, Schrier RW, Anderson RJ: Postoperative hyponatremia: a prospective study. Arch Intern Med *146*:333–336, 1986.

Feig PU, McCurdy DK: The hypertonic state. N Engl J Med *297*:1444–1454, 1977.

Laragh JH: Atrial natriuretic hormone, the renin-aldosterone axis, and blood-pressure-electrolyte homeostasis. N Engl J Med *313*:1330–1340, 1985.

Rothenberg DM, Ivankovich AD: Isotonic hyponatremia during transurethral prostate resection. Anesth Analg *68*:S240, 1989.

Shoemaker WC: Hemodynamic and oxygen transport effects of crystalloids and colloids in critically ill patients. Curr Stud Hematol Blood Transfus *53*:155–176, 1986.

Snyder NA, Fiegal DW, Arieff AI: Hypernatremia in elderly patients—a heterogeneous, morbid and iatrogenic entity. Ann Intern Med *107*:309–319, 1987.

Sterns RH, Riggs JE, Schochet SS: Osmotic demyelination syndrome following correction of hyponatremia. N Engl J Med *314*:1535–1542, 1986.

Weil MH, Henning RJ: New concepts in the diagnosis and fluid treatment of circulatory shock. Anesth Analg *58*:124–132, 1979.

Potassium

Hirsch IA, Tomlinson DL, Slogoff S, Keats AS: The overstated risk of preoperative hypokalemia. Anesth Analg *67*:131–136, 1988.

Rosa RM, Silva P, Young JB, et al: Adrenergic modulation of extrarenal potassium disposal. N Engl J Med *302*:431–434, 1980.

Vitez TS, Soper LE, Wong KC, Soper P: Chronic hypokalemia and intraoperative dysrhythmias. Anesthesiology *63*:130–133, 1985.

Calcium

Denlinger JK, Nahrwold ML, Gibbs PS, Lecky JP: Hypocalcemia during rapid blood transfusion in anesthetized man. Br J Anaesth *48*:995–1000, 1976.

Mundy GR, Ibbotson KJ, D'Souza SM, et al: The hypercalcemia of cancer: clinical implications and pathogenic mechanisms. N Engl J Med *310*:1718–1726, 1984.

Zaloga GP, Chernow B: Hypocalcemia in critical illness. JAMA *256*:1924–1929, 1986.

Magnesium

Chernow B, Bamberger S, Stoiko M, et al: Hypomagnesemia in patients in postoperative intensive care. Chest *95*:391–397, 1989.

Whang R: Magnesium deficiency: pathogenesis, prevalence and clinical implications. Am J Med *82*:24–29, 1987.

Whang R, Oei TO, Aikawa JK, et al: Predictors of clinical hypomagnesemia: hypokalemia, hypophosphatemia, hyponatremia and hypocalcemia. Arch Intern Med *144*:1794–1796, 1984.

Phosphate

Juan D: The causes and consequences of hypophosphatemia (review). Surg Gynecol Obstet *153*:589–597, 1981.

POSTOPERATIVE CENTRAL NERVOUS SYSTEM DYSFUNCTION

12

TOD B. SLOAN

One of the most distressing problems for the perioperative team is the patient who fails to recover full neurologic function after an uneventful anesthetic and surgical procedure. The neurologic problems that can occur are as complex as the nervous system itself. They range from focal or isolated difficulties such as numbness and tingling in an extremity to global or total neurologic dysfunction with alterations in consciousness.

The purpose of this chapter is to discuss many of the causes of postoperative neurologic dysfunction and to highlight the approach to assessing these patients. The general concepts of neurologic dysfunction and etiologies are discussed first, and then the approach to diagnosis and evaluation of the patient is presented. The early recognition, diagnosis, and treatment of nervous system dysfunction is critical for minimizing the amount of permanent neurologic deficit as well as the physiologic problems that may result from loss of nervous control.

ALTERATIONS IN CONSCIOUSNESS

Problems with the nervous system can be subdivided into several categories. For the purposes of diagnosis and treatment, the distinction between global and focal deficits is most important. Because alterations in the state of consciousness can be caused by either type of problem as well as by general anesthesia, a discussion of the normal mechanisms of wakefulness is necessary.

MECHANISMS OF CONSCIOUSNESS

Consciousness may be defined as that "state of alertness in which the patient is aware of his relationship in time and space, where he can demonstrate his awareness by communicating with those around him, and where he reveals memory of past events."[1] In this context the process of mentation is a product of cortical functioning. Deviations from normal cortical functioning may be the result of a variety of etiologies, including damage or alteration in the brain's environment (physiologic or chemical).

Although a full understanding of the mechanism of wakefulness in the normal brain is lacking, it is clear that normal wakefulness requires neural function in the cerebral cortices and brainstem. Pathologic processes that affect both cerebral cortices or alter either of the two brainstem-activating mechanisms can alter wakefulness.

The brainstem supports wakefulness by diffuse cortical activation, produced by the reticular formation (RF).[2] The contribution of the RF is apparent by the depression of wakefulness that occurs secondary to drugs (e.g., barbiturates) known to have a primary effect by depressing the RF.[3] Furthermore, metabolic events such as hypoglycemia and hypoxia are known to act here as well.[4]

A second mechanism supporting arousal is the cholinergic arousal system in the midbrain.[5] This particular region of the brainstem utilizes acetylcholine as its main transmitter, making it susceptible to scopolamine and atro-

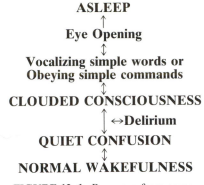

FIGURE 12–1. Recovery from coma.

pine.[6] Anticholinesterases, particularly physostigmine (which can cross the blood-brain barrier), can reverse the effects of these agents.[7]

Alterations in the cortex of these brainstem-activating systems cause depressions of consciousness. General anesthesia is a pharmacologically induced state of coma. Although this pharmacologic coma is not well understood, a variety of mechanisms appear to be involved, e.g., synaptic inhibition, synaptic excitation, selective neural depression via specific receptors, and general alterations in nervous system membrane function. It is possible that general anesthesia is in part the result of metabolic depression of nervous tissue (with the exception of stimulant anesthetics that can cause seizures.)[8]

The state of anesthetic depression appears to leave the brain in a condition of energy supply excess with reduced utilization. The anesthetized patient recovers from deep coma despite severe ventilatory or cardiovascular depression if these functions are supported. This point applies to most depressant drug ingestions as well. Recovery from coma follows patterns that are in many respects similar, regardless of whether the coma is induced by anesthetic agents. It is useful to review the normal patterns of awakening from coma (Fig. 12–1).

RECOVERY FROM COMA

The first sign of awakening from coma is eye opening, which is usually followed by the utterance of simple words or the obeying of simple commands. Although the patient is *awake,* this period is usually accompanied with a state of *clouded consciousness.* In addition to alterations in consciousness, other neurologic alterations may be present consistent with drug-induced effects. For example, pupillary size and gaze alterations may be present, and bilateral increased deep tendon reflexes may be elicited, including clonus and extensor plantar responses (positive Babinski).

During awakening from coma there may be a stage of disinhibited behavior termed *delirium.* This stage appears to occur when clouded consciousness is aggravated by physical discomfort such as a full bladder, headache, pain, or thirst. A stage of delirium may also occur during recovery from anesthesia. It may be a normal accompaniment of resolving general anesthesia (stage II), or it can be due to specific dysphoric drug effects. For example, postoperative delirium is often observed with ketamine use.

The next stage is one of *quiet confusion.* It should be noted that some patients may pass directly into this latter stage, particularly if sedative drugs are present. At this stage the patient may appear normal until questioned, when the confusion becomes obvious. For patients awakening from coma, the amnesia of the coma persists through the period of quiet confusion. From this stage, full return to *normal wakefulness* with clearing of confusion results if injury or dysequilibrium (chemical or physiologic) is not present.

With respect to awakening from general anesthesia, a variety of individual, drug-specific, and environmental factors may alter the time course and pattern of recovery. Only good clinical observation may detect when an individual patient fails to progress adequately, indicating the need for evaluation. The diagnosis of dysfunction and appropriate therapy requires the systematic evaluation of all possible causes.

DIFFERENTIATION OF FOCAL FROM DIFFUSE NEUROLOGIC PROCESSES

One of the most important distinctions when ascertaining the cause of neurologic dysfunction is to differentiate a focal (localized) process from a more diffuse process. Focal changes often are the result of localized injury and usually demonstrate a localizing phenomenon that acts as a clue to the process. Nonfocal changes are often the result of systemic derangements: The nervous system as an organ has its function altered by its chemical and physiologic environment.

Neurologic dysfunction with alteration in consciousness often is due to nonfocal processes. As discussed below, focal lesions can cause global dysfunction if they alter both cerebral cortices simultaneously.

STATES OF GLOBAL DYSFUNCTION

Global neurologic dysfunction can be divided into several categories (Table 12–1). *Clouded consciousness* is a defect of attention. These patients are easily distracted or startled and have a tendency to misjudge stimuli. This state represents generalized brain dysfunction. *Delirium* is a floridly abnormal mental state with disorientation, fear, and irritability. These patients misperceive sensory stimuli and may have visual hallucinations. They are out of touch with the environment and may be loud, talkative, offensive, suspicious, and agitated. *Obtundation* is a state of mental blunting with reduced alertness and lessened interest in the environment. *Stupor* is a state of deep sleep with unresponsiveness unless vigorously aroused. It represents a diffuse organic dysfunction. In *coma* the patient is unarousable with eyes closed and no distinguishable response to external stimuli.

Normal consciousness thus involves normal alertness as well as cognitive function (thought content). Patients may have normal thought content but be difficult to arouse, or they have normal response to the environment (appear awake) but have a disorder in thought content. Alternatively, there are patients who appear to have normal neurologic function unless detailed examination for neuropsychiatric difficulty is performed.

MECHANISMS OF GLOBAL DYSFUNCTION

The mechanisms of global dysfunction can be divided into several types (Table 12–2). Most causes of global dysfunction are systemic processes, although focal processes can cause global dysfunction as well (see below).

TABLE 12–1. STAGES OF GLOBAL NEUROLOGIC DYSFUNCTION

> Clouded consciousness
> Delirium
> Obtundation
> Stupor
> Coma

TABLE 12–2. MECHANISMS OF GLOBAL NEUROLOGIC DYSFUNCTION

> Metabolic encephalopathy
>   Altered metabolic substrates
>   Altered neurochemical environment
>   Endocrine abnormalities
>   Organ failure
>   Systemic disease
>   Seizure activity
> Drug effects
> Neurologic injury
> Hysteria

SYSTEMIC CAUSES OF GLOBAL DYSFUNCTION

The systemic processes causing global dysfunction can be divided into metabolic encephalopathy (deranged chemical, physiologic, or drug environment) and neurologic injury.

Metabolic Encephalopathy

The central nervous system (CNS) depends for its functioning on a proper physiologic and chemical environment. Adequate delivery of nutrients, effective removal of waste products, and an appropriate neurochemical microenvironment are necessary. If one or more of these parameters is altered owing to primary metabolic changes in the brain or secondary to other organ failure, global cerebral dysfunction may result (Table 12–3).

The resultant metabolic encephalopathy may cause changes in attention, alertness, ori-

TABLE 12–3. CONSISTENT FINDINGS IN METABOLIC ENCEPHALOPATHY

Failure of attention (inability to concentrate)

Altered alertness and awareness

Defects in orientation

Defects in perception

Defects in memory and thought content

Altered thought patterns

Waxing and waning level of consciousness

Retained papillary responses despite ventilatory depression, altered caloric response, or abnormal motor function

Random ocular motion (light coma) or midline resting gaze (deep coma)

Absence of focal neurologic findings

entation, grasp, memory, affect, and perception. Failure of attention is the earliest and most consistent alteration with metabolic encephalopathy. This inability to concentrate may cause a wandering thought pattern. Most metabolic derangements cause alterations in alertness and awareness. The patient, however, may fluctuate between drowsiness (inability to focus on important stimuli) and hypervigilance (distracted by unimportant stimuli). A loss of attention and awareness may help differentiate metabolic encephalopathy from dementia, where orientation and cognition tend to be lost before alertness. Severe metabolic encephalopathy usually proceeds to stupor and coma.

Several consistent findings on mental examination are present in patients with metabolic disease. Defects in orientation and perception of the environment are early, consistent findings. Memory and cognition (the content and progression of thought) are usually deranged. Affect is usually apathetic and withdrawn. When questioned, these patients have perceptual abnormalities including illusions or mistaking unknown individuals for specific, familiar people. The altered level of consciousness of metabolic encephalopathy commonly waxes and wanes depending on the level of stimulation and other environmental factors.[2,9–12]

Etiology. Causes of metabolic encephalopathy include decreased metabolic substrates, altered electrochemical environment, organ failure with endogenous toxins, endocrine abnormalities, systemic diseases (diabetes, porphyria), altered neuronal excitability, and drug effects (Table 12–4).

ALTERED METABOLIC SUBSTRATES. *Hypoglycemia* must be considered in all patients with altered consciousness. Serum glucose levels under 50 mg/dl can be associated with CNS dysfunction. However, the postanesthetic state can mask the usual effects of hypoglycemia. Several medications can lower glucose concentration, including salicylates, sulfonamides, ethanol, and antihyperglycemic medications. Rarely an insulin-producing tumor causes hypoglycemia,[13] and fatal hypoglycemia has been reported in diabetic patients given insulin or chlorpropamide.[14,15] Hypoglycemia has also been reported when hyperalimentation is abruptly withdrawn.

Thiamine deficiency may accompany decreased glucose in alcoholics. Thiamine deficiency can itself be a cause of mental derangements, particularly in alcoholics. The effects of the deficiency include delirium and stupor. When severe, Wernicke's disease can occur with irreversible damage to the neural structures around the third and fourth ventricles, which may lead to obtundation, confusion, and loss of memory. In severe cases autonomic instability, ophthalmoplegia, ataxia, dysarthria, and peripheral neuropathy occur. Because thiamine is a critical cofactor needed for metabolism of glucose, the administration of glucose with thiamine in patients deficient

TABLE 12–4. ETIOLOGY OF METABOLIC ENCEPHALOPATHY

Hypoglycemia (glucose <50 mg/dl)
  Insulin excess (exogenous, endogenous)

  Impaired gluconeogenesis

Cofactor deficiency: thiamine (Wernicke's encephalopathy), niacin, cyanocobalamin, folic acid, pyridoxine

Hyperglycemia

Hyperosmolar syndrome

Electrolyte disturbances: hyponatremia, hyper- or hypocalcemia (parathyroid disease), hypo- or hypermagnesemia, hypophosphatemia, water intoxication

Acidosis (pH <7.25) or alkalosis (metabolic or respiratory)

Hypothermia (<30°C), hyperthermia (>40°C)

Hypoxemia: anemia, methemoglobinemia, carbon monoxide poisoning

Hypercarbia

Hepatic dysfunction: porphyria, hepatic failure (ammonia), hepatolenticular degeneration

Renal dysfunction (uremia)

Endocrine dysfunction: adrenal insufficiency, pituitary insufficiency, exocrine pancreatic encephalopathy, hypothyroidism, pheochromocytoma for both (e.g., some alcoholics) may accentuate the thiamine deficiency resulting in neurologic injury.

Hyperglycemia can also produce alterations in consciousness. With glucose levels over 600 mg/dl the syndrome of hyperosmolar nonketotic hyperglycemia coma can occur.[2,16–18] With this syndrome elevated serum osmolality is present, and coma can be produced. Approximately one half of these patients have diabetes, but the syndrome can occur with severe dehydration, uremia, pancreatitis, sepsis, pneumonia, cerebral vascular accident, and large surface burns. Administration of hyperosmolar solutions (mannitol, hyperalimentation solutions) can cause the condition, or hyperosmolality may occur following peritoneal or hemodialysis or cardiac surgery. Other factors that cause an elevation in glucose (e.g., steroid administration or dextrose administration) can also contribute to the hyperosmolar state. The diagnosis is made when the glucose concentration is in excess of 600 mg/dl with elevated serum osmolarity in the absence of ketosis.[19] Azotemia and hypokalemia are commonly associated findings. Treatment consists in insulin to lower glucose and 0.5 N saline to correct dehydration.[20] Lowering the glucose too rapidly should be avoided, as it may precipitate hypovolemic shock and cerebral edema. Potassium supplementation may be required.

ALTERED NEUROCHEMICAL ENVIRONMENT. A variety of systemic chemical changes can result in an altered neurochemical environment that leads to abnormal cortical function (Table 12–4). The most common is probably *hyponatremia,* which can cause delayed awakening, mental status changes, and seizure activity. It can also cause hemiparesis and other major sequela in addition to altered mental status or coma. The more common causes of hyponatremia are water intoxication (as from transurethral prostate irrigation solutions or hyponatremic intravenous fluids) and inappropriate antidiuretic hormone (ADH) release.[2,10–12,21] A serum sodium concentration of less than 130 mM can be associated with cortical derangements (including seizure activity). The derangements are directly related to the sodium concentration or the rate of decrease.

Other electrolyte derangements associated with mental status changes include *hypo-* and *hypercalcemia* and *hypermagnesemia.*[2] Hypocalcemia due to hypoparathyroidism can cause increased intracranial pressure, diffuse electrocardiographic (ECG) alterations, and mental status changes.

Acid-base alterations have direct and indirect effects. Acidosis, due to deranged metabolism or hypoventilation, causes physiologic changes that impair cortical function. Acid-base changes can alter synaptic and axonal function as well as cerebral blood flow. In addition, the pH of the environment affects the ionization of many drugs; acidosis may alter binding to protein and the ability of the drug to penetrate cell membranes, including the blood-brain barrier.

Mental confusion is seen when cerebrospinal fluid (CSF) pH falls to 7.25 or lower. Metabolic as well as respiratory acidosis can cause these disturbances. The latter effect may be seen in diabetic patients during ketoacidosis.[22] When an acidotic patient is treated with systemic bicarbonate, the patient paradoxically may become more somnolent because the bicarbonate cannot cross the blood-brain barrier but carbon dioxide can diffuse into the CSF, which causes the CSF to become more acidotic, producing further CSF acidosis and neural alteration.

Changes in *temperature* can also alter consciousness. The direct effects of hypothermia are minimal in normal individuals when body temperature is lowered to 30° to 32°C.[23] Indirectly, hypothermia can increase the individual's sensitivity to anesthetics [the minimal alveolar concentration (MAC) is reduced 50 per cent at 28°C]. Hypothermia can also cause a reduction in enzymatic function, altering drug metabolism. The solubility of inhalational agents is increased at low temperatures, thus prolonging their action. The direct effects of hypothermia on consciousness (cold narcosis) are most pronounced in children and the elderly. Hyperthermia can also cause depressed consciousness when the core temperature exceeds 40°C (heat stroke) (see Chapter 13).

Finally, *hypoxemia* and hypercarbia impair cerebral function. Such effects amplify any residual anesthetic suppression.[24]

ENDOCRINE ABNORMALITIES. A variety of endocrine abnormalities can contribute to delayed awakening (Table 12–4). Delayed awakening during the stress of surgery and anesthesia may occur in patients with *adrenal insufficiency,*[2] as glucocorticoid deficiency causes prolonged synaptic transmission. Adrenal insufficiency can be the result of organ dysfunction (Addison's disease) or drug treatment. *Adrenal excess,* as in Cushing syndrome, can also produce delayed awakening, with excess corticoids entering the brain and producing neural dysfunction. Iatrogenic steroid excess can produce encephalopathy, delirium, psychosis, stupor, and coma; chronic excess can produce a hypokalemic metabolic alkalosis.[25]

Both *hypothyroidism* and *hyperthyroidism* can cause cerebral dysfunction. Decreased thyroid function (panhypopituitarism and hypothyroidism) can be associated not only with delayed awakening but with increased sensitivity to anesthetics and cardiac arrest. Myxedema coma in hypothyroid patients can be precipitated by anesthesia and surgery as well as by other stresses (infection, congestive heart failure, trauma, and exposure to cold).

ORGAN FAILURE. In many circumstances, failure of nonneural organs responsible for vital functioning results in mental changes. Organs of particular concern are the heart and lungs as well as those responsible for drug metabolism and excretion (kidney and liver) (Table 12–4).

Alteration in *cardiac function* clearly can cause inadequate delivery of blood and nutrients to the brain, resulting in major alterations in neural function or abnormal distribution or redistribution of drugs. *Pulmonary dysfunction* may contribute to hypoxemia (as discussed above) or alterations in carbon dioxide. Hypercapnea by itself is sufficient to produce sedation, probably via the production of cerebral acidosis.[26] Anesthetic agents that rely for part of their excretion on alveolar gas exchange have impaired excretion when there is inadequate pulmonary function, thus delaying awakening.

Renal dysfunction can produce altered neural function by several mechanisms. For those drugs depending on renal excretion or metabolism, anesthetic effect may be prolonged in the presence of renal impairment.[2,11,12] Prolongation of barbiturate anesthesia has been seen with renal failure.[27] Nonspecific factors associated with renal failure no doubt also contribute (decreased protein binding, electrolyte disturbances, and acid-base alterations). Enhanced CNS sensitivity to anesthetics in renal failure patients has also been observed and may be the result of changes in the permeability of the blood-brain barrier.[28]

Renal insufficiency can produce cerebral dysfunction as a consequence of uremia. The exact mechanism of cerebral dysfunction in uremia is not clear, but a variety of changes occur in the brain, including electrolyte imbalance, water shifts, and alterations in acid-base balance. The correction of uremia can also cause cerebral dysfunction as a consequence of dialysis dysequilibrium or dialysis encephalopathy, both of which can produce confusion, delirium, stupor, and occasionally coma. Diseases such as collagen vascular disease or diabetes, which are associated with renal failure, can cause cerebral derangements in their own right.

Altered *hepatic function* has been associated with neural dysfunction. Decreased hepatic degradation of medications can contribute to decreased consciousness. For example, mental confusion is seen with cimetidine in patients with liver dysfunction.[29] The metabolic insufficiency in liver failure compromises opioid metabolism as well as metabolism of other drugs, e.g., the benzodiazepines. Morphine has been implicated in the production of hepatic coma in patients with frank hepatic failure.

A variety of other factors are associated with decreased drug metabolism, including the extremes of age, hypothermia, and malnutrition, as well as the presence of other drugs that may compete for metabolism. The latter drugs include alcohol, barbiturates, and monoamine oxidase inhibitors.[30] The metabolism of several anesthetic agents is known to be inhibited by the presence of other drugs, e.g., methoxyflurane[31] and ketamine.[32,33]

Patients with hepatic failure or with bypass of the circulation around the liver exhibit cerebral edema that can be life-threatening. Increased serum ammonia levels and a variety of other circulating cerebral toxins are also seen with liver failure. Ammonia is a direct toxin that probably affects the chloride pump[34] and Na-K-ATPase activity,[35] as well as possibly altering the blood-brain barrier[36] and the uptake of other substances by the brain.

OTHER SYSTEMIC DISEASES. A variety of systemic illnesses can cause or contribute to cerebral dysfunction (Table 12–4). Patients with cancer widely disseminated throughout the body, metastatic to the liver with associated liver dysfunction, or disseminated to the brain can present with mental dysfunction. The cause may be an ill-defined encephalopathy due to the disease process or secondary to derangements of other organ systems affected by the disease. Cancer chemotherapeutic drugs, narcotics, or other medications taken for side effects of the disease process can also contribute to the cerebral dysfunction. Hypoglycemia is seen with some large tumors, and some tumors secrete substances that may cause dysfunction (e.g., ACTH secretion in oat cell carcinoma).

Other disease processes also may contribute to neural dysfunction. Diabetes and porphyria are such diseases. These disorders can lead directly to dysfunction. In addition, anesthetic interactions can lead to problems not seen in individuals without the disease. For example, the use of barbiturates or other enzyme-inducing agents in porphyria can result in paralysis.[37]

ALTERED NEURONAL EXCITABILITY. *Seizures* may become manifest during the recovery period after anesthesia and surgery anesthesia. They may be the result of or cause neural dysfunction. Seizures may be associated with epilepsy, structural CNS lesions, certain disease states, or epileptogenic drugs (Table 12–5).

Epilepsy is a relatively common disorder (about 1 in 100 to 200 patients), second only to stroke as a cause of neurologic dysfunction. Epileptics are more likely to have a seizure when exposed to hypoxia or hypercarbia. Hypocarbia can lower the threshold to certain anesthetics (e.g., enflurane). The pediatric patient with epilepsy is at higher risk for seizures than the adult.

Central nervous system structural lesions are associated with increased CNS excitability, as are a variety of other disease states, including cerebral trauma, cerebrovascular disease, vascular malformations, and inflammatory disease of the brain.[38] Sepsis and high body temperature tend to predispose to seizure activity. Other disease states associated with seizure activity include those leading to hyponatremia (particularly rapidly falling serum sodium levels), hypernatremia, hypomagnesemia, hypophosphatemia, hypocalcemia, hypocarbia, hypoxemia, and hyperoxia.

Among the many drugs that have been associated with seizures are enflurane,[39] amitriptyline when used with enflurane,[40] ketamine,[41,42] local anesthetics, iodinated contrast agents, anticholinesterase agents, antihistamines, a variety of antidepressants and antipsychotics, oxytocin, narcotics (including meperidine), methohexital, laudanosine (metabolite of atracurium), propanidid, and Althesin. Intoxication or withdrawal from addictive drugs or ingestion of toxins (e.g., lead or mercury) may also precipitate seizure activity.

DRUG EFFECTS. Drugs may have effects on the state of consciousness (Table 12–6), whether given intentionally as part of the anesthetic or ingested separately. Alterations in the pharmacokinetics (distribution, metabolism, and excretion) or the pharmacodynamics (sensitivity of the patient to the drug effects) of the drugs may contribute to an altered state of consciousness.

Prolonged drug effects may result from several factors. Actual overdose, caused by delivery of an excessive amount of drug to the patient, may occur. Enhanced patient sensitivity may be present, either due to individual variation or as a consequence of an abnormal neural environment such as hypoxemia. Relative

TABLE 12–5. CONDITIONS USUALLY ASSOCIATED WITH SEIZURE ACTIVITY

Drugs
  Withdrawal from barbiturates, narcotics, or ethanol
  Hypoglycemia
  Enflurane
  Methohexital
  Local anesthetic toxicity
  Meperidine
Metabolic disorders
  Hyponatremia
  Hypocalcemia
  Hypoglycemia
  Hypomagnesemia
  Sepsis
  Renal failure
  Hepatic failure
  Severe hypercarbia
  Malignant hyperthermia
  Porphyria
  Eclampsia
Neurologic disorders
  Epilepsy
  Cerebral vascular lesion
  Cerebral infection
  Intracranial injury
  Intracranial tumor

TABLE 12–6. MECHANISMS OF PROLONGED DRUG ACTION

Decreased metabolism or biotransformation

Redistribution from drug pools

Absolute drug overdose

Increased sensitivity: age, biologic variation, metabolic effects

Drug interactions

Decreased protein binding

Residual or unreversed anesthetics

Exogenous drugs

Drug withdrawal disorders: alcohol, sedatives, narcotics

overdose may occur as well, with delivery of a normal amount of drug to the patient, the effect of which is amplified by pharmacologic factors such as altered drug metabolism or distribution. Finally, there may be drug synergism, in which the effect of a normal dosage is amplified by pharmacodynamic effects of other drugs (including recreational drugs such as alcohol). Individual variability among patients may alter the metabolism of drugs. Genetic variants in metabolic enzymes may cause differences in metabolites (which may be active) or rates of metabolism of the drugs. Some variability exists with the circadian rhythm.[43] As discussed above, alterations in the organs responsible for metabolism (e.g., liver and kidney) may cause prolonged effects. Gross alteration in hepatic function is known to prolong barbiturate sleep time in animals.[44]

Age, hypothermia, and hypothyroidism[45] reduce anesthetic requirements,[46] as do certain medications (reserpine, methyldopa, and chronic dextroamphetamines).[47,48] Although many of these effects have been seen primarily in animals, it is likely that prolonged hypnosis after standard dosages of anesthetics and hypnotics also occurs in man.

For intravenous medications, the pharmacokinetics can be altered by various means. For example, the action of barbiturates may be prolonged by hypoproteinemia[44] or displacement of barbiturates from plasma protein-binding sites by other medications. The radiocontrast material sodium acetrizoate[49] and the antibiotic sulfadimethoxine[50] are known to displace thiopental, increasing the amount of drug available to the CNS.

For inhalational anesthetics, recovery depends on uptake from fatty stores and exhalation. Thus reduced cardiac output delays removal from the brain, and hypoventilation may inhibit pulmonary excretion of the drugs.[51] The latter effect is most noticeable for anesthetics with moderate solubility (e.g., halothane) and less important for agents with low solubility (nitrous oxide) or high solubility (e.g., methoxyflurane).[51]

Metabolism of drugs can produce active metabolites that may be responsible for postoperative depression. The production of bromide ion from halothane metabolism may be such a case.[52,53] In this case, the preoperative ingestion of bromide-containing medications may contribute to prolonged postoperative awakening in an additive manner.

Exogenous toxins may also contribute to altered mental states. The latter group includes alcohol, illicit drugs, and the cancer chemotherapeutic medications L-asparaginase and vincristine.[54]

Neurologic Injury

Global dysfunction can be produced by widespread neurologic injury (Table 12–7). It is usually the result of hypoxia, ischemia, hy-

TABLE 12–7. MECHANISMS OF NEUROLOGIC INJURY

Hypoxia

Cerebral ischemia: hypotension, increased ICP, anemia, venous congestion increased viscosity (polycythemia, cryoglobulinemia, macroglobulinemia, sickle cell anemia)

Hypotension

Cerebral embolus: air, calcium, fibrin, fat, aggregates of WBCs or platelets

Stroke

Cerebral edema

Hypertensive encephalopathy

Intracranial hemorrhage: rupture aneurysm, AV malformation, hypertension

Vasculitis

Infection: encephalitis, meningitis

Existing neurologic disorder: degenerative or demyelinating disease

Seizure or postictal state

Concussions

potension, increased intracranial pressure, embolism, or stroke (hemorrhagic or thrombotic).[55,56]

Cerebral hypoxic injury may result from inadequate oxygen delivery (anoxic ischemia), inadequate ventilation (e.g., drug-induced respiratory depression or residual neuromuscular blocking agents), inadequate hemoglobin (anemic ischemia), inadequate cerebral blood flow (ischemic anoxia), or excessive metabolic demands exceeding the delivered oxygen (e.g., seizures or hyperthermia).[57] The known seizure-producing potential of enflurane[58] might produce a relative hypoxemia due to an increased metabolic demand exceeding the available supply if a seizure occurs. Ketamine can cause an elevation in intracranial pressure, thereby lowering cerebral perfusion and resulting in cerebral ischemia.[59]

Reduction in cerebral blood flow can occur as the result of changes in several physiologic parameters. Such changes include a reduction of the driving pressure (mean arterial pressure, or MAP), an increase in the resistive pressure (venous or intracranial pressure), an increase in blood viscosity, or an increase in local vascular resistance (as altered abnormally by fixed atherosclerotic lesions, emboli, or vascular spasm). Cerebral dysfunction usually manifests clinically when cerebral blood flow is reduced to about one half of normal (25 ml/min/100 gm) or when the PaO_2 reaches 25 to 45 mm Hg. Ischemic lesions occur at the locations of reduced blood flow or in those regions most sensitive to reduced blood flow (caudate, putamen, globis pallidus, and the boundary zones of the cerebral cortex where the vascular distributions of the anterior, middle, and posterior cerebral arteries meet).

Cerebral ischemia can result from excessive hypotension. Patients with vascular disease (e.g., the diabetic, hypertensive, or geriatric patient) or patients in whom extremes of neck rotation or flexion are used for positioning[60] may require higher than normal perfusion pressure to overcome the obstruction to flow if the positioning problem is not corrected. Therefore relative hypotension may also result in cerebral ischemia.

Cerebral ischemia secondary to hypoxia in the operating room is most commonly thought to be secondary to the delivery of a hypoxemic gas mixture.[1] Irreversible cerebral injury may occur rapidly owing to delivery of low oxygen concentrations or moderately low concentrations over an extended period of time.

Certain situations may make the brain more easily injured during reduced oxygen delivery: cellular injury, cerebral edema, the presence of cerebral disease, aggravating metabolic derangements, and hypotension. Aging generally increases the susceptibility, whereas young patients (especially babies) may be more resistant. Repetitive bouts of hypoxia may have cumulative effects.

Cerebral edema deserves special note, as its presence may increase the susceptibility of the brain to anoxic injury. When ischemia occurs, local cerebral autoregulation and the blood-brain barrier may be disrupted, leading to edema. If the ischemia is secondary to ventilatory insufficiency, hypercarbia may be present, which also leads to cerebral edema via vasodilatation. The latter effect may produce additional ischemia if altered intracranial compliance leads to elevated intracranial pressure and reduced cerebral perfusion pressure. Thus cerebral ischemia and edema may aggravate each other, which may help to explain the delayed occurrence of anoxic injury in patients who have appeared to recover fully from an apparent anoxic event.[61]

Hysterical Neurologic Dysfunction

It should always be kept in mind that hysteria can cause a catatonic-like state. In such circumstances, all laboratory studies are normal and the patient usually has an appropriate grimace with painful stimuli.

FOCAL CAUSES OF GLOBAL DYSFUNCTION

Although global dysfunction is most commonly caused by a systemic process, focal events can alter mental status by both cerebral cortices being affected or by depression of the brainstem regions responsible for wakefulness. Thus any process capable of producing focal neurologic injury in the CNS may produce global dysfunction. To elucidate the focal process, subtle signs often must be elicited on examination, or structural studies must be done.

For example, focal supratentorial lesions can cause global dysfunction if they are large enough to result in bilateral cortical effects, such as those that result in elevated intracranial pressure. Such elevated pressure can compromise cerebral perfusion, produce herniation of the cerebral hemispheres laterally or downward on the tentorium, or compress the brainstem. Lateral herniation may occur across the midline and so affect the other cortex. With uncal herniation the occulomotor nerve is compressed between the temporal lobe and the tentorium, causing ipsilateral pupillary dilatation followed by oculoplegia and contralateral hemiplegia.

Herniation downward causes compression of the brainstem, resulting in brainstem dysfunction including Cheyne-Stokes ventilation, small reactive pupils, and bilateral extremity weakness. Downward herniation usually progresses to frank quadriplegia; immobile, fixed, and dilated pupils; ataxic or apneustic ventilation; and finally hypotension. Lesions producing downward herniation include expanding cortical lesions such as intracerebral hemorrhage, abscess, edema, expanding tumors, and large infarctions.

As a localized process, pneumocephalus and tension pneumocephalus should also be considered. The irritation of the frontal lobes by cerebral air in the supine patient may contribute to an altered mental state. If the air is under tension, it produces cerebral dysfunction akin to that associated with elevated intracranial pressure. Although not common, pneumocephalus can occur during head trauma and certain neurosurgical procedures.[62]

Similarly, focal lesions in the brainstem can cause a depression of consciousness.[55,56] Here lesions of the brainstem (ischemia, infarction, hematoma) can have direct effects on brainstem structure or may cause a secondary elevation of intracranial pressure by obstructing the ventricular drainage system (hydrocephalus). Cranial nerve dysfunction may allow localization of the lesion.

FOCAL NEUROLOGIC DYSFUNCTION

In contrast to global neurologic dysfunction, focal neurologic deficits are usually caused by focal processes (Table 12–8). These processes are identified most easily by the neurologic picture produced by injury of a specific neural entity, e.g., peripheral neuropathy. Focal lesions can be divided anatomically into CNS, spinal cord, nerve plexus, and peripheral nerve deficits. They can be further subdivided by the specific neurologic modality affected (motor deficit, sensory deficit, spinal

TABLE 12–8. CATEGORIES OF FOCAL DYSFUNCTION

Location
  Central nervous system
    Cerebral cortex
    Brainstem
    Spinal cord
  Nerve plexus
  Peripheral nerve
Type of defect
  Motor defect
  Sensory defect
  Cognitive defect
  Autonomic defect

cord deficit, cognitive deficit, and deficit of autonomic function).

Central nervous system lesions most commonly are the result of ischemic or hemorrhagic infarct or worsening of a preexisting neurologic disorder (Table 12–9). Each can be the result of several possible etiologies. Ischemia-induced infarcts can be caused by absolute hypotension, relative hypotension with a predisposing vascular abnormality, or a disease state favoring isolated injury or embolic phenomena.

The ability of *hypotension* to produce neurologic injury depends on a complex relation between local blood flow, regional metabolism, and the energy state of the neural tissue. In general, regions of the brain at greatest risk for ischemic injury include the cerebral cortex regions along the boundaries of the cerebral arteries (especially the triple boundary region at the junction of the anterior, middle, and posterior cerebral arteries) and the amygdala. Other regions at risk depend on local factors occurring in the particular patient.

It may not be possible in a given individual to determine the blood pressure below which ischemia may occur. Various vascular factors

TABLE 12–9. MECHANISMS OF FOCAL INJURY

Worsening of preexisting abnormality
Ischemic injury
  Hypotension
  Embolism
  Thrombosis
  Vascular stenosis or spasm
Fever
Seizure
Intracranial hemorrhage
Tumors
Positioning-related ischemia or pressure

in addition to blood pressure determine the actual blood flow. Local autoregulation is particularly important. Here blood pressure below about two thirds of the patient's mean arterial pressure (i.e., at about 50 mm Hg in a normotensive individual) is associated with reduced flow. Thus a chronically hypertensive individual may require a higher blood pressure to maintain blood flow above this lower limit of autoregulation. Cerebral blood flow is also reduced by the lowering of blood carbon dioxide associated with hyperventilation. The contribution of this mechanism is not clear, but the dizziness that occurs when a normal individual hyperventilates may indicate ischemia. Unfortunately, attempts to improve blood flow by physiologic manipulations such as vasodilators or hypoventilation may only shunt blood flow to a region of normal vascular responsiveness, thereby "stealing" blood from a diseased area that cannot respond to the provocative technique.

In addition to failing to respond normally to physiologic manipulations, these regions of disease may be at increased risk for injury. Abnormal vessels may become thrombosed with an associated infarct, or a vascular restriction may produce ischemia in the face of an otherwise innocuous blood pressure. In the older population, strong suspicion for cerebrovascular disease must be maintained. Patients with carotid vascular occlusive disease may not tolerate neck rotation or hypotension. Likewise, patients with vertebrovascular disease may not tolerate extended periods of neck flexion. Complete vertebrobasilar ischemia may cause loss of consciousness, and ischemia in branches of the artery may cause localized brainstem findings.

In addition to blood pressure, tissue factors play a major role. Tissues with high *metabolic rate* are at greater risk for ischemia during normal or reduced blood flow. Because the metabolic rate increases with temperature, febrile patients may be at slightly increased risk, and hypothermic patients have reduced risk. The greatest risk, however, is in tissues undergoing electrical seizure activity, where metabolic rate may increase to two to three times normal. Fortunately, during anesthesia the cerebral metabolic rate is usually decreased, and the margin of safety with ischemia is therefore increased.

Another cause of ischemic infarction that plays a major role during surgery is *embolism*. Cerebral embolism can occur in patients with any of the following risk factors: right-to-left

shunts (notably children with congenital cyanotic heart disease); extracorporeal circulation; valvular calcifications or vegetations; and atrial or ventricular thrombi. Cerebral embolization from aggressive flushing of radial arterial cannulas has been reported.[63] Fat embolism has been reported 12 to 48 hours after long bone fracture or massive trauma,[64] after closed chest massage, and in patients with fatty livers who receive massive steroid therapy.[64]

Air embolism, which can be seen in a variety of surgical circumstances where the surgical site is above the level of the heart, can also produce neurologic injury when these emboli reach the nervous system. Certainly patients with right-to-left cardiac shunts are at risk. Studies have suggested that migration to the left-sided circulation can occur in the absence of detectable shunts. Furthermore, autopsy studies have demonstrated that 15 to 20 per cent of the population have a foramen ovale that is not fully closed.[65] If right atrial pressure exceeds left atrial pressure, this "probe patent" foramen may open, allowing emboli to enter the left circulation. Such reversal of the normal pressure gradient occurs with significant air embolism and thus may contribute to neural morbidity.

The other major cause of localized neural infarction is *intracranial hemorrhage*. This problem may result from rupture of an intracranial aneurysm or vascular malformation or be due to rupture of a blood vessel secondary to hypertension. The neurologic findings with hemorrhage depend on the location of the bleed. Hypertensive bleeds within the cerebral tissue most commonly occur in the putamen, internal capsule, thalamus, cerebellar hemispheres, pons, and various locations in the white matter. With intracranial bleeding, a computed tomography (CT) scan usually reveals the blood, and the CSF from a spinal tap is often xanthochromic.

Alternatively, vascular hemorrhage can result in subdural hematomas. Although usually associated with head trauma, epidural or subdural hematomas may not be recognized preoperatively. Other factors that aggravate the cerebral dynamics can cause them to manifest postoperatively. It may be most evident with subacute or chronic hematomas, where the traumatic event is distant enough to be overlooked and the associated vague complaints are thought to have other causes. The latter may easily be true in older individuals or alcoholics, who are at a high risk for falling and in whom confusion may be part of baseline neurologic function.

Other forms of unrecognized neurologic disease may manifest as structural dysfunction when the insults of surgery, fluid and electrolyte shifts, and anesthesia are added to unrecognized, preexisting disease. Intracranial tumors can present for the first time postoperatively as edema, hemorrhage into the tumor bed, or elevated intracranial pressure secondary to surgery and anesthesia. Similarly, preexisting degenerative or demyelinating disease may manifest postoperatively as subtle findings of neurologic dysfunction, which are temporarily aggravated by anesthetic agents.

Central nervous system lesions must be differentiated from peripheral lesions on the basis of the neural distribution. *Spinal cord lesions,* although uncommon, are certainly possible. Spinal surgery is associated with an increased risk of postoperative cord dysfunction. Such dysfunction is thought to result from mechanical stress on the cord due to correction of spinal deformities, intrinsic injury to the cord, or vascular injury within the cord. An uncommon complication of the sitting position is quadriplegia or quadriparesis (thought to be associated with excessive neck flexion). Surgery on the thoracoabdominal aorta or its perforators to the cord can result in loss of motor, pain, and temperature function in the extremities because of anterior artery ischemia or infarction. The resulting anterior spinal artery syndrome is due to loss of anterior spinal cord function.

PERIPHERAL NERVE DYSFUNCTION

Peripheral nerve dysfunction following surgery and anesthesia has been described in a variety of settings. Two studies have been reported that indicate the incidence in the operative setting. One study of 30,000 patients in Sweden reported 31 patients with postoperative dysfunction, 26 of which cases involved the upper extremity.[66] Another study, involving 50,000 patients in the United States, identified 72 patients with dysfunction.[67] The latter report identified the brachial plexus as the most common injury and alcohol and diabetes as the most common preexisting medical conditions. The time of operation also plays a role, as 45 minutes appears to be the minimal time for postoperative peripheral nerve dysfunction (except for operative trauma), with

most patients having procedures in excess of 6 hours.[67]

The causes are probably multifactorial, and some patients may have postoperative dysfunction despite even the most careful positioning and preventive measures.[68,69] Many of the factors associated with peripheral nerve injury are known.

Diseases of peripheral nerves may produce a neuropathy that manifests or worsens during the operative period. Conditions associated with neuropathies include direct cervical ribs, herniated discs, nearby tissue trauma, beriberi, pellagra, pernicious anemia, alcoholic neuritis, diabetes, gout, porphyria, exposure to heavy metals (lead, arsenic, mercury, bismuth, gold, and silver), arteriosclerosis, periarteritis nodosa, arterial ischemic diseases, poliomyelitis, diphtheria, leprosy, mumps, malignancies, herpes zoster, localized infection, and neural tumors.

Subclinical neural entrapment can worsen with anesthesia and surgery.[68] Other contributing factors include direct injury by the surgical procedure, needle trauma, injection of irritant substances near the nerve, and unfavorable positioning of the patient (Table 12–10). Peripheral nerve injury has also been described following injections of horse serum or penicillin. In these cases the peripheral neuropathies accompanied by serum sickness and may be the result of perineural urticaria and edema with resulting neural ischemia.[70,71]

The surgical procedure may contribute directly, e.g., via retractor pressure on the nerve or reflex vasospasm of blood vessels supplying the nerve, or it may contribute in a fashion not yet well described, e.g., sciatic and peroneal nerve palsy following lengthy pelvic procedures.[72,73]

Based on anatomy, it is known that unfavorable positioning of the patient may contribute to some lesions isolated to peripheral nerves

TABLE 12–10. MECHANISMS OF PERIPHERAL NERVE INJURY

Surgical procedures
Vasospasm
Stretch
Pressure
Ischemia
Needle trauma
Injection of irritant substances
Tourniquet
Compartment syndrome

TABLE 12–11. TYPES OF PERIPHERAL NERVE INJURY

Type	Mechanism	Deficit
Neurapraxia	Transient pressure	Transient
Axonotmesis	Injury with sheath intact	Months
Neurotmesis	Injury with loss of sheath	Poor recovery

TABLE 12–12. FACTORS IN PERIPHERAL NERVE INJURY

Improper positioning
Hypothermia
Hypotension
Neurologic disease
Vascular occlusive disease
Serum sickness
Diabetes
Periarteritis nodosa
Alcoholism
Tourniquet
Regional anesthesia technique
Surgical injury
Preexisting neural injury

or nerve plexus.[74,75] In these cases, direct pressure, stretch, or ischemia in the involved nerve can result in postoperative dysfunction. The use of muscle relaxants may allow excessive flexion of joints and removal of protective mechanisms afforded by muscle tone.

Peripheral nerve injuries can be further grouped according to severity (Table 12–11). Ischemia secondary to external pressure or compromise of the vasa vasorum usually produces a transient neuropraxia. Here there is no axonal degeneration, but slight myelin degeneration at the site of injury may be present. Complete recovery usually occurs within 1 to 6 weeks. With more prolonged or intense injury, the nerve substance is injured and axonal (wallerian) degeneration occurs (axonotmesis) without loss of the supporting matrix. Here function is recovered when the axon grows back through its sheath and reattaches to the distal structures. The time for recovery is proportional to the amount of growth necessary (the nerve grows at the rate of about 1 mm per day after an initial latent period of about 6 weeks). Patients with neuropraxia or vitamin B deficiency are at greater risk for axonotmesis. These conditions usually improve with time, but if injury to the nerve and the nerve sheath (neurotmesis) occurs (as with surgical cutting of the nerve, severe crushing injury, or avulsion), recovery is poor unless surgical reanastomosis of the sheath is undertaken.

A variety of factors predispose to peripheral nerve injury (Table 12–12). Previously discussed are a variety of medical conditions. Hypothermia by surface cooling and deliberate hypotension in the absence of specific neural insults are associated with peripheral neuropathy.[76,77] Regional blocks are also associated with the possibility of neural injury.

Several nerves are commonly associated with postoperative dysfunction during routine procedures. In addition, certain surgical procedures or positions increase the risk for certain nerves. Nerves at special risk include the sciatic, ulnar, median, brachial plexus, and common peroneal (Table 12–13).

A simple, rapid technique has been reported to detect the function of the major nerves.[78] As shown in Table 12–14, the presence of a few simple neural functions detects the function of the major nerves to the extremities.

The brachial plexus is one of the most vulnerable neural structures owing to its long course through the shoulder. A stretch injury may occur under several circumstances when positioning assumes a nonphysiologic position. The type and direction of the force determine the portion of the plexus injured.[74,75,79] Injury can occur when the plexus is stretched or compressed against the nearby bony structures.

Stretching can occur by several mechanisms. Stretching may injure the nerve by rupturing intraneural capillaries, resulting in ischemia and intraneural hematomas. Stretch occurs when the head is turned away from the shoulder (dorsal extension and lateral flexion

TABLE 12–13. COMMON PERIPHERAL NERVE INJURY

Ulnar nerve
Sciatic nerve
Median nerve
Brachial plexus
Cervical nerve roots
Common peroneal nerve
Lateral femoral cutaneous nerve
Facial nerve
Calf compartment injury
Tourniquet injury

TABLE 12–14. METHOD FOR RAPID IDENTIFICATION OF PERIPHERAL NERVE FUNCTION

Nerve	Criteria for Pressure of Intact Nerve
Median nerve	Pinprick sensation on palmar surface of distal index finger
Ulnar nerve	Pinprick sensation on palmar surface of distal fifth finger
Radial nerve	Ability to extend the distal thumb
Peroneal nerve	Ability to dorsiflex the great toe
Posterior tibial nerve	Ability to plantarflex the great toe
Femoral nerve	
Intrapelvic portion	Ability to flex the thigh on the trunk (iliopsoas)
Extrapelvic portion	Ability to extend the leg; presence of a knee jerk
Obturator nerve	Ability to adduct the leg
Sciatic nerve	Ability to flex the leg

of the head) with the arm abducted, extended, and externally rotated. This maneuver increases the angle between the head and shoulder tip. Abduction, external rotation, and dorsal extension of the arm or allowing the arm to fall off the table stretches the plexus around the tendon of the pectoralis major. Suspension of the arm from an ether screen when the patient is in the lateral decubitus position stretches the arm around the clavicle and the tendon of the pectoralis minor. Stretch can also occur with extreme abduction of the arms in the supine position. It is aggravated when the arm is lowered below the plane of the body in the supine position. Similarly, stretch occurs with traction of the arms toward the feet, and it can occur when the weight of the arms is unsupported in the sitting position.

Compression of the plexus occurs by several mechanisms. The plexus may be pinched between the clavicle and the first rib when the Trendelenberg position is used with arm abducted and the patient slides up against a shoulder brace. The plexus may be compressed at the head of the humerus by a similar mechanism if the shoulder brace is placed too laterally. Compression may occur at the tip of the coracoid process or the tendon of the pectoralis minor when the whole shoulder girdle sags off the operating table and the arm is

abducted, extended, and externally rotated or when an ether screen is used in the lateral position to suspend the arm. In the lateral decubitus position the plexus can be injured if excessive pressure is placed on the axilla. This type of injury may be seen in children and young adults and may result in loss of function of a variety of muscle groups.

The type and direction of the injury determine the involved segment of the plexus. The most common postoperative dysfunction is usually motor or motor and sensory dysfunction of the upper roots of the plexus. Stretching the plexus by traction on the arms down toward the feet (e.g., use of wristlets to restrain the patient in the Trendelenberg position) results in the major force on the fifth and sixth cervical roots and causing an Erb-Duchenne type injury (commonly producing dysfunction to the deltoid, brachialis, and brachioradialis muscles and decreased sensation over the deltoid and radial surface of the forearm and hand). Injury to the lower roots of the plexus (C8–T1, Dejerine-Klumpke type) are more uncommon and may be associated with abduction of the arm on an armboard more than 90 degrees, particularly with a shoulder brace to prevent sliding while the patient is in the Trendelenberg position. Another mechanism is extreme abduction in the prone position with the hands together at the head of the bed. Injury to thoracic nerves can produce a Horner syndrome (a preganglionic lesion of the first thoracic root).

The facial nerve may be injured by compression from a face mask, head strap, or horseshoe head-holder if the buccal branch of the nerve emerges at the anterior edge of the parotid gland. Prolonged anterior displacement of the mandible by pressure from the angles of the jaw can also produce facial nerve pressure. Other cranial nerves may be stretched with low CSF pressure after a spinal tap. Here each cranial nerve has been reported to be involved except the tenth cranial nerve.[74] In 90 per cent of the cases the sixth cranial nerve was involved. Cranial nerves may also be injured by excessive or prolonged pressure on the face. Optic nerve injury has been described that is due to pressure on the eye, as when the patient is in the prone position or wearing a face mask. The supraorbital nerve can be injured by the pressure exerted on the brow by an endotracheal connector.

The cervical nerve roots can be injured by excessive neck rotation in the prone position. In elderly people, neutral neck positioning with the face down may help to prevent this complication.

The cubital tunnel at the elbow is thought to be the major location for ulnar neuropathy.[79] There the nerve is particularly vulnerable to pressure from contact with the operating room table. In approximately 20 per cent of cases, the nerve courses more medially, making it more susceptible.[74] A second mechanism, prolonged flexion at the elbow, can also produce pressure in the cubital tunnel.[68] Careful positioning with protection of the nerve can help prevent this injury. It includes placement of the hand with palm down when the arm is at the supine patient's side. Ulnar nerve injury is particularly common with open chest cardiac surgery (up to 20 per cent of patients), suggesting that the nerve may be injured by the mechanics of opening the chest.[80]

Studies of patients who sustained unilateral ulnar neuropathy revealed bilateral electrophysiologic abnormalities, prompting consideration of a preexisting, subclinical neuropathy in these patients.[68] If true, certain patients may be at increased risk despite normally adequate positioning. Alternatively, these patients are also at risk for entrapment postoperatively when lying in the supine position.[69] Because it is often difficult to discern when a neural injury occurs, these reports suggest that the immediate postoperative period may be a more critical period for these patients than the operative period.[69] These possibilities are supported by the observation that studies of the severity of the ulnar neuropathy had no correlation with the length or type of operation.[79]

The median nerve can be injured by needles or extravenous injections of thiopental when they are placed in the medial aspect of the antecubital fossa. The radial nerve can be injured at the wrist by excessive pressure or an intravenous cannula as it courses around the midportion of the inner surface of the humerus, particularly in the lateral position, or if the arm is allowed to sag off the operating table. The radial nerve can also be injured by an intramuscular injection given below the deltoid in the radial groove. Extravasation of intravenous thiopental at the lateral side of the wrist can cause numbness in the radial distribution of the dorsal thenar web space.

The common peroneal nerve is one of the more commonly described dysfunctional nerves in the lower extremity. It can be injured near the head of the fibula by lateral pressure on the leg. This injury occurs commonly in the lithotomy position, when the leg rests laterally on the leg supports.

The sciatic nerve may be injured preoperatively by an intramuscular injection in the buttocks. Hence intramuscular injections are usually recommended to be given in the upper, outer quadrant of the buttocks. It may also be injured by excessive hip flexion without accompanying knee flexion or pressure on the posterior hip of an emaciated patient, e.g., during a hip procedure.

The saphenous nerve may be similarly pinched against the medial tibial condyle if the foot is suspended lateral to the vertical brace that is placed medially and below the knee. The lateral femoral cutaneous nerves can be injured in the prone position by excessive pressure at the anterosuperior spine of the ilium. The femoral nerve can be injured by bladder retractors during laparotomy.

Peripheral nerves that course through the calves can be trapped in a compartment syndrome if the calves are improperly positioned on leg rests in the lithotomy position. The same compartment phenomenon can occur if casts placed on the arms or legs are applied too tightly. Similarly, pressure on the extremities by casts or tourniquets can produce nerve injury. Excessive tourniquet pressure, or application of the tourniquet for an excessive period of time (generally more than 1.5 to 2.0 hours) can cause injury, especially just below the elbow or knee where minimal muscle mass is present.

DIAGNOSIS AND MANAGEMENT OF CNS DYSFUNCTION

Evaluation of the patient with postoperative neurologic dysfunction should commence as soon as the problem is identified, as correction of physiologic derangements may minimize long-term neurologic sequelae (Table 12–15).

The initial signs of a problem may be obvious. Often a subtle deviation from normal recovery after anesthesia may be the only initial finding. Close observation during postanesthetic recovery is the key to recognition of the problem.

In many circumstances the cause is obvious. However, when the cause is not obvious (as with an unintentional relative overdose of an anesthetic), the patient should be carefully examined and the records reviewed. The diagnosis may ultimately require a careful evaluation of the patient's history, surgical proce-

TABLE 12–15. INVESTIGATION OF ALTERED MENTAL STATUS

Patient assessment
  Airway
  Ventilation
  Cardiovascular function
  Temperature
  Neurologic function

History
  Underlying neurologic disorders
  Surgical procedure
  Anesthetic management: premedication, induction, maintenance, reversal
  Nonanesthetic drugs given

Laboratory studies
  Blood gases (oxygenation, carbon dioxide, pH)
  Hemoglobin, WBCs, glucose
  BUN, creatinine, osmolality
  Na^+, K^+, Ca^{2+}, Cl^-, HCO_3^{2-}, NH_4^+, PO_4^{3-}
  Liver function, toxic drug screen
  Urine: specific gravity, culture, sensitivity tests

Consultation

Structural studies

Neurologic testing

TABLE 12–16. COMPONENTS OF BRIEF NEUROLOGIC EXAMINATION

Level of consciousness
Pupils
Ventilatory pattern
Motor activity
Peripheral nerve function
Seizure activity

---

dure, positioning, and anesthetic, as well as a detailed physical and neurologic examination. Laboratory and structural evaluations as well as consultation with specialists may also be helpful.

PATIENT EXAMINATION

A complete evaluation usually begins with a detailed history. However, prompt examination of the patient with abnormal neurologic findings is of utmost importance, so a careful assessment of the airway, ventilation, oxygenation, and cardiovascular function can be performed to provide optimal patient safety. Neurologic compromise may cause secondary alterations of vital organ function, or it may itself be due to or aggravated by vital organ dysfunction.

The vital signs and all available information from monitoring devices (e.g., ventilatory rate and volume, blood pressure, temperature, ECG, oxygen saturation) are helpful in addition to applicable laboratory studies (see below). Prompt correction of disturbances detected by physical examination (e.g., airway assessment, lung and cardiac examination, evaluation of muscular tone) is important.

Such disturbances may either cause or result from the neural dysfunction.

Although hyperthermia is rarely a cause of mental dysfunction, its presence should prompt a rapid search for signs of malignant hyperthermia, as this problem requires rapid and specific treatment (see Chapters 13 and 16).

Although hypothermia can be treated specifically by warming, an unexpected underlying cause is often overlooked. Disorders such as myxedema, hypopituitarism, and disorders of the hypothalamus should be considered, as more specific endocrine treatment may be needed. Associated metabolic depression due to drug effects (barbiturates, phenothiazines, alcohol) may also be present and need identification.

After life-threatening derangements have been identified and treated, a careful neurologic examination should be performed to identify the extent and nature of the neurologic dysfunction (Table 12–16). Of particular importance is the differentiation of peripheral (e.g., nerve, plexus, nerve root distributions) from central neurologic dysfunction. If the problem appears to be central, the differentiation of focal neurologic events from systemic effects is useful for elucidating the etiology.

Examination of the pupils represents one of the most important methods for differentiating metabolic from structural problems (Table 12–17). Metabolic coma is usually suggested by retained pupillary responses despite respiratory depression, altered caloric responses,

TABLE 12–17. PUPIL EXAMINATION

Response to light
Position
Motion
Gaze (conjugate and direction)
Caloric response
Doll's eyes

or motor abnormalities. The absence of pupillary responses strongly suggests a structural problem. The exceptions to this principle include preexisting pupillary disease (e.g., anisocoria, syphilis), asphyxia, and overdose with anticholinergics or glutethimide. To demonstrate absent pupillary responses, a magnifying glass and a strong light must be used.

A midposition (4 to 6 mm), fixed (nonresponsive to light) pupil implies a midbrain lesion. A unilaterally dilated and fixed pupil implies a third nerve lesion and may signal an impending intracranial disaster with uncal herniation. Bilaterally fixed and dilated pupils are seen with anoxic encephalopathy or intoxication with scopolamine or glutethimide. Small but reactive pupils can be the result of pontine lesions, narcotic overdose, or metabolic encephalopathy.

Ocular motion is generally random in the presence of metabolic coma, with the eyes resting in the midline as metabolic coma deepens. If the gaze is conjugate and either lateral or upward, structural disease may be present. It should be remembered that dysconjugate gaze and downward conjugate gaze are normal under anesthesia and may be seen during awakening from anesthesia; therefore these findings are not helpful in diagnosis. In the absence of depressant drugs, abnormal caloric eye responses are indicative of brainstem structural problems. Because reflex eye motion (e.g., caloric response) is sensitive to depressant drugs, assessment of this function is not particularly useful following anesthesia.

Failure to identify signs suggestive of a specific anatomic site of dysfunction generally suggests a metabolic derangement. Most patients with a metabolic encephalopathy have reactive, equal pupils of mid size. Muscle tone and tendon reflexes are symmetric, and plantar reflexes are extensor. However, systemic problems occasionally present as focal findings, e.g., the diabetic patient who presents with hemiplegia with hypoglycemia.[2] Similarly, uneven recovery from anesthesia may occur, causing transient focal findings.

Alterations in ventilation may also be useful as clues to the possible causes of dysfunction. Transient hyperpnea can be the result of hypoglycemia or anoxic injury. Patients in light coma may have posthyperventilation apnea or Cheyne-Stokes respiration. With more severe brainstem depression, transient hyperventilation may occur owing to suppression of inhibitory regions. Even more severe depression may cause depression in the reticular activating region, resulting in depressed ventilation or apnea. Anoxia, hypoglycemia, and some drugs are capable of inducing apnea without altering pupillary responses or blood pressure.

Hypoventilation may also be present as compensation for metabolic alkalosis. It may be caused by ingestion of alkalotic materials or excessive loss of acid from the body via the kidneys or gastrointestinal tract. Primary respiratory acidosis may be the result of severe pulmonary disease, neuromuscular disease, or weakness (which may be caused by inadequate neuromuscular reversal). Respiratory acidosis may also be caused by salicylism, hepatic coma, pulmonary disease, sepsis (direct endotoxin effect), or psychogenic hallucinations.

In general, hyperventilation in a comatose patient is a danger sign; the patient may be compensating for a metabolic acidosis or hypoxemia, or there may be primary respiratory stimulation. Metabolic acidosis is usually due to uremia, diabetic ketoacidosis, lactic acidosis (anoxic or spontaneous), malignant hyperthermia, or the ingestion of poisons that are acids or precursors of acids (e.g., salicylates, methanol, ethylene glycol, paraldehyde).

Motor activity should be examined grossly. Metabolic disease generally results in nonspecific disorders of strength, tone, or reflexes as well as focal or generalized seizures. Primitive reflexes (grasp, snout, routing) may be seen with light cortical depression. Decorticate and decerebrate rigidity and flaccidity can occur as the brainstem is depressed. Movement disorders of tremor, asterixis, and multifocal myoclonus are often seen with metabolic disorders. A "herky-jerky" motor pattern of residual neuromuscular blockers should not be confused with a metabolic process. Weakness in a focal pattern is uncommon in metabolic depression.

Most exogenous illicit drugs (see below regarding toxicology screening) produce similar effects on examination, with only minor variations. In general, they produce vestibular and cerebellar dysfunction with cerebral cortical dysfunction. Thus nystagmus, ataxia, and dysarthria often precede loss of consciousness. Unfortunately, recovery from anesthesia may produce some of these findings as well, confusing the picture.

Gross indications of seizure activity on examination should prompt rapid treatment to terminate the seizure. Otherwise cerebral hypermetabolism may cause cortical damage.

The normal postictal coma may cause deep unresponsiveness but rarely lasts more than 15 to 30 minutes,[25] with longer periods suggesting structural damage or an underlying metabolic derangement, e.g., hyponatremia.

Delirium can be seen on recovery from anesthesia and may be due to pain (or a full bladder) in the presence of sedative drugs. It may also be due to withdrawal from dependence on alcohol or illicit drugs or withdrawal from propanolol, digitalis, or hallucinogenic or psychotropic drugs. If the condition is not transitory, treatment with sedative reversal drugs (see below), analgesia with opioids, or bladder emptying (if indicated) should be attempted. If these measures are unsuccessful, a further search for the cause is indicated.

Other causes of delirium are cerebral infections, hepatic or renal failure, electrolyte abnormalities, hypercalcemia, head trauma, stress in a patient with dementia, porphyria, subarachnoid hemorrhage, hypoxia, thyrotoxicosis, and Cushing syndrome. Clearly, the history may be helpful, and a toxicology screen may be useful. Examination may reveal signs of hepatic failure (hepatomegaly, jaundice, asterixis), meningococcemia (pruritic rash), or other readily diagnosed conditions.

Some drugs produce specific findings, giving clues to their presence. For example, narcotic overdosage is usually associated with equal and reactive pinpoint pupils with reduced ventilatory drive. In this case, naloxone can usually reverse the effect, although naloxone reversal may be associated with pulmonary edema, hypertension, arrhythmias, and uncontrollable behavior if pain is severe. Other antagonist drugs, e.g., the mixed agonist-antagonist nalbuphine, may also be considered for reversal of narcotic effect, rather than naloxone.

Physostigmine can reverse the effects of belladonna alkaloid (e.g., atropine) overdose.[81] Patients with overdose of these agents are restless, excited, and confused. They may exhibit weakness, giddiness, and muscular incoordination. Gait and speech are disturbed, and nausea and vomiting may occur. Memory is disturbed, orientation is faulty, and the sensorium may be clouded. Mania may occur. Associated effects include dry mouth with difficulty swallowing or talking; blurred vision; photophobia; warm, dry, flushed skin; skin rash; fever; tachycardia; urinary urgency and difficulty with micturition. These effects can also be seen with overdoses of antihistamines, phenothiazines, and tricyclic antidepressants.

PATIENT HISTORY

As discussed above, the history is deferred until the examination is complete to allow rapid assessment of conditions that require immediate treatment. The most important component of the history relates to the neurologic condition. Unfortunately, a careful, detailed neurologic history is rarely documented preoperatively. If the patient cannot assist in a retrospective history evaluation, a family member may be able to help identify preexisting conditions that could contribute to the postoperative problem.

Major organ dysfunction or preexisting genetic alterations in enzyme activity can cause deviations from the normal effects of anesthetic medications. Medications taken prior to surgery may alter neurologic function or may have synergistic interactions with anesthesia medications. Preexisting neurovascular abnormalities can impair cerebral or spinal cord function or viability and set the stage for dysfunction secondary to otherwise innocuous insults, e.g., hypotension. Finally, baseline disease, particularly neurologic disease, may worsen or become unmasked after the operative experience.

Diabetes is a common disease that has many potential anesthetic implications. There are a large number of causes of mental dysfunction in diabetic patients. A history of diabetes should initiate a search for the various situations shown in Table 12–18. The autonomic

TABLE 12–18. CONDITIONS ASSOCIATED WITH DIABETES

Nonketotic hyperglycemic coma

Ketoacidosis

CNS acidosis in patients with ketoacidosis treated with bicarbonate

Cerebral edema secondary to decreased osmolarity of serum when hyperglycemia treated with insulin

Hyponatremia (SIADH)

Disseminated intravascular coagulation

Hypophosphatemia

Hypoglycemia

Uremia

Hypertensive encephalopathy

Cerebral infarction

Hypotension

Autonomic neuropathy

Lactic acidosis (usually with oral hypoglycemics)

neuropathy of diabetic patients makes them more prone to hypotension, syncope, cardiac arrest, and myocardial infarction.

SURGICAL PROCEDURES

Certain surgical procedures are associated with specific neurologic risks, and they must be considered in the evaluation. Some risks are associated with particular surgical manipulations. For example, the patient following carotid endarterectomy has an increased risk of stroke, and the patient undergoing repair of scoliosis has an increased risk of paraplegia. In general, patients undergoing surgery on the neural structures or their associated skeletal support (e.g., the spine or calvarium) or vasculature should be examined for neurologic dysfunction appropriate to known risks of these procedures.

A second form of surgical risk derives from appliances used for positioning or tourniquets used on the extremities. An extremity tourniquet may cause neural injury from direct compression and ischemia. Neurologic hazards associated with various positions utilized for surgery have been discussed.

EVALUATION OF THE ANESTHETIC TECHNIQUE

Resident anesthetic medications cause neurologic depression during the normal process of awakening from an anesthetic. An intentional or inadvertent absolute overdose may be readily recognized. However, more subtle drug interactions or alterations in metabolism may be less obvious. In addition, residual anesthetic or unreversed drug may itself cause neurologic dysfunction, thus confusing the evaluation for other causes. In this circumstance, methods that favor drug elimination (e.g., adequate ventilation in the case of an inhalational agent) or reversal of the effect (where possible, see below) may be useful.

Some anesthetic techniques may also contribute to persistent postoperative dysfunction. Regional blocks carry a risk of direct neural injury as well as secondary injury from neural compression due to a hematoma or abscess formation. Deliberate hypotensive techniques may contribute to neurologic dysfunction if the vascular supply of central structures is compromised. For example, neural compromise can occur following deliberate hypotension in patients with underlying disease (e.g.,

atherosclerotic occlusive disease) or with procedures where the structures may be compromised by the surgical instrumentation (e.g., brain retractors or spinal traction/distraction devices).

LABORATORY STUDIES

A variety of laboratory studies are useful for identifying the cause of neurologic dysfunction (Table 12–15). Basic ventilation and oxygenation can be assessed using arterial blood gases. The arterial blood gas levels, blood pH, and serum glucose level should be determined immediately, as they assist in the rapid identification of factors in need of immediate correction. The patient should also be assessed for undiagnosed hepatic, renal, or endocrine disease. Studies to be considered include serum electrolytes, calcium, magnesium, osmolality, hematocrit, blood urea nitrogen (BUN), creatinine, ammonia, phosphate, liver function studies, toxicology screen, urine specific gravity, and urine culture.

Alkalosis rarely produces cerebral dysfunction, whereas acidosis is often associated with this problem. Respiratory acidosis is far more common than metabolic acidosis, and the distortion should be apparent on the arterial blood gas assays.

Abnormalities of osmolality can often be rapidly estimated by roughly approximating serum osmolality using the following equation.

$$\text{mOsm/liter} = 2\,(\text{Na} + \text{K}) + \text{glucose}/18 + \text{BUN}/2.8$$

This value is normally 290 ± 5. Values less than 260 and above 330 are usually associated with cerebral dysfunction; however, smaller disturbances may contribute to dysfunction in the presence of other effects.

Hypoosmolar states (water intoxication) are generally due to conditions that cause hyponatremia. Treatment with hypertonic saline or diuretics (or both) can be safely accomplished if hyponatremia is the cause. It is important to rule out "false hyponatremia" caused by hyperlipidemia to ensure that the sodium level is truly low. Serum sodium values below 128 mEq/L can be associated with altered sensorium, and a rapidly falling serum sodium level or chronic values below 115 mEq/L are usually associated with seizure activity and require rapid treatment.

Hyperosmolar states may be the result of treatment with osmolar agents (mannitol, glycerol, or urea) or hypernatremia. Sodium values in excess of 160 mEq/L are often associated with depressed sensorium,[82] water depletion (diarrhea, vomiting, diabetes insipidus), or hyperglycemia. Glucose values above 800 mg/dl are usually associated with mental changes.[19] Treatment to correct the hypernatremia of hyperglycemia should be carefully accomplished, as rapid correction may lead to cerebral edema and cerebral dysfunction from the treatment.

Hypercalcemia can cause mental dysfunction and may be the result of hyperparathyroidism, immobilization, or cancer (generally metastatic to bone). Delusions, lethargy, muscle weakness, headache, stupor, coma, and seizures may occur. Hypocalcemia (calcium levels generally below 4.5 mEq/L) can be caused by uremia or hypoparathyroidism. Such a level is generally associated with muscle irritability and tetany. Delirium, stupor, coma, and seizures can also occur. When interpreting serum calcium values, it is important to recognize that a lowering of serum albumin by 1 gm/L is associated with a lowering of total serum calcium of 0.8 mEq/L, but serum ionized calcium is unchanged. Symptoms of hyper- and hypocalcemia depend on ionized calcium levels; therefore treatment strategies should be planned based on an estimate of the level of ionized rather than total calcium.

If the cause of neural dysfunction remains obscure, urine or serum toxicologic studies may identify drugs ingested preoperatively that are contributing to the dysfunction. In particular, alcohol and illicit drugs should be considered in patients having emergency surgery for trauma. Toxicology screening for commonly abused drugs may reveal the presence of amphetamines, cocaine, psychedelics, atropine-scopolamine, tricyclic antidepressants, phenothiazines, lithium, benzodiazepines, sedatives, barbiturates, alcohol, and opiates.

Diagnostic and Structural Studies

Structural studies such as CT scans or magnetic resonance imaging may be useful to differentiate and elucidate focal lesions. Contrast enhancement may be useful. The CT scan can demonstrate a hyperdense lesion immediately when intracranial hemorrhage is present. Follow-up angiography may allow elucidation of an associated aneurysm or atriovenous malformation (AVM). If the lesion is an ischemic infarct, however, the CT scan may not show a lucent area for 4 to 5 days unless the infarct is massive (which may be seen a few hours after injury).

Because the heart is the major source of intrinsic embolic events, echocardiography may be a useful diagnostic tool.

Electroencephalograms obtained acutely are rarely useful because the patterns may be nonspecific and suppressed by anesthetic agents. Documentation of seizure activity is useful, and repeated serial studies may allow observation of the course and prognosis of a discrete lesion. Similarly, other forms of electrophysiologic testing (electromyography and somatosensory evoked potentials) may be useful for identifying discrete abnormalities and may supplement the neurologic examination.

Consultation

If the underlying cause remains unidentified or unresolved, consultation with a neurologist or neurosurgeon is important. The consultant's assistance allows a carefully guided evaluation and optimal treatment.

Treatment

Supportive care must be administered initially to prevent further sequelae and to ensure an optimal environment for neural recovery. Problems of an acute nature (airway, ventilation, oxygenation, blood pressure, and perfusion) must be corrected immediately (Table 12–19).

Hypoglycemia, a frequent cause of metabolic coma in patients, is readily and easily reversed by the intravenous injection of 25 gm of glucose. Therefore intravenous glucose should be given when hypoglycemia may be a

TABLE 12–19. TREATMENT OF ALTERED NEUROLOGIC FUNCTION

Airway management
Ensurance of ventilation and oxygenation
Circulatory support
Drug therapy
   Consider glucose and thiamine
   Consider naloxone (Narcan) and physostigmine
   Terminate seizures if present
Supportive therapy
Specific treatment if cause known

contributory factor—after a pretreatment blood sample for glucose determination is obtained. Thiamine should be given with the glucose if malnutrition or chronic alcoholism is suspected.

Certain life-threatening conditions must be specifically treated. If hypothyroidism is suspected, the presence of myxedema coma should be ruled out, as it can be fatal rapidly. Treatment with triiodothyronine or thyroxine can be life-saving. Hypoventilation, hyponatremia, hypothermia, and hypotension are usually associated with myxedema coma. These problems must also be treated with supportive therapy.

Hypothermia should be treated by warming. Acidosis should be corrected by ventilatory support if it is respiratory and sodium bicarbonate if it is metabolic in origin (being sure that adequate ventilatory support is available when the carbon dioxide load produced by the bicarbonate occurs).

The management of seizures includes basic management of the airway and ventilation as well as the use of such agents as short-acting barbiturates to terminate the seizure. Long-acting agents may cloud recovery and make subsequent neurologic evaluation difficult. If the seizure is the result of local anesthetic toxicity, hyperventilation raises the seizure threshold, thereby reducing the duration of the seizure. Conversely, hyperventilation may aggravate seizure activity due to epilepsy.

Other conditions must be dealt with specifically. Increased intracranial pressure must be treated by hyperventilation, diuresis, and steroids. Sedation may be needed for withdrawal from alcohol, narcotics, or barbiturates.

Few anesthetic reversal agents are available, and each has associated hazards and should be used with caution. Of particular importance are neostigmine, pyridostigmine, and edrophonium chloride (Tensilon) for reversing residual nondepolarizing muscle relaxants. With the reversal, atropine or glycopyrrolate should be given simultaneously to prevent muscarinic effects and severe bradycardia. Physostigmine can be used to reverse the central action of anticholinergics (notably scopolamine) and may have some value in reversing other tranquilizers.[83] Naloxone can be used to reverse residual narcotic effects. Pulmonary edema and severe tachycardia and hypertension are associated with the use of naloxone (Narcan). Soon to be available is a drug for the reversal of the benzodiazepines, flumazenil.[84]

Clearly, many problems require consultation and more specific treatment. This point is particularly true of focal cerebral events and those related to cortical structural abnormalities.

For central insults, certain techniques may be useful. If the intracranial pressure is elevated because of a mass lesion such as a hematoma, methods to lower the pressure and to optimize cerebral perfusion are important, and neurosurgical drainage may be required. Pneumocephalus can often be lessened by ventilating the patient with 100 per cent oxygen, but neurosurgical treatment of hyperbaric treatment may be needed. If a lesion is due to ischemic or embolic infarction, anticoagulation or hypervolemic hypertension may be indicated. Evidence suggests that certain drugs such as calcium channel blockers may play a role in minimizing the effects of ischemic lesions in the future. Anticoagulation may also be utilized for transient ischemic attacks, reversible ischemic neurologic deficits, or stroke in progress.

If an infarct has a hemorrhagic component, anticoagulation may be contraindicated. If a hemorrhagic event is related to an intracranial aneurysm or AVM, management to prevent rebleeding or reduce associated vascular spasm is critical; neurosurgical ablation may also be required.

SUMMARY

The identification of neurologic problems following anesthesia and surgery may permit diagnosis and treatment of physiologic abnormalities causing or produced by the dysfunction. Life-threatening consequences can often be altered. Maintenance of essential functions and provision of supportive care are essential, as a thorough and detailed evaluation of the patient is performed. Early intervention and consultation can help minimize the neurologic consequences.

References

1. Haugen FP: The failure to regain consciousness after general anesthesia. Anesthesiology 22:657–666, 1961.
2. Denlinger JK: Prolonged emergence and failure to regain consciousness. In Orkin FK, Cooperman LH, eds. Complications in Anesthesiology. Philadelphia, Lippincott, 1983.
3. Larabee MG, Posternak JM: Selective action of anesthetics on synapses and axons in mammalian sympathetic ganglia. J Neurophysiol 15:91–98, 1952.
4. Arduini A, Arduini MG: Effect of drugs and metabolic alterations on brain stem arousal mechanism. J Pharmacol Exp Ther 110:76–82, 1954.

5. Krnjevic K: Central cholinergic pathways. Fed Proc 28:113–117, 1973.

6. Krnjevic K: Chemical transmission and cortical arousal. Anesthesiology 28:100–109, 1967.

7. Duvoison RC, Katz R: Reversal of central anticholinergic syndrome in man by physostigmine. JAMA 206:1963–1967, 1968.

8. Nahrwold ML, Cohen PL: Anesthetic and mitochondrial function. In Cohen PJ, ed. Clinical Anesthesia Series, Vol. 1: Metabolic Aspects of Anesthesia. Philadelphia, Davis, 1975, pp. 25–44.

9. Cassem EH: Approach to the patient with mental and emotional complaints. *In* Braunwald E, Isselbacher KJ, et al, eds. Harrison's Principles of Internal Medicine, 11 ed. New York, McGraw-Hill, 1987.

10. Plum RF, Brennan RW: Differential diagnosis of altered states of consciousness. *In* Youmans JR, ed. Neurological Surgery, Vol. 2. Philadelphia, Saunders, 1982.

11. Stone WM: States of Altered Consciousness Neurology: The Physician's Guide. New York, Thieme-Stratton, 1984.

12. Seibert CP: Recognition management and prevention of neuropsychological dysfunction after operation. Int Anesthesiol Clin 24:39–54, 1986.

13. Schnelle N, Molnar GD, Ferris DO, et al: Circulating glucose and insulin in surgery for insulinomas. JAMA 217:1072–1076, 1971.

14. Schen RJ, Khazzam AS: Postoperative hypoglycemic coma associated with chlorpropamide. Br J Anaesth 47:899–893, 1975.

15. Enderby GEH: A report on mortality and morbidity following 9,107 hypotensive anesthetics. Br J Anaesth 33:109–114, 1961.

16. Bedford RF: Hyperosmolar hyperglycemic nonketotic coma following general anesthesia: report of a case. Anesthesiology 35:652–656, 1971.

17. Wulfson HD, Dalton B: Hyperosmolar hyperglycemic nonketotic coma in a patient undergoing emergency cholecystectomy. Anesthesiology 41:286–293, 1974.

18. Toker P: Hyperosmolar hyperglycemic nonketotic coma: a case of delayed recovery from anesthesia. Anesthesiology 41:284–287, 1974.

19. Arieff AI, Carroll HJ: Nonketotic hyperosmolar coma with hyperglycemia: clinical features, pathophysiology, renal function, acid-base balance, plasma-cerebrospinal fluid equilibria and the effects of therapy in 37 cases. Medicine (Baltimore) 51:73–82, 1972.

20. Gerich JE, Mertin MN, Recant L: Clinical and metabolic characteristics of hyperosmolar nonketotic coma. Diabetes 20:228–232, 1971.

21. Arieff AI: Hyponatremia, convulsions, respiratory arrest and permanent brain damage after elective surgery in healthy women. N Engl J Med 314:1539–1534, 1986.

22. Ohman JL Jr, Marliss EB, Aoki TT, et al: The cerebrospinal fluid in diabetic ketoacidosis. N Engl J Med 284:283–287, 1971.

23. Jones JP Jr, Engleman EP, Najarian JS: Systemic fat embolism after renal homotransplantation and treatment with corticosteroids. N Engl J Med 273:1453–1457, 1965.

24. Kafer ER: Cardiorespiratory effects of hypoxia. Anesthesiol Intensivmed Prax 180:33–39, 1985.

25. Plum F, Posner JB: The Diagnosis of Stupor and Coma, 3rd ed. Philadelphia, Davis, 1982.

26. Eisele JH, Egere EL II, Muallem M: Narcotic properties of carbon dioxide in the dog. Anesthesiology 28:856–859, 1967.

27. Dundee JW, Richards RK: Effect of azotemia upon the action of intravenous barbiturate anesthesia. Anesthesiology 15:333–338, 1954.

28. Freeman RB, Sheff MG, Maher JF, et al: The blood-cerebrospinal fluid barrier in uremia. Ann Intern Med 56:233–238, 1962.

29. Schentag JJ, Cerra FB, Calleri GM, et al: Age, disease, and cimetidine disposition in healthy subjects and chronically ill patients. Clin Pharmacol Ther 29:737–741, 1981.

30. Schmidt KF, Roth RH Jr: Interaction of psychotropic drugs with agents employed in clinical anesthesia. Clin Anesth 3:60–65, 1967.

31. Berman ML, Lowe HJ, Bochantin J, et al: Uptake and elimination of methoxyflurane as influenced by enzyme induction in the rat. Anesthesiology 27:118–123, 1966.

32. Cohen ML, Chan S, Way WL, et al: Distribution in the brain and metabolism of ketamine in the rat after intravenous administration. Anesthesiology 39:370–374, 1973.

33. White PF, Johnston RR, Pudwell CR: Interaction of ketamine and halothane in rats. Anesthesiology 42:179–184, 1975.

34. Meyer H, Lux HD: Action of ammonium on a chloride pump: removal of hyperpolarizing inhibition in an isolated neuron. Pflugers Arch 350:18, 1974.

35. Skou JC: Further investigations on a Mg^{2+} + Na^+-activated adenosine triphosphate possible related to the active, linked transport of Na^+ and K^+ across the nerve membrane. Biochim Biophys Acta 42:6–23, 1960.

36. Laursen H, Westergaard E: Enhanced permeability to horseradish peroxidase across cerebral vessels in the rat after portacaval anastomosis. Neuropathol Appl Neurobiol 3:29–44, 1979.

37. Dean G: Porphyria. Br Med J 2:1291–1298, 1953.

38. Brown TR: Epilepsy in neurology. *In* Feldman RG, ed. The Physician's Guide. New York, Thieme-Stratton, 1984, pp. 52–64.

39. Nicoll JMV: Status epilepticus following enflurane anesthesia. Anaesthesia 41:927–929, 1986.

40. Sprague DH, Wolf S: Enflurane seizures in patients taking aminotriptyline. Anesth Analg 61:67–71, 1982.

41. Thompson GE: Ketamine-induced convulsions. Anesthesiology 37:662–667, 1972.

42. Burrowes FA, Seeman RG: Ketamine and myoclonic encephalopathy of infants (Kinsbourne syndrome). Anesth Analg 61:873–879, 1982.

43. Munson ES, Martucci RW, Smith RE: Circadian variations in anesthetic requirement and toxicity in rats. Anesthesiology 32:507–513, 1970.

44. Saidman LJ: Uptake, distribution and elimination of barbiturates. *In* Eger EI II, ed. Anesthetic Uptake and Action. Baltimore, Williams & Wilkins, 1974, pp. 228–248.

45. Babad AA, Eger EI II: The effects of hyperthyroidism and hypothyroidism on halothane and oxygen requirements in dogs. Anesthesiology 29:1087–1092, 1968.

46. Eger EI II: MAC. *In* Eger EI II, ed. Anesthetic Uptake and Action. Baltimore, Williams & Wilkins, 1974, pp. 1–25.

47. Miller RD, Way WL, Eger EI II: The effects of alpha-methyldopa, reserpine, guanethidine and iproniazid on minimum alveolar anesthetic requirement [MAC]. Anesthesiology 24:665–669, 1963.

48. Johnston RR, Way WL, Miller RD: Alteration of anesthetic requirement by amphetamine. Anesthesiology 36:357–361, 1972.

49. Lasser EC, Elizondo-Martel G, Granke RC: Potentiation of pentobarbital anesthesia by competitive protein binding. Anesthesiology 24:665–669, 1963.

50. Ghonein MM, Pandya HB, Kelley SE: Binding of thiopental to plasma proteins: effects on distribution in the brain and heart. Anesthesiology 45:635–640, 1976.

51. Stoelting RK, Eger EI II: The effects of ventilation and anesthetic solubility on recovery from anesthesia. Anesthesiology 30:290–296, 1969.

52. Tinker JH, Gandolfi AJ, Van Dyke RA: Elevation of plasma bromide levels in patients following halothane anesthesia. Anesthesiology 44:194–199, 1976.

53. Johnstone RE, Kennell EM, Behar M, et al: Increased serum bromide concentration after halothane anesthesia in man. Anesthesiology 42:498–503, 1975.

54. Weiss HD, Walker MD, Weirnik PH: Neurotoxicity of commonly used antineoplastic agents. N Engl J Med 291:75–86, 1974.

55. Ropper AH, Martin JB: Coma and related disturbances of consciousness. In Braunwald E, Isselbacher KJ, et al, eds. Harrison's Principles of Internal Medicine, 11th ed. New York, McGraw-Hill, 1987.

56. Pryse-Phillips W, Murray TJ: Reduction in consciousness level. In Essential Neurology, 3rd ed. New York, Medical Examination Publishing, 1986, p. 169.

57. Carrora JJ: Diagnosis, prognosis and treatment of hypoxic coma. Adv Neurol 26:1–13, 1985.

58. Kruczek M, Albin MS, Wolf S, Berton JM: Post operative seizure activity following enflurane anesthesia. Anesthesiology 53:175–176, 1980.

59. Hougaard K, Hansen A, Brodersen P: The effect of ketamine on regional cerebral blood flow in man. Anesthesiology 41:562–566, 1974.

60. Toole JF: Effects of change of head, limb and body position on cephalic circulation. N Engl J Med 279:307–311, 1968.

61. Plum F, Posner JB, Hain RR: Delayed neurological deterioration after anoxia. Arch Intern Med 110:56–62, 1962.

62. Toung T, Donham R, Lehrer A, et al: Tension pneumocephalus after posterior fossa craniotomy; report of four additional cases and review of postoperative pneumocephalus. Neurosurgery 12:164–168, 1983.

63. Lowenstein E, Little JW III, Lo HH: Prevention of cerebral embolism from flushing radial-artery cannulas. N Engl J Med 285:1414–1419, 1971.

64. Patrick RT, Devloo RA: Embolic phenomena of the operative and postoperative period. Anesthesiology 22:715–719, 1961.

65. Jones HR Jr, Caplan LR, Come PC, et al: Cerebral emboli of paradoxical origin. Ann Neurol 13:314–319, 1983.

66. Dhuner K: Nerve injuries following operations: a survey of cases occurring during a six-year period. Anesthesiology 11:289–293, 1950.

67. Leffert RD: Brachial-plexus injuries. N Engl J Med 291:1059–1067, 1974.

68. Alvine FG, Schurrer ME: Postoperative ulnar-nerve palsy: are there predisposing factors? J Bone Joint Surg [Am] 69:255–259, 1987.

69. Grundberg AB: Letter to the editor. J Bone Joint Surg [Am] 69:951, 1987.

70. MacGibbon JB: Neurological complications following the administration of sera. Am J Med Sci 230:520–524, 1955.

71. Doyle JB: Neurologic complications of serum sickness. Am J Med Sci 185:484, 1933.

72. Herrera-Ornelas L, Tolls RM, Petrelli NJ, et al: Common peroneal nerve palsy associated with pelvic surgery for cancer. Dis Colon Rectum 29:392–397, 1986.

73. Burkhart FL, Daly JW: Sciatic and peroneal nerve injury: a complication of vaginal operations. Obstet Gynecol 28:99–102, 1966.

74. Britt BA, Gordon RA: Peripheral nerve injuries associated with anaesthesia. Can Anaesth Soc J 11:514–536, 1964.

75. Nicholson MJ, Eversole UH: Nerve injuries incident to anaesthesia and operation. Anesth Analg 36:19–32, 1957.

76. Stephens J, Appleby S: Polyneuropathy following induced hypothermia. In Transactions of the American Neurological Association, 80th Meeting, 1955, p. 102.

77. Swan H, Virtue R, Blount SG Jr, Kircher LT Jr: Hypothermia in surgery: analysis of 100 clinical cases. Ann Surg 142:382–386, 1955.

78. Livingston KE: Simple method of rapid identification of major peripheral nerve injuries. Lahey Clin Bull 5:118–121, 1947.

79. Miller RG, Camp PE: Postoperative ulnar neuropathy. JAMA 242:1636–1639, 1979.

80. Seyfer AE, Grammer NY, Bogumill GP, et al: Upper extremity neuropathies after cardiac surgery. J Hand Surg [Am] 10:16–19, 1985.

81. Bready LL: Delayed emergence. In Bready LL, Smith RB, eds. Decision Making in Anesthesiology. Toronto, BC Decker, 1987, p. 166.

82. Sridhar CB, Calvert GD, Ibbertson HK: Syndrome of hypernatremia hypodipsia and partial diabetes insipidus: a new interpretation. J Clin Endocrinol Metab 38:890–901, 1974.

83. Hill GE, Stanley TH, Sentker CR: Physostigmine reversal of postoperative somnolence. Can Anaesth Soc J 24:707–715, 1977.

84. Brogden RN, Goa KL: Flumazenil: a preliminary review of its benzodiazepine antagonist properties, intrinsic activity and therapeutic use. Drugs 35:448–467, 1984.

13 MANAGING PERIOPERATIVE HYPOTHERMIA AND HYPERTHERMIA

ROBERT A. NATONSON

The importance of a patient's body temperature to overall health has been recognized by physicians for centuries, even before it was understood or accurately measured. Today, monitoring body temperature is a primary means of assessing the well-being of patients and their progress postoperatively.

Despite large variations in ambient temperature, human body temperature rarely fluctuates more than 2°C. Such precise control is accomplished through a variety of behavioral and physiologic mechanisms.

During the perioperative period, factors such as premedication, anesthesia, and the stress of surgery interact in complex ways to disrupt normal thermoregulation. Alterations in temperature beyond normal physiologic limits may adversely affect virtually all body functions, especially the cardiovascular, respiratory, and central nervous system. In addition, prolonged postoperative decreases in body temperature have been linked to increased mortality after surgery.[1] As the number of high risk patients increases and longer procedures are attempted, understanding normal thermoregulation and the effects of temperature alterations becomes even more essential.

This chapter discusses the physiology of temperature regulation, the merits and shortcomings of various methods for measuring temperature, and the causes, consequences, and treatment of mild to moderate hypothermia or hyperthermia.

PHYSIOLOGY OF TEMPERATURE CONTROL

NORMAL HUMAN THERMOREGULATION

Humans are homeotherms; that is, they maintain a body temperature of approximately 37°C. To maintain homeothermy, a complex and highly sensitive temperature regulation system is required. In humans this system consists of peripheral and central mechanisms that sense the body's temperature and a control system that effects a response. The hypothalamus functions as the primary control center.

Physiologists describe human thermoregulation in terms of a two-compartment model: the body's shell and its core. The core temperature, which is of primary importance, is the mean temperature of the body's vital organs, including the contents of the skull, thorax, and abdomen. Core structures account for 70 per cent of total body heat.[2] The shell consists of skin, subcutaneous fat tissue, and superficial muscle. Shell temperature, which is often different from core temperature, can vary with changes in regional blood flow and environmental conditions.

MECHANISMS OF HEAT LOSS

Core temperature is determined by the balance between heat gain and heat loss. Heat

202

exchange between the body and environment follows a thermal gradient: The body loses heat at low ambient temperatures and may gain heat when ambient temperatures are higher. Heat loss from the body is more common than heat gain during usual operating room conditions.

There are four primary mechanisms of heat loss: radiation, convection, evaporation, and conduction. To understand how heat is lost from the body and the advantages of some therapeutic measures over others in maintaining normothermia, it is important to review these heat-loss mechanisms (Table 13–1).

Radiation involves energy transfer via electromagnetic waves, with no direct contact between objects. The human body has an effective radiating surface of about 85 per cent; opposing surfaces, such as the inner thighs, most often radiate heat to each other rather than to the environment. Radiant heat loss is proportional to the fourth power of surface area exposed and accounts for 40 to 50 per cent of the body's total heat loss in the operating room.[3]

Convection refers to heat transfer by air movement, i.e., by collisions between air molecules and molecules on the body's surface. Wind chill is a result of this heat loss mechanism. Air velocity, ambient temperature, and exposed surface area primarily determine convective heat loss, which can account for up to 35 per cent of total heat loss in the operating room.[4]

Evaporation occurs primarily through perspiration but also from the respiratory tract and open body cavities. Vaporization of water requires heat—about 0.6 kcal/gm of water—which is supplied by the body.[5] Evaporation is the major means by which the body prevents hyperthermia in warm environments: an increase of 0.7°C above the body's set point leads to a fourfold increase in sweat production, and sweating can cause a 10-fold increase in evaporative heat loss in humans. Unlike the other three mechanisms, evaporation can exchange heat *against* a thermal gradient. It can produce a net heat loss even when ambient temperatures are higher than skin temperatures. Up to 25 per cent of total heat loss is due to evaporation.[6]

Conduction is the transfer of heat by direct contact with a stable medium: a cold preparation on exposed skin, for example, or the use of cool intravenous and irrigating solutions. Muscles, fat, and skin act as natural insulators to decrease conducted heat loss from the warmer tissues in the core. In a room at 22°C conduction accounts for about 10 per cent of total heat loss.[2] Immersion in cold water dramatically increases conductive loss.

MECHANISMS OF HEAT GAIN

There are four primary mechanisms of heat gain: basal metabolism, voluntary movement, shivering, and nonshivering thermogenesis.

Basal metabolism accounts for all the net body heat production for humans in a neutral environment. At rest, major organs supply 50 to 60 per cent of the body's heat and muscles about 20 per cent. The heat formed from metabolism must be eliminated to maintain body temperature within normal limits.

Voluntary movement can greatly increase heat production. During exercise, for example, up to 90 per cent of the body's heat may be generated by muscles.

Shivering can increase the rate of heat production by as much as 400 to 500 per cent.[7] Mechanical work does not occur during shivering, so the energy produced by involuntary muscle contractions primarily creates heat. Shivering is not effective over the long term because it increases convective and radiative heat loss through increased blood flow and muscle activity.[5] Shivering ceases altogether at a body temperature of 33°C. Metabolic rate then drops progressively with temperature, decreasing to 50 per cent of normal at 28°C.[8] In addition to increasing oxygen consumption,[9,10] shivering increases cardiac work,[11,12] decreases PO_2,[9,12] and increases demand on ventilation.[11] Thus patients with decreased cardiac or pulmonary reserves may be placed at risk (Table 13–2).

Nonshivering thermogenesis is an effective mechanism of heat production most common in neonates, where it occurs primarily through the metabolism of brown fat. Brown adipose tissue is highly vascular and distributed around the body's core, so that heat generated

TABLE 13–1. FOUR MECHANISMS OF HEAT LOSS

Mechanism	Amount of Total Heat Loss in OR (%)
Radiation	Up to 50
Convection	Up to 35
Evaporation	Up to 25
Conduction	Up to 10

TABLE 13–2. CONSEQUENCES OF SHIVERING

Increased O_2 consumption
Increased CO_2 production
Increased ventilatory demand
Increased myocardial work
Decreased arterial oxygen saturation

by lipid metabolism can be efficiently distributed to the brain, heart, and spinal cord. The amount of metabolic activity in this tissue is dictated by the temperature of the interior hypothalamus and controlled via the sympathetic nervous system.[13]

CONTROL OF BODY TEMPERATURE

Although temperature homeostasis in humans is not fully understood, the following description integrates the latest knowledge about this process. First, cutaneous thermoreceptors sense an environmental temperature change. At ambient temperatures above 44°C heat-sensitive receptors increase their firing rate, whereas temperatures below 24°C stimulate cold-sensitive receptors.[5]

Information from these peripheral receptors is relayed via the lateral spinothalamic tract to the anterior hypothalamus, which contains central sensors that respond to the temperature of blood flowing around them. Together, the anterior and posterior hypothalamus establish a reference temperature—the set point—which is affected by age, exercise, medication, anesthetics, and other factors. When a difference is detected between body temperature and the set point, the posterior hypothalamus initiates the appropriate heat-generating or heat-conserving response, which is controlled either neurally or hormonally.

Input from peripheral and central sensors is not processed equally. Central sensors are dominant and exert an overriding control over peripheral sensors. For example, if body temperature is at the set point, and blood going to the hypothalamus is cooled, shivering and vasoconstriction are observed. If core temperature rises above the set point, even with a decrease in skin temperature the heat production does not rise, once again demonstrating the concept of central sensor dominance.

Peripheral input does play a role as evidenced by the fact that when core temperature does fall but skin temperature remains above 33°C heat production is minimal. A person who is sweating because of an elevation in core temperature above the set point abruptly stops sweating when skin temperature drops below 29°C.

Using information from the hypothalamus, the cerebral cortex coordinates behavioral responses, seeking warmer environments or putting on more clothing when body temperature falls, for example. In addition, vasoconstriction occurs within seconds. When body temperature rises, cortical centers stimulate heat-dissipating behaviors, including moving to cooler climates and shedding clothing.

MEASURING BODY TEMPERATURE

Measuring core temperature is of primary importance for monitoring perioperative body temperature changes. Not all sites accurately reflect core temperature. In addition, temperature values from various body sites can differ considerably from one another. It is important to understand the advantages and shortcomings of each site and whether values obtained provide an accurate indication of core temperature (Table 13–3). Other factors to consider when choosing a site include proximity to major arteries, insulation of the site from the external environment, absence of inflammation or pathology, the patient's age and condition, and the length and type of surgical procedure.[14]

ESOPHAGEAL TEMPERATURE

The temperature of mixed venous blood reflects the general thermal status of body tissues. Esophageal temperature at the level of the heart is perhaps the closest to mixed venous blood temperature and is therefore gen-

TABLE 13–3. TEMPERATURE MONITORING SITES

Reflective of Core Temperature	Reflective of Shell Temperature
Esophagus	Mouth
Nasopharynx	Axilla
Tympanic membrane	Skin
Bladder	
Rectum	

erally considered the best measurement to obtain.

When measuring esophageal temperature, the position of the probe is critical. Distal esophageal temperature is considered reflective of core temperature. Readings are several degrees cooler if the probe is placed more cephalad rather than more caudad in the esophagus. Whitby and Duncan[15] found that an esophageal probe must be positioned in the lower one fourth of the esophagus to eliminate the influence inspired gases might have on the measured temperature.

NASOPHARYNGEAL TEMPERATURE

Positioning a probe in the nasopharynx posterior to the soft palate provides an estimate of hypothalamic temperature. However, careful placement of the probe is paramount to minimize the risk of trauma. Leakage of air around the endotracheal tube cuff can affect temperature readings.[16]

TYMPANIC MEMBRANE TEMPERATURE

Tympanic membrane thermistors closely approximate hypothalamic temperature.[17] In fact, tympanic membrane temperature has been recommended as the most reliable measurement of core temperature.[18] Readings can be influenced by cerumen, and the canal or membrane can be easily injured if the thermistor is not inserted carefully.[5]

BLADDER TEMPERATURE

In a study of patients on cardiopulmonary bypass, Moorthy et al.[19] found that nasopharyngeal and esophageal temperatures were similar to each other during both rapid cooling and rewarming. Bladder temperatures changed more slowly than the above, and rectal temperatures were the slowest to change. The investigators concluded that monitoring bladder temperature avoids the inconvenience and contamination of rectal monitoring and better represents the steady-state core temperature.

In another study, Cork et al.[20] found that bladder temperature measured with Foley catheters compared favorably with rectal, nasopharyngeal, and esophageal probes. They concluded that Foley catheter sensors are useful alternatives to esophageal, rectal, nasopharyngeal, and tympanic membrane probes. Other researchers,[21–23] using tympanic membrane temperature as a standard for core temperature, demonstrated that nasopharyngeal, esophageal, and bladder temperature measurements were most accurate. These investigators further recommended using one or more of those sites rather than risking injury to the tympanic membrane. Ilsley et al.,[24] however, found a bladder temperature-measuring device unsuitable for clinical use owing to fragile leads and puckering of the urinary catheter surface from traction on the thermistor lead.

RECTAL TEMPERATURE

Rectal temperature is usually a few tenths of a degree higher than arterial blood temperature. Rectal probes have been used to measure core temperature, mostly because of convenience. Rectal temperatures can be affected by cool blood returning from the legs, insulation by feces, and heat-producing organisms in the bowel. For these reasons, many researchers question how accurately rectal temperature reflects core temperature.

ORAL TEMPERATURE

Oral temperature poorly reflects blood temperature. The popularity of its measurement results purely from convenience. Oral temperature tends to be 0.30 to 0.65°C below rectal temperature. Indeed, oral temperature may be clinically misleading. In a study of patients in an emergency department, Tandberg and Sklar[25] found that the difference between oral and rectal temperatures increased progressively with increasing respiratory rates. Oral readings ranged from 2° to 3°C below rectal values in many patients with tachypnea, presumably owing to respiratory cooling of the mouth. These investigators stated that such misleading readings may mask the presence of fever and thus of serious disease.

AXILLARY TEMPERATURE

The accessibility of the axilla is both a benefit and a detriment. Although it is convenient for measuring temperature, it is also more influenced by environmental factors than are other sites. For this reason, axillary temperature is perhaps best used to monitor general trends in body temperature. Axillary probes typically read 0.5°C below oral temperatures and 1°C below rectal temperature.[5] These probes are sensitive to muscle temperature and quickly sense temperature increases such as those seen with malignant hyperthermia and its markedly increased muscle metabolic rate and heat production. However, axillary temperature is considered to be a poor measure of core temperature.

SKIN TEMPERATURE

Despite their convenience, skin probes (either liquid crystal strips or flat metal disks) have several shortcomings, the most important of which may be accuracy.[20] As discussed previously, skin temperature often correlates poorly with core temperature. During anesthesia, liquid crystal strips may be used when exact core temperatures are not needed. However, core temperatures are recommended for most patients, especially infants: patients undergoing major abdominal, neurosurgical, or cardiovascular procedures and anyone with a history of thermoregulation difficulty.[7]

HYPOTHERMIA

Hypothermia occurs when systemic heat loss lowers core body temperature below 36°C.[26] It can be divided into three stages (Table 13–4). Hypothermia is a common occurrence intraoperatively and postoperatively. Vaughan et al.[11] found, for example, that 195 of 198 patients in their study had an average core body temperature of 35.6 ± 0.6°C within 5 minutes of recovery room admission. Hypothermia readily occurs because the conditions associated with surgery and anesthesia typically inhibit the body's heat-generating mechanisms and favor its heat-loss mechanisms.

CAUSES OF PERIOPERATIVE HYPOTHERMIA

A number of factors can contribute to reducing the body's core temperature during the perioperative period. The most common are discussed below.

TABLE 13–4. STAGES OF HYPOTHERMIA

Stage	Core Body Temperature (°C)
Mild	36–32
Moderate	32–30
Severe	≤30

Preexisting Medical Conditions

Thermoregulation may be impaired by preexisting medical conditions, including hypothyroidism, decreased metabolic rate, hypoadrenalism, circulatory failure, and central nervous system disorders. In addition, a decrease in muscle mass and activity, which are major sources of heat production, often accompany conditions of paralysis and chronic arthritis.[27]

Preoperative Medications and Conditions

Narcotics, sedatives, and other preoperative medications are associated with disruption of normal thermoregulation. Many patients become poikilotherms after receiving these drugs; that is, their body temperature closely mimics environmental temperature. Ozuna and Foster[28] found that several patients in their study experienced a reduction in oral temperature even before they reached the operating room. This temperature drop was related to the use of preoperative medications, which not only depress central heat-regulating mechanisms but also cause vasodilation.

Lack of clothing and extended waiting periods in cold rooms or hallways also contribute to reductions in the patient's body temperature during the preoperative period. Neonates and the elderly are particularly sensitive. The ability to generate heat depends in large part on body mass. Heat loss correlates with the ratio of surface to body mass. Neonates have a surface area/mass ratio three times greater than that of adults[29] as well as an inability to shiver, so they have difficulty thermoregulating in cold environments. Old age may also be a liability for hypothermia owing to the elderly's decreased muscle mass, decreased ability to vasoconstrict in response to heat conservation, and decreased ability to increase metabolic rate in order to generate greater heat production.

Operating Room Conditions

The ambient temperature and humidity, the number of room air exchanges, and the presence of laminar airflow systems can contribute to the loss of body heat in the operating room (OR). The temperature in most ORs is 20°C or less, mainly to inhibit bacterial growth and to keep surgical personnel comfortable.[7] Consequently, patient hypothermia is prevalent in these cool rooms.[30] It has been suggested that hypothermia is likely to occur when OR temperatures are 20°C or less and unlikely when rooms are above this temperature.[31]

However, there is conflicting evidence about the effects of ambient temperature. Joachimsson et al.[32] reported that even when room temperature was kept above 21°C patients undergoing minor abdominal surgery lost heat and had core temperatures below the preinduction value at the end of the operation.

Anesthesia

Anesthetics interfere with thermoregulation by inhibiting afferent input, allowing set point temperature to drift, or interfering with efferent responses. Under normal conditions, ventilatory heat loss corresponds to 12 per cent of the total body heat production at rest.[33] However, this loss increases during anesthesia, as heat production decreases and patients often are hyperventilated. Because cold, unhumidified anesthetic gases are delivered directly to the lungs via an endotracheal tube, the natural heating and humidifying system in the nose is bypassed, further increasing evaporative loss. Volatile anesthetics are also potent vasodilators that facilitate blood flow to the skin, which contributes to both radiative and conductive heat loss.

The solubility and potency of inhalation agents increase as temperature decreases. This statement means that, as body temperature decreases for the same anesthetic concentration given, the patient's depth of anesthesia is greater and a longer time is required for the anesthetic to be eliminated. As a result, the patient recovers more slowly. As previously mentioned, anesthetized patients tend to become poikilotherms owing to disruption of thermoregulation. The degree of this disruption is proportional to the depth of anesthesia such that deeply anesthetized patients have a greater degree of body temperature alteration.

Muscle relaxants abolish shivering by virtue of their ability to eliminate motor activity, thus causing the body to lose its natural ability to generate heat. Epidural or spinal anesthetics have been shown to produce greater heat loss than do general anesthetics primarily because of their marked vasodilating action resulting from the sympathetic blockade caused by these anesthetic techniques. In summary, anesthetics can interfere with thermoregulation by preventing vasoconstriction, abolishing shivering, depressing metabolic rate, and prohibiting appropriate behavioral responses.

Other Factors

Other important factors that contribute to perioperative heat loss include the use of unwarmed intravenous and irrigating fluids and blood, and the exposure of major body cavities during surgery to the ambient atmosphere of the OR.

For example, Workhoven[34] examined the effect of warmed and room-temperature intravenous fluids on shivering in 44 parturients undergoing epidural anesthesia for elective cesarean section. Of those administered 1 liter of room-temperature balanced salt solution, 64 per cent shivered, compared to only 14 per cent in the warmed (30° to 33.9°C) fluid group. Workhoven concluded that room-temperature fluids may increase the incidence of shivering, whereas warmed fluids may lower the incidence and thus make elective cesarean section safer and more satisfying for the parturient.

PHYSIOLOGIC CONSEQUENCES OF HYPOTHERMIA

Hypothermia affects virtually every body function. Some important physiologic consequences of hypothermia are shown in Table 13–5.

The consequences of hypothermia usually become most apparent during the postoperative period. The impact of low core temperature can vary from restlessness, discomfort, and a cold, pale cyanotic periphery to such physiologic responses as reduced peripheral blood flow with risk of thrombosis, increased carbon dioxide production and oxygen consumption, and hypoxemia. Postoperatively, three major complications are of concern: shivering, peripheral vasoconstriction, and delayed drug clearance.

TABLE 13–5. MAJOR PHYSIOLOGIC CONSEQUENCES OF HYPOTHERMIA

Core Body Temperature (°C)	Physiologic Responses
≤33	Can be well tolerated with no detrimental effect. Intestinal motility can decrease, and ileus can occur.[5]
33	Beginning of the danger zone. Impaired cerebration begins if the patient is conscious. Shivering ceases. Respiratory rate begins to fall.
32	Cardiac output begins to decline.[35] Hyperglycemia can occur.[36] Some cold agglutinins are triggered. Platelet count falls.
31	Cardiac conduction abnormalities can appear.[37]
30	Cardiac output has decreased up to 40%.[5] Ventricular arrhythmias may appear. Loss of consciousness and pupilary dilatation supervene.[38] Glomerular filtration rate decreases to 50% of normal.[5] Blood viscosity has increased.
28	Ventricular fibrillation commonly occurs.[39] Patient becomes comatose and areflexic.[40] Metabolic rate falls to 50% of normal.[8]
24	Respiratory drive ceases.

SHIVERING

As discussed earlier, shivering can produce a 500 per cent increase in metabolic rate.[9] Under these conditions, increased oxygen consumption and greater carbon dioxide production can increase the ventilatory requirements. If these requirements are not met, the PCO_2 increases. If the body cannot meet the metabolic demands of shivering, mixed venous oxygen saturation decreases and arterial hypoxemia can occur, especially if any significant intrapulmonary shunting coexists.[41] The increased demand for blood flow by these active muscles can increase sharply, requiring cardiac output and cardiac work to increase. The resulting increase in myocardial oxygen consumption, especially when associated with a decrease in arterial oxygen, can result in myocardial ischemia, particularly in the elderly or in patients with coronary artery disease.[5]

PERIPHERAL VASOCONSTRICTION

Vasoconstriction, a particularly deleterious consequence of postoperative hypothermia, may be responsible for unexplained hypertension in the recovery room. Because vasoconstriction can increase systemic vascular resistance and myocardial work, the potential for myocardial ischemia increases. In addition, vasoconstriction can mask hypovolemia, and so sudden reductions in blood pressure can occur as the patient warms and vasodilates.[5]

DELAYED DRUG CLEARANCE

Delayed drug clearance as a consequence of hypothermia is particularly significant in elderly patients, who may already have impaired drug-clearing mechanisms and decreased metabolic rate. For example, the maximum rate of renal excretion of a drug can decline by 10 per cent for every 0.6°C fall in body temperature.[42] In addition, elderly hypothermic patients are more likely to have residual paralysis due to muscle relaxants that is difficult to reverse pharmacologically.

Prolonged postoperative hypothermia has been linked to increased mortality after surgery. Slotman et al.[1] evaluated the effects of hypothermia on postsurgical morbidity and mortality in 100 patients (Fig. 13–1). Hypothermia intraoperatively and at time zero was not significantly associated with mortality. However, the mortality of patients who remained hypothermic at 2, 4, and 8 hours significantly increased compared to normothermic patients. The investigators concluded that the physiologic stress of prolonged hypothermia may be the prime determinant of mortality

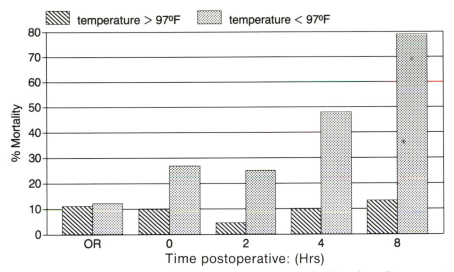

FIGURE 13–1. Temperature and mortality during and after surgery in 100 patients. Per cent mortality of those with temperatures greater than and less than 97°F during surgery and 0, 2, 4, and 8 hours postoperatively is depicted.

in critically ill surgical patients. Table 13–6 summarizes the consequences of hypothermia, by system.

PREVENTION AND TREATMENT OF HYPOTHERMIA

Medical personnel must recognize their role as patient advocates when monitoring a patient's body temperature. Because little can be done to increase heat production in the anesthetized patient, most efforts to prevent hypothermia are directed at limiting heat loss. Identification of patients at risk is the first priority. Table 13–7 lists surgical and patient conditions most commonly associated with hypothermia.

Minimizing Heat Loss

The greatest heat loss generally occurs during the first hour of anesthesia. In operating rooms at 21°C or less, mean body temperature has been shown to fall 1.3°C during the first hour but only 0.3°C during the second hour and 0.1°C during the third.[43] This loss may occur because of an initial redistribution of body heat from the core to the shell. As a result, heat loss increases, as the gradient between

TABLE 13–6. PHYSIOLOGIC CONSEQUENCES OF HYPOTHERMIA

Cardiovascular consequences
    Myocardial depression
    Ventricular arrhythmias
    Increased blood viscosity
    Decreased effective blood volume
    Increased pulmonary and systemic vascular resistance

Neurologic consequences
    Decreased cerebral blood flow
    Impaired mentation
    Hypothalamic dysfunction

Renal consequences
    Decreased renal perfusion
    Increased renin secretion
    Decreased tubular reabsorption, producing "cold diuresis"
    Acute tubular necrosis

Gastrointestinal consequences
    Decreased intestinal motility/ileus
    Susceptibility to ulcerative changes

Metabolic consequences
    Increased oxygen consumption
    Metabolic acidosis
    Decreased insulin production: hyperglycemia
    Electrolyte imbalances
    Altered hepatic clearing of substrates and drugs

Pulmonary consequences
    Depressed alveolar ventilation
    Alveolar edema
    Increased deadspace ventilation

TABLE 13–7. RISK FACTORS FOR PERIOPERATIVE HYPOTHERMIA

Patient factors
Age, especially neonates and patients ≥65 years
Burn victims
Major vascular or abdominal surgery
Paget's disease
Paraplegics and quadriplegics
Trauma victims
Exfoliative dermatitis
Surgical factors
Duration >3 hours
Blood loss
Major body cavities exposed
Infusion of cold fluids

skin and the environment is at its greatest during this period. Consequently, because of increased heat loss during the first hour, preventive measures against hypothermia should be initiated early.

There are several methods of minimizing heat loss perioperatively, as discussed in the following sections. Although all have been shown to be effective in certain situations, any one method alone may not be enough to adequately minimize heat loss. Consequently, combining these techniques as appropriate may be the most effective way of preventing hypothermia.[44]

Raise Ambient Temperature

Raising ambient temperature is perhaps the most effective way of minimizing heat loss. Morris[31] showed that a "critical ambient temperature" of 21°C exist for adults, regardless of whether surgery involves exposure of major body cavities. Patients in rooms below this temperature typically become hypothermic, whereas those in rooms above this temperature tend to maintain normothermia even after 2 hours of surgery. However, because OR personnel may not be comfortable if the ambient temperature is increased, maintaining room temperature at 22° to 24°C only until the patient is draped may be a reasonable compromise.[5]

Humidify Inspired Gases

A relation between warming and humidifying inspired gases and increased mean nasopharyngeal temperatures exists. Stone et al.[45] showed that heating and humidifying gases to 37°C and 100 per cent relative humidity effec-

tively maintains normothermia and warms hypothermic adults. Moreover, humidification of gases can reduce hourly heat loss up to 15 per cent.[46] On the other hand, several other studies have demonstrated that humidifying gases alone may not be adequate for controlling hypothermia.[32,44,47]

There are two ways to humidify gases: heat-moisture exchanges or electrically heated humidifiers. The most efficient heat-moisture exchangers provide absolute humidity of 28 to 32 mg $H_2O \cdot L^{-1}$ at 6 $L \cdot min^{-1}$.[48] These devices can collect mucus, which can cause increased resistance to airflow secondary to moisture trapping.[5]

Electrically heated humidifiers have been shown to be beneficial in clinical practice,[49] although bacterial contamination and electrical hazards such as overheating are potential shortcomings of these devices.[5]

It is important to remember that inspired temperatures must be monitored carefully with these devices. Inspired gas temperatures exceeding 43.3°C can lead to tracheal hyperemia and burns.[50]

Blood and Fluid Warmers

It has been demonstrated that 2 U of blood infused at 4°C can lower core temperature by 0.5°C.[5] In fact, rapid infusion of 10 U of blood has resulted in cardiac arrest due to hypothermia.[5]

An ideal blood warmer provides blood at temperatures above 32°C and at flow rates above 150 $ml \cdot min^{-1}$.[51] In addition to avoiding hypothermia, warming blood has other advantages, including venodilatation and a reduction in its viscosity by more than twofold.[51]

On the other hand, warming fluids and blood alone is often inadequate for controlling hypothermia. For example, low flow rates and long extension tubing allow the temperature of the fluid to approach room temperature. Despite the advantages of warming blood discussed above, there are disadvantages, including the potential of hemolysis at temperatures above 45°C. If the infusion rate of warmed blood is too slow, the risk of bacterial contamination increases because bacteria grow more readily in a warm environment.[51]

Warming Blankets

A warming blanket (thermal mattress heated by water that circulates at temperatures up to 41°C) can reduce conductive heat loss from the patient to the underlying mattress. However, in procedures lasting up to 3 hours, Morris and Kumar[52] found no difference in the esophageal temperatures of control patients and patients on warming blankets. Potential reasons for this finding include the small surface area of the body exposed to the blanket, the fact that sheets were interposed for safety, and the possibility that peripheral vasoconstriction impaired the blanket's effectiveness as a heat exchanger. In addition, it is important to remember that third-degree thermal burns can occur if these devices are improperly used.[53]

Reflective Blankets

The effectiveness of reflective blankets (metallized plastic sheeting) is controversial. A reflective blanket alone may[4] or may not[54] be able to halt the development of hypothermia.

Rewarming the Core

Research has shown that, after a severe reduction in body temperature, core rather than shell rewarming may be most beneficial. In theory, rapid external rewarming may cause the cold acidotic blood that has pooled in the periphery to shunt centrally. This action can further lower core temperature and pH and precipitate arrhythmias. This phenomenon is called "afterdrop." Therefore active core rewarming may be safer than external rewarming if core temperature is less than 32°C.[8]

Core rewarming techniques include instillation of body-temperature saline at nasogastric, peritoneal, or thoracic sites. The goal of therapy should be a maximal temperature rise of 0.5°C per hour to avoid rapid return to the central circulation of blood from cold extremities.

POSTOPERATIVE EVALUATION

During the postoperative period the patient's risk status and core temperature dictate management procedures. Generally, minimizing continuing heat loss and providing external heat are the primary considerations in the recovery room. Care must be taken when rewarming patients postoperatively because peripheral vasodilation in a patient who has lost blood can lead to acute hypotension.

If core temperature is 33° to 36°C, a healthy patient can be extubated. However, the el-

derly or patients with cardiac or respiratory problems may require elective ventilation with paralysis to prevent shivering. Appropriate management methods include warming infusions, warming blankets, and an overhead radiant warmer.

At core temperature below 33°C, reduced cardiac output, arrhythmias, and central nervous system impairment become increasingly likely. Patients with this core temperature should be electively ventilated with warmed humidified gases and have their electrocardiogram monitored. Warming blankets and other external measures should be utilized and, if necessary, core rewarming measures implemented as well.

HYPOTHERMIA—SUMMARY

Patient hypothermia is a serious but preventable consequence of surgery. Medical personnel can have a significant impact in the prevention or reversal of inadvertent hypothermia by becoming aware of the causative factors, the patients at risk, and the preventive measures available. Some rewarming methods are more effective than others, but minimizing heat loss is best accomplished when several techniques are used simultaneously.

HYPERTHERMIA

By definition, hyperthermia occurs at any core body temperature above normal. Severe, clinically significant hyperthermia results when core temperature exceeds 40°C (104°F). Though not as common perioperatively as hypothermia, hyperthermia is nevertheless a serious complication of surgery.

Postoperative fever should be distinguished from other hyperthermic syndromes. There is a fundamental difference between fever and specific hyperthermic states. In nonfever hyperthermic states, body temperature rises above normal despite the body's heat-dissipating mechanisms (e.g., vasodilation and sweating). Therefore excessive heat gain, secondary to either internal or external factors, exceeds the body's cooling capabilities with a consequent rise in body temperature.

In contrast, fever results from a resetting to a higher temperature from the normal set point. Until the body reaches its new set point temperature, heat-generating mechanisms (shivering, vasoconstriction) are activated.

Once the new set point temperature is reached, there is an equilibrium between heat generation and heat loss. Unlike hyperthermia, with fever there is no physiologic activity to bring body temperature back to normal.

Whereas physical cooling is an appropriate therapy for most hyperthermias, such measures used to treat fever may be resisted physiologically and may distress the patient.[56]

CAUSES OF PERIOPERATIVE HYPERTHERMIA

There are many factors that can contribute to raising core body temperature during the perioperative period.

Blood transfusions
Warm environment
Drug-induced fever
Use of anticholinergics
Infection
Overuse of techniques to prevent hypothermia
Endocrine disorders
Hypothalamic injury
Malignant hyperthermia

In addition, hyperthermia may occur with hypothalamic injury, severe infection, or endocrinopathy. It often follows blood transfusions, even when the donor blood is sterile and properly matched.[57] Overuse of heating methods to prevent hypothermia can actually result in hyperthermia.

Drug-induced hyperthermia is also common. Hyperthermia resulting from heat stress can occur during anesthesia, for instance, particularly if high doses of atropine or other anticholinergics are used for premedication.[58] Atropine, along with its central thermoregulating inhibitory effect, blocks the cholinergic innervation of sweat glands and, by preventing heat loss from sweating, leads to a rise in body temperature. (*Note:* Atropine-induced hyperthermia is different from the fever that results from drug reactions; see below.)

A serious, though rare, form of drug-induced hyperthermia is malignant hyperthermia, in which a genetic defect predisposes patients, given certain triggering agents (i.e., succinylcholine or volatile anesthetics), to develop catastrophic hyperthermia.[59,60] Thyroid storm and pheochromocytoma may be difficult to distinguish from malignant hyperthermia in the anesthetized patient, and they may also produce hyperthermic conditions. Malignant hyperthermia is discussed in detail in Chapter 16.

NEUROGENIC HYPERTHERMIA

Neurogenic hyperthermia occurs when increased body temperature results from lesions in the centromedial forebrain around the third ventricle. This condition has been observed with cranial trauma, cerebral emboli, neurosurgical intervention, expansive intracranial tumors, and thromboses of the cerebral venous sinuses. Rudy[61] suggested that prostaglandins released from the injured tissue act on the surviving tissues of the anterior hypothalamus preoptic region. This report supports evidence that prostaglandins play an important role in the development of fever.

Neurogenic hyperthermia is resistant to traditional antipyretic treatment. However, indomethacin, which is rarely used as an antipyretic, has been shown to be effective in treating this condition.[62]

FEVER

As mentioned, fever is a form of hyperthermia in which body temperature rises above normal in a regulated way. During fever, thermoregulation occurs as if the set point temperature had been reset upward. The patient may seek heat, for example, and may undergo a rise in metabolic rate and vasoconstriction and a reduction in sweating. All of these responses produce an increase in body temperature.

Fever has been shown to be beneficial in many ways. It appears to play a major role in the body's defense against infection. Survival of those with infection correlates with the presence of moderate fever. Furthermore, leukocyte function and antibody production are enhanced by elevated body temperature. Mackowiak[63] reported that high body temperature reduces bacterial growth rate and may increase resistance to viral infections by interrupting virus reproduction.

Fever is a response to circulating pyrogens in the body. These pyrogens are released by leukocytes that have been activated by viruses, bacteria, fungi, antigens, or tissue debris. The pyrogens are believed to induce the release of prostaglandins, which appear to play a crucial role in the initiation of fever. Fever has been shown to be associated with increased hypothalamic levels of prostaglandins E_1 and E_2.[55] Prostaglandins in turn act on the neurons in the preoptic area of the hypothalamus, a process that causes core body temperature to be reset higher.

Postoperative fevers are common. Possible causes are as follows.

Atelectasis
Dehydration
Wound infection
Blood transfusion reaction
Abscess formation
CNS damage
Fat emboli following bone trauma
Pneumonia
Urinary tract infection
Drug reaction
Phlebitis/deep vein thrombosis
Malignancy
Pulmonary emboli
Silent aspiration

A slight rise in core body temperature is part of the normal inflammatory response to the surgical insult. Patients often have temperatures of 38.9°C during the first 24 to 48 hours after open heart surgery, for example, because of the inflammatory response to tissue damage.[64]

Fever during the first 24 hours after surgery is generally caused by poor respiratory ventilation and resulting atelectasis, which is associated with tachypnea and abnormal auscultatory findings. Pneumonia can result if atelectasis is allowed to progress. Another possible cause is undetected silent aspiration of gastric contents during the perioperative period.

Fever commonly results from blood transfusion reactions, which occur during or immediately after the transfusion. Reactions frequently result from major incompatibility between donor and recipient, leukocyte reactions, or contamination. The cause of fever is often easier to determine in conscious postoperative patients who are receiving or have just received a transfusion because of the presence of other signs and symptoms. See Chapter 15 for further discussion on transfusion reactions.

Drug reactions are often overlooked as a cause of fever, yet they can account for 10 per cent of fevers in hospitalized patients.[65] Symptoms of drug-induced fever include a maculopapular rash on the soles and palms, bradycardia, negative blood cultures, and a patient who feels well despite a high temperature.

Generalized sepsis or localized infections may be responsible for fever as well. The evaluation, appropriate cultures and laboratory tests, and therapy are discussed in Chapter 21.

THERAPY

Hyperthermia

Primary therapy for hyperthermia includes cooling and decreasing thermogenesis. Cooling by either evaporative or direct external methods has proved effective. Evaporative cooling may be accomplished by placing a nude patient in a cool room, wetting the skin with cool water, and using fans to enhance evaporation.

Direct external cooling involves immersing the patient in ice water or packing the patient in ice. Although highly effective, direct external cooling is inconvenient for patient monitoring and management. Consequently, evaporative cooling may be most beneficial, especially for patients at high risk of cardiovascular collapse.

If these methods fail to reduce body temperature, peritoneal lavage with iced saline, gastric lavage or hemodialysis or cardiopulmonary bypass, with external cooling of the blood, may be required.

Malignant Hyperthermia

For a detailed description of therapeutic measures for malignant hyperthermia, see Chapter 16.

Fever

Although physical cooling is an appropriate therapy for other hyperthermias, attempts to cool a febrile patient may be resisted by the thermoregulatory system.[56] Consequently, the first course of action is to restore normothermia with the use of antipyretic drugs. Aspirin and other antipyretics are useful because they have the ability to prevent prostaglandin synthesis in the hypothalamus. Antipyretics may be the only therapy necessary for febrile adults and most children, although sponging with tepid water may be of additional assistance. Note that cold water and alcohol should be avoided: Cold water causes shivering, and alcohol has dangerous fumes and can be absorbed through the skin.

Certain measures may be used to manage the febrile patient.

1. Use antipyretics, if indicated.[63,66]
2. Sponge or bathe with tepid water.[67]
3. Keep the environment cool.
4. Cover the patient with a loincloth or a wet sheet.[67]

5. Use a hypothermia blanket for sustained fever.
6. Monitor the fluid and electrolyte balance, as fluid needs increase during fever.

Note: For a detailed discussion of antibiotic therapy for infectious causes of fever, see Chapter 21.

SUMMARY

Although less common perioperatively than hypothermia, hyperthermia is nevertheless a serious complication of surgery. It is important to note that there is a fundamental difference between specific hyperthermic states and fever. Consequently, therapeutic measures that are effective for most hyperthermias may not be appropriate for fever. It is important that medical personnel become aware of this distinction and its implications for therapy.

CONCLUSION

Many factors can disrupt normal thermoregulation during the perioperative period. However, careful temperature monitoring and early therapeutic intervention can have a significant positive impact in patients at risk for perioperative hypothermia or hyperthermia. By understanding the physiology of temperature control, the causes of body temperature alterations, and appropriate treatment options, medical personnel can utilize this information to truly benefit many patients as they journey through this stressful perioperative period.

ACKNOWLEDGMENT. The author thanks Ken Ganzer for his assistance in preparing this manuscript.

References

1. Slotman FJ, Jed EH, Burchard KW: Adverse effects of hypothermia in postoperative patients. Am J Surg *149*:499, 1985.
2. Moss J: Accidental severe hypothermia. Surg Gynecol Obstet *162*:501–513, 1986.
3. Brengelman G: Temperature regulation. *In* Ruch TC, Patton HD (eds): Physiology and Biophysics: Digestion, Metabolism, Endocrine Function and Reproduction, 20th ed. Philadelphia, Saunders, 1979, p. 109.
4. Bourke DL: Intraoperative heat conservation using a reflective blanket. Anesthesiology *60*:151–154, 1984.
5. Morley-Forster PK: Unintentional hypothermia in the operating room. Can Anaesth Soc J *33*:516–527, 1986.
6. Saidman LJ, Harvard ES, Eger EI: Hyperthermia during anesthesia. JAMA *190*:1029–1032, 1964.
7. Fallacaro MD, Fallacaro NA, Radel TJ: Inadvertent hypothermia. AORN J *44*:54–61, 1986.
8. Reuler JB: Hypothermia: pathophysiology, clinical settings and management. Ann Intern Med *89*:519–527, 1978.
9. Bay J, Nunn JF, Prys Roberts C: Factors influencing arterial PO_2 during recovery from anaesthesia. Br J Anaesth *40*:398–407, 1968
10. Roe C: The influence of body temperature on early postoperative oxygen consumption. Surgery *60*:85–92, 1966.
11. Vaughan MS, Vaughan RW, Cork RC: Postoperative hypothermia in adults: relationship of age, anesthesia and shivering to rewarming. Anesth Analg *60*:746–751, 1981.
12. Prys Roberts C: Postanesthesia shivering. In Artusio JF (ed): Clinical Anesthesia. Philadelphia, Davis, 1968, p. 358.
13. Elder PT: Accidental hypothermia. *In* Shoemaker WC, Thompson WL, Holbrook (eds): Textbook of Critical Care. Philadelphia, Saunders, 1984, pp. 85–93.
14. Blainey CG: Site selection in taking body temperature. Am J Nurs *74*:1859–1861, 1974
15. Whitby JD, Dunkin LJ: Temperature differences in the oesophagus. Br J Anaesth *40*:991–995, 1968.
16. Whitby JD, Dunkin LJ: Cerebral oesophageal and nasopharyngeal temperatures. Br J Anaesth *43*:673–676, 1971.
17. Rawson RO, Hammel HT: Hypothalamic and tympanic membrane temperatures in rhesus monkeys. Fed Proc *22*:283, 1963.
18. Benzinger M: Tympanic thermometry in surgery and anesthesia. JAMA *209*:1207–1211, 1969.
19. Moorthy SS, Winn BA, Jallard MS, et al: Monitoring urinary bladder temperature. Heart Lung *14*:90–93, 1985.
20. Cork RC, Vaughan RW, Humphrey LS: Precision and accuracy of intraoperative temperature monitoring. Anesth Analg *62*:211–214, 1983.
21. Burgess GE, et al: Continuous monitoring of skin temperature using a liquid-crystal thermometer during anesthesia. South Med J *71*:516–518, 1978.
22. Vaughan MS, Cork RC, Vaughan RW: Inaccuracy of liquid crystal thermometry to identify core temperature trends in postoperative adults. Anesth Analg *61*:284–287, 1982.
23. Lacoumenta S, Hall GM: Liquid crystal thermometry during anesthesia. Anesthesia *39*:54–56, 1984.
24. Ilsley AH, Rutten AJ, Runciman WB: An evaluation of body temperature measurement. Anaesth Intens Care *11*:31–39, 1983.
25. Tandberg D, Sklar D: Effect of tachypnea on the estimation of body temperature by an oral thermometer. Med Intell *308*:945–946, 1983.
26. Flacke JW, Flacke WE: Inadvertent hypothermia: frequent, insidious and often serious. Semin Anesth *2*:183, 1983.
27. Heymann AD: The effect of incidental hypothermia on elderly surgical patients. Gerontology *32*:46–48, 1977
28. Ozuna JM, Foster C: Hypothermia and the surgical patient. Am J Nurs *79*:646–648, 1978.
29. Kanto WP, Calvert LJ: Thermoregulation of the newborn. Am Fam Physician *16*:157–163, 1977.
30. Morris RH, Wilkey BR: The effects of ambient temperature on patient temperature during surgery not involving body cavities. Anesthesiology *32*:102–107, 1970.
31. Morris RH: Influence of ambient temperature on pa-

tient temperature during intraabdominal surgery. Ann Surg *173*:230–233, 1971.

32. Joachimsson PO, Hedstrand U, Tabow F, et al: Prevention of intraoperative hypothermia during abdominal surgery. Acta Anesthesiol Scand *31*:330–337, 1987.

33. Caldwell PRB, Gomez DM, Fritts HW: Respiratory heat exchange in normal subjects and in patients with pulmonary disease. J Appl Physiol *26*:82–88, 1969.

34. Workhoven MN: Intravenous fluid temperature, shivering and the parturient. Anesth Analg *65*:496–498, 1986.

35. Rose JC, McDermott TF, Lilienfield LS, et al: Cardiovascular function in hypothermic anesthetized man. Circulation *15*:512–517, 1957.

36. Curry DL, Curry KP: Hypothermia and insulin secretion. Endocrinology 87:750–755, 1970.

37. Boyan CP, Howland WS: Blood temperature: a critical factor in massive transfusion. Anesthesiology *22*:559–563, 1961.

38. Hervey GR: Hypothermia. Proc R Soc Med Lond [Biol] *66*:1053–1057, 1973.

39. Welton DE, Mattox KL, Miller RR, et al: Treatment of profound hypothermia. JAMA *240*:2291–2292, 1978.

40. Paton BC: Accidental hypothermia. Pharmacol Ther *22*:377, 1983.

41. Jones HD, McLaren CAB: Postoperative shivering and hypoxaemia after halothane, nitrous oxide and oxygen anaesthesia. Br J Anaesth *37*:35–41, 1965.

42. Holdcroft A: Body temperature control. In Anaesthesia, Surgery and Intensive Care. London, Ballière Tindall, 1980, p. 80.

43. Morris RH: Operating room temperature and the anesthetized, paralyzed patient. Arch Surg *102*:95–97, 1971.

44. Shanks CA, Ronai AK, Schafer MF: The effects of airway heat conservation and skin surface insulation on thermal balance during spinal surgery. Anesthesiology *69*:956–958, 1988.

45. Stone DR, Downs JB, Paul WL, et al: Adult body temperature and heated humidification of anesthetic gases during general anesthesia. Anesth Analg *60*:736–741, 1981.

46. Shanks CA: Humidification and loss of body heat during anaesthesia. 1. Quantification and correlation in the dog. Br J Anaesth *46*:859–862, 1974.

47. Hendrickx HHL, Trahey GE: Paradoxical inhibition of decrease in body temperature by use of heated and humidified gases. Anesth Analg *61*:393–394, 1982

48. Weeks DB, Ramsey FM: Laboratory investigation of six artificial noses for use during endotracheal anesthesia. Anesth Analg *62*:758–763, 1983.

49. Tausk HC, Miller R, Roberts RB: Maintenance of body temperature by heated humidification. Anesth Analg *55*:719–723, 1976.

50. Klein EF Jr, Graves SE: Hot pot tracheitis. Chest 65:225–226, 1974.

51. Russell WJ: A review of blood warmers for massive transfusion. Anaesth Intens Care 2:109–130, 1974.

52. Morris RH, Kumar A: The effect of warming blankets on maintenance of body temperature of the anesthetized, paralyzed adult patient. Anesthesiology *36*:408–411, 1972.

53. Crino MH, Nagel EL: Thermal burns caused by warming blankets in operating room. Anesthesiology *29*:149–150, 1968.

54. Radford P, Thurlow AC: Metallized plastic sheeting in the prevention of hypothermia during neurosurgery. Br J Anaesth *51*:237–239, 1979.

55. Curley FJ, Irwin RS: Disorders of temperature control. Part 1. Hyperthermia. J Intens Care Med *1*:5–14, 1986.

56. Mitchell D, Laburn HP: Pathophysiology of temperature regulation. Physiologist *28*:507–517, 1985.

57. Roe CF: Temperature regulation and energy metabolism in surgical patients. Prog Surg *12*:96–127, 1973.

58. Fraser JG: Iatrogenic benign hyperthermia in children. Anesthesiology *48*:375, 1978.

59. Aldrete JA: Advances in the diagnosis and treatment of malignant hyperthermia. Acta Anaesthesiol Scand 25:477–483, 1981.

60. Haber J, Hammer DJ, Butler B: Malignant hyperthermia. JAPA *73*:442, 1983.

61. Rudy TA: Studies of fever associated with cerebral trauma and intracranial hemorrhage in experimental animals. *In* Lipton JM (ed): Fever. New York, Raven Press, 1980, pp. 165–175.

62. Benedek G, Toth-Daru P, Janaky J, et al: Indomethacin is effective against neurogenic hyperthermia following cranial trauma or brain surgery. Can J Neurol Sci *14*:145–148, 1987.

63. Mackowiak PA: Direct effects of hyperthermia on pathogenic microorganisms teleologic implications with regard to fever. Rev Infect Dis *3*:508, 1981.

64. Gurevich I: Infectious complications in open heart surgery. Heart Lung *13*:47–55, 1984.

65. Cunha BA, Digamon-Beltran M: Implications of fever in the critical care setting. Heart Lung *13*:460, 1984.

66. Bernheim HA, Block LH, Atkins E: Fever pathogenesis, physiology, and purpose. Ann Intern Med *91*:261, 1979.

67. Castle M, Watkins J: Fever: understanding a sinister sign. Nursing *9*(2): 27, 1979.

14 POSTOPERATIVE ENDOCRINE PROBLEMS

SALLY A. KRAFT, FREDERICK G. MIHM,
and THOMAS W. FEELEY

This chapter reviews the pathophysiology, diagnosis, and treatment of several common endocrine disorders seen following surgery and anesthesia. The chapter first focuses on abnormalities of glucose metabolism, as the high prevalence of diabetes mellitus brings many patients with this disorder to surgery. Thyroid abnormalities are then reviewed followed by sections on adrenocortical insufficiency, pheochromocytoma, and carcinoid.

ABNORMALITIES OF GLUCOSE METABOLISM

HYPERGLYCEMIA

Surgical stress and trauma initiate a number of metabolic responses that result in elevated serum glucose levels. These responses serve to enhance survival by promoting glucose availability to the brain, which requires glucose as an energy substrate. Other beneficial effects of hyperglycemia may include initial restitution of intravascular volume secondary to increased osmolality and delivery of energy substrate to injured tissue.[1]

Hyperglycemia is common during the perioperative period and generally does not require treatment in the nondiabetic patient. However, the metabolic responses promoting hyperglycemia may cause decompensation in the diabetic patient and could potentially result in life-threatening diabetic ketoacidosis (DKA) or hyperosmolar hyperglycemia nonketotic syndrome (HHNS). Physicians caring for patients during the postoperative period must be able to identify the hyperglycemic patient who requires immediate intervention and initiate therapeutic modalities.

DKA AND HHNS

Diabetes mellitus is the most common endocrine disorder, affecting 2 to 5 per cent of the population.[2] It is estimated that 50 per cent of diabetic persons will undergo a surgical procedure in their lifetime.[3] Multiple factors during the perioperative period predispose the diabetic patient to metabolic decompensation including infection, dehydration, and reduced caloric intake, as well as physiologic responses to the stress of surgery. DKA and HHNS represent the extremes of decompensated diabetes and are fatal if not recognized and appropriately treated.

Pathophysiology

The pathophysiology of DKA and HHNS is similar (Fig. 14–1). Both conditions arise from a relative insulin deficiency. With DKA, a myriad of metabolic derangements arising from insulin deficiency result in two abnormalities of central importance: hyperglycemia and ketogenesis. Hyperglycemia causes glucosuria and an osmotic diuresis, and ketogenesis produces metabolic acidosis. With HHNS, hyperglycemia is the predominant abnormality; ketogenesis, if present, is mild. The metabolic perturbations of DKA are outlined first.

With DKA, hepatic glycogenolysis and gluconeogenesis result in hyperglycemia. Early in this process, glucose produced by the liver comes from the breakdown of glycogen stores. Glycogen is rapidly depleted, and sustained hepatic glucose production continues by gluconeogenesis. Decreased insulin concentrations result in an increased glucagon/insulin ratio in portal venous blood, which is a major stimulus for hepatic glucose production.

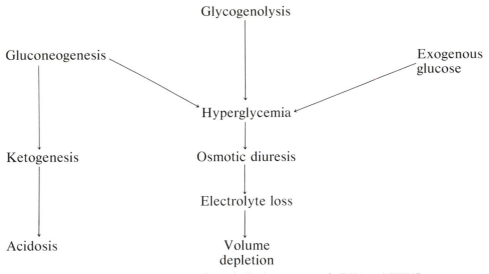

FIGURE 14–1. Overview of metabolic derangements in DKA and HHNS.

Glucagon modulates the rate of gluconeogenesis by reducing the hepatic enzyme fructose 2,6-diphosphate.[4] Peripheral proteins are broken down to amino acids, which are used by the liver to produce glucose at an average rate of 42 mg/min.[5] Glucagon, epinephrine, growth hormone, norepinephrine, and cortisol are secreted in response to stress and are referred to as counterregulatory hormones. Secretion of these hormones results in increased glucose production and diminished glucose clearance. Insulin-dependent diabetics exhibit an exaggerated hyperglycemic response to these hormones, further increasing plasma glucose concentrations in DKA.[6]

Elevated plasma glucose levels exceed the renal glucose threshold, resulting in glucosuria and an osmotic diuresis. Typically, patients with DKA have a 5- to 10-liter water deficit and average sodium and potassium deficits of 500 mEq and 300 to 1000 mEq, respectively.[5] Chloride, magnesium, and phosphorus are also lost. Volume depletion exacerbates hyperglycemia by reducing renal glucose clearance.

Ketoacidosis results from excess production of ketones in the liver and decreased metabolism of ketones in the periphery. Fatty acids are mobilized from adipocytes during insulin deficiency. An increased glucagon/insulin ratio induces hepatic enzymatic changes, which promote oxidation of fatty acids rather than reesterification to triglycerides.[4] Hepatic levels of carnitine are increased, and the concentration of malonyl coenzyme A is decreased, promoting the oxidation of fatty acids

and increased production of acetoacetic acid and β-hydroxybutyric acid.[7] These strong acids dissociate at physiologic pH and are buffered by the bicarbonate system to acetoacetate and β-hydroxybutyrate. Continued acid production overwhelms buffering capacity, and acidemia develops.

In summary, insulin deficiency and an elevated glucagon/insulin ratio result in increased hepatic glucose production, hyperglycemia, and subsequent osmotic diuresis. Increased ketogenesis results in metabolic acidosis. Release of counterregulatory hormones further promotes hepatic glucose production and induces an insulin-resistant state. Untreated, these metabolic derangements progress to a fatal outcome.

The pathophysiology of HHNS is similar to that of DKA except that significant ketogenesis does not develop. Patients who develop HHNS typically have mild diabetes and a "relative" insulin deficiency, rather than the absolute deficiency present in insulin-dependent diabetics. It has been postulated that hepatic insulin concentrations may be high enough to prevent ketogenesis but not high enough to prevent increased hepatic glucose production.[8] Trace ketones may be present with HHNS, but significant metabolic acidosis is ascribed to lactic acidosis or increased concentrations of other organic acids.[9]

Clinical Features

Although the pathophysiologic changes of DKA and HHNS are similar, clinical presentations of these two entities tend to differ. Classically, the patient with DKA is younger and has previously been diagnosed with insulin-requiring diabetes. Conversely, only 32 to 66 per cent of patients with HHNS are known diabetics prior to the onset of HHNS,[10,11] and in general these patients have mild diabetes that can be controlled by diet alone or an oral hypoglycemic drug.[12] In general, the patient with HHNS is older, the average age ranging from 57 to 69 years.[12] Onset of DKA is usually abrupt; common precipitating factors include infection, myocardial infarction, trauma, and failure to receive insulin during stress.[7] Onset of HHNS is generally insidious, developing over days to weeks. Acute infection is a common precipitant of HHNS, and surgery has been reported to precipitate HHNS.[10] Drugs precipitating HHNS have been recognized and include thiazide diuretics, phenytoin, steroids, and total parenteral nutrition and enteral feedings.[9,11] The mortality rate associated with DKA is 6 to 10 per cent[4] but is significantly higher with HHNS (17 to 50 per cent),[10,13] probably reflecting the elderly population with this disorder.

The clinical features of classic DKA or HHNS are usually dramatic and easy to recognize, but during the postoperative period many of the classic signs and symptoms may be altered by the preceding surgery and anesthetic. Hypovolemia, present with both DKA and HHNS, will have been treated to some extent by intraoperative fluid administration. Vomiting, which has been reported to occur in as many as 69 per cent of patients with DKA,[14] could be ascribed to a number of causes in the postoperative patient. Neurologic changes are common with both DKA and HHNS but are also common during the acute postoperative

period. Neurologic changes in patients presenting with DKA are usually mild. Forty per cent of patients are fully conscious and an equal per cent are stuporous,[7] although only 5 to 10 per cent of patients are comatose.[4,7] With HHNS, most of the patients are lethargic or confused, and the incidence of coma varies between 27 and 50 per cent.[13] Mild neurologic changes are common during the postoperative period and may not be recognized as symptoms of an underlying disease. It is of note that focal neurologic disturbances are relatively common with HHNS, occurring in as many as 20 per cent of these patients.[12] Seizures can occur and may be generalized or focal. It is important to recognize this complication, as phenytoin impairs insulin release and could exacerbate the metabolic abnormalities.[9] Seizures resolve with appropriate therapy for HHNS.[12]

Though clinical features of DKA or HHNS may be atypical during the postoperative period, laboratory examinations can be helpful for defining these syndromes (Table 14–1). Hyperglycemia is present to varying degrees. With HHNS, hyperglycemia may be dramatic, with plasma glucose concentrations averaging 1000 mg/dl.[13] The average glucose concentration in DKA patients is 500 mg/dl but may be nearly normal.[13] Acidosis is severe in those with DKA (mean arterial pH 7.07), but it tends to be mild, if present at all, in HHNS patients (mean pH 7.26).[8] The anion gap—($[Na]$ + $[K]$ − ($[Cl]$ + [total CO_2]))—is elevated (>12) in patients with DKA owing to the accumulation of acetoacetic and β-hydroxybutyric acids.

Serum ketones are present in DKA patients at 1:2 or higher dilutions[7] but are generally absent in HHNS patients or present in only

TABLE 14–1. LABORATORY EXAMINATIONS FOR THE DIFFERENTIAL DIAGNOSIS OF DKA AND HHNS

Diagnosis	Plasma Glucose	pH	Serum Ketones	Anion Gap	Osmolality
DKA	+ +	− − −	+ + +	+ +	+
HHNS	+ + +	−	N or +	N	+ + +
Alcoholic ketoacidosis	N or −	+ or −	+	+	N
Salicylate intoxication	N or −	+ or −	N or +	+	N
Starvation	N	N	+	+	N
Lactic acidosis	N	− − −	N	+	N

+ = increased; − = decreased; N = normal.

trace amounts. The nitroprusside reagent reacts with acetoacetate and not β-hydroxybutyrate. With severe DKA, the β-hydroxybutyrate/acetoacetate ratio is increased, and the apparently small degree of ketonemia may appear inconsistent with the severe acidemia. As acidemia is corrected, this ratio decreases and the reaction may become stronger; hence the laboratory measurement of ketonemia may worsen as the patient improves clinically.[2]

Serum sodium levels may be reduced secondary to hyperglycemia or hypertriglyceridemia. A general rule of thumb is that there is an expected serum sodium decrease of 1.6 mEq/L for every 100 mg/dl increment in serum glucose above a baseline 100 mg/dl.[15] Serum potassium in DKA patients may be normal or high owing to the acidosis promoting a shift of potassium from the intracellular to the extracellular space. A low serum potassium level in the setting of significant acidosis is an ominous sign, suggesting massive potassium losses.

Serum osmolality is usually elevated above 350 mOsm/kg in patients with HHNS, whereas patients with DKA generally have lower osmolalities.[13] Serum osmolality is calculated by the following formula.[16]

$$mOsm/kg \ H_2O = 2 \times sodium \\ + glucose/18 + BUN/2.8$$

where BUN = blood urea nitrogen. (Normal serum osmolality 286 ± 4 mOsm/kg of water.)

Patients with DKA usually present earlier in the course of their disease owing to the consequences of acidosis. In the elderly population with HHNS, the clinical course tends to be insidious, and a prolonged period may pass before the patient comes to medical attention. This protracted period of ongoing osmotic diuresis leads to the development of the extreme hyperosmolar state in these patients.

Differential Diagnosis

History, clinical features, and laboratory values should help differentiate DKA from HHNS (Table 14–1). Alcoholic ketoacidosis may present in a manner similar to that of DKA. Patients usually do not have significant blood alcohol levels, as ketoacidosis typically occurs after a chronic alcoholic has recently discontinued alcohol consumption. Serum glucose is generally not elevated in alcoholic ketoacidosis. Salicylate poisoning can resemble DKA, as the patient may have an increased anion gap acidosis with positive serum ketones.[5] However, glucose values are usually

normal in this condition. A report of intraoperative ketoacidosis developing in a malnourished patient illustrated similarities to patients with DKA.[17]

Treatment

The treatment of DKA and HHNS is similar. Occasionally, it is difficult to differentiate the patient with DKA from the patient with HHNS, but therapeutic strategies are common for both diseases. The goals of therapy are clear: correction of fluid, electrolyte, and metabolic abnormalities resulting from hyperglycemia and/or ketogenesis (Table 14–2).

Correction of hypovolemia and replacement of free water deficits are of paramount importance. Intravascular volume depletion exacerbates hyperglycemia by stimulating release of counterregulatory hormones and reducing renal glucose clearance. Rehydration, even in the absence of insulin administration, decreases serum glucose.[18] Typically, patients with DKA or HHNS have large fluid deficits, and intraoperative fluid administration may not have corrected these deficits. The volume of fluid required for resuscitation can be guided by clinical parameters (pulse, blood pressure, urine output) in the patient without cardiovascular, renal, or pulmonary disease but may require invasive monitoring of the central venous pressure or pulmonary artery pressure in the patient with concomitant disease. Debate continues as to the correct intravenous solution to use during resuscitation. In patients who are hypotensive owing to intravascular depletion, we recommend normal saline to replace the intravascular volume. Correction of free water deficit should occur more

TABLE 14–2. INITIAL TREATMENT OF DKA OR HHNS

1. Fluid: If patient is hypotensive, use normal saline or colloid to stabilize. After hypotension is corrected, replace free water deficit with 0.45% NaCl. Add dextrose when serum glucose equals 250 mg/dl.

2. Insulin: Regular insulin 10 U IV, then 0.1 U/kg/hr. Monitor serum glucose q1–2h. When plasma glucose equals 250 mg/dl, decrease insulin infusion to 1–3 U/hr.

3. Potassium: *If initial K^+ > 5.5 mEq/dl,* do not give potassium but monitor q1–2h. Anticipate decrease in K^+. Add 20–40 mEq to 1 liter of IV fluid as potassium falls and urine output is adequate.
   If initial K^+ < 3.5 mEq/dl, begin potassium administration immediately, 20–40 mEq/hr. Monitor q1–2h.

slowly over the following 24 to 48 hours with 0.5 N saline.

Insulin must be given by a dependable route. Intramuscular and subcutaneous absorption can be erratic: subcutaneous insulin absorption varies 25 per cent on a day-to-day basis even in nonstressed diabetic patients.[19] We recommend intravenous insulin for the acutely ill patient. Insulin binding by plastic tubing is not a significant problem, and albumin does not need to be added to the infusion. The goal of insulin therapy is to reduce the serum glucose concentration to 250 mg/dl and to continue insulin administration until the acidosis has cleared. Blood glucose measurements must be made frequently (every 1 to 2 hours) while the patient is being treated with an insulin infusion. Urine glucose assays are not adequate; serum must be used. Bedside glucose meters provide accurate glucose measurements reliably and quickly.

For patients with DKA or HHNS a typical insulin dosage is as follows: 10 U of regular insulin intravenously followed by an infusion of 0.1 U/kg/hr. The glucose concentration should fall by at least 10 per cent per hour. If plasma glucose levels do not respond to the initial insulin dose, the infusion rate should be doubled. Individual patient response should be appreciated. Dextrose should be added to the intravenous fluid when the serum glucose is 250 mg/dl and the insulin infusion decreased at that time to 1 to 3 U/hr.

Potassium supplementation is required in almost every case of DKA. If the serum potassium is low on initial evaluation, potassium therapy should be started immediately at an initial rate of 20 to 40 mEq/hr.[4] If the initial potassium level is higher than 5.5 mEq/dl, fluid and insulin therapy should be initiated and potassium levels checked frequently (every 1 to 2 hours). Potassium concentrations typically fall as the acidosis is corrected and glucose metabolism is normalized. Hyperchloremic acidosis commonly occurs in DKA patients owing to the retention of chloride and excretion of ketone salts.[20] By replacing some of the potassium deficit with potassium phosphate, rather than potassium chloride, exogenous chloride is decreased. Although phosphate stores are frequently depleted in DKA, phospate replacement has not been shown to have clinical benefit.[21]

Bicarbonate therapy in DKA remains controversial. One prospective study[22] examining the use of bicarbonate in patients with DKA and initial arterial pH values of 6.9 to 7.4 found that bicarbonate did not affect recovery or outcome. Certainly, if cardiac decompensation occurs in an acidotic patient, bicarbonate therapy is justified, otherwise in a patient with DKA and an arterial pH of more than 7.1, routine use of bicarbonate is not recommended.

The most common complication of treatment is hypoglycemia. It is imperative that glucose measurements be made frequently and accurate bedside methods utilized to prevent time lags secondary to "laboratory turnaround." Hypokalemia is another frequent therapeutic mishap, and potassium supplementation should be started early in anticipation of the fall in the serum potassium level as DKA is treated. Cerebral edema is rare in both conditions but has a high mortality if it does occur. Maintaining serum glucose concentrations at approximately 250 mg/dl may prevent this complication by preventing too vigorous a correction in serum osmolality.

Hyperglycemia not due to DKA or HHNS is common during the postoperative period due to the normal metabolic responses to stress. After ketoacidosis and HHNS have been ruled out, the decision to treat hyperglycemia is based on several factors. Patients previously treated with insulin certainly require insulin postoperatively. In general, if patients are not able to eat, intravenous solutions should contain dextrose, and short-acting regular insulin should be used to allow flexible control. Subcutaneous insulin can be used in the stable patient, but intravenous delivery should be utilized if patients are critically ill in order to avoid erratic absorption from the subcutaneous depot. In uncomplicated diabetic patients, blood glucose should be checked every 4 to 6 hours and insulin administered as outlined in Table 14–3. In unstable patients requiring intravenous insulin, blood glucose levels must be checked every 1 to 2 hours. A plasma glucose concentration of

TABLE 14–3. REGULAR INSULIN DOSAGE FOR STABLE DIABETIC PATIENTS

Plasma Glucose (mg/dl)	Regular Insulin (U)
200–250	5
250–350	10
350–400	15
>400	Assess patient; rule out DKA or HHNS

150 to 250 mg/dl is a reasonable goal, as tighter control exposes the patient to the risks of hypoglycemia.

Patients with mild diabetes treated preoperatively with oral hypoglycemic agents or diet alone may require insulin during the postoperative period, particularly if undergoing a major surgical procedure or if the postoperative course is complicated. The route of administration (subcutaneous, intramuscular, or intravenous) depends on the condition of the patient. If the patient has undergone a minor surgical procedure and will soon be resuming a normal diet and oral hypoglycemic agent, plasma glucose concentrations up to 250 mg/dl are well tolerated and do not require therapy. Plasma concentrations above this level may simply require removal of glucose from intravenous fluids or subcutaneous insulin until oral therapy has been resumed.

HYPOGLYCEMIA

Hypoglycemia is defined as a plasma glucose concentration of less than 50 mg/dl. Hemorrhagic shock, pancreatitis, sepsis, renal failure, and alcoholism have been associated with hypoglycemia.[23] In one review, hypoglycemia was documented in 1.2 per cent of hospitalized adults over a 6-month period.[24] Failure to diagnose and treat hypoglycemia may result in irreversible central nervous system damage (see Chapter 12). During the postoperative period, special vigilance is required, as medications may mask the signs and symptoms of hypoglycemia.

Although hypoglycemia can occur in any patient, several factors identify a population at high risk. Patients with diabetes are at particular risk as a result of inappropriate insulin doses.[24] Fasting prior to surgery places diabetic patients at greater risk if insulin doses have not been appropriately modified. Renal insufficiency, which commonly results from diabetic nephropathy, is frequently associated with hypoglycemia due to several mechanisms, including increased insulin half-life.[24] Patients receiving total parenteral nutrition (TPN) frequently require concomitant insulin therapy and are at risk for hypoglycemia if the insulin dose is incorrect. Also, acute discontinuation of TPN can result in hypoglycemia, a complication that can be avoided by tapering the TPN infusion over several hours or administering a 10 per cent dextrose solution when the TPN has finished. Many drugs can cause hypoglycemia, including alcohol, salicylates, haloperidol, propanolol, and propoxyphene.[25]

Clinical Features

The most dramatic signs and symptoms of hypoglycemia relate to the central nervous system (CNS), reflecting the dependence of the brain on glucose as an energy source. Headache, diplopia, confusion, lethargy, seizures, and coma may result from neuroglucopenia.[26] Hemiplegic hypoglycemia presents as hemiparesis, which responds to glucose.[27] Systemic manifestations of hypoglycemia reflect adrenergic stimulation and include tachycardia, tremor, anxiety, and diaphoresis.

During the postoperative period, the symptoms and signs of hypoglycemia may be attributed to other factors. Neurologic manifestations of hypoglycemia may be ascribed to the effects of medications. Tachycardia and anxiety are nonspecific and may result from any number of factors during this period. The population at increased risk for developing hypoglycemia (including patients with diabetes, renal insufficiency, or liver disease, those receiving TPN, or those who are malnourished) should be watched closely and blood glucose levels checked if any suspicion is raised.

Treatment

Documenting hypoglycemia should take only minutes with a bedside glucose measurement. Blood can be sent to the laboratory for a more accurate glucose determination, but treatment of hypoglycemia should be made in response to clinical signs and bedside measurements; it should not be withheld to await laboratory confirmation. Artifactual hypoglycemia may be observed in patients with leukemia, during hemolytic crisis, or in those with polycythemia vera.[28] The risks of glucose administration are negligible, but the consequences of delayed therapy may be significant.

Treatment consists in glucose administration and correcting any identified etiologies, e.g., discontinuing an insulin infusion. An infusion of 10 per cent dextrose should be started immediately. If this fluid is not readily available, 25 to 50 ml of 50 per cent dextrose should be given intravenously. Blood glucose monitoring should be performed frequently to ensure normoglycemia.

ABNORMALITIES OF THYROID FUNCTION

Thyroid hormones regulate cellular metabolic activity and have profound effects on the cardiovascular, pulmonary, and neurologic systems. Insufficiency or excess of thyroid hormone may progress to the life-threatening decompensated conditions of myxedema coma or thyroid storm. Thyroid disease is the second most common endocrine disorder (after diabetes mellitus),[29] and the thyroid is the endocrine gland that most frequently undergoes surgery.[30] It is important for physicians caring for surgical patients to be able to recognize and treat thyroid emergencies, even though they occur in their severe form only rarely. Surgical stress can precipitate both thyroid storm and myxedema coma, conditions that are life-threatening if not diagnosed and treated.

Thyroid hormones have widespread effects on metabolic processes and organ systems. Thyroid hormones affect protein, carbohydrate, and lipid metabolism. Of special importance is the interaction of thyroid hormones and the sympathetic nervous system. Hyperthyroidism produces a clinical state similar to that produced by excess catecholamines; patients exhibit tremor, tachycardia, diaphoresis, and elevated temperature. In contrast, hypothyroid patients appear catecholamine-deficient. Thyroid hormones affect both the number of α- and β-adrenergic receptors and receptor responsiveness. The effects of thyroid hormones on the sympathetic nervous system are complex, varying among species and even among tissues within one species.[31]

Thyroid hormones have important effects on the cardiovascular system. Cardiac output is increased in hyperthyroidism secondary to increased stroke volume and heart rate, whereas it is diminished in hypothyroid states. Thyroid-induced changes in the sympathoadrenal system contribute to the cardiovascular manifestations of thyroid disease. Exogenous thyroid hormone has been shown in animals to increase the number of myocardial β-adrenergic receptors.[32] Thyroid hormone also has direct chronotropic and inotropic effects on the heart.[33]

Respiratory muscle weakness has been documented in both hypo- and hyperthyroid states.[34,35] Hypothyroid patients have a decreased ventilatory drive in response to hypercapnia or hypoxia. Pleural effusions occur commonly in hypothyroid patients and may cause pulmonary dysfunction. Dyspnea is a common symptom in hyperthyroid patients probably due to decreased vital capacity resulting from respiratory muscle weakness and decreased pulmonary compliance.[36]

Patients undergoing major surgery have significant alterations in thyroid function tests.[37] Total triiodothyronine (T_3) and total thyroxine (T_4) concentrations fall acutely after major surgery and recover to baseline levels over 6 to 9 days. Reverse T_3 falls immediately after surgery, but levels are significantly increased on the first postoperative day and return to normal over 1 week. Basal thyroid-stimulating hormone (TSH) levels decrease immediately after surgery. This decrease in TSH has also been demonstrated in hypothyroid patients undergoing major surgical procedures; hence a normal TSH level during the postoperative period does not rule out hypothyroidism. These alterations in thyroid hormone levels may represent adaptive mechanisms resulting in decreased metabolic demands during stress.

HYPERTHYROIDISM

Thyroid storm represents the extreme state of decompensated thyrotoxicosis. Despite treatment, this disease has a mortality rate of at least 20 per cent.[38] Thyrotoxic patients inadequately prepared for surgery are at high risk for developing thyroid storm during the postoperative period. Even hyperthyroid patients who are well controlled preoperatively are at risk, as the stress of surgery or infection may precipitate thyroid storm. Patients with unrecognized thyrotoxicosis are particularly prone to postoperative complications owing to inadequate control of their disease preoperatively. Though patients with the classic signs and symptoms of Graves disease are easy to identify, thyrotoxicosis in the critically ill or elderly patient may be difficult to recognize preoperatively. Apathetic hyperthyroidism describes the elderly thyrotoxic patient who presents with slowed mentation, blunted affect, and absence of increased motor activity.[39] Postoperative thyroid storm may be the first clinical indication that thyrotoxicosis exists in these patients.

Signs of thyrotoxicosis include tachycardia, fever, arrhythmias, vasodilatation, and a widened pulse pressure. With thyroid storm, the CNS is always affected, with symptoms ranging from agitation and psychosis to coma.[40] Gastrointestinal symptomatology may include abdominal pain, jaundice, vomiting, or hepatomegaly, and it may mimic a surgical abdomen.

Treatment

Therapy is aimed at reducing the synthesis and release of thyroid hormone and inhibiting their peripheral effects (Table 14–4). General supportive measures include peripheral cooling, antipyretics, and meperidine to block shivering. Acetaminophen should be used, as salicylates displaced thyroid hormones from binding proteins. Intravenous fluid intake should be increased to replace increased insensible losses from tachypnea and diaphoresis.

Propranolol is traditionally used for β-blockade because it has been shown to decrease conversion of T_4 to T_3. Nadolol also has this property.[41] Propranolol can be given intravenously with continuous cardiac monitoring in doses of 1 to 2 mg every 5 to 10 minutes until the pulse has fallen to 90 to 110 beats/min in the afebrile patient. In febrile patients, tachycardia may persist until temperature is reduced. Patients in whom a β-blocker is contraindicated (bronchospasm, cardiac failure) may be treated with reserpine (2.5 mg IV q4–6h) or guanethidine (50 to 150 mg PO).[42,43]

Antithyroid drugs block thyroid hormone biosynthesis by diverting oxidized iodide away from thyroid hormone synthesis.[44] Propylthiouracil (PTU) is used in preference to methimazole for thyroid storm because PTU blocks peripheral monodeiodination of T_4 to T_3. PTU is generally given orally, although it can be given intravenously in an alkaline solution.[42] The oral dose of PTU is 300 mg q6h. Methimazole can be given orally or per rectum in doses of 80 to 100 mg daily divided in four to six doses. Blood levels of T_3 are reduced by 50 per cent 1 day after PTU administration.[43]

Iodide is given after PTU or methimazole therapy to prevent iodide utilization by the thyroid. Iodide blocks the release of thyroid hormone. Potassium iodide 10 drops PO q8h or sodium iodide 1 to 2 mg IV over 24 hours should be used.[42] In addition, glucocorticoids are frequently given to decrease peripheral conversion of T_4 to T_3.

HYPOTHYROIDISM

The diagnosis of hypothyroidism spans a wide spectrum of clinical disease, from the asymptomatic to the critically ill myxedematous patient. Typically, this disease follows a slowly progressive course, and patients who have physiologically adapted to the thyroid-deficient state generally have no difficulties during surgery. However, the stress of surgery can precipitate myxedema coma, and hypothyroid patients can decompensate acutely during the postoperative period. Several minor complications may be anticipated in the hypothyroid patient who is well compensated, however the development of myxedema coma is associated with a high mortality.

Correction of the thyroid-deficient state is desirable prior to surgery, but two retrospective studies showed no increase in mortality when patients with mild to moderate hypothyroidism undergo surgical procedures.[45,46] In these studies, hypothyroid patients did have increased episodes of intraoperative hypotension, postoperative gastrointestinal and neuropsychiatric complications, and a tendency for prolonged time to extubation. None of these complications had serious clinical effects, and

---

TABLE 14–4. MANAGEMENT OF THYROID STORM

Clinical features
    Tachycardia, fever, agitation, coma, abdominal pain, vomiting, dyspnea

Treatment
1. Propranolol 1–2 mg IV with continuous cardiac monitoring. Repeat every 5 minutes until pulse rate drops to 90–110.
2. PTU 300 mg PO q6h.
3. Saturated solution of potassium iodide (SSKI) 10 drops PO q8h or NaI 1–2 mg IV over 24 hr.
4. Hydrocortisone 200 mg IV q8h.
5. General supportive therapy with acetaminophen, IV fluids, peripheral cooling.

the investigators concluded that surgery is not contraindicated in patients with mild to moderate hypothyroidism.

In contrast, myxedema coma is a disease with a mortality rate of 50 per cent despite treatment.[47] Myxedema coma may be precipitated by surgery, cold exposure, infection, phenothiazines, narcotics, and anesthetics.[38] Pulmonary and cardiovascular failure are the most common life-threatening problems; neurologic dysfunction, deficient thermogenesis, and metabolic and coagulation abnormalities are frequently present.

Myxedema represents a decompensated state of hypothyroidism and produces a number of clinical signs and symptoms, which are helpful for making the diagnosis. Nervous system dysfunction is an essential feature of this disease.[40] Although coma represents the extreme situation, psychosis may be present and herald the onset of coma.[38] Classically, deep tendon reflexes are "hung up" with delayed relaxation time. Bradycardia is a frequent finding, and the respiratory rate may be depressed. Deficient thermogenesis results in peripheral vasoconstriction and diastolic hypertension. Hypothermia is usually present unless concurrent infection elevates the temperature, in which case the patient may have a "normal" temperature.

Several laboratory tests reflect the altered physiology in the hypothyroid patient, although these tests tend to be nonspecific. Hyponatremia results from impaired water excretion. Arterial blood gases may reveal hypoxia or respiratory acidosis due to alveolar hypoventilation. Elevated creatine phosphokinase enzymes (muscle fraction), hypercholesterolemia, hypertriglyceridemia, and increased serum glutamic oxaloacetic acid (SGOT) may be present. Confirmatory laboratory data are not readily available. Thyrotropin (TSH) levels are normally elevated in hypothyroidism, but during the postoperative period TSH may be temporarily decreased to normal limits. Because the laboratory confirmation of hypothyroidism cannot be made quickly or reliably during the postoperative period, the decision to treat patients with thyroid replacement depends on the history and clinical presentation.

Treatment of myxedema coma consists of thyroid replacement and correction of metabolic and physiologic aberrations (Table 14–5). There is debate as to the best schedule for thyroid replacement. Many have recommended an initial "loading dose" of 300 to 500 μg L-thyroxine intravenously followed by 50 to 100 μg daily.[2,38,40,48] Patients should begin to improve after 24 hours. Others have pointed out that peripheral conversion of T_4 to T_3 is reduced in severe illness and have recommended 50 μg T_3 intravenously daily.[49]

A difficult dilemma occurs when presented with a myxedematous patient with known or suspected coronary artery disease. Thyroid replacement can precipitate angina or myocardial infarction. The risks and benefits of thyroid replacement in this situation must be considered. Although coronary arteriography and coronary artery bypass surgery have been performed on hypothyroid patients without evidence of increased risk, none of these patients was myxedematous.[50] A conservative approach in these patients would be to initiate therapy with 50 μg L-thyroxine intravenously.

Glucocorticoids are routinely given when treating myxedema coma. Reasons for administering steroids include the possibility that pituitary insufficiency may be the cause of hypothyroidism; therefore these patients would be

TABLE 14–5. MANAGEMENT OF MYXEDEMA COMA

Clinial features
Hypothermia, psychosis, coma, bradycardia

Laboratory findings
Hyponatremia, hypoxia, respiratory acidosis, elevated CPK, increased SGOT, hypoglycemia

Treatment
1. L-Thyroxine 100 μg IV, further loading dose to be determined in consultation with an endocrinologist. L-Thyroxine 50 μg IV if coronary artery disease is present.
2. Hydrocortisone 50–100 mg IV q8h. Fluids should contain glucose. If hyponatremia is present, restrict free water.
3. Avoid narcotics, sedatives, digitalis, rapid warming.

deficient in pituitary adrenocorticotropic hormone (ACTH), which stimulates cortisol secretion. Corticosteroids are also given because of the association of autoimmune thyroid disease with autoimmune adrenal disease. A blood sample for determining serum cortisol can be obtained prior to administering hydrocortisone 50 to 100 mg IV q8h, and the decision to continue corticosteroid therapy is then based on the result of the initial serum cortisol level when it is available.

Hypothyroid patients routinely have a decreased blood volume secondary to peripheral vasoconstriction.[48] These patients are susceptible to hypovolemic shock with vasodilation or circulating volume loss. This problem may be dramatically demonstrated if warming blankets are placed on myxedematous patients in an attempt to treat hypothermia. Intravenous solutions should provide glucose; and if hyponatremia is present, free water should be restricted. Close attention to respiratory parameters is required. These patients have markedly increased sensitivity to narcotics and sedatives, and these drugs should be avoided or administered in reduced doses. Hypothyroid patients are particularly prone to digitalis toxicity.

ADRENOCORTICAL INSUFFICIENCY

Acute adrenal insufficiency is fatal if not recognized and treated appropriately. Although it occurs uncommonly during the postoperative period, predisposing factors are common in the surgical patient, and there is a significant potential for this acute medical emergency to arise during the perioperative period. Knowledge of these risk factors and recognition of clinical signs and symptoms facilitate the difficult diagnosis of acute adrenal insufficiency and prompt life-saving therapy to be initiated.

The adrenal cortex synthesizes glucocorticoids, mineralocorticoids, and androgens. The primary mineralocorticoid is aldosterone; its secretion is regulated primarily by the renin-angiotensin axis and by potassium balance. ACTH has limited effects on aldosterone secretion.[51] Aldosterone has its major effects on the renal tubule, increasing sodium reabsorption and increasing excretion of potassium and hydrogen ion.

The prototypical glucocorticosteroid is cortisol. Basal cortisol secretion is 25 to 30 mg within a 24-hour period and may increase to as high as 300 mg/day during stress.[51] Glucocorticoids have widespread effects on multiple organ systems. Glucocorticoids increase plasma glucose concentrations by enhancing hepatic gluconeogenesis, inhibiting insulin secretion, and decreasing peripheral glucose utilization. Glucocorticoids cause accelerated protein catabolism and mobilization of fatty acids. The cardiovascular effects of glucocorticoids are illustrated by the glucocorticoid-deficient state, resulting in decreased cardiac work and contractility and decreased blood volume. Renal effects of glucocorticoid deficiency include reduced renal plasma flow, decreased glomerular filtration rate, and impaired water excretion. Cortisol diminishes the leukocyte response to inflammation and alters cell-mediated immunity.

Surgical stress has repeatedly been shown to cause an increase in cortisol secretion. The degree of surgical stress is correlated with the degree of cortisol secretion. Minor surgical procedures do not result in the significantly increased concentrations of plasma cortisol concentrations associated with moderate and major surgical procedures.[52] The cortisol response appears rather short-lived (assuming no ongoing stress) with return to baseline, in most cases, by 24 hours and return to baseline in all cases by the fifth postoperative day.[52]

Probably the most common cause of adrenocortical insufficiency during the postoperative period is exogenous glucocorticoid therapy. Exogenous steroids in supraphysiologic doses (>7.5 mg prednisone daily) suppress the hypothalamic-pituitary-adrenal axis.[53] Any patient who has received more than 2 weeks of glucocorticoid therapy during the preceding year should be considered potentially adrenocortically deficient. Although these patients may not have symptoms at baseline, they may be unable to mount an adequate glucocorticoid response to surgical stress. It is of note that topical steroids with occlusive dressings and inhaled steroids have been associated with hypothalamic-pituitary suppression.[51]

Other etiologies of adrenocortical insufficiency include intrinsic adrenal gland dysfunction (Addison's disease), most commonly resulting from destruction of the gland by an autoimmune process. Frequently autoimmune Addison's disease is associated with other diseases also thought to be autoimmune in origin, including hypoparathyroidism, insulin-dependent diabetes mellitus, pernicious anemia, and autoimmune thyroid diseases.[54] Adrenal gland replacement with metastatic carcinoma, most frequently that of the breast, colon, or lung, may result in adrenal insufficiency.[55] Adrenal hemorrhage in association with septicemia may cause fatal cardiovascular collapse, although in some cases the fatal outcome is due to septic shock, and plasma cortisol levels are actually elevated.[56]

Bilateral adrenal hemorrhage has been the subject of review.[57] The incidence is difficult to ascertain, with autopsy reports ranging from 0.14 to 1.10 per cent.[58] The three major risk factors for adrenal hemorrhage are thromboembolic disease, coagulopathy (secondary to anticoagulants or intrinsic coagulation defects), and the postoperative state. The use of anticoagulants is the most common cause of adrenal hemorrhage. Interestingly, clotting studies may be within the therapeutic range at the time of adrenal hemorrhage.[57]

The diagnosis of adrenal insufficiency is difficult because the clinical features are nonspecific and diagnostic laboratory examinations are not immediately available. Hypotension is a characteristic finding but may not be prominent if intravascular volume was augmented by intraoperative fluids. Furthermore, hypotension may not occur until catastrophic cardiovascular collapse develops.[57] Postoperative hypotension may be incorrectly attributed to inadequate intraoperative fluid replacement or ongoing volume losses ("third space" sequestration, hemorrhage). Anorexia, nausea, pain, and fever are symptoms of adrenocortical insufficiency,[55] but they commonly occur during the postoperative period for a variety of reasons. In patients with bilateral adrenal hemorrhage, pain was the only consistent feature and was present in the abdomen, flank, lower chest, or back.[57]

Preoperative and intraoperative therapies may obscure characteristic laboratory values. Hyponatremia and hyperkalemia (serum sodium/potassium ratio <30) are associated with adrenal insufficiency but may not be present owing to previously administered intravenous fluids.[59] Hypoglycemia and metabolic acidosis are laboratory abnormalities commonly associated with adrenocortical insufficiency, which may have been corrected by prior fluid and electrolyte administration.

Diagnostic laboratory studies are not routinely available on a "stat" basis, and treatment should not be withheld for the results of these tests. A serum cortisol level of less than 20 μg/dl in a patient in severe stress suggests adrenal failure.[59] The definitive test is the demonstration of decreased cortisol response to exogenous ACTH (cosyntropin, Cortrosyn). To perform this test, 250 μg of synthetic ACTH is given intravenously, and blood samples for plasma cortisol assays are obtained 30 and 60 minutes later. A normal response is generally regarded as an increase in cortisol of 7 μg/dl or more above baseline and an absolute increase of more than 18 μg/dl. Confirmatory testing can be done after initial resuscitation is completed, as dexamethasone administration does not interfere with the plasma cortisol radioimmunoassay.

Immediate treatment is mandatory for acute adrenal insufficiency. Normal saline infusion for volume repletion must be adjusted based on the patient's intravascular volume status. Hypoglycemia is a potential complication, and intravenous glucose should be provided and plasma glucose levels frequently monitored. A serum sample should be obtained for a cortisol level and then intravenous hydrocortisone 200 mg or intravenous dexamethasone 10 mg given acutely. Hydrocortisone is the synthetic equivalent of cortisol and has sufficient mineralocorticoid activity when given in 100 mg or higher doses so that mineralocorticoid supplementation is not needed acutely.[51] Hydrocortisone should be given in 100 mg doses every 6 hours or by continuous infusion until a definitive diagnosis is made.

Numerous protocols have been outlined describing glucocorticoid replacement in the patient with known adrenal insufficiency undergoing a surgical procedure. A simple protocol recommends hydrocortisone 100 mg IV q6h beginning prior to surgery and continuing through the day of surgery, tapering by 50 per cent per day if the postoperative course is uneventful. Studies now question the need for supraphysiologic doses of glucocorticoids in patients undergoing minimal or moderate surgical procedures.[52,60] Continuing physiologic glucocorticoid replacement may be all that is necessary in these circumstances.

PHEOCHROMOCYTOMA

Pheochromocytomas occur in fewer than 0.1 per cent of hypertensive patients.[61] Approximately 10 per cent of pheochromocytomas are malignant, but both benign and malignant tumors are associated with significant morbidity and mortality owing to the excessive catecholamine state. Surgical excision is the therapy of choice, and perioperative care

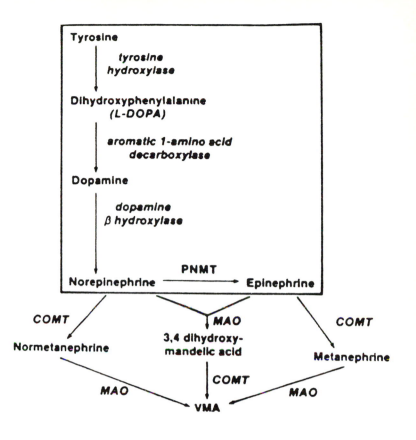

FIGURE 14–2. Synthesis and metabolism of catecholamines. PNMT = phenylethanolamine-*N*-methyltransferase; MAO = monoamine oxidase; COMT = catechol-*O*-methyltransferase; VMA = vanillylmandelic acid. (From Levine SN, McDonald JC: The evaluation and management of pheochromocytomas. Adv Surg *17*:281, 1984, with permission.)

can be challenging. Advances in the pharmacologic control of the hyperadrenergic state have been associated with a decrease in mortality from 45 per cent to 3 per cent or less.[62]

Pheochromocytomas are tumors arising from the chromaffin cells of the sympathoadrenal system. These tumors synthesize and secrete catecholamines (Fig. 14–2). Most tumors secrete a combination of norepinephrine and epinephrine. Catechol-*o*-methyltransferase metabolizes epinephrine and norepinephrine to metanephrine and normetanephrine, respectively. Additional oxidation by monoamine oxidase produces vanillylmandelic acid. These metabolites are the basis for diagnostic studies.[61]

Several features of pheochromocytomas follow a "10 per cent rule." Ten per cent are inherited as an autosomal dominant trait, either independently or associated with other endocrinopathies or neuroectodermal disorders. In adults, 10 per cent of pheochromocytomas are extraadrenal, whereas in children this incidence is 30 per cent. Overall, bilateral tumors occur in only 10 per cent of patients; but when a pheochromocytoma is inherited as part of a multiple endocrine neoplasia (MEN) syndrome, the incidence of bilateral tumors is almost universal.[63] Ten per cent of pheochromatocytomas are malignant. There are no morphologic features that distinguish benign from malignant tumors except the presence of local invasion or metastatic spread.

Clinical manifestations generally are a result of catecholamine hypersecretion. Symptoms frequently occur in paroxysms, usually lasting less than 1 hour, and may be precipitated by physical activity, change in position, abdominal pressure, induction of anesthesia, or a number of pharmacologic agents.[61] Signs and symptoms are outlined in Table 14–6. Ninety-five per cent of patients have either head-

TABLE 14–6. FREQUENCY OF SIGNS AND SYMPTOMS OF PHEOCHROMOCYTOMA

Signs and Symptoms	Approximate % of Patients
Headache	80
Sweating	70
Persistent hypertension	66
Palpitations	60
Pallor	40
Tremor	40

aches, palpitations, or increased sweating, alone or in combination.[64] Hypertension is sustained in 50 to 60 per cent of patients with pheochromocytomas. Cardiomyopathy has been reported to occur in 20 to 30 per cent of patients with pheochromocytoma.[65] Multiple etiologies for myocardial disease include hypertension, ischemia, and the direct cardiac effect of excess catecholamines.[66]

After surgical excision of a pheochromocytoma, the three most common problems during the postoperative period are hypotension, hypertension, and hypoglycemia. Hypotension may result from a number of causes, including residual α- or β-blockade, decreased sensitivity to catecholamines, hemorrhage, hypovolemia, or adrenal insufficiency if both adrenal glands are removed. Circulating blood volume is reduced in many patients with these tumors secondary to catecholamine-induced vasoconstriction.[67] One goal of preoperative treatment with α-blockade is to allow spontaneous restoration of the circulating plasma volume by blocking the vasoconstrictive effect of the catecholamines. However, intravascular volume may not be fully restored, and the initial response to hypotension during the postoperative period should be volume replacement, unless the patient appears volume-replete or overloaded. Because of the significant incidence of myocardial disease in patients with pheochromocytoma, myocardial dysfunction should be considered in the differential diagnosis of hypotension in these patients. It has been demonstrated that central venous pressure correlates poorly with pulmonary artery occlusive pressure in these patients, and use of the central venous pressure alone to guide volume replacement may lead to inappropriate decisions regarding fluid replacement.[68] If a patient develops hypotension after surgical removal of a pheochromocytoma and does not respond to an initial trial of volume replacement, consideration should be given to insertion of a pulmonary artery catheter, as well as further studies to elucidate the cause of hypotension (hematocrit, electrocardiogram, review of drugs administered preoperatively and intraoperatively).

Hypertension may occur during the postoperative period for all the same reasons it occurs in any postoperative patient, including pain, hypoxia, hypercapnia, and hypervolemia. In particular, β-blocker withdrawal and remaining pheochromocytoma may present as postoperative hypertension. Plasma and urinary catecholamine levels are often elevated during the first postoperative week, and some degree of hypertension may persist on this basis.[69] Even in the population of patients from whom all tumor has been resected, 25 per cent remain hypertensive postoperatively.[70] If hypertension persists despite the correction of reversible causes, sodium nitroprusside infusion with continuous arterial monitoring provides rapid and titratable blood pressure control. If patients have confirmed remaining tumor, or if the patient is suspected de novo of having a pheochromocytoma, initial control of hypertension should be with a direct vasodilator (e.g., nitroprusside), which is then replaced with an α-blocking agent. β-Blockers used before adequate α-blockade may result in vasoconstriction due to unopposed α-stimulation. The short-acting agent esmolol is ideal for titrating β-blockade in these patients.[62]

Hypoglycemia is a rare postoperative complication following pheochromocytoma removal.[71] Catecholamines produce hyperglycemia by promoting hepatic glucose production, suppressing insulin secretion, and creating an insulin-resistant state. Upon sudden removal of the tumor there is rebound hyperinsulinemia, resulting in hypoglycemia. Furthermore, glycogen stores are depleted by catecholamine-induced glycogenolysis, so glycogen stores are inadequate to supply glucose needs. β-Blockade potentiates hypoglycemia by preventing skeletal muscle glycogenolysis.[71] During the postoperative period, intravenous solutions should provide glucose, and blood glucose levels should be monitored.

Infrequently, patients may have undiagnosed pheochromocytoma and undergo surgery only to have complications arise during the perioperative period secondary to excess catecholamine secretion. Though it is a rare occurrence, the mortality among these patients is high.[72] These patients may have a clinical presentation consistent with a hyperadrenaline state: hypertension, tachycardia, arrhythmias, hyperpyrexia, dilated pupils, hyperglycemia. The constellation of all, or some, of these signs and symptoms may be similar to that of patients presenting with thyrotoxicosis, malignant hypertension, uncontrolled diabetes mellitus, sepsis, alcohol withdrawal, or the carcinoid syndrome.[61] If a pheochromocytoma is considered to be a potential cause of postoperative deterioration, the use of β blockers to control hypertension is contraindicated before α-blockade has been initiated.

CARCINOID TUMORS

Carcinoid tumors arise from enterochromaffin cells. Although these tumors are histologically similar to carcinomas, their more benign clinical course prompted the descriptive term "carcinoid." One of the most dramatic complications that may occur perioperatively results from the secretion of large amounts of neurohumors resulting in a carcinoid crisis, a rare life-threatening complication that is difficult to treat. The perioperative management of patients with carcinoid tumors can be challenging, but new therapeutic modalities appear promising.

Biochemically, carcinoid tumors are known to produce more than 20 neurohumors, including serotonin, histamine, peptides of the tachykinin family, substance P, prostaglandins, catecholamines, and kallikrein-bradykinin.[73] Serotonin production (Fig. 14–3), originally identified during the 1950s, was thought to be the cause of the humoral symptoms associated with carcinoid tumors. It is now recognized that serotonin alone is not responsible for all the manifestations of these tumors, although its metabolism is the basis for the single most useful diagnostic test. Most carcinoid tumors take up and metabolize tryptophan to serotonin (Fig. 14–3). After secretion, serotonin is converted to 5-hydroxyindoleacetic acid (5-HIAA) and excreted in the urine. Increased urinary 5-HIAA levels are present in almost all patients with the carcinoid syndrome.[74]

The carcinoid syndrome refers to the manifestations of the neurohumors secreted and may include flushing, diarrhea, bronchospasm, and cardiac valvular disease. Fewer than 25 per cent of patients with carcinoid tumors have the carcinoid syndrome.[75] The appearance of the carcinoid syndrome is associated with extensive hepatic metastatic disease in more than 90 per cent of cases.[76] Hormones responsible for the carcinoid syndrome are inactivated by the liver; thus the syndrome occurs when tumors secrete their mediators directly into the systemic circulation, as occurs with bronchial tumors, ovarian tumors, or hepatic metastases.

Diarrhea is the most common symptom and may be due to hypermotility from serotonin, partial small bowl obstruction, or mesenteric vascular insufficiency.[77] Flushing is typically diffuse, involving the face and upper trunk, and it usually lasts several minutes. Bronchial carcinoids may produce prolonged flushing episodes accompanied by hypotension and bronchoconstriction.[74] About 20 per cent of patients with the carcinoid syndrome have evidence of cardiac disease.[74] The endocrine-mediated plaque-like thickening of the valves may cause stenosis or incompetence. The pulmonic and tricuspid valves are predominantly involved. It has been postulated that the mo-

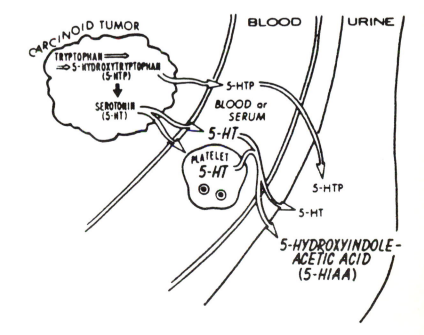

FIGURE 14–3. Synthesis and metabolism of serotonin by carcinoid tumors. (From Feldman JM: Carcinoid tumors and syndrome. Semin Oncol *14*:237, 1987, with permission.)

noamine oxidase present in the lung deactivates the mediators prior to delivery to the left side of the heart.

Carcinoid tumors may secrete large amounts of neurohumors, resulting in life-threatening episodes called carcinoid crises. Carcinoid crises have been reported to occur in association with anesthesia, surgery, or aggressive chemotherapy.[78,79] Catecholamines stimulate mediator release and physiologic events that induce endogenous catecholamine release (stress, pain, hypothermia, hypercapnia), may precipitate a carcinoid crisis.[73] Drugs that cause histamine or serotonin release and pharmacologic adrenergic agents may also induce crisis.

The hypotension associated with the carcinoid crisis may be severe and refractory to routine therapy. Adrenergic agonists or calcium infusions may worsen the situation by increasing mediator release. Multiple pharmacologic agents have been used in the past with only moderate success, but more recent reports describing the use of a somatostatin analogue have demonstrated the efficacy of this agent in reversing life-threatening carcinoid crisis.[73]

Somatostatin is a naturally occurring peptide that blocks release of growth hormone and thyrotropin, reduces hormonal and exocrine secretions in the gut,[78] and prevents the release of active mediators from carcinoid tumors.[73] Somatostatin has a plasma half-life of less than 2 minutes, with necessitates administration by intravenous infusions, but the analogue SMS 201-995 has a prolonged half-life in circulation (90 to 115 minutes), which makes it useful in long-term as well as short-term therapy.[76] In one report[78] 100 mg IV provided dramatic reversal of life-threatening hypotension from a carcinoid crisis. In patients undergoing surgical procedures who have a known carcinoid tumor, this agent should be available for treatment of carcinoid crisis if it should occur.

SUMMARY

A wide variety of endocrine problems can arise during the postoperative period. When endocrine dysfunction has been diagnosed preoperatively, specific clinical problems can be anticipated and therapy directed to prevent these complications. However, in patients with unrecognized or de novo endocrine disease, surgical stress may precipitate a number of life-threatening endocrine emergencies requiring immediate recognition and treatment. Perioperative therapy (medications, intravenous fluid administration) may alter clinical and laboratory presentations, making diagnoses difficult.

Hyperglycemia is common during the postoperative period due to the physiologic response to stress. In diabetic patients untreated hyperglycemia produces an osmotic diuresis, resulting in dehydration, and ketogenesis produces metabolic acidosis. Intravascular volume repletion, correction of electrolyte deficiencies, and insulin administration are the mainstays of therapy. Blood glucose must be assessed frequently (every 1 to 2 hours), and frequent electrolyte monitoring is needed as well. Hypoglycemia may occur in a number of clinical settings; particular vigilance is indicated in the diabetic patient subjected to fasting and insulin adjustments preoperatively. Hypoglycemia can be documented and treated in minutes but may be overlooked in the post anesthesia care unit (PACU) if neurologic changes due to neuroglucopenia are incorrectly ascribed to the effects of anesthetic agents.

Thyroid storm and myxedema coma are rare, but each may be precipitated by surgery. Patients at greatest risk of thyroid storm are hyperthyroid patients requiring emergent surgical intervention and patients with unrecognized hyperthyroidism who are not prepared for the stress of surgery. Antithyroid drugs and β-blockade should be started as soon as the decompensated thyrotoxic state is recognized. Mild to moderate hypothyroidism may be a cause of hypoventilation during the postoperative period. Myxedema coma has a mortality of 50 per cent despite treatment and should be considered in the differential diagnosis of the patient with bradycardia, hypothermia, and neurologic changes.

Acute adrenal insufficiency should be suspected in a patient with unexplained hypotension who has received supraphysiologic doses of steroids during the preceding year. A serum sample should be obtained for a cortisol level and therapy started empirically with intravenous hydrocortisone. This life-threatening condition can be avoided by preoperative administration of corticosteroids.

Pheochromocytoma and carcinoid are rare endocrine tumors that secrete vasoactive and neuroactive substances. The common problems seen following removal of pheochromocytoma are hypotension, hypertension, and hypoglycemia. Carcinoid tumors secreting a large amount of neurohumors can result in carcinoid crisis with profound, vasopressor-resistant shock.

References

1. Gann DS, Amaral JF: Endocrine and metabolic responses to injury. *In* Schwartz SI, Shires GT, Spencer FC (eds): Principles of Surgery, 5th ed. New York, McGraw-Hill, 1989, pp. 1–68.

2. Molitch ME: Endocrinology. *In* Molitch ME (ed): Management of Medical Problems in Surgical Patients. Philadelphia, Davis, 1982, pp. 151–218.

3. Goldman DR: Surgery in patients with endocrine dysfunction. Med Clin North Am 71:499–509, 1987.

4. Foster DW, McGarry JD: The metabolic derangements and treatment of diabetic ketoacidosis. Engl J Med 309:159–169, 1983.

5. Kern EFO, Simmons DA, Martin DB: Diabetic ketoacidosis and hyperglycemic nonketotic coma. *In* Geelhoed GW, Chernow B (eds): Endocrine Aspects of Acute Illness. New York, Churchill Livingstone, 1985, pp. 285–305.

6. Cryer PE, White NH, Santiago JV: The relevance of glucose counterregulatory systems to patients with insulin-dependent diabetes mellitus. Endocr Rev 7:131–139, 1986.

7. Kitabachi AE, Murphy MB: Diabetic ketoacidoses and hyperosmolar hyperglycemic nonketotic coma. Med Clin North Am 72:1545–1563, 1988.

8. Boehm TM: Hyperglycemia in critical care medicine. Crit Care Q 6:48–62, 1983.

9. Zaloga GP, Chernow B: Insulin, glucagon, and growth hormone. *In* Chernow B, Lake CR (eds): The Pharmacologic Approach to the Critically Ill. Baltimore, Williams & Wilkins, 1983, pp. 562–585.

10. Wachtel TJ, Silliman RA, Lamberton P: Predisposing factors for the diabetic hyperosmolar state. Arch Intern Med 147:499–501, 1987.

11. Bivins BA, Hyde GL, Sachotello CR, Griffen WO Jr: Physiopathology and management of hyperosmolar hyperglycemic nonketotic dehydration. Surg Gynecol Obstet 154:534–540, 1982.

12. Crapo LM, Reaven G: Hyperosmolar nonketotic diabetic coma. Med Grand Rounds 2:344–356, 1983.

13. Khardori R, Soler NG: Hyperosmolar hyperglycemic nonketotic syndrome. Am J Med 77:899–904, 1984.

14. Johnston DG, Alberti KGMM: Diabetic emergencies: practical aspects of the management of diabetic ketoacidosis and diabetes during surgery. Clin Endocrinal Metab 9:437–460, 1980.

15. Katz MA: Hyperglycemia-induced hyponatremia—calculation of expected serum sodium depression. Engl J Med 289:843–844, 1973.

16. Gennari FJ: Serum osmolality: uses and limitations. N Engl J Med 310:102–105, 1984.

17. Sorisky A, Devlin JT: Intraoperative ketoacidosis and malnutrition. Ann Intern Med 109:337–338, 1988.

18. Waldhausl W, Klienberger G, Korn A, et al: Severe hyperglycemia: effect of rehydration on endocrine derangements and blood glucose concentration. Diabetes 28:577–584, 1979.

19. Skyler JS: Insulin pharmacology. Med Clin North Am 72:1337–1354, 1988.

20. Adrogue HJ, Wilson H, Boyd AE III, et al: Plasma acid-base patterns in diabetic ketoacidosis. N Engl J Med 307:1603–1610, 1982.

21. Fisher JN, Kitabachi AE: Randomized study of phosphate therapy in the treatment of diabetic ketoacidosis. J Clin Endocrinol Metab 57:177–180, 1983.

22. Morris LR, Murphy MB, Ketabachi AE: Bicarbonate therapy in severe diabetic ketoacidosis. Ann Intern Med 105:836–840, 1986.

23. Chernow B: Hormonal and metabolic consideration in critical care medicine. *In* Shoemaker WC, Thompson WL, Holbrook PR (eds): Textbook of Critical Care. Philadelphia, Saunders, 1984, pp. 646–664.

24. Fischer KF, Lees JA, Newman JH: Hypoglycemia in hospitalized patients: causes and outcomes. N Engl J Med 315:1245–1250, 1986.

25. Seltzer HS: Drug-induced hypoglycemia: a review based on 473 cases. Diabetes 21:955–966, 1972.

26. Malouf R, Brust J: Hypoglycemia: causes, neurological manifestation and outcome. Ann Neurol 17:421–430, 1985.

27. Gale E: Hypoglycaemia. Clin Endocrinol Metab 9:461–475, 1980.

28. Service FJ: Hypoglycemia. Endocrinol Metab Clin North Am 17:601–616, 1988.

29. Hay ID, Klee GG: Thyroid dysfunction. Endocrinol Metab Clin North Am 17:473–509, 1988.

30. Weber CA, Clark OH: Surgery for thyroid disease. Med Clin North Am 69:1097–1115, 1985.

31. Bilezikian JP, Loeb JN: The influence of hyperthyroidism and hypothyroidism on alpha- and beta-adrenergic receptor systems and adrenergic responsiveness. Endocr Rev 4:378–404, 1983.

32. Williams L, Lefkowitz R, Watanabe A, et al: Thyroid hormone regulation of beta-adrenergic receptor number. J Biol Chem 252:2787–2789, 1977.

33. Skelton CL: The heart and hyperthyroidism. N Engl J Med 307:1206–1208, 1982.

34. Laroche CM, Cairns T, Moxhan J, Green M: Hypothyroidism presenting with respiratory muscle weakness. Am Rev Respir Dis 138:472–474, 1988.

35. Mier A, Brophy C, Wass J, Green M: Respiratory muscle function in hyperthyroidism before and after treatment. Thorax 41:716, 1986 (abstract).

36. Ingbar SH: The thyroid gland. *In* Wilson JD, Foster DW (eds): Williams Textbook of Endocrinology, 7th ed. Philadelphia, Saunders, 1985, pp. 682–815.

37. Zaloga GP, Chernow B, Smallridge RC, et al: A longitudinal evaluation of thyroid function in critically ill surgical patients. Ann Surg 201:456–464, 1985.

38. Hoffenberg R: Thyroid emergencies. Clin Endocrinol Metab 9:503–512, 1980.

39. Hurley JR: Thyroid disease in the elderly. Med Clin North Am 67:497–516, 1983.

40. Nicoloff JT: Thyroid storm and myxedema coma. Med Clin North Am 69:1005–1017, 1985.

41. Cooper DS, Ridgway EC: Clinical management of patients with hyperthyroidism. Med Clin North Am 69:953–971, 1985.

42. Forfar JC, Caldwell GC: Hyperthyroid heart disease. Clin Endocrinol Metab 14:491–508, 1985.

43. Mackin JF, Canary JJ, Pittman CS: Thyroid storm and its management. N Engl J Med 291:1396–1398, 1974.

44. Cooper DS: Antithyroid drugs. N Engl J Med 311:1353–1362, 1984.

45. Weinberg AD, Brennan MD, Gorman CA, et al: Outcome of anesthesia and surgery in hypothyroid patients. Arch Intern Med 143:893–897, 1983.

46. Ladenson PW, Levin AA, Ridgway ECH, Daniels GH: Complications of surgery in hypothyroid patients. Am J Med 77:261–266, 1984.

47. Senior RM, Birge SL: The recognition and management of myxedema coma. JAMA *217*:61–65, 1971.

48. Murkin JM: Anesthesia and hypothyroidism: a review of thyroxine physiology, pharmacology, and anesthetic implications. Anesth Analg *61*:371–383, 1982.

49. Ladenson PW, Goldenheim PD, Ridgway EC: Rapid pituitary and peripheral tissue responses to intravenous L-triiodothyronine in hypothyroidism. J Clin Endocrinol Metab *56*:1252–1259, 1983.

50. Myerowitz PD, Kamienski RW, Swanson DK, et al: Diagnosis and management of the hypothyroid patient with chest pain. J Thorac Cardiovasc Surg *86*:57–60, 1983.

51. Chin R Jr, Chernow B: Corticosteroids. *In* Chernow B, Lake CR (eds): The Pharmacologic Approach to the Critically Ill. Baltimore, Williams & Wilkins, 1983, pp. 510–529..

52. Chernow B, Alexander HR, Smallridge RC, et al: Hormonal responses to graded surgical stress. Arch Intern Med *147*:1273–1278, 1987.

53. Goldmann DR: Surgery in patients with endocrine dysfunction. Med Clin North Am *71*:499–509, 1987.

54. Neufeld M, Maclaren NK, Blizzard RM: Two types of autoimmune Addison's disease associated with different polyglandular autoimmune (PGA) syndromes. Medicine (Baltimore) *60*:355–362, 1981.

55. Steer M, Fromm D: Recognition of adrenal insufficiency in the postoperative patient. Am J Surg *139*:443–446, 1980.

56. Burke CW: Adrenocortical insufficiency. Clin Endocrinol Metab *14*:947–976, 1985.

57. Rao RH, Vagnucci AH, Amico JA: Bilateral massive adrenal hemorrhage: early recognition and treatment. Ann Intern Med *110*:227–235, 1989.

58. Jacobson SA, Blute RD Jr, Green DF, et al: Acute adrenal insufficiency as a complication of urological surgery. J Urol *135*:337–340, 1986.

59. Zaloga GP, Chernow B: The use of hormones as therapeutic agents. Semin Respir Med *7*:39–51, 1985.

60. Udelsman R, Ramp J, Gallucci WT, et al: Adaptation during surgical stress—a reevaluation of the role of glucocorticoids. J Clin Invest *77*:1377–1381, 1986.

61. Sheps SG, Jiang NS, Klee GG: Diagnostic evaluation of pheochromocytoma. Endocrinol Metab Clin North Am *17*:397–414, 1988.

62. Nicholas E, Deutschman CS, Allo M, Rock P: Use of esmolol in the intraoperative management of pheochromocytoma. Anesth Analg *67*:1114–1117, 1988.

63. Lips KJM, Van Der Stuye Veer J, Struyrenberg A, et al: Bilateral occurrence of pheochromocytoma in patients with the multiple endocrine neoplasia syndrome type 2A (Sipple's syndrome). Am J Med *70*:1051–1060, 1981.

64. Levine SN, McDonald JC: The evaluation and management of pheochromocytomas. Adv Surg *17*:281–313, 1984.

65. Gilsanz FJ, Luergo C, Conejero P, et al: Cardiomyopathy and pheochromocytoma. Anaesthesia *38*:888–891, 1983.

66. Imperato-McGinley J, Gautier T, Ehlers K, et al: Reversibility of catecholanine induced dilated cardiomyopathy in a child with a pheochromocytoma. N Engl J Med *316*:793–797, 1987.

67. Hull CJ: Phaeochromocytoma: diagnosis, preoperative preparation and anaesthetic management. Br J Anaesth *58*:1453–1468, 1986.

68. Mihm FL: Pulmonary artery pressure monitoring in patients with pheochromocytoma. Anesth Analg *62*:1129–1133, 1983.

69. Cryer PE: Phaeochromocytoma. Clin Endocrinol Metab *14*:2303–220, 1985.

70. Sanaan NA, Hickley RC: Pheochromocytoma. Semin Oncol *14*:297–305, 1987.

71. Channa AB, Mofti AB, Taylor GW, et al: Hypoglycaemia encephalopathy following surgery on phaeochromocytoma. Anaesthesia *47*:1298–1301, 1987.

72. Sellevoldf OFM, Raeder J, Stenseth R: Undiagnosed phaeochromocytoma in the perioperative period. Acta Anaesthesiol Scand *29*:474–479, 1985.

73. Roy RC, Carter RF, Wright PD: Somatostatin, anaesthesia, and the carcinoid syndrome. Anaesthesia *42*:627–632, 1987.

74. Roberts LJ: Carcinoid syndrome and disorders of systemic mast-cell activation including systemic mastocytosis. Endocrinol Metab Clin North Am *17*:415–436, 1988.

75. Mason RA, Steane PA: Carcinoid syndrome: its relevance to the anaesthetist. Anaesthesia *31*:228–242, 1976.

76. Goden P, Comi RJ, Maton PN, Go VLW: Somatostatin and somatostatin analogue (SMS 201-995) in treatment of hormone-secreting tumors of the pituitary and gastrointestinal tract and non-neoplastic diseases of the gut. Ann Intern Med *110*:35–50, 1989.

77. Thompson GB, van Heerden JA, Martin JK Jr, et al: Carcinoid tumors of the gastrointestinal tract: presentation, management and prognosis. Surgery *98*:1054–1062, 1985.

78. Marsh HM, Martin JK Jr, Kvols LK, et al: Carcinoid crisis during anesthesia: successful treatment with a somatostatin analogue. Anesthesiology *66*:89–91, 1987.

79. Oates JA: The carcinoid syndrome. N Engl J Med *315*:702–704, 1986.

ALLERGIC AND TRANSFUSION REACTIONS 15

MICHAEL E. WEISS and JERROLD H. LEVY

Anaphylaxis is an acute, severe, life-threatening reaction that may be fatal. The first reported death from anaphylaxis was recorded in 2600 BC. Written in hieroglyphics, it tells the story of Menes, who died after a fatal Hymenoptera sting.[1] In 1902 Portier and Richet reported that a second injection of a sea anemone extract, which had initially caused only mild symptoms, resulted in a fatal systemic reaction in dogs.[1] Richet coined the word "anaphylaxis" from the Greek *anna* ("contrary to") and *phylaxis* ("protection"). Thus the term was initially used to describe a phenomenon in which repeated exposure to a foreign protein produced an adverse reaction rather than the intended immunization or prophylaxis. Around that same time (1906), the Viennese investigator Clemens Von Pirquet coined the word "allergy" from the Greek *alos* ("other") and *ergon* ("work").[1]

The term anaphylaxis has been employed to denote an immunoglobin E (IgE) antibody-mediated reaction that results in a severe, abrupt event manifested by cutaneous (urticaria/angioedema), respiratory (asthma, laryngeal edema), gastrointestinal (nausea, vomiting, abdominal pain, diarrhea), or cardiovascular (hypotension, tachycardia, cardiovascular collapse) pathophysiologic alterations. The same clinical manifestations may occur consequent to non-IgE-mediated reactions and have previously been termed anaphylactoid or "pseudoallergic" reactions. For simplicity, throughout the rest of this chapter the term anaphylaxis refers to the clinical syndrome described above, without implying a specific mechanism.

CLASSIFICATION OF ALLERGIC REACTIONS

Gell and Coombs classified four types of immunopathologic reaction[2] (Table 15–1).

Type I reactions—immediate hypersensitivity. These reactions result from the interaction of antigens with preformed antigen-specific IgE antibodies that are bound to tissue mast cells or circulating basophils via high affinity IgE receptors. Cross-linking two or more IgE receptors by antigen leads to the release of both preformed and newly generated mediators. Release of these mediators can lead to urticaria, laryngeal edema, and bronchospasm with or without cardiovascular collapse.

Type II reactions—cytotoxic antibodies. These reactions result when IgG or IgM antibody reacts with a cell-bound antigen, i.e., blood group antigens, penicillin determinants bound to red blood cells (RBCs). The antigen–antibody interaction activates the complement system, resulting in cell lysis. Type II reactions may also be complement-independent. IgG or IgM antibody may bind to cell membrane-bound antigen, resulting in neutrophil or macrophage attachment and activation via an IgG or IgM Fc receptor. This opsonization can result in injury to the antigen-laden cell. Examples of type II reactions include ABO-incompatible transfusion reactions, drug-induced hemolytic anemia or thrombocytopenia, rhesus (Rh) disease of the newborn, and Goodpasture syndrome.

Type III reactions—immune complexes (Arthus reaction). Antigen-specific IgG or IgM

233

TABLE 15–1. CLASSIFICATION OF IMMUNOPATHOLOGIC REACTIONS ACCORDING TO GELL AND COOMBS

Type of Reaction	Description	Antibody	Cells	Other	Clinical Reactions
I	Anaphylactic (reagenic); immediate hypersensitivity	IgE	Basophils, mast cells		Anaphylaxis, urticaria
II	Cytotoxic or cytolytic	IgG, IgM	Any cell with isoantigen	C', RES	Coombs + hemolytic anemia; drug-induced nephritis; transfusion reaction; Rh disease
III	Immune complex disease	Soluble immune complexes (Ag-Ab)	None directly	C'	Serum sickness; drug fever; glomerulonephritis
IV	"Delayed" or cell-mediated hypersensitivity	None known	Sensitized T lymphocytes		Contact dermatitis
V	Idiopathic		? ? ? ?	? ? ? ?	Maculopapular eruptions; eosinophilia; Stevens-Johnson syndrome; exfoliative dermatitis

C' = complement; RES = reticuloendothelial system; Ag-Ab = antigen antibody; (?) = immunopathologic mechanism is in doubt.
Reproduced with permission from Gell PGH, Coombs RRA: Classification of allergic reactions responsible for clinical hypersensitivity and disease. *In* Gell PGH, Coombs RRA, Hachmann PJ (eds): Clinical Aspects of Immunology, 3rd ed. Oxford, Blackwell Scientific Publications, 1975, pp. 761–781.

antibodies form circulating complexes with antigens. The complexes lodge in tissue sites, fix complement, and attract polymorphonuclear leukocytes, which attempt to phagocytize the immune complexes. The release of potent enzymes from the phagocytic cells results in tissue damage. Immune complex reactions typically appear 7 to 14 days after the contin-

ual exposure of antigen. Examples include serum sickness and possibly drug fever.

Type IV reactions—cell-mediated hypersensitivity. These reactions are not mediated by an antibody but, rather, T lymphocytes that are specifically sensitized to recognize a particular antigen. After being modified by antigen-processing cells (i.e., macrophages,

TABLE 15–2. CLASSIFICATION OF ALLERGIC REACTIONS BASED ON THEIR TIME OF ONSET

Reaction Type	Onset (hr)	Clinical Reactions
Immediate	0–1	Anaphylaxis Hypotension Laryngeal edema Urticaria/angioedema Wheezing
Accelerated	1–72	Urticaria/angioedema Laryngeal edema Wheezing
Late	>72	Morbilliform rash Interstitial nephritis Hemolytic anemia Neutropenia Thrombocytopenia Serum sickness Drug fever Stevens-Johnson syndrome Exfoliative dermatitis

Reproduced with permission from Levine BB: Immunologic mechanisms of penicillin allergy: a haptenic model system for the study of allergic diseases of man. N Engl J Med *275*:1115–1125, 1966.

Langerhans cells), the modified antigen is presented in association with MHC class II molecules to the T lymphocyte. The sensitized T lymphocyte recognizes the processed antigen through an antigen-specific T cell receptor. The T cell is thus triggered to release substances known as cytokines, which orchestrate the immune response by recruiting and stimulating proliferation of other lymphocytes and mononuclear cells, ultimately causing tissue inflammation and injury. Examples of cell-mediated immune reactions are tuberculin skin testing, contact dermatitis (i.e., poison ivy), and graft versus host disease.

Some reactions have obscure pathogenesis and are called *idiopathic reactions* (Table 15–1).

Levine proposed classifying adverse reactions to an antigen such as penicillin according to the time of onset[3] (Table 15–2). Immediate reactions occur within the first hour after antigen administration; the reaction may involve anaphylaxis, laryngeal edema, urticaria, or wheezing. Accelerated reactions occur 1 to 72 hours after antigen presentation and most commonly involve urticaria. Late reactions begin more than 72 hours after the onset of therapy: Anaphylaxis does not occur in the course of continuous antigen therapy; maculopapular eruptions are most common, but type II, III, and IV reactions also occur within this time frame. Allergic reactions may also be classified according to their predominant clinical manifestations, as seen in Table 15–3.

MAST CELL ACTIVATION

Of allergic drug reactions, anaphylaxis (involving mast cell or basophil mediator release) may be the most important clinically because of its potential for sudden onset with catastrophic outcomes. Tissue mast cells and circulating basophils may be triggered to release their mediators by both IgE and non-IgE mechanisms (Fig. 15–1).

IgE-Mediated Anaphylaxis

Antigenic molecules (usually proteins) capable of stimulating IgE antibody production may cause IgE-mediated anaphylaxis on reexposure. Haptens are molecules that are too small to stimulate immune responses in and of themselves. However, haptens may bind to endogenous proteins such as serum albumin and become antigenic (i.e., capable of stimulating antibody production). IgE antibodies, once produced, become fixed to tissue mast cells or circulating basophils, both of which contain high affinity IgE receptors.[4] This attachment takes place via the Fc region of the IgE molecule, which allows the Fab region of the IgE antibody to bind antigen. Reexposure to antigens or haptens that are functionally multivalent (have two or more antigenic sites) is required to cross-link IgE antibodies bound to mast cells or basophils. Cross-linking of IgE antibodies causes the direct bridging of IgE receptor molecules on mast cell and basophil cell membranes, which induces activation of membrane-associated enzymes, causing complex biochemical cascades that lead to an influx of extracellular calcium and mobilization of intracellular calcium with subsequent release of preformed granule-associated mediators and the generation of new mediators from cell membrane phospholipids.[5,6] Examples of IgE antibody-mediated allergic reactions include insulin, chymopapain, muscle relaxants, and penicillin (hapten).

COMPLEMENT-MEDIATED REACTIONS

Activation of the complement system results in the membrane attack unit (C5b

TABLE 15–3. CLASSIFICATION OF ALLERGIC REACTIONS ACCORDING TO THEIR PREDOMINANT CLINICAL MANIFESTATIONS

Anaphylaxis
    Laryngeal edema
    Hypotension
    Bronchospasm

Cutaneous reactions
    Urticaria/angioedema
    Vasculitis
    Stevens-Johnson syndrome
    Exfoliative dermatitis
    Contact sensitivity
    Fixed drug eruption
    Toxic epidermal necrolysis
    Morbilliform rash

Destruction of formed elements of blood
    Hemolytic anemia
    Neutropenia
    Thrombocytopenia

Serum sickness
Drug fever
Systemic vasculitis

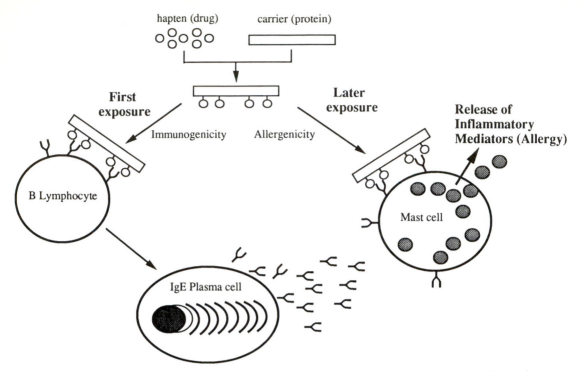

FIGURE 15–1. Drug hapten combining with a carrier molecule to induce IgE antibody production against the drug. On subsequent exposure, the drug combines with IgE antibody on the mast cell surface, leading to an anaphylactic reaction.

through C9) and the generation of low-molecular-weight peptides C3a, C4a, and C5a (known as the anaphylatoxins).[7] The anaphylatoxins are capable of causing mast cell and basophil mediator release, directly increasing vascular permeability, contracting smooth muscles, aggregating platelets, and stimulating macrophages to produce thromboxane.[7,8] The complement cascade may be activated through either the classic pathway or the alternative pathway. Complement activation through the classic pathway can be initiated through IgG or IgM antibody binding to antigens such as in hemolytic ABO-incompatible blood transfusion reactions. Heparin–protamine complexes have also been shown in vitro[9] and in vivo[10,11] to activate complement via the classic pathway. Injection of preformed immune complexes or IgG aggregates can activate complement and mimic clinical anaphylaxis.[12] Patients lacking IgA antibody may develop IgG anti-IgA antibodies after receiving multiple transfusions, which may result in complement activation and anaphylactic reactions.[13] Complement activation via the alternative pathway may be stimulated by lipopolysaccharides (endotoxins),[14] Althesin,[15] radiocontrast media,[16] and membranes used for cardiopulmonary bypass and dialysis.[17]

PHARMACOLOGIC (NONIMMUNOLOGIC) MAST CELL ACTIVATORS

Certain agents can cause mast cell mediator release by a nonimmunologic mechanism. The exact mechanism of nonimmunologic mediator release is poorly understood, but release is noncytotoxic. Agents thought to induce nonimmunologic release include opiates (especially morphine)[18,19] and neuromuscular blocking agents such as *d*-tubocurarine.[20] Evidence suggests that the neuromuscular blocking agents such as atracurium and succinylcholine may induce mast cell mediator release via IgE antibodies directed against quaternary or tertiary ammonium ion epitopes.[21,22]

PRESUMED ABNORMALITIES OF ARACHIDONIC ACID METABOLISM

Anaphylactic responses caused by aspirin and structurally unrelated nonsteroidal antiinflammatory drugs (NSAIDs) have been estimated to occur in approximately 1 per cent of individuals.[23] The incidence of aspirin sensitivity (intolerance) in adult patients with

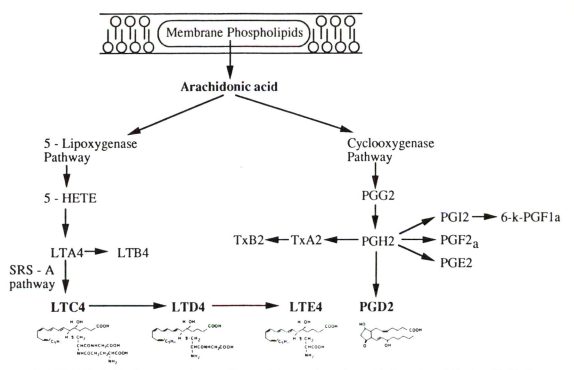

FIGURE 15–2. Newly generated vasoactive mediators produced by metabolism of arachidonic acid. Mediators in boldface type are the predominant products by human mast cells.

asthma ranges from 10 to 20 per cent and occurs most commonly during middle age.[23] Aspirin-sensitive patients frequently have asthma, rhinitis, sinusitis, and nasal polyps. Intolerance to aspirin may result in severe bronchospasm (usually occurring in asthmatic patients) or urticaria and angioedema (usually seen in normal individuals or in patients with rhinitis).[23] Aspirin and NSAIDs inhibit cyclooxygenase, the first enzyme in the metabolic pathway that converts arachidonic acid to prostaglandin and thromboxane (Fig. 15–2). It has been suggested that the cyclooxygenase blockade could lead to a decrease in bronchodilating prostaglandins or cause shunting of arachidonic acid to the 5-lipoxygenase pathway, resulting in production of the vasoactive leukotrienes.[23]

MEDIATORS OF ANAPHYLACTIC REACTIONS

Any of the mechanisms described above may lead to mast cell or basophil mediator release. Mediators released include those preformed and stored in granules as well as those newly generated upon appropriate stimulation. Release of these mediators may cause various pathophysiologic responses that may result in life-threatening anaphylactic reactions. The various preformed and newly generated mediators released by mast cells or basophils, their biologic actions, and their physiologic manifestations are shown in Table 15–4.

ANAPHYLAXIS

CLINICAL MANIFESTATIONS

Individuals vary in terms of the time of onset and manifestations of anaphylaxis. In general, symptoms begin soon (within minutes) after introduction of the causative agent, although they may be delayed for up to 1 to 2 hours. Along with other symptoms, patients frequently describe a sense of impending doom. The primary anaphylactic target organs in humans are the cutaneous, gastrointestinal, respiratory, and cardiovascular systems (Table 15–5). Involvement of the respiratory and cardiovascular systems are of primary importance. In a large series of patients with fatal anaphylactic reactions, 70 per cent died from respiratory complications and 24 per cent from cardiovascular complications.[24]

1. *Cutaneous manifestations.* Initial signs and symptoms may include erythema, flush-

TABLE 15–4. BIOLOGIC ACTIONS AND PHYSIOLOGIC MANIFESTATIONS OF MAST CELL MEDIATORS

Mediators	Biologic Action	Physiologic Manifestations
Preformed		
Histamine	Smooth muscle contraction	Bronchospasm, abdominal pain, diarrhea, nausea, vomiting
	Vasodilation	Tachycardia, hypotension
	Increases vasopermeability	Edema, urticaria/angioedema, influx of inflammatory cells
	Stimulates mucus secretion	Excessive respiratory and gastrointestinal secretions, inspissation
ECF-A	Eosinophil chemotaxis	Inflammation
NCA	Neutrophil chemotaxis	Inflammation
Neutral proteases	Cleave amino acids from proteins	?
	?Stimulate mucus secretion	
Proteoglycans (heparin and chondroitin sulfate)	Anticoagulant	?
Newly generated		
PGD$_2$	Smooth muscle contraction	Bronchospasm, abdominal pain, diarrhea, nausea, vomiting
	Vasodilation	Tachycardia, hypotension
	Stimulates mucous secretion	Excessive respiratory and gastrointestinal secretions, inspissation
	Enhances basophil mediator release	Potentiates reactions
	Inhibits platelet aggregation	?
LTC$_4$/D$_4$/E$_4$ (SRS-A)	Smooth muscle contraction	Bronchospasm, abdominal pain, diarrhea, nausea, vomiting
	Vasodilation	Tachycardia, hypotension
	Increases vasopermeability	Edema, urticaria/angioedema, influx of inflammatory cells
	Stimulates mucus secretion	Excessive respiratory and gastrointestinal secretions, inspissation
PAF	Smooth muscle contraction	Bronchospasm, abdominal pain, diarrhea, nausea, vomiting
	Vasodilation	Tachycardia, hypotension
	Increases vasopermeability	Edema, urticaria/angioedema, hypotension
	Decreases inotropy of heart	Hypotension
	Neutrophil stimulation	?
	Platelet aggregation	?

ing, and pruritus (especially of the palms, soles, and groin), which often progress to urticaria and angioedema.

2. *Gastrointestinal manifestations.* Gastrointestinal findings include nausea, cramping abdominal pain, vomiting, and intense diarrhea, which may be bloody.

3. *Respiratory manifestations.* Upper respiratory tract involvement may involve laryngeal edema, which may progress to asphyxia. This finding is of grave importance and must be carefully assessed. Early symptoms of laryngeal edema include hoarseness, dysphonia, or a "lump in the throat." Lower respiratory tract involvement is often expressed as chest tightness, shortness of breath, coughing, or wheezing.

4. *Cardiovascular manifestations.* Cardiovascular signs may include hypotension and tachycardia with symptoms of light-headedness, faintness, and syncopy. Cardiovascular complications include myocardial infarction, dysrhythmia, and cardiovascular collapse.

5. *Miscellaneous manifestations.* Other signs and symptoms reported in association with anaphylaxis include nasal, ocular, and palatal pruritus, sneezing, diaphoresis, disorientation, and incontinence. Some subjects

TABLE 15–5. CLINICAL MANIFESTATIONS OF ANAPHLAXIS, BY SYSTEM

Cutaneous
    Pruritis
    Flushing
    Erythema
    Urticaria/angioedema

Gastrointestinal system
    Nausea
    Abdominal pain
    Diarrhea
    Vomiting

Respiratory system
    Laryngeal edema
    Hoarseness
    Dysphonia
    "Lump in throat"
    Chest tightness
    Dyspnea
    Cough
    Wheezing
    Cyanosis
    Increase in peak airway pressure

Cardiovascular system
    Light-headedness
    Faintness
    Syncopy
    Tachycardia
    Hypotension
    Dysrhythmia

Signs in boldface type are most likely to occur in intubated patients.

have spontaneous recrudesce of anaphylaxis 8 to 24 hours later (equivalent to late-phase reactions).

INTRAOPERATIVE/PERIOPERATIVE ANAPHYLAXIS

Evaluation and treatment of patients who develop anaphylaxis in the operating room is challenging even for the experienced physician. During the perioperative period, multiple medications are frequently given in close succession, making temporal relations more difficult to interpret. Patients are frequently unconscious and draped, potentially masking early signs and symptoms of anaphylaxis. Anesthetics themselves alter mediator release, possibly delaying early recognition of the syndrome.[5] Often the only observed manifestation of anaphylaxis during anesthesia is cardiovascular collapse,[26] a relatively late event in the syndrome. With suspected anaphylactic reactions in patients undergoing hemodynamic monitoring, cardiovascular changes are characterized by decreases in systolic, diastolic, and mean arterial pressures. Systemic vascular resistance also decreases, and cardiac output and stroke volume increase. Sudden decreases in pulmonary compliance may be manifested by an increase in airway pressures during positive pressure ventilation. Cyanosis (associated with oxygen desaturation) may be noted.

DIFFERENTIAL DIAGNOSIS

Anaphylaxis is most easily confused with a vasovagal reaction (Table 15–6), which usually occurs when a patient collapses after an injection or painful situation. With vasovagal reactions, the patient looks pale and complains of nausea before syncopy but does not note pruritus or become cyanotic. Respiratory difficulty does not occur, and symptoms are relieved almost immediately once the patient is supine. The syndrome is usually accompanied by profuse diaphoresis and bradycardia, without flushing, urticaria, angioedema, pruritus, or wheezing. The differential diagnosis of sudden collapse also includes dysrhythmia, myocardial infarction, aspiration of food or a foreign body, pulmonary embolism, seizure disorder, hypoglycemia, and stroke.

In the presence of laryngeal edema, especially when accompanied by abdominal pain, the diagnosis of hereditary angioedema should be considered. Globus hystericus and fictitious asthma need to be considered when respiratory symptoms are present.

Serum sickness may present with urticaria similar to anaphylaxis. However, it generally occurs 6 to 21 days after the antigenic stimula-

TABLE 15–6. DIFFERENTIAL DIAGNOSIS OF ANAPHYLAXIS

Vasovagal reaction
Dysrhythmia
Myocardial infarction
Overdose of medication or illicit drugs
Pulmonary embolism
Seizure disorder
Cerebral vascular accident
Aspiration
Globus hystericus
Fictitious asthma
Hereditary angioedema
Physical or idiopathic urticaria
Serum sickness
Carcinoid tumors
Systemic mastocytosis

tion and is frequently associated with fever, lymphadenopathy, arthralgias, arthritis, nephritis, and neuritis. Other conditions that can mimic anaphylaxis include overdose of medication, cold urticaria (especially if generalized), idiopathic urticaria, carcinoid tumors, and systemic mastocytosis.

TREATMENT

It is essential that anaphylactic reactions be recognized early, as death may occur within minutes.[27] The longer initial therapy is delayed, the greater is the incidence of fatality.[24] Morbidity and mortality from anaphylactic reactions are primarily associated with compromised cardiovascular and respiratory function. Therefore close monitoring of vital signs, focusing on blood pressure and airway patency and ventilation, is most important when assessing the severity of the reaction and response to therapy. Treatment of anaphylactic reactions can be divided into initial and secondary therapies (Table 15–7).

Initial Therapy

1. When possible, steps should be taken to interrupt further administration and absorption of the offending agent. Intravenous infusions of suspected allergens should be stopped immediately. If the antigen had been given subcutaneously (i.e., insulin or immunotherapy), a venous tourniquet should be placed proximal to the site and aqueous epinephrine 1 : 1000 (0.01 ml/kg, with a maximum dose 0.3 to 0.5 ml) should be injected directly into the antigen source in order to reduce the local circulation and systemic absorption of antigen.

2. Maintain the airway and administer 100 per cent oxygen; adequate oxygenization should be monitored using arterial blood gas assays. If the patient is not already intubated and there is any suggestion of airway compromise secondary to laryngeal edema, the patient should be intubated immediately. If laryngospasm or laryngeal edema is present, aerosolized epinephrine (three inhalations of 0.16 to 0.20 mg epinephrine per inhalation) or by a nebulizer (8 to 15 drops of 2.25 per cent epinephrine in 2 ml normal saline) may be use-

TABLE 15–7. MANAGEMENT OF ANAPHYLAXIS

Initial therapy
    1. Stop administration or reduce absorption of offending agent. If antigen given SC:
        a. Venous tourniquet proximal to site.
        b. Epinephrine 1:1000 into antigen site.
    2. Maintain airway and administer 100% O_2.
        a. Aerosolized epinephrine
        b. Cricothyrotomy
    3. Rapid intravascular volume expansion: 25–50 ml/kg (2–4 liters) of crystalloid for hypotension.
    4. Administer epinephrine
        a. 0.1 ml/kg of 1:1000 SC or IM (maximum dose 0.3–0.5 ml)—may repeat every 15 minutes.
        b. 0.1 ml/kg of 1:10,000 (100 μg/ml) IV (maximum dose 5 ml)—titrate as needed.
        c. 10 ml of 1:10,000 endotracheal administration.
    5. Discontinue all anesthetic agents.
    6. Consider use of MAST.

Secondary therapy
    1. Administer antihistamine.
        a. Diphenhydramine 1 mg/kg IV or IM (maximum dose 50 mg).
        b. Ranitidine 1 mg/kg IV (maximum dose 50 mg).
    2. Administer glucocorticoids.
        a. Hydrocortisone 5 mg/kg initially, then 2.5 mg/kg q4–6h.
        b. Methylprednisolone 1 mg/kg initially, then q4–6h.
    3. Administer aminophylline.
        a. Loading dose 5–6 mg/kg.
        b. Continuous infusion 0.4–0.9 mg/kg/hr (check blood level).
    4. Administer continuous catecholamine infusion.
        a. Epinephrine 0.02–0.05 μg/kg/min (2–4 μg/min).
        b. Norepinehrine 0.05 μg/kg/min (2–4 μg/min).
        c. Dopamine 5–20 μg/kg/min.
    5. Administer sodium bicarbonate 0.5–1.0 mg/kg initially, then titrate using arterial blood gas assays.

ful. If the laryngospasm or laryngeal edema is refractory to these measures or is progressing too rapidly, a needle catheter cricothyrotomy or emergency surgical cricothyrotomy may be necessary.

3. At the first signs of a severe reaction, intravenous access should be established (if not already in place), and blood pressure should be maintained with the administration of isotonic crystalloid (normal saline) or colloidal solutions. Rapid administration of normal saline or lactated Ringer's solution (25 to 50 ml/kg—2 to 4 liters in an adult) is important for the initial therapy of these reactions. Military antishock trousers (MAST suit) can be useful for patients suffering from hypotension secondary to anaphylaxis.[28,29] The MAST suit provides profusion to vital organs and may be helpful for obtaining peripheral venous access in the upper extremities.[29]

4. Epinephrine 1 : 1000 is the mainstay of initial treatment and should be given in a dose of 0.01 ml/kg SC or IM (maximum dose 0.3 to 0.5 ml). Treatment may be repeated every 15 to 20 minutes as necessary. In cases of severe hypotension or laryngospasm a 0.1 ml/kg dose of 1 : 10,000 epinephrine (100 μg/ml) should be given intravenously (maximum dose 0.5 to 1.0 ml). Depending on the patient's condition, the dosage may need to be higher, although risks include cardiac arrhythmias, myocardial infarction, or stroke. If an intravenous line is not in place, 0.5 ml of 1 : 1000 epinephrine can be given intramuscularly, or 10 ml of 1 : 10,000 epinephrine can be administered through the endotracheal tube. However, for a patient in shock, the absorption of intramuscular or subcutaneous epinephrine is unreliable.

5. Discontinue all anesthetic agents. Anesthetic agents have negative inotropic properties, may decrease systemic vascular resistance, and may interfere with the reflex compensatory response to hypotension. Halothane also sensitizes the heart to catecholamines, which are required for severe anaphylactic reactions.

Secondary Treatment

Once a patient's condition has begun to stabilize, administration of other pharmacologic agents may be warranted.

1. An antihistimine such as diphenhydramine 1 mg/kg IV or IM (up to 50 mg) is helpful for symptomatic relief of itching. Although there is no evidence demonstrating the effectiveness of H_2-receptor antagonists in the treatment of anaphylaxis, ranitidine 1 mg/kg IV may be useful when hypotension is persistent, as peripheral vasodilation may be exacerbated by the effects of histamine on endothelial H_2 receptors. Intravenous cimetidine has been reported to cause short-term hypotension and therefore should probably be avoided.[30]

2. Glucocorticoids may be useful for preventing potential late-phase reactions but have no immediate effects. Hydrocortisone 5 mg/kg (up to 200 mg initial dose) and then 2.5 mg/kg q6h or methylprednisolone 1 mg/kg initially and then q6h as indicated may be given.

3. For persistent bronchospasm, aminophylline administered intravenously in a loading dose (5 to 6 mg/kg) followed by a continuous infusion (0.4 to 0.9 mg/kg/hr) may be helpful.

4. For persistent hypotension, catecholamine infusions may be used. Epinephrine may be useful if both hypotension and bronchospasm persist. The suggested starting dose of epinephrine is 0.02 to 0.05 μg/kg/min (2 to 4 μg/min) and should be titrated to maintain tissue perfusion. If more than 8 to 10 μg/min is required, tachycardia may be a significant side effect and norepinephrine may be more effective. The suggested starting dose for norepinephrine is 0.05 μg/kg/min (2 to 4 μg/min) and should be titrated to maintain tissue perfusion. Dopamine may be used to maintain blood pressure. A dose of 5 to 20 μg/kg/min may be helpful for maintaining cardiac output and improving coronary, cerebral, renal, and mesenteric blood flow.

5. If acidosis is suspected, sodium bicarbonate (0.5 to 1.0 mg/kg) should be administered initially. Acid-base status must be monitored using arterial blood gas levels to guide further therapeutic interventions.

Response to therapy is usually prompt; but despite all of the above measures, some patients do not respond quickly. In one study where the efficacy of immunotherapy for insect sting allergy was assessed by deliberate sting challenge, investigators found that even when they were totally prepared to treat anaphylaxis in an intensive care unit setting severe, persistent hypotension occurred that was protracted and difficult to treat.

Treatment of anaphylaxis may be complicated by the increased use of β-adrenergic blocking agents (i.e., propranolol).[31] How best to treat patients experiencing anaphylaxis who are taking β-blocking drugs is not clear. A limited number of studies have suggested that in addition to the above mentioned measures, use of the MAST suit and administration of atropine or glucagon may be of benefit.[12]

DETERMINING THE CAUSE OF ALLERGIC REACTIONS

Patients who have suffered anaphylactic reactions to drugs administered in the operating room require evaluation to identify the causal agents and to guide selection and use of future medications. The evaluation starts with a detailed history, including concurrent illness and prior allergic and anesthetic encounters. It is helpful to prepare a flow diagram of the patient's reaction depicting temporally the clinical manifestations of the reaction and the medications received including indications, when initiated, doses, and duration of therapy. Equally important information includes previous exposure to the same or structurally related medications, the effect of drug discontinuation, the response to treatment, and any prior diagnostic testing or rechallenge. Medications should be considered with regard to their known propensity for causing anaphylaxis. The proximity of drug administration to the onset of acute reactions should also be documented. In general, agents that have been used for long, continuous periods of time before the onset of an acute reaction are less likely to be implicated than agents recently introduced or reintroduced. However, during the perioperative period, it is common for patients to receive many medications in close temporal proximity, making a diagnosis by history alone difficult.

SPECIFIC ALLERGIC REACTIONS DURING THE PERIOPERATIVE PERIOD

PENICILLIN ANTIBIOTICS

Penicillin antibiotics constitute the most common medications causing allergic drug reactions. Available data do not permit exact conclusions as to the true frequency of allergic reactions to penicillin, but such reactions are reported to occur in 0.7 to 8.0 per cent of penicillin treatment cases in various studies.[32] Anaphylactic reactions occur in 0.004 to 0.015 per cent of penicillin treatment cases.[32] Fatal-

ity due to penicillin anaphylaxis occurs about once in every 50,000 to 100,000 treatment cases,[32] resulting in 400 to 800 deaths per year.[33] All four types of immunopathologic reaction described by Gell and Coombs have been seen with penicillin[2] (Table 15–1). Some reactions to penicillin have an obscure pathogenesis and have been labeled idiopathic. Among them are the common maculopapular rash, eosinophilia, Stevens-Johnson syndrome, exfoliative dermatitis, and toxic epidermal necrolysis (Table 15–1). For reasons presently unknown, ampicillin induces rashes with much greater frequency than penicillin.[34] Pseudoanaphylactic reactions have been observed after intramuscular or inadvertent intravenous injection of procaine penicillin. These reactions are most likely due to a combination of a toxic and embolic phenomena from procaine.[35] IgE-mediated reactions may be the most important allergic reaction to penicillin clinically because of the risk of life-threatening anaphylaxis.

Penicillin (molecular weight 356 daltons) is a low-molecular-weight chemical and as such most first covalently combine with tissue macromolecules (presumably proteins) to produce multivalent hapten–protein complexes, which are required for both induction of an immune response and elicitation of an allergic reaction.[36] During the 1960s Levine and Parker showed that the β-lactam ring in penicillins spontaneously opens under physiologic conditions, forming the penicilloyl group.[37] More recent evidence suggests that this reaction may be facilitated by low-molecular-weight molecules in serum.[38] The penicilloyl group has been designated the *major determinants* because about 95 per cent of the penicillin molecules that irreversibly combine with proteins form penicilloyl groups.[3] This reaction occurs with the prototype benzylpenicillin and virtually all semisynthetic penicillins. Benzylpenicillin can also be degraded by other metabolic pathways to form additional antigenic determinants.[39] These derivatives are formed in small quantities and stimulate a variable immune response and hence have been termed the *minor determinants*. Therefore for penicillin and other β-lactams, IgE antibodies can be produced against a number of haptenic derivatives labeled the major and minor determinants. Anaphylactic reactions to penicillin are usually mediated by IgE antibodies directed against minor determinants, although some anaphylactic reactions have occurred in patients with only penicilloyl-specific IgE antibodies.[3,39,40] Accelerated and late urticarial reactions are generally mediated by penicilloyl-specific IgE antibody (major determinant).[3]

Parenteral administration of penicillin produces more allergic reactions than orally administered penicillin. Evidence suggests that it may be more related to dose than route of administration. When equivalent doses of penicillin are given orally, the incidence of allergic reactions is not different from that of intramuscular procaine penicillin.[41] Individuals with a history of penicillin reactions have a four- to sixfold increased risk for subsequent reactions to penicillin compared to those without such a history.[42] However, most serious and fatal allergic reactions to penicillin and β-lactam antibiotics occur in individuals who have never had a prior allergic reaction. Sensitization of these individuals may have resulted from their last therapeutic course of penicillin or (less likely) from occult environmental exposures.

Approximately 10 to 20 per cent of hospitalized patients claim a history of penicillin allergy. However, studies have shown that many of these patients have been either incorrectly diagnosed as allergic to penicillin or have lost their sensitivity. The most useful single piece of information when assessing an individual's potential for an immediate IgE-me-

diated reaction is the skin test response to major and minor penicillin determinants[43] (Fig. 15–3). Because the minor determinants are labile and cannot be readily synthesized in multivalent form, skin testing for minor determinant specificities is usually accomplished using a mixture, collectively called the minor determinant mixture (MDM). At the present, an MDM is not commercially available in the United States. If one uses benzylpenicillin diluted to a concentration of 10,000 U/ml (10^2 M) as the sole minor determinant reagent, about 5 to 10 per cent of skin test reactive patients are missed.[44,45] Although some of those missed are at risk for serious, anaphylactic reactions,[46] this substance is a reasonable alternative to MDM for use in patients *without* an impressive history of IgE-mediated reactions. For patients whose histories are more suggestive of an IgE-mediated anaphylactic reaction, referral to a center with access to MDM is advised.

When therapeutic doses of penicillin are given to patients with a history of penicillin allergy but a negative skin test, IgE-mediated reactions occur rarely and are almost always mild and self-limited. About 1 per cent of skin test-negative patients develop accelerated urticarial reactions, and approximately 3 per cent develop other mild reactions.[47] Penicillin anaphylaxis has not been reported in skin test-

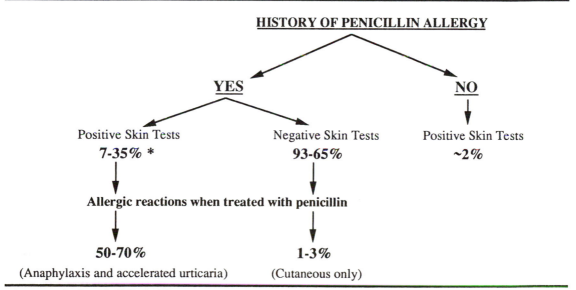

FIGURE 15–3. Prevalence of positive and negative skin tests and the subsequent allergic reactions in patients treated with penicillin (based on studies using both PPL nd MDM as skin test reagents).

negative patients. Therefore negative skin tests indicate that penicillin antibiotics may be safely given. A limited number of patients with positive skin tests have been treated with therapeutic doses of penicillin, and the risk of an anaphylactic or accelerated allergic reaction ranges from 50 to 70 per cent in these patients.[47] Therefore if skin tests are positive, equally effective, non-cross-reacting antibiotics should be substituted when available.

If alternative drugs fail, induce unacceptable side effects, or are clearly less effective, administration of penicillin should be considered using a desensitization protocol. Infections with which this situation most commonly arises are subacute bacterial endocarditis due to enterococci, brain abscess, bacterial meningitis, overwhelming infections with staphylococci or *Pseudomonas* organisms (e.g., osteomyelitis or sepsis), *Listeria* infections, neurosyphilis, and syphilis during pregnancy. Use of a desensitization protocol for penicillin skin test-positive patients markedly reduces the risk of anaphylaxis.

Acute penicillin desensitization should be performed only in an intensive care setting. Any remedial risk factors should be corrected. All β-adrenergic antagonists, e.g., propranolol or even timolol ophthalmic drops, should be discontinued. Asthmatic patients should be under optimal control. An intravenous line should be established, baseline electrocardiography (ECG) and spirometry performed, and continuous ECG monitoring instituted. Premedication and antihistamines or steroids is not recommended, as these drugs have not proved effective for suppressing severe reactions but may mask early signs of reactivity that would otherwise result in modification of the protocol.[48,49]

Protocols have been developed for penicillin desensitization using both the oral and parenteral routes[50,51] and are not discussed in detail here. Approximately one third of patients undergoing desensitization have a transient allergic reaction during desensitization or subsequent treatment. These reactions are usually mild and self-limited in nature, although they may be severe. Once desensitized, the patient's treatment with penicillin must not lapse or the risk of an allergic reaction increases.

CEPHALOSPORINS

Like penicillins, cephalosporins possess a β-lactam ring, but the five-membered thiazolidine ring is replaced by the six-membered dihydrothiazine ring. Shortly after the cephalosporins came into clinical use, allergic reactions including anaphylaxis were reported and the question of cross-reactivity between cephalosporins and penicillins was raised.[52] Studies in both animals and man have clearly demonstrated cross-reactivity between penicillins and cephalosporins using immuno- and bioassays to evaluate IgG, IgM, and IgE antibodies.[53–55] Primary cephalosporin allergy in non-penicillin-allergic patients have been reported, but the exact incidence is not clear.[56,57] Studies have been limited because the haptenic determinants involved in cephalosporin allergy are unknown. The incidence of clinically relevant cross-reactivity between the penicillins and the cephalosporins, although unknown, is probably small; but it cannot be discounted on statistical grounds because life-threatening anaphylactic cross-reactivity has occurred. Therefore patients with positive skin tests to any penicillin reagent should not receive cephalosporin antibiotics unless alternative drugs are clearly less desirable. If cephalosporin drugs are to be used, they should be administered using a modified desensitization protocol.

β-LACTAM ANTIBIOTICS

Two new classes of β-lactam antibiotics are the carbapenems (imipenem) and monobactams (aztreonam). Initial studies suggest significant cross-reactivity between penicillin determinants and imipenem, indicating the prudence of withholding carbopenems from penicillin skin test-positive patients.[58] Initial investigations suggest weak cross-reactivity between aztreonam and other β-lactam antibiotics and indicate that aztreonam may be administered safely to most if not all penicillin-allergic subjects.[59,60]

VANCOMYCIN

Hypotension is the most serious immediate adverse effect associated with the use of vancomycin. Direct myocardial depression[61] and nonimmunologically mediated histamine release[62] have been reported as the mechanism of vancomycin-induced hypotension. In humans hypotension occurs most commonly when the drug is rapidly infused or when it is administered in a concentrated solution.[61] Vancomycin-associated hypotension most commonly occurs during the perioperative period and may be related to the concomitant use of other drugs that cause vasodilation or have a negative inotropic effect.[61] In addition to hypotension, vancomycin can produce the "red neck syndrome," alternatively called the "red man's syndrome," which consists of an intense erythematous discoloration of the upper trunk, arms, and neck sometimes associated with pruritus. Vancomycin has also been associated with the sudden development of throbbing pain or spasm in the chest or parasternal muscles without evidence of myocardial ischemia. To minimize the risk of reactions, vancomycin should be infused over a period of at least 60 minutes and in a dilute solution (500 mg/dl). Preoperatively, the first infusion of vancomycin should be administered with supervision. Reactions should be treated by discontinuation of vancomycin infusion, administration of an antihistamine, and the use of medications that have a positive inotropic effect rather than a pure vasoconstrictor effect if hypotension persists.

SULFONAMIDES

Sulfonamides are frequently responsible for drug-induced skin eruptions (usually exanthematous) and drug fever, often appearing between the seventh and tenth days of treatment. Less common reactions include vasculitis, a pulmonary reaction, the Stevens-Johnson syndrome, and urticaria. The introduction of trimethoprim-sulfamethoxazole, which is effective for treating a variety of infections, has been responsible for the resurgence of the widespread use of sulfonamides. The incidence of reactions from trimethoprim-sulfamethoxazole in hospitalized patients is between 3 and 6 per cent.[63] The incidence of reactions is approximately 10 to 15 times higher among patients with the acquired immunodeficiency syndrome (AIDS).[64] The reason for the increased incidence of reactions in patients with AIDS is unknown. The immunochemistry of sulfonamide allergy in man is not completely understood, although there is evidence to suggest that some sulfonamide reactions are mediated through IgE antibody.[65] It appears that hepatic metabolism is required to convert the native sulfonamide to its immunogenic metabolite.[66] Isolated examples of desensitization to sulfamonides have been reported using different desensitization protocols,[67,68] although severe reactions have been induced by oral desensitization to trimethoprim-sulfamethoxazole.[69]

MUSCLE RELAXANTS

Anaphylactic reactions, including cardiovascular collapse, tachycardia, urticaria, and bronchospasm, may follow the administration of muscle relaxants.[70] Certain muscle relaxants (e.g., *d*-tubocurarine) produce nonimmunologic histamine release.[26] Evidence presented by Vervloet and colleagues[71] and Baldo et al.[21,22] suggests that anaphylactic reactions to myorelaxants are caused by an IgE-mediated mechanism. Extensive in vitro cross-reactivity has been reported between the muscle relaxants and other compounds that contain quarternary and tertiary ammonium ions.[21] These compounds occur widely in many drugs, foods, cosmetics, disinfectants, and industrial materials. The clinical significance of this in vitro cross-reactivity is unclear, although it has been postulated that patients may become sensitized through environmental contact with these various compounds.[21] Because the muscle relaxants contain two ammonium ions, they appear to be functionally divalent, capable of cross-linking cell surface IgE and initiating mediator release from mast cells and basophils without haptenizing to carrier molecules.[71] Muscle relaxants with a rigid backbone between the two ammonium ions (e.g., pancuronium and vercuronium) appear to be less active than flexible molecules in initiating mediator release.[72]

Atopy does not appear to be a risk factor for the occurrence of anaphylactic reactions to muscle relaxants.[73] It is of interest that 90 to 95 per cent of anaphylactic reactions to muscle relaxants occurs in females,[74] the reason for which is unclear.

Although the incidence of allergic reactions caused by muscle relaxants is unknown, it appears that reactions are less common in the United States than in France or Australia (personal observation). Skin testing and the radio allergosorbent test (RAST) can be used to evaluate the presence of IgE antibody directed against muscle relaxants.[21,67] However, more studies are needed to determine the predictive value of these tests.

BARBITURATES

Acute allergic reactions have been reported after the administration of thiobarbiturates, and most of these reactions have been associated with thiopental administration.[26] Proposed mechanisms for thiobarbiturate reactions include nonimmunologically induced

TABLE 15–8. CLASSIFICATION OF LOCAL ANESTHETICS

Group I: Benzoic Acid Esters	Group II: Amides (Others)
Amydricaine (Alypin)	Antihistamines[a]
Butacaine (Butyn)	Bupivacaine (Marcaine)
Benzocaine	Dibucaine (Nupercaine)
Chlorprocaine (Nesacaine)	Dicyclonine (Dyclone)
Cyclomethycaine (Surfacaine)	Lidocaine (Xylocaine)
Isobucaine (Kincain)	Mepivacaine (Carbocaine)
Meprylcaine (Oracaine)	Oxethazine (Oxaine)
Metabulethamine (Oracaine)	Phenacaine (Holocaine)
Piperocaine (Metycaine)	Pramoxine (Tronothane)
Procain (Novocaine)	
Tetracaine (Pontocaine)	

[a] Antihistamines have minor anesthetic effect.

mediator release and IgE-mediated reactions.[26] Positive immediate skin tests to thiopental have been reported in patients who had anaphylactic reactions following induction of general anesthesia.[75] A thiopental RAST has been reported,[76] although the predictive value of skin testing and RAST to thiopental is uncertain at present.

LOCAL ANESTHETICS

Despite patients commonly reporting adverse reactions to local anesthetics and being advised that they are "allergic" to these agents, true allergic reactions to injected local anesthetics are rare. Reactions to local anesthetics are often the result of vasovagal reactions, toxic reactions (probably due to inadvertent intravenous injection), side effects from epinephrine, or psychomotor responses including hyperventilation. Toxic symptoms often involve the central nervous and cardiovascular symptoms and may produce slurred speech, euphoria, dizziness, excitement, nausea, emesis, disorientation, or convulsions.[77]

Vasovagal reactions are usually associated with bradycardia, sweating, pallor, and rapid involvement in symptoms when the patient is supine. Sympathetic stimulation, due to epinephrine or anxiety, may result in tremor, diaphoresis, tachycardia, and hypertension. Rarely, symptoms of reactions to local anesthetics are consistent with IgE-mediated reactions, e.g., urticaria, bronchospasm, and anaphylactic shock. However, acceptable documentation of IgE-mediated reactivity against local anesthetics in such patients is lacking, with few exceptions.[78] IgE-mediated sensitivity has, on rare occasions, also been reported for the parabens, preservatives used in local anesthetics.[79]

Local anesthetics are divided into two chemical groups (Table 15–8). Group I consists of chemicals containing benzoate esters, which may cross-react with each other but not with group II drugs. Group II agents include mostly amides, which do not substantially cross-react with each other.

Evaluation of a patient with a history of an adverse reaction to local anesthetics should include a complete history of the episode, skin

TABLE 15–9. PROTOCOL FOR EVALUATION OF LOCAL ANESTHETIC ALLERGY: JOHNS HOPKINS

Step[a]	Route	Volume (ml)	Dilution
1	Intradermal	0.02	1:1000[b]
2	Intradermal	0.02	1:100
3	Intradermal	0.02	1:10
4	Intradermal	0.02	Undiluted
5	Subcutaneous	0.30	Undiluted

[a] Administer at 15-minute intervals.
[b] If history is strongly suggestive of IgE-mediated reaction, start with puncture at 1:1000 dilution.

TABLE 15–10. PROTOCOL FOR EVALUATION OF LOCAL ANESTHETIC ALLERGY: NORTHWESTERN UNIVERSITY

Step[a]	Route	Volume (ml)	Dilution
1	Puncture		Undiluted
2	Subcutaneous	0.1	Undiluted
3	Subcutaneous	0.5	Undiluted
4	Subcutaneous	1.0	Undiluted
5	Subcutaneous	2.0	Undiluted

[a] Administer at 15-minute intervals.

testing, and an incremental drug challenge. The protocol used at Johns Hopkins is listed in Table 15–9. A more aggressive protocol is used at Northwestern (Table 15–10). The local anesthetic tested should be appropriate for the proposed procedure and one that would not be expected to cross-react with the drug implicated in the previous reaction. If the previous drug is unknown, a group II anesthetic (frequently lidocaine) should be chosen. In a patient with a history suggestive of an IgE-mediated reaction or one suggesting possible paraben sensitivity, preparations without paraben should be used for testing, challenge, and treatment. Preparations without epinephrine should be used for skin testing because they may mask a positive skin test[80] and may induce toxic effects.

NARCOTICS

Narcotics cause nonimmunologically mediated histamine release from skin mast cells. Most opiate-induced reactions are self-limiting cutaneous reactions, restricted to hives and pruritus or mild hypotension treated by fluid administration. Evidence suggests that IgE antibodies may be induced that bind epitopes contained in opiate narcotics.[81-83] However, the pharmacologic release of mediators induced by opiates is a far more common clinical occurrence than reactions induced by morphine-specific IgE antibody. As codeine and morphine routinely cause positive skin responses secondary to nonimmunologic skin mast cell stimulation, skin tests must be interpreted cautiously and must be accompanied by skin testing of normal control subjects.

RADIOCONTRAST MEDIA

The incidence of reactions induced by radiocontrast medium (RCM) injections is between 5 and 8 per cent.[16] Vasomotor reactions (nausea, vomiting, flushing, or warmth) occur in 5 to 8 per cent of patients.[16] Anaphylactoid reactions (urticaria, angioedema, wheezing, dyspnea, hypotension, or death) occur in 2 to 3 per cent of patients receiving intravenous or interarterial infusions.[70] Fatal reactions following radiocontrast media administration occurs in about 1 : 50,000 intravenous procedures,[70] and it has been estimated that as many as 500 deaths per year are due to RCM administration. Most reactions begin 1 to 3 minutes after intravascular administration. Patients with a previous anaphylactic reaction to RCM have approximately a 33 per cent (range 17 to 60 per cent) chance of a repeat reaction upon reexposure.[70]

The etiology(ies) of adverse reactions to RCM are unknown at present. Histamine liberation appears to be a feature of some reactions,[16] although elevations in plasma histamine have occurred without hemodynamic changes or anaphylactic reactions.[16] Activation of serum complement, which follows the intravascular injection of RCM,[80] may occur by the classic or the alternative pathway. Therefore it has been suggested that production of anaphylatoxins with subsequent mast cell and basophil mediator release is the cause of RCM reactions. Yet RCM is capable of inducing nonimmunologic histamine release from mast cells and basophils in the absence of complement activation.[16] It has been suggested that the hypertonicity of RCM results in nonimmunologic mediator from mast cells and basophils.[16] Although it appears clear that the vasomotor reactions (pain, nausea, vomiting, and warmth) and histamine release in vitro are caused by hyperosmolarity, it is unclear if hyperosmolarity is the cause of anaphylactic reactions in humans. There is no evidence that IgE-mediated mechanisms play a role in RCM reactions.

A patient who requires RCM administration and who has had a previous RCM reaction has

TABLE 15–11. PREMEDICATION OF PATIENTS WITH PREVIOUS RADIOCONTRAST MEDIA REACTION

Premedication	Repeat Reaction Rate
a. No premedication	**a.** 33% (17–60%)
b. Prednisone (50 mg PO) 13, 7, and 1 hr before	
c. Diphenhydramine (50 mg IM or PO) 1 hr before	**b&c.** 9% (reactions mild)
d. Ephedrine (25 mg PO) 1 hr before	**b,c,d.** 3.1% (historical controls)
e. ?Ranitidine	

an increased (35 to 60 per cent) risk for a reaction on reexposure[16] (Table 15–11). Pretreatment of these high risk patients with prednisone 50 mg at 13, 7, and 1 hour before RCM administration along with diphenhydramine 50 mg 1 hour before RCM administration reduces the risk of reactions to 9 per cent.[84] Almost all reactions in pretreated patients are of no clinical importance (e.g., mild urticaria).[16] The addition of ephedrine 25 mg 1 hour before RCM administration (in patients without angina, arrhythmia, or other contraindications for ephedrine administration) resulted in a reaction rate of 3.1 per cent.[16] It might be expected that the addition of an H_2-receptor antagonist (e.g., cimetidine or ranitidine) might further decrease the incidence of RCM reactions. To date, however, no study has shown a benefit from the addition of H_2-receptor antagonists to RCM pretreatment regimens. One study showed that steroid pretreatment before the administration of hyperosmolar RCM is as effective (and less expensive) than the use of newer, nonhyperosmolar RCM.[85]

ASPIRIN

Reactions to aspirin (acetylsalicylic acid, ASA) appear to be limited to the skin (urticaria, angioedema) or the respiratory system (bronchospasm, rhinitis, sinusitis). ASA-induced bronchospasm is rare in nonasthmatics. It occurs in approximately 10 per cent of asthmatics more than 10 years of age; in 30 to 40 per cent of asthmatics with nasal polyps, rhinitis, and sinusitis; and in 60 to 85 per cent of asthmatics who give a history of ASA-induced reactions.[23] These reactions may be severe, are difficult to treat, and may produce death.

Aspirin-induced reactions are not IgE-mediated, and the mechanism is incompletely understood at present. A working hypothesis suggests that aspirin (and other NSAIDs) inhibit cyclooxygenase, shunt arachidonic acid metabolism through the 5-lipoxygenase pathway and so produce increased amounts of leukotrienes, C_4, D_4, and E_4. Essentially all NSAIDs except benoxaprofen cross-react with ASA and should be avoided by ASA-sensitive asthmatics.[23]

If ASA or other NSAIDs are required for treatment of a disease in a patient with a history of aspirin sensitivity, ASA desensitization may be indicated.[86] During the desensitization process the patient invariably experiences worsening of asthmatic symptoms. Thus the procedure should be undertaken only by experienced personnel in a setting where severe asthmatic reactivity and anaphylaxis can be treated immediately. Desensitization induces a refractory state that allows the patient to tolerate ASA or NSAIDs without experiencing adverse reactions so long as daily administration continues.

INSULIN

Insulin consists of two polypeptide chains joined by disulfide bonds. The most common commercial preparations contain both bovine and porcine insulin. Bovine insulin differs from human insulin in three amino acids; porcine insulin differs from human insulin in only one amino acid. These differences may account for the immunogenicity of commercial insulins. Changes in tertiary structure may also contribute to insulin immunogenicity. This alteration in tertiary structure is thought in part to be the cause of allergic reactions to recombinant human insulin.[87]

Although, most patients receiving daily injections of insulin develop antibodies to insulin during the first few weeks of therapy,[88] estimates of insulin allergy in patients receiving insulin range from 5 to 10 per cent. Most of these reactions are local.

Local reactions, usually mild, consist of erythema, induration, burning, and pruritus at the injection site.[80] These reactions usually occur within the first 1 to 4 weeks after initiation of insulin injections. Reactions almost always disappear in 3 to 4 weeks with continued insulin administration. Occasionally they persist and may precede a systemic reaction.[80] Stopping insulin treatment because of local reactions may increase the risk of systemic reactions if insulin treatment is later resumed. Most local allergic reactions can be treated with H_1-receptor antagonists. Evidence exists that local allergic reactions coincide with antiinsulin IgE antibody production and that symptoms disappear with the concomitant production of antiinsulin IgG antibodies.[80]

Systemic allergic reactions to insulin, characterized by generalized urticaria, angioedema, bronchospasm, and hypotension, are rare. If a systemic allergic reaction to insulin occurs, insulin should not be discontinued. The next dose should be reduced to approximately one third of the previous dose and then slowly increased (by 2 to 5 units per treatment) until adequate doses are achieved. In patients with a history of a systemic allergic reaction to insulin in whom insulin therapy has been discontinued, desensitization may be cautiously attempted if insulin therapy is required. The least allergenic insulin may be selected by comparative cutaneous testing of bovine, porcine, and human insulin. Desensitization protocol schedules have been reported.[70]

PROTAMINE

Protamine sulfate is a polycationic (strongly basic) small protein (molecular weight 43,000 daltons). Protamine is extracted from salmon milt and is used medicinally to reverse heparin anticoagulation and to regard the absorption of certain insulins (NPH and PZI). The use of intravenous protamine has increased with the advent of cardiopulmonary bypass technology, cardiac catheterization, hemodialysis, and plasmaphoresis. This increase in intravenous protamine use has resulted in increasing reports of adverse reactions.

Adverse reactions to intravenous protamine administration include rash, urticaria, bronchospasm, pulmonary vasoconstriction, and systemic hypotension leading at times to cardiovascular collapse and death.[89]

Diabetic patients receiving daily subcutaneous injections of insulins containing protamine have a 40- to 50-fold increased risk for life-threatening reactions when given protamine intravenously.[90,91] Another group putatively at increased risk for protamine reactions are men who have undergone vasectomy. With disruption of the blood-testis barrier, studies have shown that 20 to 33 per cent of such men develop hemagglutinating autoantibodies against protamine-like compounds.[92] It has been postulated that these autoantibodies may cross-react with medicinal protamine, causing adverse reactions.[93] Although protamine reactions in vasectomized men have been described,[94] no study has systematically evaluated the prevalence of antibodies directed against medicinal protamine in this population.

Another group at theoretic risk for protamine reactions are fish-allergic individuals. Because protamine is produced from the matured testis of salmon or related species of fish belonging to the family Salmonidae or Clupeidae, it has been suggested that individuals allergic to fish may have serum antibodies directed against protamine. Conversely, commercial protamine preparations may be contaminated with fish proteins to which fish-allergic patients may react. To date, evidence supporting the increased risk for protamine reactions in fish-allergic patients is lacking and is limited to case reports.[94]

Finally, previous exposure to intravenous protamine given for reversal of heparin anticoagulation may increase the risk for a reaction on subsequent protamine administration.[89] No systematic study has been done to evaluate the human immune response to protamine following intravenous administration.

Skin testing with protamine does not appear to be useful for discriminating between subjects with significant serum antiprotamine IgE antibody and control subjects. It has been suggested that protamine is an incomplete or univalent antigen that first must combine with a tissue macromolecule or possibly heparin to become a complete, multivalent antigen capable of eliciting mediator release. Thus it appears likely that more than one mechanism

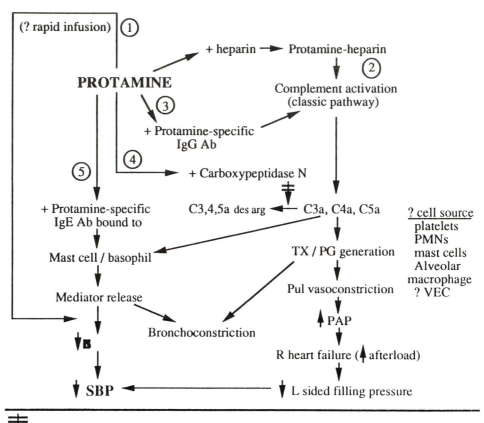

$\mp{\downarrow}$, inhibition; TX, thromboxane; PG, prostaglandins; PAP, pulmonary artery pressure; VEC, vascular endothelial cells; Ab, antibody; SVR, sytemic vascular resistance; SBP, systemic blood pressure.

FIGURE 15–4. Possible mechanisms for protamine reactions: 1) high concentration of protamine inducing direct nonimmunologic mediator release; 2) complement activation from protamine–heparin complexes; 3) complement activation from protamine and complement-fixing IgG antibody; 4) protamine-inhibiting carboxypeptidase N; and 5) protamine and protamine IgE antibody-inducing mast cell/basophil mediator release.

may be responsible for the adverse reactions associated with protamine (Fig. 15–4).

CHYMOPAPAIN

Chymopapain is injected intradiscally for chemonucleolysis of herniated lumbar intervertebral discs. The incidence of anaphylaxis to chymopapain is about 1 per cent, whereas the incidence of fatal anaphylaxis appears to be about 0.14 per cent.[95] Women appear to be three times more likely to develop anaphylaxis than do men.[80] Chymopapain is obtained from a crude fraction called papain from the papaya tree. Exposure to chymopapain may occur in meat tenderizers, cosmetics, beer, and soft contact lenses.[17] Evidence suggests that chymopapain reactions may be IgE-mediated.[70,95] In vivo skin tests and in vitro immunoassays have been used to detect antichymopapain IgE antibody,[95] but more studies are required to determine the predictive value of these tests.

STREPTOKINASE

Streptokinase is a protein derived from group C β-hemolytic streptococci. It is used as a thrombolytic agent to lyse acute thrombi obstructing coronary arteries and retinal veins. The incidence of allergic reactions to streptokinase is unknown, with reports ranging from 1.7 per cent to 18 per cent.[96] In vivo skin tests and in vitro immunoassays have been used to detect IgE antibodies to streptokinase. Protocols have been recommended for skin testing before streptokinase thrombolytic therapy,[97] but relatively few patients have been evaluated and the predictive value of these tests remains to be determined. The use of recombinant tissue plasminogen activator (rTPA) as a thrombolytic agent may make the use of streptokinase less common, although a randomized, prospective study showed that rTPA was no better than streptokinase for preserving myocardial function after an acute myocardial infarction.[98]

MANNITOL

The administration of mannitol or other hyperosmotic agents may cause direct, nonimmunologic histamine release from circulating basophils and mast cells.[26] There is no evidence that mannitol causes immunologically mediated reactions. It is thought that slow infusion helps to avoid this problem.

METHYLMETHACRYLATE

Methylmethacrylate (bone cement) is used during orthopedic surgery to attach the prosthetic joint to raw bone. Cardiopulmonary complications to methylmethacrylate include hypotension, hypoxemia, noncardiogenic pulmonary edema, and cardiac arrest. Many reasons have been postulated for these physiologic manifestations, none of which is allergic in nature.[26]

TRANSFUSION REACTIONS

Transfusion reactions can be classified as hemolytic or nonhemolytic. The clinical manifestations of classic hemolytic transfusion reactions are produced by the interaction of antibodies with red blood cell antigens, whereas nonhemolytic transfusion reactions result from leukoagglutinin reactions or IgA deficiency.[26]

HEMOLYTIC TRANSFUSION REACTIONS

Hemolytic reactions can be defined as the occurrence of increased red blood cell destruction after transfusion. Following transfusion of ABO-incompatible blood, where IgG or IgM antibodies from the donor or recipient react with red blood cells, complement is activated, causing cell lysis and liberation of complement anaphylatoxins. Reactions may appear within 24 hours of transfusion or may develop 4 to 10 days later. Manifestations of acute reactions include hemoglobinuria, pain (lumbar, sternal, or intravenous), restlessness, rigors, dyspnea, flushing, and shock.[26] Hypotension, urticaria, bronchospasm, or bleeding may be the only sign(s) in an intubated patient. Disseminated intravascular coagulation results after tissue thromboplastin release from the erythrocyte stroma or activation of Hageman factor.[26] Careful blood banking, quality control, and attention to detail when administering blood have made acute hemolytic transfusion reactions far less common than in the past. Delayed hemolytic reactions from weakly reactive antibodies are also rare. The therapy for acute hemolytic reactions is as follows.

1. Immediately stop the transfusion to prevent additional incompatible red blood cell administration. The compatibility of transfused blood must be reevaluated by the blood bank.
2. Rapidly assess and treat the reaction according to its severity. If the patient develops anaphylaxis, therapeutic interventions (as previously described) should be followed.
3. Maintain renal blood flow with intravenous furosemide and mannitol once the patient has been resuscitated and is hemodynamically stable.
4. Replace coagulation factors if severe bleeding occurs.

NONHEMOLYTIC TRANSFUSION REACTIONS

Allergic reactions may also result from antibodies directed to antigens on the white blood cells, platelets, or plasma proteins. These reactions may range from urticaria, fever, and pruritus to life-threatening bronchospasm, hypotension, angioedema, and acute respiratory distress.[26] Transfusion-associated respiratory distress is an example of fluid overload producing hypervolemia or cardiogenic pulmonary edema in patients with ventricular dysfunction. However, pulmonary edema may also be allergic, occurring in patients with normal ventricular function but resulting from altered capillary permeability. This form of acute respiratory failure is called noncardiogenic pulmonary edema as it results from acute lung injury. Allergic reactions to blood products can liberate a spectrum of inflammatory mediators, producing endothelial damage, increased capillary permeability, and resultant perivascular edema in the lung.[26] The following section discusses the pathophysiology of allergy-mediated nonhemolytic transfusion reactions.

LEUKOCYTE-ASSOCIATED REACTIONS

If fresh blood containing viable leukocytes is administered to recipients with antileukocyte antibodies, or if the donor blood contains leukoagglutinins directed against viable recipient granulocytes, the aggregated leukocytes are metabolically active and capable of inducing inflammatory injury.[26] In such a manner, activated granulocyte aggregates are trapped in the pulmonary microcirculation, producing acute lung injury. The attachment of an IgG antibody to the granulocyte surface may serve as a direct trigger to the cell, causing it to aggregate; alternatively, the antibody attaching to the granulocyte surface may activate the complement cascade.

The activated, aggregated granulocytes sequester in the pulmonary vasculature to microvascular occlusion from white blood cell emboli.[26] Acute lung injury results from vascular inflammation and pulmonary endothelial damage following the release of leukocyte products, including arachidonic acid metabolites, oxygen free radicals, and proteolytic enzymes. Clinical findings include hypoxemia, noncardiogenic pulmonary edema, and pulmonary hypertension, often characterized as the adult respiratory distress syndrome.[26] Fatal reactions have also been reported. The treatment of severe leukoagglutinin reactions is supportive and includes hemodynamic support and mechanical ventilation with positive end-expiratory pressure. Any blood product

containing plasma (i.e., fresh frozen plasma, cryoprecipitate, platelets, whole blood, or packed red blood cells) can produce such a reaction. Patients with a history of leukoagglutinin reactions should receive saline-washed red blood cells when subsequent increases in oxygen-carrying capacity are required.

One in every 700 to 850 subjects is believed to have IgA deficiency. Selective IgA deficiency is defined as: 1) a serum IgA concentration below 0.05 mg/ml; 2) normal levels of other immunoglobulins; and 3) otherwise normal cell-mediated immune function.[26] Patients with IgA deficiency develop IgE and complement-fixing IgG antibodies to IgA.[26] Anaphylactic reaction can occur when these patients are given only a few milliliters of whole blood, fresh frozen plasma, or packed red blood cells replete with IgA.[26] Therefore frozen, washed, packed red blood cells or blood from other IgA-deficient donors should be administered when transfusions are required. A registry of IgA-deficient donors can be obtained from the Red Cross. Collagen vascular disease and other autoimmune disorders such as rheumatoid arthritis or systemic lupus erythematosus are associated with IgA deficiency. Unfortunately, most IgA-deficient individuals are asymptomatic and present for evaluation following transfusion reactions.

References

1. Ovary Z: The history of immediate hypersensitivity. Hosp Pract February:99–109, 1989.
2. Gell PGH, Coombs RRA: Classification of allergic reactions responsible for clinical hypersensitivity and disease. *In* Gell PGH, Coombs RRA, Hachmann PJ (eds): Clinical Aspects of Immunology, 3rd ed. Oxford, Blackwell Scientific Publications, 1975, pp. 761–781
3. Levine BB: Immunologic mechanisms of penicillin allergy: a haptenic model system for the study of allergic diseases of man. N Engl J Med 275:1115–1125, 1966.
4. Metzger H, Alcaraz G, Hohman R, et al: The receptor with high affinity for immunoglobulin E. Annu Rev Immunol 4:419–470, 1986.
5. Ishizaka T: Mechanisms of IgE-mediated hypersensitivity. *In* Middleton E Jr, Reed CE, Ellis EF, et al (eds): Allergy: Principles and Practice, 3rd ed. St. Louis, Mosby, 1988, pp. 71–93.
6. Siraganian RP: Histamine secretion from mast cells and basophils. Trends Pharmacol Sci 432–437, 1983.
7. Ghebrehiwet B: The complement system: mechanisms of activation, regulation, and biological functions. *In* Kaplan AP (ed): Allergy. New York, Churchill Livingstone, 1985, pp. 131–152.
8. Yancey KB, Hammer CH, Harvath L, et al: Studies of human C5a as a mediator of inflammation in normal human skin. J Clin Invest 75:486–495, 1985.

9. Rent R, Ertel N, Eisenstein R, Gewurz H: Complement activation by interaction of polyanions and polycations. I. Heparin-protamine induced consumption of complement. J Immunol *114*:120–124, 1975.
10. Kirklin JK, Chenoweth DE, Naftel DC, et al: Effects of protamine administration after cardiopulmonary bypass on complement, blood elements, and the hemodynamic state. Ann Thorac Surg *41*:193–199, 1986.
11. Best N, Sinosich MJ, Teisner B, et al: Complement activation during cardiopulmonary bypass by heparin-protamine interaction. Br J Anaesth *56*:339, 1984.
12. Wasserman SI, Marquardt DL: Anaphylaxis. *In* Middleton E Jr, Reed CE, Ellis EF, et al (eds): Allergy: Principles and Practice, 3rd ed. St. Louis, Mosby, 1988, pp. 1365–1376.
13. Vyas GN, Perkins HA, Fudenberg HH: Anaphylactoid transfusion reactions associated with anti-IgA. Lancet *2*:312, 1968.
14. Fearon DT, Ruddy S, Schur PH, McCabe WR: Activation of the properdin pathway of complement in patients with gram-negative bacteremia. N Engl J Med *292*:937–940, 1975.
15. Watkins J, Clark A, Appleyard TN, et al: Immune mediated reactions to Althesin (alphaxalone). Br J Anaesth *55*:231, 1976.
16. Greenberger PA: Contrast media reactions. J Allergy Clin Immunol *74*:600–605, 1984.
17. Craddock PR, Fehr J, Brigham KL, et al: Complement and leukocyte-mediated pulmonary dysfunction in hemodialysis. N Engl J Med *296*:769–774, 1977.
18. Hermens JM, Ebertz JM, Hanifin JM, Hirshman CA: Comparison of histamine release in human mast cells by morphine, fentanyl, and oxymorphone. Anesthesiology *62*:124–129, 1985.
19. Ebertz JM, Hermens JM, McMillan JC, et al: Functional differences between human cutaneous mast cells and basophils: a comparison of morphine-induced histamine release. Agents Actions *18*:455–462, 1986.
20. North FC, Kettelkamp N, Hirshman CA: Comparison of cutaneous and in vitro histamine release by muscle relaxants. Anesthesiology *66*:543–546, 1987.
21. Baldo BA, Fisher MM: Substituted ammonium ions as allergenic determinants in drug allergy. Nature *306*:262–264, 1983.
22. Harle DG, Baldo BA, Fisher MM: Detection of IgE antibodies to suxamethonium after anaphylactoid reactions during anaesthesia. Lancet *1*:930–932, 1984.
23. Stevenson DD: Adverse reactions to aspirin and non-steroidal anti-inflammatory drugs. Presented at the 12th International Congress of Allergology and Clinical Immunology 1985, pp. 20–25.
24. Barnard JH: Studies of 400 Hymenoptera sting deaths in the United States. J Allergy Clin Immunol *52*:259, 1973.
25. Kettelkamp NS, Austin DR, Cheek DBC, et al: Inhibition of d-tubocurarine-induced histamine release by halothane. Anesthesiology *66*:666–669, 1987.
26. Levy JH: Anaphylactic Reactions in Anesthesia and Intensive Care. Boston, Butterworth, 1986.
27. James LP, Austen KF: Fatal systemic anaphylaxis in man. N Engl J Med *270*:597, 1964.
28. Bickell WH, Dice WH: Military antishock trousers in a patient with adrenergic-resistant anaphylaxis. Ann Emerg Med *13*:189, 1984.
29. Loehr MM: Suit up against anaphylaxis. Emerg Med April:127–128, 1985.
30. Parrillo JE: Intravenous cimetidine administration commonly produces a decrease in arterial pressure in critically ill patients. Update Crit Care Med *1*(7):5, 1986.
31. Jacobs RL, Geoffrey WR Jr, Fournier DC, et al: Potentiated anaphylaxis in patients with drug-induced beta-adrenergic blockade. J Allergy Clin Immunol *68*:125–127, 1981.
32. Idsoe O, Guthe T, Willcox RR, De Weck AL: Nature and extent of penicillin side-reactions, with particular reference to fatalities from anaphylactic shock. Bull WHO *38*:159–188, 1968.
33. Sheffer AL: Anaphylaxis. J Allergy Clin Immunol *75*:227–233, 1985.
34. Shapiro S, Siskin V, Slone D, et al: Drug rash with ampicillin and other penicillins. Lancet 1969.
35. Galpin JE, Chow AW, Yoshikawa TT, Guze LB: "Pseudoanaphylactic" reactions from inadvertent infusion of procaine penicillin G. Ann Intern Med *81*:358, 1974.
36. Eisen HN: Hypersensitivity to simple chemicals. *In* Lawrence HS (ed): Cellular and Humoral Aspects of the Hypersensitive States. New York, Hoeber, 1959, pp. 111–126.
37. Levine BB: Immunochemical mechanisms involved in penicillin hypersensivity in experimental animals and in human beings. Fed Proc *24*:45–50, 1965.
38. Sullivan TJ: Facilitated haptenation of human proteins by penicillin. J Allergy Clin Immunol *83*:255, 1989 (abstract).
39. Levine BB, Redmond AP: Minor haptenic determinant-specific reagins of penicillin hypersensitivity in man. Int Arch Allergy *35*:445–455, 1969.
40. Levine BB, Redmond AP, Fellner MJ, et al: Penicillin allergy and the heterogeneous immune responses of man to benzylpenicillin. J Clin Invest *45*:1895–1906, 1966.
41. Adkinson NF Jr, Wheeler B: Risk factors for IgE-dependent reactions to penicillin. *In* Kerr JW, Ganderton MA (eds): XI International Congress of Allergology and Clinical Immunology. London, Macmillan Press, 1983, pp. 55–59.
42. Sogn DD: Prevention of allergic reactions to penicillin. J Allergy Clin Immunol *78*:1051–1052, 1987.
43. Parker CW: The immunochemical basis for penicillin allergy. Postgrad Med J *40*:141–155, 1964.
44. Sullivan TJ, Wedner HJ, Shatz GS, et al: Skin testing to detect penicillin allergy. J Allergy Clin Immunol *68*:171–180, 1981.
45. Parker CW: Drug therapy (first of three parts). N Engl J Med *292*:511–514, 1975.
46. Gorevic PD, Levine BB: Desensitization of anaphylactic hypersensitivity specific for the penicilloate minor determinant of penicillin and carbenicillin. J Allergy Clin Immunol *68*:267–272, 1981.
47. Weiss ME, Adkinson NF Jr: Immediate hypersensitivity reactions to penicillin and related antibiotics. Clin Allergy *18*:515–540, 1988.
48. Mathews KP, Hemphill FM, Lovell RG, et al: A controlled study on the use of parenteral and oral antihistamines in preventing penicillin reactions. J Allergy *27*:1–15, 1956.
49. Sciple GW, Knox JM, Montgomery CH: Incidence of penicillin reactions after an antihistaminic simultaneously administered parenterally. N Engl J Med *261*:1123–1125, 1959.
50. Sullivan TJ, Yecies LD, Shatz GS, et al: Desensitization of patients allergic to penicillin using orally administered beta-lactam antibiotics. J Allergy Clin Immunol *69*:275–282, 1982.
51. Adkinson NF Jr: Penicillin allergy. *In* Lichtenstein LM, Fauci A (eds): Current Therapy in Allergy, Im-

munology and Rheumatology. Ontario, Canada, B. S. Decker, 1983, pp. 57–62.

52. Grieco MH: Cross-allergenicity of the penicillins and the cephalosporins. Arch Intern Med 119:141–146, 1967.

53. Petz L: Immunologic cross-reactivity between penicillins and cephalosporins: a review. J Infect Dis 137:S74–S79, 1978.

54. Shibata K, Atsumi T, Itorivchi Y, Mashimo K: Immunological cross-reactivities of cephalothin and its related compounds with benzylpenicillin (penicillin G). Nature 212:419–420, 1966.

55. Abraham GN, Petz LD, Fudenberg HH: Immunohaematological cross-allergenicity between penicillin and cephalothin in humans. Clin Exp Immunol 3:343–357, 1968.

56. Abraham GN, Petz LD, Fudenberg HH: Cephalothin hypersensitivity associated with anticephalothin antibodies. Int Arch Allergy 34:65–74, 1968.

57. Ong R, Sullivan T: Detection and charactertization of human IgE to cephalosporin determinants. J Allergy Clin Immunol 81:222, 1988.

58. Saxon A, Beall GN, Rohr AS, Adelman DC: Immediate hypersensitivity reactions to beta-lactam antibiotics. Ann Intern Med 107:204–215, 1987.

59. Adkinson NF Jr, Swabb EA, Sugerman AA: Immunology of the monobactam aztreonam. Antimicrob Agents Chemother 25:93–97, 1984.

60. Adkinson NF Jr, Wheeler B, Swabb EA: Clinical tolerance of the monobactam aztreonam in penicillin allergic subjects. Presented at the 14th International Congress of Chemotherapy, Kyoto, Japan, June 1988 (abstract WS-26-4).

61. Southorn PA, Plevak DJ, Wright AJ, Wilson WR: Adverse effects of vancomycin administered in the perioperative period. Mayo Clin Proc 61:721–724, 1986.

62. Verburg KM, Bowsher RR, Israel KS, et al: Histamine release by vancomycin in humans. Fed Proc 44:1247, 1985.

63. Jick H: Adverse reactions to trimethoprim-sulfamethoxazole in hospitalized patients. Rev Infect Dis 4:326, 1982.

64. Gorden FM, Simon GL, Wofsy CB: Adverse reactions to trimethoprim-sulfamethoxazole in patients with the acquired immunodeficiency syndrome. Ann Intern Med 100:495, 1984.

65. Carrington DM, Earl HS, Sullivan TJ: Studies of human IgE to a sulfonamide determinant. J Allergy Clin Immunol 79:442–447, 1987.

66. Rieder MJ, Uetrecht J, Shear NH, et al: Diagnosis of sulfonamide hypersensitivity reactions by in vitro "rechallenge" with hydroxylamine metabolites. Ann Intern Med 110:286–289, 1989.

67. Smith RM, Iwamoto GK, Richerson HB, Flaherty JP: Trimethoprim-sulfamethoxazole desensitization in the acquired immunodeficiency syndrome. Ann Intern Med 106:335, 1987.

68. Finegold I: Oral desensitization to trimethoprim-sulfamethoxazole in a patient with acquired immunodeficiency syndrome. J Allergy Clin Immunol 78:905–908, 1986.

69. Sher MR, Suchar C, Lockey RF: Anaphylactic shock induced by oral desensitization to trimethoprim/sulfmethoxazole (TMP-SMZ). J Allergy Clin Immunol 77:133, 1986.

70. Patterson R, DeSwarte RD, Greenberger PA, Grammer LC: Drug allergy and protocols for management of drug allergies. N Engl Reg Allergy Proc 4:325–342, 1986.

71. Vervloet D, Arnaud A, Senft M, et al: Leukocyte histamine release to suxamethonium in patients with adverse reactions to muscle relaxants. J Allergy Clin Immunol 75:338–342, 1985.

72. Didier A, Cador D, Bongrand P, et al: Role of the quaternary ammonium ion determinants in allergy to muscle relaxants. J Allergy Clin Immunol 79:578–584, 1987.

73. Charpin D, Benzarti M, Hemon Y, et al: Atopy and anaphylactic reactions to suxamethonium. J Allergy Clin Immunol 82:356–360, 1988.

74. Charpin J, Vervloet D, Nizankovska E: Adverse reactions due to muscle relaxants. 1983.

75. Dolovich J, Evans S, Rosenbloom D, et al: Anaphylaxis due to thiopental sodium anesthesia. Can Med Assoc J 123:292–294, 1980.

76. Harle DG, Baldo BA, Smal MA, et al: Detection of thiopentone-reactive IgE antibodies following anaphylactoid reactions during anaesthesia. Clin Allergy 16:493–498, 1986.

77. Schatz M: Skin testing and incremental challenge in the evaluation of adverse reactions to local anesthetics. J Allergy Clin Immunol 606:616–1984, 1989.

78. DeShazo RD, Nelson HS: An approach to the patient with a history of local anesthetic hypersensitivity: experience with 90 patients. J Allergy Clin Immunol 63:387–394, 1989.

79. Nagel JE, Fuscaldo JT, Fireman PL: Paraben allergy. JAMA 237:1594, 1977.

80. DeSwarte RD: Drug allergy. In Patterson R (ed): Allergic Diseases: Diagnosis and Management, 3rd ed. Philadelphia, Lippincott, 1989, pp. 505–661.

81. Harle DG, Baldo BA, Coroneos NJ, Fisher MM: Anaphylaxis following administration of papaveretum: case report, implication of IgE antibodies that react with morphine and codeine and identification of an allergenic determinant. Anesthesiology 71:489–494, 1989.

82. Zucker-Pinchoff B, Ramanathan S: Anaphylactic reaction to epidural fentanyl. Anesthesiology 71:599–601, 1991.

83. Bennett MJ, Anderson LK, McMillan JC, et al: Anaphylactic reaction during anaesthesia associated with positive intradermal skin test to fentanyl. Can Anaesth Soc J 33:71–74, 1986.

84. Kelly JF, Patterson R, Lieberman P, et al: Radiographic contrast media studies in high risk patients. J Allergy Clin Immunol 62:181–184, 1978.

85. Lasser EC, Berry CC, Talner LB, et al: Pretreatment with corticosteroids to alleviate reactions to intravenous contrast material. N Engl J Med 317:845–849, 1987.

86. Stevenson DD: Diagnosis, prevention, and treatment of adverse reactions to aspirin (ASA) and nonsteroidal anti-antiflammatory drugs (NSAID). J Allergy Clin Immunol 74:617–622, 1984.

87. Patterson R, Lucena G, Metz R, et al: Reaginic antibody against insulin: demonstration of antigenic distinction between native and extracted insulin. J Immunol 103:1061, 1969.

88. Findeberg SE, Galloway JA, Fineberg NS, et al: Immunologic aspects of insulin. Am J Med 31:882, 1961.

89. Sharath MD, Metzger WJ, Richerson HB, et al: Protamine-induced fatal anaphylaxis. J Thorac Cardiovasc Surg 90:86–90, 1985.

90. Stewart WJ, McSweeney SM, Kellett MA, et al: Increased risk of severe protamine reactions in NPH insulin-dependent diabetics undergoing cardiac catheterization. Circulation *70*:788–792, 1984.
91. Gottschlich GM, Gravlee GP, Georgitis JW: Adverse reactions to protamine sulfate during cardiac surgery in diabetic and non-diabetic patients. Ann Allergy *61*:277–281, 1988.
92. Samuel T: Antibodies reacting with salmon in human protamines in sera from infertile men and from vasectomized men and monkeys. Clin Exp Immunol *30*:181, 1977.
93. Watson RA, Ansbacher R, Barry M, et al: Allergic reaction to protamine: a late complication of elective vasectomy? Urology *22*:493, 1983.
94. Knape JTA, Schuller JL, De Haan P, et al: An anaphylactic reaction to protamine in a patient allergic to fish. Anesthesiology *55*:324–325, 1981.
95. Grammer LC, Patterson R: Proteins: chymopapain and insulin. J Allergy Clin Immunol *74*:635–640, 1984.
96. McGrath KG, Patterson R: Anaphylactic reactivity to streptokinase. JAMA *252*:1314–1317, 1984.
97. Dykewicz MS, McGrath KG, Davison R, et al: Identification of patients at risk for anaphylaxis due to streptokinase. Arch Intern Med *146*:305–307, 1986.
98. White HD, Rivers JT, Maslowski AH, et al: Effect of intravenous streptokinase as compared with that of tissue plasminogen activator on left ventricular function after first myocardial infarction. N Engl J Med *320*:817–821, 1989.

16 PERIOPERATIVE PEDIATRIC CARE

STEVEN C. HALL

In a study of perioperative morbidity and mortality in children, postoperative complications were seen in more than 24 per cent of all patients. Although most of these complications were minor, this figure still represents a higher rate of complications than is seen with adults.[1] The care of children during the postoperative period therefore demands a high degree of attention to the patient because of the frequency of complications, coupled with a thorough knowledge of the unique characteristics of children of different ages.

POST ANESTHESIA CARE UNIT

A properly staffed and equipped post anesthesia care unit (PACU) is an integral part of acute pediatric postoperative care. The unit and its personnel must be capable of providing care for the wide diversity of problems associated with the pediatric patient. It entails stabilizing the unconscious or semiconscious patient, recognizing and initiating therapy of complications, preventing complications (e.g., hypothermia) by prospective activity, and readying the patient for discharge.

If the PACU accepts pediatric patients, there must be proper equipment readily available for the different ages of children (Table 16–1). Each bedside must have oxygen (preferably humidified), a self-inflating resuscitation bag, and suction immediately available. The self-inflating bag should have the capability of administering 100 per cent oxygen. If newborns are brought to the PACU, an oxygen–air blender should be available to allow enriched, but controlled, air–oxygen mixtures to be administered. Blood pressure cuffs, pulse oximeter probes, temperature probes, masks, oral airways, laryngoscopic blades, and endotracheal tubes must be present in sizes accommodating all ages. The unit's emergency cart should have the same pediatric-sized airway equipment stocked, along with infant defibrillator paddles. It is also useful to have a list of drug doses by weight available for resuscitation drugs, muscle relaxants, inotropic and vasopressor drips, and antiseizure medication to allow personnel to determine appropriate doses quickly for any size child. Lastly, heating lights, intravenous fluid pumps, fluid warmers, cart pads, pediatric intravenous equipment, and electrocardiography equipment should be available.

One special piece of equipment that is increasingly being found in the resuscitation carts in pediatric hospitals is a bone marrow needle. This needle is especially useful for intraosseous administration of fluids and drugs in patients with poor venous access.[2] Usually used only in an emergency setting, the intraosseous route allows access with infusion characteristics similar to those of the intravenous route. The preferred site in children usually is the flat surface of the anterior tibia about an inch inferior to the epiphyseal plate.

It is the responsibility of the anesthesia staff to assist in the education of nursing care in the PACU. It is useful to have a designated medical director to coordinate the unit's activities. Periodic lectures and case discussions are an opportunity to continually upgrade the knowledge of the PACU staff. Although cardiopulmonary resuscitation (CPR) and advanced cardiac life support (ACLS) training are now commonly a part of nursing staff development, pediatric life support courses are offered and should be strongly considered. Nursing should be included in the quality assurance activities of the anesthesia department in that complications that occur or are treated in the PACU should be discussed with the nursing staff. Such discussion allows the entire staff to benefit from the experience. Lastly, protocols should be established and explained to deal with pediatric conditions, e.g., postintubation croup, patient-controlled

TABLE 16–1. SPECIAL EQUIPMENT FOR PEDIATRIC POST ANESTHESIA CARE (ADDED TO REGULAR ADULT SETUP)

Airway equipment
    Full range of pediatric-sized masks and oral and nasal airways
    Self-inflating bag capable of administering 100% oxygen
    Laryngoscope with variety of pediatric blades
    Uncuffed endotracheal tubes (2.5–6.5 mm i.d.)
    Cuffed endotracheal tubes (5.5–8.0 i.d.)
    Stylets for all sizes of endotracheal tubes
    Tracheostomy set
    Suction catheters of all sizes
    Oxygen/air blender with appropriate mask sizes
    Ultrasonic mist generator
    Racemic epinephrine
    Albuterol inhaler

Cardiac equipment
    Full range of blood pressure cuff sizes
    Doppler probe and monitor
    Pediatric and neonatal pulse oximeter probes
    Pediatric fluid metrisets
    Pediatric intravenous catheters (20, 22, 24 gauge)
    Pediatric defibrillation paddles
    Bone marrow needles
    Cut-down tray
    Blood warmer
    Heating lights

Written list of drug doses for pediatric patients

analgesia, malignant hyperthermia syndrome, and discharge criteria. The staff should also have clearly defined procedures for care of the immunocompromised child and the child with a highly contagious disease (e.g., chickenpox).

NORMAL EMERGENCE

When the pediatric patient arrives in the PACU the anesthesia personnel ensure that the patient is stable, with a patent airway and unlabored ventilation. Monitoring is then applied or instituted. Pulse oximetry is useful for all patients and should be used in the PACU. Pulse, blood pressure, respiratory rate, and temperature are periodically measured and the mental status assessed. Preprinted flow sheets make recording this information systematic and the patient's progress easy to follow. After initial vital signs are noted, the anesthesia personnel should give the report to the nursing staff, which should also include the surgery performed, anesthetics used, any underlying medical problems, allergies, intraoperative complications, and an estimate of anticipated postoperative complications. Special attention is directed to fluid administration and loss,

postoperative analgesic requirements, and an estimate of the length of the recovery period.

For the pediatric patient, recovery is usually rapid and uneventful. Most children are awake enough to leave the unit within 30 to 45 minutes. The most common complications requiring intervention are related to the airway and may be as simple as soft tissue or tongue upper airway obstruction manifested by snoring and mild retractions. This problem can be relieved by pulling the mandible forward using finger pressure behind the ramus, placing a roll under the child's shoulders, or positioning the child in the lateral position. As the child awakens, soft tissue obstruction should rapidly resolve. If it does not, investigation is warranted.

EMERGENCE DELIRIUM

Occasionally, a child demonstrates agitation or delirium on emergence. This can be due to potentially hazardous and treatable conditions that should be evaluated first. Hypoxemia, hypoventilation, acidosis, hypotension, and increased intracranial pressure are potential causes of agitation that should be considered. Once life-threatening conditions are eliminated as a cause of agitation, the possibility of pain or fear should be appreciated. Pain should be treated as aggressively as it is with adult patients. For the child without appreciable pain, awakening in a strange environment may be enough to induce agitation. Usually, comforting by the nursing staff is sufficient to relieve it. An alternative is parental presence at this point to help calm the child. In some institutions, parents are brought to the PACU by the surgeon; they view and comfort their child and then leave. In other institutions the parents are allowed to be present with the stable child throughout most of the PACU stay. If parents are allowed to visit, the nursing staff must be prepared and enthusiastic about parental presence.

Agitation may be related to agents given in the operating room. Although ketamine has been implicated as a cause of agitation in adults, the reaction is less commonly seen in children, who usually respond to recovery in a quiet, dim environment. Scopolamine has also been mentioned as a cause of delirium. Although treatment with physostigmine (0.02 to 0.05 mg/kg) has been suggested as a specific antidote for scopolamine, most children pass through their excitement phase quickly without the need for therapeutic intervention.

DELAYED EMERGENCE

Delayed emergence (Table 16–2) is unusual in children, though it is common to have the child awaken, cry, and then nap intermittently. It is especially true of infants and young children. However, if there is concern about delayed emergence, patients should be evaluated by asking three important questions.

1. *Is there any evidence that life-threatening conditions are present?* The ABCs of basic life support (*a*irway, *b*reathing, *c*ardiac status) are evaluated. Hypoxemia and hypoventilation can result from airway obstruction, pneumothorax, hypothermia, and metabolic disturbances. Hypotension occurs for a variety of reasons, but the most common cause in children is hypovolemia. Blood loss, third space loss, or incomplete correction of preoperative dehydration can be responsible. Because hypotension is a late sign of hypovolemia in children, it should be treated promptly and aggressively. An initial bolus of 10 ml of balanced salt solution per kilogram is appropriate, followed by crystalloid or colloid infusions as indicated by the clinical situation. A commonly overlooked cause of delayed emergence in children is hypothermia. Infants and young children develop hypothermia easily, with resulting hypoventilation, hypotension, and delayed emergence. Periodic temperature monitoring should be accompanied by heat loss-preventing measures, including heating lights and warm blankets for infants. Newborns are best nursed in incubators or beds with radiant lights.

2. *Is there evidence that drug therapy is the cause of the delayed emergence?* Heavy premedication, use of fixed agents intraoperatively (narcotics, barbiturates, ketamine), and use of "deep" levels of inhalational agents occasionally are responsible for delayed emergence, but these factors should be obvious to the anesthesiologist. Examination of the child may point to these factors as well. The sweet smell of halothane on the breath may be an indication that the child is still partially anesthetized by this agent, just as constricted pupils may point to prolonged narcotic activity. The presence of jerky, uncoordinated movements or poor muscle tone suggest incomplete reversal of neuromuscular blockade, which should be ruled out by applying a blockade monitor and checking train-of-four responses. For the infant and newborn, blockade monitors often do not give easily interpreted results. One physical sign that correlates well with return of adequate muscle strength is hip lift. If an infant is able to lift its hips off the bed, it has enough muscular power to produce a normal vital capacity. In most cases, delayed emergence secondary to drug administration improves with time. However, if hypoventilation, airway obstruction, or hypotension occurs, it should be treated aggressively.

3. *Are there medical or surgical conditions in this particular patient that could influence*

TABLE 16–2. CAUSES OF DELAYED AWAKENING OF THE PEDIATRIC PATIENT

Hypoxemia–hypoventilation
Hypovolemia
Hypothermia
Residual anesthetic agent
Residual muscle relaxant
Endocrine problems
Increased intracranial pressure
Low gestational age

emergence? The patient with diabetes, for instance, should be evaluated for hypo- and hyperglycemia, whereas the child who has just had intracranial surgery should be evaluated in conjunction with the neurosurgical service.

There is wide variability in children's response to anesthetic agents. Some children awaken immediately, whereas others are slow to respond, taking longer to become completely alert. Young children tend to wake up and then nap for the rest of the day. Although there is great emphasis in our system on having children "street ready" as quickly as possible after surgery, it should be remembered that the normal response of some children to the stresses of hospitalization and surgery is to nap and resist efforts aimed at arousal.

NAUSEA AND VOMITING

Postoperative nausea and vomiting comprise probably the most common acute complication of pediatric anesthesia.[1] The incidence varies widely, with figures as low as 11 per cent and as high as 85 per cent being given for children, in contrast with the rate of 5 per cent commonly associated with adults.[4-6] Not only is vomiting a particularly unpleasant experience for the child, it may place the child at risk for aspiration, dehydration, and delay of discharge. Risk factors implicated in a high incidence of vomiting include longer procedures, the type of surgery (especially strabismus operations), the premedication and anesthetic agents used (especially narcotics), the nature and age of the child (greatest tendency between 5 and 10 years of age), and oral intake upon awakening. Some children vomit only when forced to drink fluids during the postoperative period, whereas others develop active vomiting. The degree of intervention indicated depends on the nature of the vomiting.

Patients with a known history of vomiting or those who undergo operations associated with a high incidence of vomiting may benefit from prophylactic antiemetic therapy. The standard model for evaluating therapy has been strabismus surgery because of the high incidence of vomiting after these repairs. A variety of agents have been used and recommended, with droperidol and metoclopramide being used most often currently.

Droperidol 75 μg/kg given during surgery or before emergence has been shown to decrease the incidence after strabismus surgery, though this dose may be accompanied by prolonged somnolence.[4] There has been disagreement about the efficacy of lower doses of droperidol in terms of reducing vomiting. Some of the studies are difficult to compare because of significant differences in the rates of vomiting among untreated patients (controls).

Metoclopramide 0.15 mg/kg treatment of children undergoing strabismus surgery produced a reduction in vomiting.[6] Although it was decreased in both incidence and intensity, it was not eliminated. However, the advantage of metoclopramide is its ability to decrease gastric motor activity and vomiting without sedation or other adverse reactions. Finding an effective drug without side effects continues to be an area of active investigation.

It is the clinical impression of many institutions that children often vomit once in the PACU but do not develop protracted or severe vomiting if they are left in a quiet state without having oral fluids forced on them. Often if one waits until the child is thirsty enough to request fluids, feeding can proceed without vomiting. However, if active vomiting in the PACU does not improve after intravenous hydration and a period of nothing by mouth, antiemetic therapy with droperidol or a phenothiazine such as prochlorperazine is usually started. The role of metoclopramide in this setting has not been investigated. If, despite therapy, active vomiting continues, overnight admission for intravenous hydration is recommended. On the other hand, when the child is discharged, the parents must be advised to notify the child's physician if vomiting persists. Rarely, it has been necessary for the patient to come to the hospital's emergency room for evaluation and intravenous hydration.

AIRWAY OBSTRUCTION

As mentioned earlier, upper airway obstruction is common during emergence and usually responds to a jaw thrust or positioning in the lateral position. The child who is still partially anesthetized may require more aggressive intervention because the relative large tongue of children continues to obstruct the airway. Nasal airways are occasionally helpful but must be used with caution because of potential bleeding from friable nasal mucosa or hypertrophied adenoid tissue. The proper-size oral airway is one in which the tip ends just before the angle of the mandible; one that is smaller cannot effectively hold the soft tissue forward, and a larger one risks obstructing the airway and inducing laryngospasm. The size can easily be judged by placing the airway next to the child's face to check landmarks before insertion. Children do not tolerate oral airways as they awaken and develop pharyngeal reflexes. The airway must be removed at this point to prevent induction of laryngospasm.

If laryngospasm develops, with its characteristic, high-pitched whistle, treatment must start immediately. Positive airway pressure with 100 per cent oxygen relieves the obstruction in most cases. All staff assigned to the PACU not only must be taught the proper use of a self-inflating bag but most also understand that if laryngospasm is detected positive pressure by mask must be started immediately by whoever is at the bedside. If positive pressure by mask does not result in rapid improvement of the obstruction, intravenous succinylcholine is given. A full intubating dose is usually not necessary, nor is intubation needed if the airway clears completely after partial paralysis is induced. Controlled ventilation is used so long as partial paralysis is present. If laryngospasm recurs after the succinylcholine wears off, the oral pharynx should be resuctioned to ensure that blood, secretions, or foreign material is not touching and irritating the vocal cords.

Some patients demonstrate recurrent upper airway obstruction, even after awakening. This problem is most common in infants with congenital micrognathia, such as Pierre Robin or Treacher Collins syndrome. Until about 3 months of age these infants have incomplete muscular control of their tongue, leading to airway obstruction even when awake. Placing the child in the prone position occasionally is effective, but more aggressive measures, e.g., a nasopharyngeal airway, may be needed. In these patients and other infants undergoing extensive cleft palate repairs, the surgeon may elect to place and leave a silk suture through the tongue to facilitate pulling the tongue forward and clearing the airway. Rarely, tongue or palatal swelling is so severe that an artificial airway is needed.[7] These patients require prolonged observation in an intensive care setting.

POSTINTUBATION CROUP

Postintubation croup is more common in children than in adults, being seen in 1 to 6 per cent of pediatric cases. In the preadolescent patient, the narrowest area of the airway is at the level of the cricoid. Pressure on this mucosa can result in significant swelling and relative obstruction of airflow. One millimeter of edema can reduce airflow in the newborn by as much as 75 per cent.[8] Edema in this area becomes progressively less significant in older children. For this reason, postintubation croup is uncommon after 4 years of age. Factors that increase the likelihood of croup include traumatic or repeated intubations, coughing or "bucking" on the tube, intubation for over an hour, surgery in a position other than supine, and an endotracheal tube fit that prevents an air leak until pressures above 25 cm H_2O are used.[9] Children with congenital narrowing of the larynx, e.g., those with Down syndrome or congenital subglottic stenosis, are also at risk.

Postintubation croup usually becomes symptomatic within the first hour after extubation, although it may develop later. It has been determined that the maximum edema usually occurs at 4 hours after extubation and resolves by 24 hours.[9] It characteristically presents with a "barky" cough, retractions, and tachypnea. Cyanosis or duskiness, a soft voice, and patient distress are signs of advanced airway obstruction. Although postintubation croup usually resolves without endangering the patient, the child is at risk for progressive airway obstruction and hypoxemia. For this reason, symptomatic therapy is usually given (Table 16–3).

The initial therapy is humidified oxygen by face mask. Nebulized racemic epinephrine (0.5 ml of 2.25 per cent epinephrine in 2.5 ml saline) is commonly administered by face mask to vasoconstrict the laryngeal mucosa.

TABLE 16–3. POSTINTUBATION CROUP THERAPY

Pulse oximeter monitoring
Humidified oxygen, preferably mist
Racemic epinephrine
    Nebulized
    Dose: 0.25–0.50 ml of 2.25%
    Watch for rebound in 60 minutes
    Can be repeated

Steroids
    Controversial
    Dexamethasone 0.5–1.0 mg/kg
    Effect seen in 3–4 hours

Airway support
    Intubation if respiratory distress worsens
    Observation in intensive care setting

The older method of administration by positive pressure ventilation does not offer any benefits. Racemic epinephrine has traditionally been used (even though only the *l*-isomer is active) because of supposed decreased cardioactive side effects, though the lesser side effects may be related more to dilution and poor absorption. Although tachycardia, circumoral pallor, and arrhythmias can be seen with racemic epinephrine, they are rarely troublesome. After racemic epinephrine administration, improvement is usually noticed immediately. Because of the limited length of action of the vasoconstriction, the patient must be reexamined after an hour to see if there has been a "rebound" recurrence of the edema and obstruction. Although a single treatment is usually adequate, racemic epinephrine administration can be repeated at hourly intervals, only rarely being limited by the development of tachycardia. However, children who require multiple administrations of racemic epinephrine may be at high risk for progressive obstruction, necessitating reintubation. These patients need constant observation until the condition resolves.

Another treatment commonly used is steroid administration. The efficacy of this modality is controversial. The bulk of research has been on viral laryngotracheobronchitis, not postintubation croup.[10] Studies have indicated that dexamethasone decreases signs of viral croup but must be given in large doses. Dexamethasone 0.5 to 1.0 mg/kg may be most effective if given prior to airway manipulation, e.g., rigid bronchoscopy, in the patient at risk for croup. The studies with viral croup indicate that it takes 4 to 6 hours before maximum effect is seen.

Rarely, postintubation croup is severe enough to warrant prolonged observation in the hospital by personnel equipped to provide immediate airway support. If reintubation is required, it is best to use an endotracheal tube a half-size smaller than normal to minimize pressure on the inflamed area. These patients require prolonged management in an intensive care unit. In patients who continue to have a barky cough but are without other signs of respiratory distress, it may be difficult to diagnose the difficulty. The cough is obvious proof of some abnormality of the airway, but the lack of other signs indicates that the swelling is mild. Discharge to home is reasonable if both the physicians and parents are in agreement that the croup is mild and does not represent a threat to the child. The parents should be instructed to observe the child frequently through the night and to bring the child immediately back to the hospital if there are any signs of respiratory distress. A cool mist vaporizer is often recommended for the child's room. If there is any doubt by either the medical staff or the parents about the advisability of discharge, the child should be admitted for overnight observation.

ASTHMA

Wheezing may be evidence of several underlying conditions, such as aspiration pneumonitis, retained secretions, heart failure, or an upper respiratory tract infection. Asthma is probably responsible for most wheezing episodes in the PACU. Asthma or "wheeziness" is relatively common in children, being diagnosed in up to 10 per cent of all patients sometime during childhood. The range of disease runs from a single episode of bronchospasm during a respiratory tract infection to recurrent, life-threatening disease. When evaluating a child with wheezing in the PACU it is useful to know the child's history. Useful information includes the frequency and severity of wheezing attacks, their response to medications, and baseline medications.

Physical examination focuses on three specific areas. First, is expiratory wheezing heard over all lung fields, or is it localized? If the wheezing is localized, the possibility of aspiration, pneumonia, unilateral atelectasis, or a foreign body should be considered. Second, is there evidence of the use of accessory muscles? Accessory muscle use and retractions are correlated with more severe obstruction. Third, does gas exchange appear adequate? A child with a prolonged expiratory phase, severe retractions, barely audible breath sounds, or cyanosis demands immediate aggressive therapy, whereas a child with wheezing but no other signs can be approached in a more deliberate fashion.

Pulse oximetry should be used for continuous monitoring of arterial oxygen saturation during evaluation and treatment. Chest roentgenograms are necessary only for the child with suspected new lung pathology or who is unresponsive to therapy.

Therapy for bronchospasm involves both specific and general measures (see Chapter 5). Supplemental oxygen is given to all patients until the wheezing is under control. The mainstay of specific therapy usually starts with β_2-

adrenergic agonists, e.g., albuterol.[12] Albuterol 0.5 per cent can be easily given to the child by aerosol inhalation. If the child is cooperative and knows how to use a metered-dose inhaler, he or she can self-administer the albuterol. These agents are easy to give and are associated with few complications. If the β_2-agonists are not adequate, intravenous aminophylline can be started. A loading dose of 5 mg/kg over 30 minutes followed by an infusion of 0.7 to 1.2 mg/kg/hr is given with continuous ECG monitoring. Patients who have received chronic steroid therapy may benefit from an additional dose of hydrocortisone 1–2 mg/kg, though evidence for such benefit is sparse.

Rarely, bronchospasm, with inadequate ventilation and hypoxemia, is life-threatening. Subcutaneous or intravenous epinephrine 5 μg/kg or subcutaneous terbutaline 5 μg/kg can produce immediate relief of bronchoconstriction. Terbutaline has the advantages of producing fewer cardiovascular side effects and having longer action. With severe cases, an infusion of isoproterenol 0.1 μg/kg/min is added, with the infusion increased to effect but decreased if arrhythmias or a heart rate of more than 200 beats/min results.[13] With severe cases, arterial blood gas monitoring is mandatory. Intubation, neuromuscular relaxation, sedation, and controlled ventilation are used if the patient develops respiratory failure despite aggressive therapy.

HYPOVENTILATION

Hypoventilation during the postoperative period may occur for a variety of reasons. The first step when evaluating the child is to ensure a clear airway. Soft tissue swelling, croup, secretions, vomitus, or laryngospasm may be responsible. After a clear airway is ensured, the second step is to determine the adequacy of ventilation. If it is thought that ventilation is inadequate, bag-and-mask ventilation is immediately started. *Diagnostic efforts are begun only after the patient's safety has been ensured.*

A rational approach to investigating possible causes of hypoventilation starts with basic vital signs. Hypoventilation may be secondary to decreased cardiac output (low blood pressure or pulse) or hypothermia. Pulse oximetry should be part of the basic vital sign measurements and supplemental oxygen started if saturations are low. Physical examination may reveal mechanical impairment, e.g., a

pneumothorax. Of special note is a distended abdomen, especially in the infant. Because newborns and young infants are primarily "diaphragm breathers," gastric distension can impair diaphragmatic movement and ventilation.

The pattern of ventilation is important and should be examined closely. Narcotics usually produce slow, deep inspirations and are associated with constricted pupils. Small doses of naloxone should be titrated to induce increased ventilation and arousability, without eliminating all analgesia. Because the narcotic action may outlast the intravenous naloxone, the patient should be closely observed for the need for additional doses. The volatile agents are easy to detect on the breath of the child. With a little experience, it is easy to determine if the amount of exhaled agent is large enough to consider it the main cause of the hypoventilation. Because the child progressively eliminates the volatile agent by breathing, this condition is usually self-limited. Inadequate reversal of neuromuscular blockade produces a different clinical picture. The child often shows signs of being awake and distressed but shows uncoordinated breathing efforts and "jerky" movements of the extremities. As mentioned earlier, the ability of an infant to lift his or her hips off the bed is a sign of adequate muscular strength. For older children, a blockade monitor can quickly ascertain adequate reversal.[14] If it is unclear that reversal is adequate, it is reasonable to give an additional half-dose of the reversal medication (neostigmine 0.035 mg/kg or atropine 0.02 mg/kg).

Lung auscultation can detect bronchospasm, secretions, rales, and absent breath sounds over a lobe or lung. If there is evidence of pulmonary pathology, e.g., absent breath sounds, a chest film should be obtained immediately to confirm the presence of atelectasis, pleural effusion, aspiration pneumonitis, or pulmonary edema. Treatment of these conditions is the same as in adults.

It should be reemphasized that if breathing is determined to be inadequate, the first objective is to establish adequate ventilation. Only after this goal has been accomplished can diagnosis and definitive therapy proceed.

PAIN

Traditionally, pain has been undertreated in children for a variety of reasons, including a perception that children do not feel pain "as much'' as adults. This assumption is not true. Children experience pain just like adults but may manifest their distress in different ways. It is important that PACU personnel become adept at assessing pain in children of all ages and addressing these problems.

For young patients, the most obvious manifestations of pain are tachycardia, hypertension, and restlessness. Infants may cry, moan, frown, or become withdrawn, refusing to interact with the PACU staff. Occasionally, the child writhes, becomes rigid, or pulls at the surgical area. Although nonverbal pain scores for use in young children have been developed, they are not widely used. Two special components of pediatric pain should be mentioned. The child who has just arrived in the PACU and who suddenly becomes active and combative may be experiencing pain, not just emerging from general anesthesia. The second special consideration in children is that older children often admit to significant pain if asked but do not volunteer this information. It is important to not only observe for signs of pain but also to ask children about their comfort level.[15]

Efficient pain control starts in the operating room. Some procedures are relatively noninvasive and are usually associated with minimal postoperative pain; they may be treated with acetaminophen orally or per rectum. However, many patients benefit from intraoperative administration of analgesics to smooth the intraoperative and postoperative courses. Intravenous narcotic analgesics are especially effective when the titrated doses are large enough to provide the patient with analgesia but small enough so they do not cause delayed emergence or hypotension.[16] There is increasing interest in the role of regional anesthesia for postoperative pain relief. Intraoperative regional blocks, e.g., caudal or epidural administration of long-acting local anesthetic (usually bupivacaine), have the advantage of significant postoperative pain relief without the disadvantages of sedation or nausea and vomiting seen occasionally with narcotics. These blocks can be given at either the beginning or the end of the operative period and can provide several hours of postoperative relief.[17]

In the PACU analgesia is most commonly provided by narcotics. Intravenous titration of such drugs can provide analgesia without excessive sedation or hypoventilation and is preferable to intramuscular administration. Except for the neonatal period, pediatric patients probably react to narcotics in a fashion similar to that in adults. The particular drug chosen is more a matter of tradition and personal preference than science. As with older patients, small doses of morphine 0.025 mg/kg, meperidine 0.5 mg/kg, or fentanyl 1 μg/kg can be used under close monitoring. The goal is to produce a calm, comfortable, but arousable state without the respiratory rate or blood pressure falling below normal.

Patient-controlled analgesia (PCA) with narcotic analgesics, usually morphine, has become increasingly popular in children.[19] The age at which this modality is appropriate has been lowered as more experience is gained. In many pediatric centers, cooperative children under 10 years of age have successfully benefited from this technique. PCA works best when the child has been familiarized with the machine before surgery and dosage starts in the PACU under the supervision of the nursing staff.

SPECIAL CONSIDERATIONS FOR THE NEWBORN

Among pediatric patients, the newborn is anatomically, physiologically, and pharmacologically the most different from adults. Postoperative care of these fragile patients demands the highest level of vigilance and attention to detail. Practical experience has taught us that localizing signs are not as common in newborns as in the older child. The newborn who does not cry or become vigorous after stimulation is viewed with suspicion, as lethargy may be an early warning of decreased cardiac output, acidosis, hypercarbia, hypoglycemia, or sepsis. Special considerations are directed toward avoiding or rapidly recognizing and correcting hypoxemia, hypoventilation, hypothermia, and hypotension.

Newborns and young infants are more prone to the rapid development of hypoxemia (Table 16–4). Anatomically, their upper airway is more prone to obstruction because of a relatively short neck, large tongue, increased anteroposterior diameter of the skull, and abundant soft tissue. They also have decreased number of alveoli, a decreased functional residual capacity/minute ventilation ratio, a higher metabolic rate, and lower hemoglobin delivery capacity than older infants and children. For these reasons, the newborn and young infant are more at risk for airway obstruction, hypoventilation, and hypoxemia

TABLE 16–4. SPECIAL CONSIDERATIONS FOR THE NEWBORN: THE FIVE H's

Hypoxemia
   Decreased functional residual capacity/minute ventilation reserve
   Airway obstructs easily

Hyperoxia
   Normal arterial saturation 92–96%
   Prolonged exposure to high oxygen saturation implicated in retinal damage

Hypoventilation
   Unusually sensitive to anesthetics, muscle relaxants
   Abdominal distension, hypothermia contribute to hypoventilation

Hypothermia
   Unusually susceptible to rapid falls in temperature
   Responses include metabolic acidosis, hypoventilation, and bradycardia
   Active measures to prevent hypothermia mandatory

Hypotension
   Hypovolemia a common cause
   Anesthetic overdose, hypothermia, sepsis can contribute
   Cardiac output is heart rate-dependent; bradycardia must be aggressively treated

during the intraoperative and postoperative periods.[20] Caring properly for these patients requires constant attention to providing a clear airway and unimpeded ventilation, which entails careful monitoring (physical examination, pulse oximetry) and technical expertise when positioning the child to maintain adequate ventilation. The staff must be trained and facile with bag-and-mask maintenance of the airway and ventilation.

Although oxygen administration is routinely done in children, there is concern about excessive oxygen administration in newborns. The newborn, especially the preterm infant under 1500 gm and 34 weeks' gestation, is at risk for oxygen toxicity of the eye, retrolental fibroplasia or, as it is now being called, the retinopathy of prematurity (ROP).[21,22] Although the exact cause of the condition and safe levels of administered oxygen in the premature neonate are not yet completely accepted, it is prudent to keep the preductal (blood obtained from the right radial or superficial temporal arteries) PO_2 values at 50 to 70 mm Hg in the term newborn and at 40 to 60 mm Hg in the preterm infant. These values correlate with arterial oxygen saturation (SaO_2) levels of 92 to 96 per cent. The length of time a newborn must be exposed to enriched oxygen before toxicity develops has not yet been established.

However, there is evidence that hypoxemia, as well as hyperoxia, may be an etiologic factor in the development of ROP. Hypoxemia should be as much a concern as hyperoxia.

The definition of hypotension varies by age. Hypotension in the newborn is defined by a systolic pressure of less than 50 to 60 mm Hg and in the preterm newborn as less than 40 to 50 mm Hg. Although hypovolemia is the most common cause of hypotension in the newborn, hypoxemia, acidosis, and hypothermia can also be responsible. If the patient does not respond to fluid challenges of 10 ml/kg of balanced salt solution or colloid, other causes should be suspected. The stroke volume is fixed in newborns, resulting in cardiac output being directly related to heart rate. Thus augmentation of heart rate with atropine or, in those with severe hypotension, epinephrine helps to increase cardiac output.

Hypothermia is a constant risk in the newborn. Newborns rely primarily on increased metabolic rate to respond to any cold stresses. Such nonshivering thermogenesis results in metabolic acidosis, increased oxygen consumption and decreased oxygenation of vital tissues, hypoventilation, and decreased cardiac output. The newborn who slowly but steadily becomes less responsive in the PACU may be cooling. Frequent temperature measurements are mandatory. Hypothermia should be prevented by maintaining a neutral thermal environment for the baby, using elevated room temperature, heating lights and blankets or an incubator, warmed fluids and gases, and protective skin covering, e.g., cellophane film (Saran Wrap).

Most newborns who undergo surgery have significant, life-threatening lesions. These patients usually go directly to the neonatal intensive care unit after surgery, bypassing the PACU. However, if a newborn is admitted, it is important to consider not only the general principles of neonatal care but also the special problems associated with the surgical condition. For instance, the newborn with a repair of a myelomeningocele is at risk for hydrocephalus and increased intracranial pressure.

NEW FRONTIERS: APNEA IN THE PRETERM INFANT

The preterm newborn is often the graduate of a prolonged stay in a neonatal intensive care unit. These infants may have residual cardiac, pulmonary, or neurologic disease that can alter postoperative management. They may require supplemental oxygen because of underlying lung disease (bronchopulmonary dysplasia). Even in the absence of known complications, there is an increased risk for postoperative respiratory complications, primarily apnea and bradycardia, in ex-preterm infants. All preterms show periodic breathing, but apneic spells lasting longer than 20 seconds or associated with bradycardia are considered to be potentially life-threatening. The cause of these spells appears related to a weak central respiratory drive and undeveloped musculature, and it is inversely related to postconceptual age.[23] It is important to monitor patients at risk for these apneic spells for at least 12 hours postoperatively with an electronic apnea monitor in a setting that has close nursing observation. However, the determination of which patient is at risk for postoperative apnea is controversial.[24–26]

The studies currently available are difficult to compare to each other. Not all the studies are prospective; the definitions of apnea are disparate; the observations or measurements are not uniform; studies within the same institution have found different rates of apnea in different studies; surgical procedures and anesthetic regimens varied; and the oldest postconceptual age observed differed significantly among studies. Nonetheless, it is important to draw conclusions to guide clinical practice.

Most studies have shown that a history of apnea or lack thereof does *not* correlate with apneic spells during the postoperative period.[24] Thus it has not been possible to predict which patients are at risk. The incidence decreases significantly with increasing postconceptual age, but the exact age at which the infant is beyond risk is controversial. Different institutions have developed recommendations based on their own experiences. Such recommendations have included overnight observation in all ex-preterm infants under 44 week postconceptual age, under 46 weeks' postconceptual age (only if there is a history of apnea),[27] and under 60 weeks' postconceptual age.[24] In our institution, we have found that some parents are not aware of the exact number of weeks preterm their child was at birth. For this reason, ex-preterm infants are admitted for observation and monitored overnight if they are younger than 6 months old. For example, with an infant born at 30 weeks' gestation, this rule ensures that the infant is 56 week postconceptual age before discharge on the day of surgery is allowed.

There is currently a great deal of research aimed at defining more accurately which patients are at risk and if any therapeutic interventions, e.g., intravenous caffeine or regional anesthesia, are useful for preventing complications.[26,28] Although there is not universal agreement about which ex-preterms need overnight observation and monitoring, it is important to recognize the problem and establish a consistent policy for one's institution.

DISCHARGE FROM THE PACU

There is great variation in the rate at which children recover from general anesthesia. It is not uncommon for healthy children having short procedures to be awake, alert, and ready to leave in less than a half-hour. On the other hand, some children, especially those undergoing extensive surgical procedures, take longer to reach a degree of recovery adequate for discharge to less intense nursing care and observation of the hospital ward.

Because discharge from the PACU is not the same as ultimate discharge from the hospital, the criteria for discharge from the PACU may vary, depending on the place to which the child goes from the PACU. For instance, a

THE CHILDREN'S MEMORIAL HOSPITAL
POST ANESTHESIA CARE UNIT RECORD

ADMITTED
DISCHARGED
PROCEDURE
AIRWAY
O_2
RECEIVED FROM
DISCHARGED BY
ADMIT V. S.

Temperatures
E/R°C 200
160
120
PULSE = o
B.P. = V/Λ
RESP. = X
80
40
0

FLUID BALANCE ON LEAVING P.A.C.
IN
OUT
INTRAVENOUS
MEDICATIONS
LABORATORY
DRAINS

NURSING OBSERVATIONS/RECOVERY ROOM SCORES

		ON ADMISSION	5 MIN	15 MIN	30 MIN	DISCHG
AWAKE	FULLY AWAKE					
	AROUSABLE					
	NOT RESPONDING					
VENTILATION	CAN COUGH OR CRY					
	BREATHING EASILY					
	AIRWAY REQUIRES ATTENTION					
MOVEMENT	MOVING PURPOSEFULLY					
	MOVING INVOLUNTARY					
	NOT MOVING					

FORM 509

FIGURE 16–1. PACU record.

child discharged to an intensive care unit (ICU) may well have significant cardiovascular or pulmonary compromise that would be unacceptable for discharge to a hospital ward. Criteria should be exceptionally stringent if the patient is discharged to a holding area or outpatient surgical area that is lightly staffed. In any case, an anesthesiologist should usually be responsible for discharge from the PACU. If there are special postoperative considerations based on the perioperative course, it is the responsibility of the anesthesiologist to contact the other physicians caring for the child. It is the responsibility of the PACU nurse to report directly to the hospital ward, ICU, or holding area nurse receiving the patient. The report should include a brief narrative of the child's perioperative course, including vital signs, medications given, fluids given and currently running, postoperative laboratory work, and any complications (Fig. 16–1).

Criteria for discharge from the PACU have several aspects. Stable vital signs, intact reflexes, and return to a reasonable level of consciousness and responsiveness are the keystones of adequate emergence from anesthesia and surgery. There should be no signs of respiratory distress, cardiovascular instability, active bleeding, or active vomiting. Using a scoring system for respiratory, cardiac, and central nervous system criteria is a useful way of quantifying the recovery process. With the increased use of pulse oximetry, a higher incidence of desaturation has been found in patients in the PACU.[29,30] Therefore a useful objective measure of the child's ability to maintain an airway and oxygenate is stable saturation on room air. Children who have received racemic epinephrine should be observed at least an hour for signs of rebound croup, and those who have been given narcotics should be observed for at least a half-hour to ensure that there is both adequate analgesia and no discernible ventilatory depression. Children who had an intraoperative regional block may still show evidence of motor or sensory blockade. Institutions vary as to whether these children can be transferred to a ward or outpatient holding area before all evidence of the block is gone. There should be a clear policy about whether these children can be adequately nursed on a hospital ward or outpatient area.

Rarely, children spend extensive periods in the PACU, sometimes because of unexpected complications that require extensive therapy, e.g., an asthma attack. Patients may also spend longer periods in the PACU because of the lack of immediate availability of ICU or hospital bed accommodations. The PACU has been used as a modified intensive care setting for overnight observation because of the ability of the nursing staff to care properly for acutely ill patients. If the PACU is used in this capacity, the nursing staff must have the same training, equipment, and personnel backup that is provided for the ICU. Just as importantly, there must be protocols in place to ensure that when the PACU is used as an ICU alternative there are modifications made to nursing staffing to prevent inadequate coverage of other patients or "burnout" due to excessively long hours with acutely ill patients.

SUMMARY

Recovery from anesthesia usually proceeds in an uncomplicated, rapid fashion in children. Young infants, children with significant medical problems, and patients undergoing extensive surgery often experience longer stays. The nursing and medical staff must be attuned to the problems and needs of the pediatric patient, with special attention to the airway, ventilation, temperature, pain relief, and fluids. Careful attention to detail minimizes complications and ensures a speedy recovery.

References

1. Cohen MM, Cameron CB, Duncan PG: Pediatric anesthesia morbidity and mortality in the perioperative period. Anesth Analg 70:160–167, 1990.
2. Spivey WH: Intraosseous infusions. J Pediatr 111:639–643, 1987.
3. Patel RI, Hannallah RS: Anesthetic complications following pediatric ambulatory surgery: a 3-yr study. Anesthesiology 69:1009–1012, 1988.
4. Nicolson SC, Kaya KM, Betts EK: The effect of preoperative oral droperidol on the incidence of postoperative emesis after paediatric strabismus surgery. Can J Anaesth 35:364–367, 1988.
5. McConachie IW, Day A, Morris P: Recovery from anaesthesia in children. Anaesthesia 44:986–990, 1989.
6. Broadman LM, Ceruzzi W, Patane PS, et al: Metoclopramide reduces the incidence of vomiting following strabismus in children. Anesthesiology 72:245–248, 1990.
7. Patane PS, White SE: Macroglossia causing airway obstruction following cleft palate repair. Anesthesiology 71:995–996, 1989.

8. Borland LM (ed): The pediatric airway. Int Anesthesiol Clin 26:1–88, 1988.

9. Koka BV, Jeon ISA, Andre JM, et al: Postintubation croup in children. Anesth Analg 56:501–505, 1977.

10. Kairys SW, Olmstead EM, O'Connor GT: Steroid treatment of laryngotracheitis: a meta-analysis of the evidence from randomized trials. Pediatrics 83:683–693, 1989.

11. Super DM, Cartelli NA, Brooks LJ, et al: A prospective randomized double-blind study to evaluate the effect of dexamethasone in acute laryngotracheitis. J Pediatr 115:323–329, 1989.

12. Schuh S, Parkin P, Rajan A, et al: High- versus low-dose, frequently administered, nebulized albuterol in children with severe, acute asthma. Pediatrics 83:513–518, 1989.

13. Tendler C, Grossman S, Tenenbaum J: Medication dosages during pediatric emergencies: a simple and comprehensive guide. Pediatrics 84:731–735, 1989.

14. Gwinnutt CL, Meakin G: Use of the post-tetanic count to monitor recovery from intense neuromuscular blockade in children. Br J Anaesth 61:547–550, 1988.

15. Lloyd-Thomas AR: Pain management in paediatric patients. Br J Anaesth 64:85–104, 1990.

16. Yaster M, Deshpande JK: Management of pediatric pain with opioid analgesics. J Pediatr 113:421–429, 1988.

17. Rice LJ, Pudimat MA, Hannallah RS: Timing of caudal block placement in relation to surgery does not affect duration of postoperative analgesia in paediatric ambulatory patients. Can J Anaesth 37:429–431, 1990.

18. Casey WF, Rice LJ, Hannallah RS, et al: A comparison between bupivacaine instillation versus ilioinguinal/iliohypogastric nerve block for postoperative analgesia following inguinal herniorrhaphy in children. Anesthesiology 72:637–639, 1990.

19. Rodgers BM, Webb CJ, Stergios D, Newman BM: Patient-controlled analgesia in pediatric surgery. J Pediatr Surg 23:259–262, 1988.

20. Motoyama EK, Davis PJ. Smith's Anesthesia for Infants and Children, 5th ed. St. Louis, Mosby, 1990.

21. Lucey JF, Dangman B: A reexamination of the role of oxygen in retrolental fibroplasia. Pediatrics 73:82–96, 1984.

22. Merritt JC, Sprague DH, Merritt WE, et al: Retrolental fibroplasia: a multifactorial disease. Anesth Analg 60:109–111, 1981.

23. Barrington KJ, Finer NN: Periodic breathing and apnea in preterm infants. Pediatr Res 27:118–121, 1990.

24. Kurth CD, Spitzer AR, Broennle AM, et al: Postoperative apnea in preterm infants. Anesthesiology 66:483–488, 1987.

25. Cox RG, Goresky GV: Life-threatening apnea following spinal anesthesia in former premature infants. Anesthesiology 73:345–348, 1990.

26. Welborn LG, Hannallah RS, Fink R, et al: High-dose caffeine suppresses postoperative apnea in former preterm infants. Anesthesiology 71:347–349, 1989.

27. Liu LMP, Cote CJ, Goudsouzian NG, et al: Life-threatening apnea in infants recovering from anesthesia. Anesthesiology 59:506–510, 1983.

28. Welborn LG, Rice LJ, Hannallah RS, et al: Postoperative apnea in former preterm infants: postoperative comparison of spinal and general anesthesia. Anesthesiology 72:838–842, 1990.

29. Patel R, Norden J, Hannallah RS: Oxygen administration prevents hypoxemia during post-anesthetic transport in children. Anesthesiology 69:616–618, 1988.

30. DeSoto H, Patel RI, Soliman IE, Hannallah RS: Changes in oxygen saturation following general anesthesia in children with upper respiratory infection signs and symptoms undergoing otolaryngological procedures. Anesthesiology 68:276–279, 1988.

ORTHOPEDICS 17

JOHN KERCHBERGER

Orthopedic anesthesia may be viewed as an amalgam of several specialty areas, including trauma, geriatrics, and regional anesthesia. Therefore orthopedic patients may present with a wide variety of problems during the post anesthetic period. Although the issues related to recovery from regional anesthesia, pain relief, and medical management of concomitant pathology of major organ systems of patients during the postoperative period are covered elsewhere in this text, unique problems are encountered when caring for orthopedic patients. This chapter reviews postoperative management of patients who have common orthopedic procedures.

COMMON OPERATIONS IN ORTHOPEDIC SURGERY

FEMORAL NECK FRACTURES

Femoral neck fractures occur frequently in elderly patients owing to their risk posed by advancing osteoporosis, chronic illness, and confusion. The postoperative assessment and care of these patients should take these factors into consideration as well as the decline in cardiovascular and respiratory reserve seen in the elderly.[1]

Their postoperative management depends to a large degree on the type of anesthetic used intraoperatively. A general, regional, or combination anesthetic technique may have been used. Controversy exists regarding the postoperative benefits of general versus regional anesthesia for surgical repair of hip fractures.[2] For instance, although long-term mortality may not be different when comparing these two techniques, regional anesthesia may offer improved survival during the immediate postoperative period.[3]

Patients who have undergone repair of hip fractures under general anesthesia should be expected to have a decreased functional residual capacity and decreased PaO_2 postopera-

tively.[4] These patients may require endotracheal intubation and mechanical ventilation until they have sufficient strength, adequate gas exchange, and the ability to protect their airway from aspiration. Patients who have had spinal anesthesia should not have significant alterations in PaO_2 or $PaCO_2$ unless the amount of sedation required for the surgical procedure was sufficient to depress ventilation.

Significant alterations in fluid balance may occur if the patient received sufficient intraoperative fluids to worsen preexisting congestive heart failure. Even in the presence of careful intraoperative fluid management, postoperative fluid assessment in these patients may be challenging because they may present with either hypo- or hypervolemia.

Several possible etiologies for hypovolemia exist. Preoperatively, a hematoma forms at the fracture site that may sequester a large volume of blood. The patient may also be receiving chronic diuretic therapy for hypertension or congestive heart failure, or the patient may be malnourished and dehydrated preoperatively due to poor tolerance of oral fluids.

The intraoperative estimate of blood loss may be inadequate. For instance, blood loss may be difficult to estimate when a fracture table is used because a portion of the blood is spilled onto the vertical sterile drapes. Blood loss may also be appreciable if a hemiarthroplasty is performed because the reaming out of the femoral canal for the femoral prosthesis results in additional bleeding. Postoperatively, the patient may continue to lose blood, which may be difficult to assess owing to a bulky dressing on the thigh.

Unfortunately, these patients may also be subject to volume overload if the anesthesiologist overestimates the blood loss, particularly as the patient's cardiovascular reserve for dealing with excess intravascular volume may be limited. The patient who has uncompensated congestive heart failure preoperatively is at highest risk for this complication. For these reasons, the usual parameters for fluid assessment (e.g., pulmonary rales, S3 heart sound, urine, wound drains output, and estimated blood loss) may not be sufficient to guide postoperative fluid management. In cases of doubt, measurement of either central venous pressures (assuming an absence of significant left ventricular dysfunction) or pulmonary artery pressures may be helpful for guiding fluid management. A systemic arterial catheter is also useful when assessing a hemodynamically unstable patient. Arterial catheters allow immediate assessment of the effect of vasopressors and suggest the diagnosis of hypovolemia if the arterial trace oscillates with respiration. Moreover, arterial catheters can be used to guide a decision on whether the patient requires additional blood transfusions or, if there is evidence of hypovolemia with an adequate hemoglobin, colloid or crystalloid replacement. Patients with ischemic heart disease or diminished cardiovascular reserve may require a blood transfusion if they have a hemoglobin level of less than 9 to 10 gm/dl to maintain adequate tissue oxygen delivery.[1]

Postoperative confusion is another problem that occurs in patients with femoral neck fractures and elderly patients in general. Confused patients have prolonged hospital stays and a higher incidence of postoperative complications, including urinary tract infections, incontinence, and pressure sores.[5]

Several studies have attempted to elucidate the mechanisms of this problem in patients who have undergone pelvic floor surgery[6] total hip arthroplasty,[7] and femoral neck fractures.[5] Factors that appear to contribute to confusion after general anesthesia include preoperative use of anticholinergic drugs (including tricyclic antidepressants), a history of depression, and postoperative hypoxemia.[5] Surprisingly, Berggren et al. found that the incidence of postoperative confusion was not influenced by the anesthetic technique, even though patients who had received general anesthesia and were confused had a significant decline in PaO_2 measured 30 minutes after anesthesia.[5] Patients who received epidural anesthesia and experienced postoperative confusion did not demonstrate a similar decline in arterial oxygenation.

In any event, one is left with the dilemma in the post anesthesia care unit (PACU) of how to assess and care for the confused patient. One should first ensure that the patient is not hypoxic. The fastest measure by which to assess oxygenation is to use a pulse oximeter. If oximetry is not an option, blood gas analysis should be performed, and supplemental oxygen should be administered at an FIO_2 of 1.0 until the results are available. If the patient is hypoventilating with no prospects for immediate recovery, endotracheal intubation with mechanical ventilatory support should be begun if not already present. In addition to determining the PaO_2, arterial blood gas samples should be sent to determine blood glucose and electrolyte levels, as both hypoglycemia and hyponatremia are associated with confusion. If anticholinergics were given intraoperatively, one could also consider administering a 1 mg intravenous dose of physostigmine. Physostigmine, an anticholinesterase, can reverse the central nervous system (CNS) effects of anticholinergics by crossing the blood-brain barrier and increasing the availability of acetylcholine for neurotransmission.

If the patient remains confused after this assessment, one should consider supportive measures, such as restraining the patient from disconnecting the intravenous catheters and surgical drains or pulling at the operative dressing. Pain medication should be given as needed and the patient reassured and oriented frequently by the medical staff. A neurologic examination should be performed and perhaps neurologic consultation requested to rule out the possibility of subarachnoid hemorrhage or other intracranial event that could cause confusion.

Pain management for hip fracture patients is a function of the intraoperative anesthetic technique. Patients who have a functioning epidural catheter may benefit from continuous infusion of either a low concentration of bupivacaine (0.125 to 0.250 per cent) or a mixture of bupivacaine and narcotic (0.1 per cent bupivacaine with either 0.1 mg/ml morphine sulfate or 10 μg/ml fentanyl citrate).[8] An infusion of a bupivacaine–fentanyl solution at 3 to 8 ml/hr is usually adequate. The low systemic levels of narcotic analgesics or local anesthetics resulting from an epidural infusion may help minimize adverse drug interactions in patients requiring multiple medications for chronic illness.

One specific concern for orthopedic patients with long bone and pelvic fractures as well as crush injuries is the fat embolization syndrome (FES). Respiratory insufficiency and neurologic deficits are the primary abnormalities seen with FES.

This syndrome is believed to be caused by release of fat from fat cells in bone marrow and embolization of the fat into the central venous circulation and pulmonary vasculature. The release of fat is associated with a rise in serum free fatty acids. These free fatty acids have been implicated in toxicity to type II alveolar cells and are associated with the release of vasoactive substances, including histamine and serotonin. The result of the presence of these substances in the pulmonary vasculature is a breakdown of the alveolar capillary membrane, interstitial hemorrhage, and edema.[9] Additionally, the release of fat globules is associated with subclinical evidence of disseminated intravascular coagulation (DIC), probably initiated by activation of the extrinsic clotting cascade.

The incidence of FES in trauma cases ranges from 1 to 5 per cent of those with long-bone fractures[10] and 5 to 10 per cent of patients with pelvic injuries.[11] FES is less common in children owing to decreased fat content in developing long-bone marrow, and it may be more common in patients with diseases that increase the fat content of the bone, e.g., osteoporosis and extremity immobilization. The clinical importance of this syndrome is reflected by an associated mortality that was reported to be as high as 15 per cent during the 1960s.[11] With early diagnosis and ventilatory support, however, mortality can be dramatically reduced.[12]

The early clinical diagnosis of FES is based on observation of dyspnea, sinus tachycardia, and fever with no known source. Mental status changes are seen ranging from disorientation, confusion, and agitation to stupor and coma. These changes may be due primarily to hypoxemia, although systemic emboli through a patent foramen ovale to the cerebral circulation may also contribute. Focal and generalized seizures have been reported as well. Their etiology should be differentiated from possible concurrent head trauma. Although respiratory insufficiency is usually the predominant feature of FES, there are cases of mental status changes from fat emboli without evidence of hypoxemia.[13]

When the syndrome is in an advanced state, petechiae may be seen across the thorax and in the conjunctiva, and cotton spots may appear in the retina. The onset of symptoms is variable but usually occurs 12 to 72 hours after injury. There are reports of patients dying intraoperatively, whereas others succumb to FES several days after surgery.[14] Therefore it is important to be alert for symptoms of FES early during the postoperative period.

The hallmark of abnormal laboratory findings in FES is hypoxemia detected by arterial blood gas analysis. Respiratory alkalosis may be noted early in the course of the syndrome as well. A patient's chest roentgenogram upon admission is often initially normal, assuming no thoracic trauma is present. As the patient becomes symptomatic, the chest film usually reveals patchy bilateral parenchymal infiltrates.

A decrease in the hemoglobin or hematocrit may be due to red blood cell sequestration at the site of the wound or in the lung. The platelet count also falls during the first few days after injury because of platelet and fibrin adherence to fat globules. Even so, patients rarely have important clinical coagulopathies as a result of FES, unless they develop DIC. Serum lipase levels are also reported to be elevated, but this test is nonspecific and the elevated levels seen in trauma cases often do not correlate with clinically evident FES. Fat in the urine and sputum are also not specific diagnostic indicators. The electrocardiogram may indicate signs of right heart strain, particularly if flow across the pulmonary vasculature is sufficiently obstructed. A computed tomographic scan of the head usually shows diffuse brain swelling with compressed ventricles and flattened sulci.[15]

Prevention of FES entails early immobilization and prompt operative correction of fractures. Supplemental oxygen and ventilatory support are the mainstay of treatment. Mechanical ventilation with positive end-expiratory pressure may be required to maintain adequate oxygen-carrying capacity. High frequency ventilation has been applied in the treatment of FES and was shown to provide adequate oxygenation and allow patients to tolerate mechanical ventilation without heavy sedation or muscle relaxation.[16] Although the maintenance of adequate oxygenation may not immediately resolve neurologic deficits,[15] these deficits often clear after the respiratory insufficiency has been treated. Most patients recover completely if adequate ventilatory support is given.

Finally, one should be aware of the high risk of deep venous thrombosis (DVT) in patients who have suffered a hip fracture. Approximately, 48 to 50 per cent of these patients have evidence of DVT and as many as 3.5 per cent suffer fatal pulmonary emboli.[17] Low dose warfarin therapy administered perioperatively,[18] as well as spinal anesthesia when compared with general anesthesia, appears to reduce the incidence of DVT in this setting.[19] A discussion of perioperative prevention and therapy for DVT and pulmonary emboli can be found in the section on total hip arthroplasty.

TOTAL HIP ARTHROPLASTY

Patients requiring total hip arthroplasty (THA) range from an American Society of Anesthesiologists (ASA) class I patient with avascular necrosis of the hip joint to an elderly arthritic patient who shares the same complex medical problems as patients described in the previous section. In contrast to patients who have suffered femoral neck fractures, postoperative management of elective total hip arthroplasty patients may be more straightforward, as there should be adequate time preoperatively to optimize medical therapy of concurrent chronic illness.

Postoperative airway and fluid management should be consistent with the principles outlined in the previous section. As with patients who have sustained femoral neck fractures, patients who have had a total hip arthroplasty under general anesthesia may have significantly lower PaO_2 values on the first postoperative day than those who receive epidural anesthesia.[17] These patients may also be at risk for fat emboli syndrome.[20] It is therefore important to monitor these patients for adequate oxygenation using pulse oximetry or blood gas analysis and to provide supplemental oxygen in the PACU.

The next consideration for patients who have undergone total hip arthroplasty is positioning. Because of the application of balanced suspension early during the postoperative period, these patients are usually transported to the PACU in their hospital bed instead of on a gurney. This practice decreases the number of transfers from bed to bed and thereby decreases the likelihood of dislocating the hip. Prior to returning to the hospital ward, radiography of the hip is usually performed to ensure that the hip has not dislocated. The incidence of hip dislocation is about 3 per cent, with 5 per cent of these dislocations occurring on postoperative day 1.[21] The operative hip is stabilized in the PACU by placing it in balanced suspension (Fig. 17–1), which maintains the leg in an elevated and abducted position.[22]

Patients in balanced suspension should be evaluated for evidence of hematoma and motor or sensory loss. Evaluation of motor and sensory levels of anesthetic are particularly important if a regional anesthetic technique has been used perioperatively. Bromage[23] has described a method to measure the intensity of motor blockade, defining a complete motor block as the inability to move the feet or knees. The ability to move only the feet is considered an almost complete motor block, the ability to move the knees as a partial motor block, and full flexion of knees and feet as no motor block (Fig. 17–2). Although it may be difficult to assess upper lumbar sensory levels for an epidural block on the operative side due to the bulky dressing, it is usually possible to assess sensory block by testing the patient's foot response to cold, pinprick, or touch.

It is important to establish bilateral intact motor and sensory function following anesthesia because of the possibility of sciatic nerve injury to the leg during total hip replacement. The incidence of sciatic injury following total hip arthroplasty is reported to be 0.7 to 3.5 per cent for primary hip replacement and up to 7.5 per cent for revisions.[24,25] Nerve injury is thought to be related to compression or traction of the nerve or to lengthening of the operated leg, which causes a stretch injury to the sciatic nerve.[26,27] A delayed sciatic nerve palsy has been attributed to migration of the trochanteric wire.[28]

Measures to predict or prevent the development of postoperative nerve injuries, e.g., somatosensory evoked potential monitoring,[29] have been suggested. Unfortunately, these attempts have not produced uniformly successful results. It is important to be vigilant for signs of sciatic nerve injury, which include unexplained sensory loss to the foot or decreased strength of plantar extension and flexion of the foot on the operative side. Because epidural or spinal anesthesia can mask sensory and motor changes, the patient should remain in the recovery room until it is evident that the nerve blockade is regressing appropriately.

Pain management of these patients may be accomplished with parenteral narcotics or via intrathecal or epidural routes for narcotics or local anesthetics (see Chapter 19). Side effects of the chosen pain management techniques are also important during the postoperative period. Nausea, vomiting, pruritus, and respiratory depression may be experienced with parenteral, intrathecal, and epidural narcotics. A

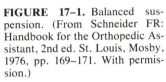

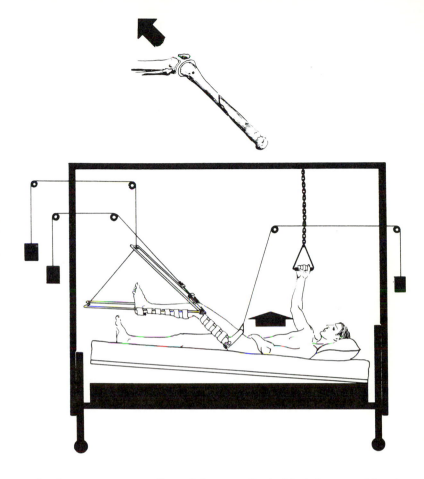

FIGURE 17–1. Balanced suspension. (From Schneider FR: Handbook for the Orthopedic Assistant, 2nd ed. St. Louis, Mosby, 1976, pp. 169–171. With permission.)

particular concern for patients who have undergone total hip arthroplasty is the development of urinary retention. These patients have the added risk of bacteremia and bacterial seeding of the prosthetic hip joint, resulting in a deep wound infection, if the patient requires urinary catheterization.[30] An immediate or late deep wound infection of the prosthesis

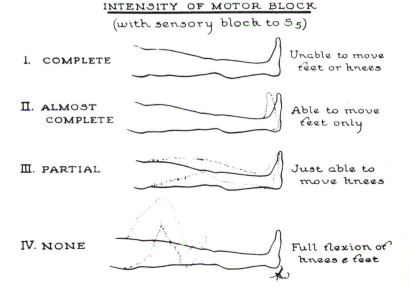

FIGURE 17–2. Assessment of motor block following spinal or epidural anesthesia (see text). (From Bromage PR: A comparison of the hydrochloride and carbon dioxide salts of lidocaine and prilocaine in epidural analgesia. Acta Anaesth Scand [Suppl] 16:55, 1965. With permission.)

INTENSITY OF MOTOR BLOCK
(with sensory block to S_5)

I. COMPLETE — Unable to move feet or knees

II. ALMOST COMPLETE — Able to move feet only

III. PARTIAL — Just able to move knees

IV. NONE — Full flexion of knees & feet

has serious consequences for the patient. Treatment includes removal of the prosthesis and débridement of the wound plus 6 weeks of intravenous antibiotics. Walts et al.[31] found that use of epidural morphine significantly increased the need for urinary catheterization independent of the intraoperative anesthetic technique. Others have reported that a preoperative low peak urinary flow rate[32] or a history of urinary obstruction[33] predisposes patients to postoperative urinary retention.

One treatment that may help prevent urinary retention is administration of 10 mg of phenoxybenzamine orally during the immediate postoperative period.[34] Phenoxybenzamine reduces the incidence of urinary retention by relaxing the bladder's sphincter.

At my institution the orthopedic services prefer that patients who undergo epidural anesthesia have a urinary catheter inserted intraoperatively in anticipation of retaining the epidural catheter for postoperative pain management. They have not experienced an increase in failed total hip arthroplasties due to prosthetic infection—perhaps because of the perioperative antibiotic prophylaxis each patient received. Because the rate of infected prostheses is low, a large number of patients would have to be studied to demonstrate a significant difference in the rate of infection between having or not having a urinary catheter. Until such a study is conducted, it is not known if the benefits of postoperative epidural narcotics outweigh the risks of postoperative deep wound infections.

Although the risk of a postoperative wound infection is low, patients who have undergone total hip anthroplasty appear to be at high risk for developing DVT of the lower extremities.[35] In the absence of perioperative anticoagulation, 45 to 70 per cent of patients who have undergone total hip anthroplasty may develop a DVT. Possible causes for this increased risk of DVT include venostasis due to patient immobilization[36] and postoperative hypercoagulability seen as a response to surgical stress. Epidural anesthesia has been reported to decrease the risk of DVT,[37] probably owing to an increase in blood flow to the lower extremities or a decrease in stress response to surgery. Low dose warfarin also decreases the risk of DVT without causing excessive postoperative bleeding.[38] Fixed-dose subcutaneous heparin has not been consistently shown to decrease the rate of DVT in orthopedic patients; however, an adjusted dose of heparin, based on maintaining an activated partial thromboplas-

tin time between 31.5 and 36.0 seconds, effectively decreased the incidence of DVT.[39] Other anticoagulants that prevent DVT, e.g., intravenous dextran or oral aspirin therapy, have not been used as frequently. Both low-molecular-weight dextran (dextran 40) and high-molecular-weight dextran (dextran 70) are effective in preventing DVTs by decreasing blood viscosity and inhibiting platelet aggregation.[40,41] Some patients, however, suffer from potentially serious side effects, e.g., congestive heart failure due to volume overload, and a small risk of an allergic response to dextran 70. Finally, although aspirin might prevent DVTs by inhibiting platelet aggregation, the results of clinical trials on the value of aspirin for DVT prophylaxis have been contradictory.[35]

In addition to pharmacologic prophylaxis for the prevention of DVT, graduated compression stockings have been studied. They may decrease the risk by limiting venous stasis without the potential bleeding complications seen with anticoagulants. Unfortunately, although several studies have suggested a reduction in DVTs with the use of leg compression stockings[42,43] the NIH Consensus Conference could not recommend the sole use of graduated pressure stockings to prevent DVT.[44] Although the initiation of a DVT often begins intraoperatively, diagnosis is usually delayed until after the patient has been transferred from the recovery room to the floor. Part of the reason for this delay is the difficulty of making a diagnosis of DVT based on clinical findings, as the signs and symptoms of lower extremity swelling, erythema, and tenderness not only take time to develop but are also nonspecific and unreliable. Therefore, the diagnosis of DVT depends on laboratory studies. The pathophysiology of thromboembolism has been reviewed elsewhere.[45,46]

Even though the diagnosis of DVT is most commonly made after discharge from the PACU, pulmonary emboli are occasionally encountered intraoperatively[47,48] or immediately postoperatively. A multicenter trial found that the average time to develop a pulmonary embolus was 14 days postoperatively,[49] although one patient in this study died from a pulmonary embolus on the first postoperative day. It is necessary therefore to be able to diagnose and have a treatment protocol for the management of pulmonary embolus early during the postoperative period.

Clinical diagnosis of pulmonary embolus is difficult because of the highly variable presentations of the disease. The most frequent symptoms include dyspnea, pleuritic chest pain, and apprehension. The most frequent signs are tachypnea and rales. Wheezing is not frequent, even though localized bronchoconstriction occurs distal to the occluded pulmonary artery. It is mediated by a release of serotonin, prostaglandins, and histamine from the embolized thrombus.[45] Some degree of hemoptysis occurs in 20 to 30 per cent of patients, although coughing is infrequent.[50] Fever up to 40°C may be experienced by one half of the patients.[45]

A number of other medical problems, e.g., atelectasis, asthma, congestive heart failure, acute myocardial infarction, aspiration pneumonitis, and postoperative splinting, may mimic or mask these symptoms. Because of the morbidity and mortality associated with pulmonary emboli, pulmonary embolus should be included in the differential diagnosis of any patient complaining of chest pain and dyspnea.

Chest roentgenograms are abnormal in most patients with acute pulmonary embolus. Sixty-per cent have an elevated hemidiaphragm, an infiltrate, or both.[45] Forty-per cent exhibit a pleural effusion on lateral chest films.[51] Unfortunately, 20 to 30 per cent of chest films are interpreted as normal, so the sensitivity and specificity of this test is not high.

Arterial blood gas examination indicates a PaO_2 of more than 80 mm Hg in up to 15 per cent of patients.[50,52] In the presence of increased deadspace, patients may be able to maintain normal oxygenation by hyperventilating. However, the alveolar–arterial oxygen gradient is usually increased and the $PaCO_2$ decreased in association with a normal PaO_2. No venous blood studies are useful for the diagnosis of pulmonary embolus.[45]

Electrocardiographic changes are common but consist primarily of transient nonspecific ST-T wave changes.[53] Sinus tachycardia is usually present and is not commonly associated with atrial dysrhythmias. Right heart strain patterns are observed only in the presence of massive single or multiple diffuse pulmonary embolism.

Because none of the previously mentioned diagnostic tests can reliably establish the presence of a pulmonary embolus, the use of ventilation/perfusion (V/Q) lung scans and pulmonary angiography are required for a definitive diagnosis. V/Q scans involve a two-step process. Ventilation scans involve inhalation of

an inert radioactive gas such as xenon 133. A scintillation detector then records areas of radioactivity in the lung. Normal ventilation scans show a uniform wash-in and wash-out of the radioactivity throughout the lungs.

Perfusion scans require intravenous injection of a radionuclide-labeled albumin solution. In areas of normal pulmonary perfusion, the radiolabeled albumin is detected immediately. Areas of poor perfusion due to emboli, hypoxic pulmonary vasoconstriction, or vasoconstriction of any other etiology demonstrate a lack of radioactivity. A normal perfusion study virtually eliminates the diagnosis of a pulmonary embolus.[54] If perfusion defects are seen, however, the nuclear medicine specialist must examine the patient's chest roentgenogram and ventilation scan for evidence of pulmonary infiltrates or areas of decreased ventilation that match the perfusion defect.

Isolated perfusion defects without a matching ventilation defect or a small subsegmental perfusion and ventilation defect are termed low probability for pulmonary embolus. Intermediate probability V/Q scans have multiple subsegmental perfusion defects and no ventilation defects. Pulmonary emboli are considered highly probable only in the presence of segmental perfusion defects with no matching ventilation defect. Unfortunately, ventilation perfusion scans for both low and intermediate probability require further evaluation if the clinical setting suggests a pulmonary embolus. The reason for this further assessment is that even a low probability reading has a more than 20 per cent probability for a true pulmonary embolus.[55] Additionally, patients with postoperative atelectasis, pneumonia or pneumonitis, and chronic obstructive pulmonary diseases or asthma are difficult to evaluate for isolated perfusion defects because of hypoxic pulmonary vasoconstriction.

In the absence of a normal or high probability V/Q scan, the patient should proceed to pulmonary angiography. This procedure is particularly appropriate if a surgical embolectomy is contemplated or if the patient is a candidate for thrombolytic therapy (e.g., urokinase, streptokinase, or tissue plasminogen activator). The importance of making a definitive diagnosis stems from the associated morbidity and mortality of these therapies. For instance, the mortality rate for surgical embolectomy ranges from 10 to 30 per cent.[56]

Morbidity associated with thrombolytic therapies is much lower than surgical embolectomy but includes the risk of intracranial hemorrhage in 1 per cent of patients.[57] Most importantly, thrombolytic therapy is considered by most to be at least relatively contraindicated during the immediate postoperative period because of the likelihood of lysing clots at the surgical site.[58] A lysed clot in the hip and thigh could result in substantial blood loss, hematoma formation, wound dehiscence, and an associated risk of hepatitis from additional blood transfusions. Protocols for the administration of tissue plasminogen activator during the perioperative period have been reported.[59] This protocol does not, however, apply to patients in the PACU.

If there is clinical suspicion of a pulmonary embolus while the patient is in the PACU, and the suspicion is confirmed by a positive pulmonary angiogram, the physician has few options. An excellent review of the diagnosis and therapy of perioperative pulmonary thromboembolic (PTE) events by Dehring and

Arens[46] provided an outline for rational management (Figs. 17–3 and 17–4). If the patient is hemodynamically unstable, a surgical consultation for emergency embolectomy is appropriate. Emboli in the central but not the peripheral pulmonary arterial tree are amenable to embolectomy.

Several maneuvers may help in the management of hemodynamically unstable patients prior to definitive surgical treatment. Because the primary hemodynamic problem is right ventricular failure secondary to pulmonary artery obstruction, attempts should be made to improve right ventricular myocardial perfusion and decrease right ventricular afterload. Oxygen should be administered to optimize oxygen-carrying capacity and tissue delivery. Careful administration of fluids by titrating the central venous pressures to 12 to 15 cm H_2O should improve left ventricular filling and cardiac output.[46] α_1-Agonists are useful for im-

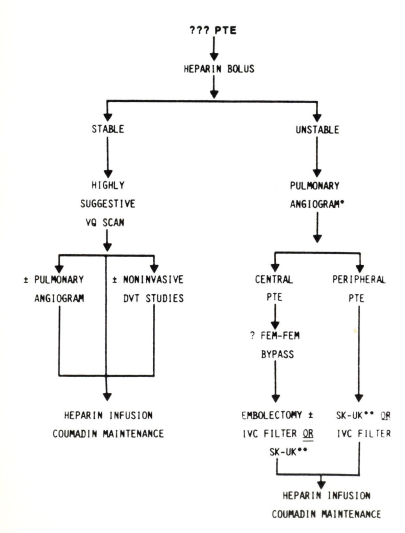

FIGURE 17–3. Management of pulmonary thromboembolism (PTE) in patients with no contraindications to anticoagulants. * VQ scan useful if negative. ** PTT must be normal in patients after streptokinase-urokinase (SK-UK). (From Dehring DJ, Arens JF: Orthopedic concerns. Anesthesiology 73:146–164, 1990. With permission.)

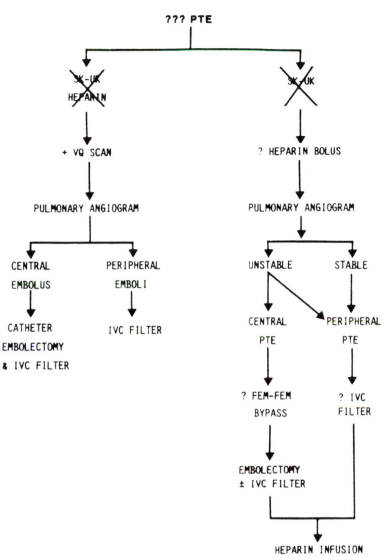

FIGURE 17–4. Management of pulmonary thromboembolism (PTE) in patients with contraindications to anticoagulants. Patients with contraindications to either streptokinase-urokinase (SK-UK) and heparin or contraindications just to SK-UK are indicated by the large X through the anticoagulants.

proving right ventricular coronary perfusion. For instance, a 100 μg bolus of norepinephrine followed by a norepinephrine infusion of 0.08 to 0.16 μg/kg/min has been shown to improve right ventricular coronary perfusion.[60] Intra-aortic balloon pumps in dogs have also been shown to improve right ventricular perfusion by elevating diastolic pressures.[61] Case reports have detailed the use of hydralazine in patients with pulmonary emboli to decrease right ventricular afterload.[62] Although patients improved in these anecdotal reports, no controlled studies of hydralazine for pulmonary emboli are available.

Hemodynamically stable patients with the diagnosis of a pulmonary embolus immediately postoperatively have only limited thera-peutic options. Heparin may be cautiously administered to the patient with vigilant observation of the surgical site for bleeding. The usual dose of heparin is a 5000 U bolus followed by a heparin infusion at 1000 U/hr. Insertion of an inferior vena cava filter (e.g., Greenfield filter)[63] in total hip arthroplasty patients also may prevent recurrent pulmonary emboli without risking the bleeding complications of heparin.

Finally, there are a number of rarely encountered postoperative complications of total hip arthroplasty. They include various complications resulting from erosions of methylmethacrylate into the pelvis. Erosions into the common iliac vein, external iliac artery,[64] and femoral artery[65] have been reported. Intraoperative perforations may present postoperatively as an ischemic limb or hematoma at the surgical site. These complications may also surface as arteriovenous fistulas months to years after surgery. Bladder compression by encroachment of the methylmethacrylate into the bladder[66,67] has also been reported as a late postoperative complication.

TOTAL KNEE ARTHROPLASTY

Management of patients who have undergone a total knee arthroplasty is similar to that for the total hip arthroplasty patient in the PACU. After the initial assessment, issues of postoperative bleeding and pain control are again important. The large dressing and bandage covering the operative knee may obscure substantial blood loss, and the surgical drainage system should be frequently observed regarding the volume of blood. Autotransfusion devices connected to wound drains, e.g., the Solcotrans, may lessen the risk of transfusion reaction or a viral infection associated with heterologous blood transfusions. Epidural analgesia during the postoperative period provides intense pain relief, especially when surgeons choose to use a continuous passive motion device. Neurologic deficits after total knee arthroplasty are unusual.

As in the case of surgical procedures around the hip, patients undergoing total knee arthroplasty are at risk for DVT.[68,69] There are also case reports of fat emboli after total knee arthroplasty.[70] Thromboembolism and fat emboli syndrome have been discussed in previous sections of this chapter.

SCOLIOSIS

Scoliosis may be broadly categorized into idiopathic and nonidiopathic types. Nonidiopathic scoliosis is associated with a number of other syndromes including neuromuscular diseases (e.g., spinal muscle atrophy, muscular dystrophy, Friedreich's ataxia, and myelomeningocele) and congenital heart disease, myelodysplasias, and Marfan syndrome. The anesthetic implications of scoliosis associated with these conditions have been reviewed elsewhere.[71,72] In addition to these specific concerns about other medical problems, patients who have undergone scoliosis repair require careful monitoring during the post anesthetic period for respiratory and cardiovascular problems. Before discussing the postoperative management of scoliosis patients, a brief review of the pulmonary and cardiovascular sequelae of scoliosis is necessary.

The lateral spinal curvature seen in scoliosis (especially when in combination with kyphosis) causes impaired pulmonary function. This curvature results in restrictive lung disease by decreasing the chest wall compliance and impairing the ability of intercostal muscles to expand the thoracic cage. Pulmonary function testing in these patients reveals reductions in vital capacity, total lung capacity, and functional residual capacity.[71] As the disease progresses, hypoxemia and later hypercarbia develop as patients are unable to compensate for the increased work of breathing. In addition to the predisposition to ventilatory failure, patients eventually develop cor pulmonale and progressive pulmonary hypertension secondary to chronic hypoxemia.

During the acute postoperative period, the alveolar-arterial oxygen gradient and vital capacity worsen, so it is important to anticipate those patients in whom this additional respiratory impairment will precipitate ventilatory failure. Patients who are likely to require ventilatory support include those who have preoperative vital capacities of less than 30 to 40 per cent of predicted values.[71] Preoperative hypercarbia also predisposes patients to inadequate postoperative ventilation. Patients with nonidiopathic scoliosis are reported to be at increased risk for a range of pulmonary complications if they are more than 20 years of age, mentally retarded, undergoing anterior spinal fusion, and have preoperative hypoxemia or obstructive lung disease (determined by preoperative pulmonary function testing).[73]

Patients who are at risk for postoperative respiratory failure should remain intubated in the PACU until they have clearly awakened from anesthesia, are normothermic, are hemodynamically stable, and have had their muscle relaxants fully reversed. The decision on the appropriate timing for extubation may be difficult and should be based on comparison of postoperative blood gases, and pulmonary tests of strength with preoperative pulmonary function tests and clinical judgment.

These patients should also be monitored for signs of hypovolemia and anemia in the PACU, as substantial blood loss often occurs intraoperatively. Patients with evidence of right ventricular failure may require a pulmonary artery catheter to evaluate adequacy of left ventricular filling without overloading the right ventricle.

Spinal stabilization surgery may also cause postoperative neurologic deficits, including paraplegia due to compression of the spinal cord or impairment of the spinal cord's vascular supply by the realigned vertebrae. Therefore frequent neurologic evaluation of the lower extremities for motor or sensory deficits is necessary. Deficits have occurred in the presence of a normal wake-up test[74] and normal intraoperative somatosensory evoked potential monitoring.[75] These deficits may take hours or days to develop because of progressive spinal cord edema.[76]

Finally, several unusual and late-occurring complications may appear after scoliosis repair. Chylothorax has been seen after anterior spinal correction.[77] The chylothorax appeared to be due to direct injury to the lymphatic system, and it resolved spontaneously with conservative therapy. Another unusual complication is iliofemoral thrombosis following posterior spinal correction.[78] This problem occurs only in the left common iliac vein presumably due to compression of the vein when it crosses the right iliac artery during prone positioning of the patient.

ARTHROSCOPY

Many of the concerns for arthroscopic surgical patients are addressed in Chapter 20. In addition to the usual concerns, nerve injury in patients who have undergone knee arthroscopy has been reported in a large series by Sherman et al.[79] They noted that about 0.5 per cent of these patients developed postoperative hyperesthesias or paresthesias of the saphenous nerve underneath the knee. Similar paresthesias have been encountered following medial meniscectomy.[80]

Several studies have examined the risks and benefits of regional anesthesia versus general anesthesia in outpatients. For knee arthroscopy, epidural anesthesia resulted in a shorter stay in the PACU and outpatient recovery room. These stays were accompanied by lower incidences of pain, nausea, and vomiting.[81]

Spinal anesthesia for outpatients has also been evaluated. For knee arthroscopy, patients undergoing spinal anesthesia spent more time in the PACU but experienced less pain, nausea, and vomiting. There was a 5 per cent

incidence of postural headache when a 25 gauge spinal needle was used in patients. None of these patients required an epidural blood patch.[82] In another study, 27 gauge spinal needles were used in outpatients; 2.1 per cent of 242 patients reported a spinal headache, and again no patient required an epidural blood patch.[83]

It appears that spinal anesthesia may be considered for outpatients. It is important to advise these patients about the potential for a postoperative headache. The patient should be instructed concerning how to contact the anesthesiologist if a headache should occur. Treatment of spinal headaches may begin conservatively with bed rest and oral fluid replacement. In the case of severe postural headache, the patient may not be able to maintain adequate oral fluid consumption and should return to the hospital for parental fluid replacement and evaluation for either parenteral caffeine therapy or epidural blood patch placement.

References

1. Barash PG, Cullen BF, Stoelting RK: Clinical Anesthesia. Philadelphia, Lippincott, 1989, pp. 1163–1184.
2. Goucke CR: Mortality following surgery for fractures of the neck of the femur. Anaesthesia *40*:583–586, 1985.
3. McKenzie PJ, Wishart HY, Smith G: Long-term outcome after repair of fractured neck of femur. Br J Anaesth *56*:581–584, 1984.
4. Davis FM, Laurenson VG: Spinal anesthesia or general anesthesia for emergency hip surgery in the elderly. Anesth Intens Care *9*:352–358, 1981.
5. Berggren D, Gustafson Y, Eridsson B, et al: Postoperative confusion after anesthesia in elderly patients with femoral neck fractures. Anesth Analg *66*:497–504, 1987.
6. Chung F, Meier R, Lautenschlager E, et al: General or spinal anesthesia: which is better in the elderly? Anesthesiology *67*:422–427, 1987.
7. Riis J, Lomholt B, Haxholdt O: Immediate and long-term mental recovery from general versus epidural anesthesia in elderly patients. Acta Anaesthesiol Scand *27*:44–49, 1983.
8. Lubenow TR, Wong J, McCarthy RJ, Ivankovich AD: Prospective evaluation of continuous epidural narcotic-bupivacaine infusion in 1500 postoperative patients. Reg Anesth *14*:32, 1989.
9. Gossling HR, Ellison LH, DeGraff AC: Fat embolism. J Bone Joint Surg [Am] *56A*:1327, 1974.
10. Wildsmith JAW, Masson AHB: Severe fat embolism: a review of 24 cases. Scott Med J *23*:141–148, 1978.
11. Peltier LF: Fat embolism: a perspective. Clin Orthop *232*:263–270, 1988.
12. Guenter CA, Braum H: Fat embolism syndrome: changing prognosis. Chest *79*:143, 1981.
13. Findlay JM, DeMajo W: Cerebral fat embolism. J Trauma *8*:812–820, 1968.

14. Gresham GA: Fat embolism. Forensic Sci Int *31*:175–180, 1986.

15. Jacobsen DM, Terrence CF, Reinmith OM: The neurologic manifestations of fat embolism. Neurology *36*:847–851, 1986.

16. Lee A, Simpson D: High frequency jet ventilation in fat embolism syndrome. Anaesthesia *41*:1124–1127, 1986.

17. Covert CR, Fox GS: Anesthesia for hip surgery in the elderly. Can J Anaesth *36*:311–319, 1989.

18. Morris GK, Mitchell JRA: Warfarin sodium in the prevention of deep venous thrombosis and pulmonary embolism in patients with fractured neck of femur. Lancet *2*:869–872, 1976.

19. McKenzie PJ, Wishart HY, Gray I, Smith G: Effects of anaesthetic technique on deep vein thrombosis. Br J Anaesth *57*:853–857, 1985.

20. Splengler DM, Costenbader M, Bailey R: Fat embolism syndrome following total hip arthroplasty. Clin Orthop *121*:105–107, 1976.

21. Woo RYG, Morrey BF: Dislocations after total hip arthroplasty. J Bone Joint Surg [Am] *64*:1295–1306, 1982.

22. Schneider FR: Handbook for the Orthopedic Assistant, 2nd ed. St. Louis, Mosby, 1976, pp. 169–171.

23. Bromage PR: Epidural Anesthesia. Philadelphia, Saunders, 1978, p. 144.

24. Weber ER, Daube JR, Coventry MB: Peripheral neuropathies associated with total hip arthroplasty. J Bone Joint Surg [Am] *58*:66–69, 1976.

25. Zechmann JP, Reckling FW: Association of preoperative hip motion and sciatic nerve palsy following total hip arthroplasty. Clin Orthop *241*:197–199, 1989.

26. Edwards BN, Tullos HS, Noble PC: Contributing factors and etiology of sciatic nerve palsy in total hip arthroplasty. Clin Orthop *218*:136–141, 1987.

27. Johanson NA, Pellici PM, Tsairis P, Salvati EA: Nerve injury in total hip arthroplasty. Clin Orthop *179*:214–222, 1983.

28. Asnis SE, Hanley S, Shelton PD: Sciatic neuropathy secondary to migration of trochanteric wire following total hip arthroplasty. Clin Orthop *196*:226–228, 1985.

29. Porter SS, Black PL, Reckling FW, Mason J: Intraoperative cortical somatosensory evoked potentials for detection of sciatic neuropathy during total hip arthroplasty. J Clin Anesthesiol *1*:170–175, 1983.

30. Irvine R, Johnson BL, Amstatz HC: The relationship of genitourinary tract procedures and deep sepsis after total hip arthroplasty. Surg Gynecol Obstet *139*:701–706, 1974.

31. Walts LF, Kaufman RD, Moreland JR, Weiskopf M: Total hip arthroplasty: an investigation of factors related to postoperative urinary retention. Clin Orthop *194*:280, 1985.

32. Redfern TR, Orth MCH, Mackin DG, et al: Urinary retention in men after total hip arthroplasty. J Bone Joint Surg [Am] *68*:1435–1438, 1986.

33. Walton JK, Robinson RG: An analysis of a male population having total hip replacement with regard to urological assessment and postoperative urinary retention. Br J Urol *54*:519, 1982.

34. Tammela T, Kontturi M, Puranen J: Prevention of postoperative urinary retention after total hip arthroplasty in male patients. Ann Chir Gynaecol *76*:170–172, 1987.

35. O'Meara PM, Kaufman EE: Prophylaxis for venous thromboembolism in total hip arthroplasty: a review. Orthopedics *13*:173–178, 1990.

36. McKenzie PJ, Loach AB: Local anaesthesia for orthopedic surgery. Br J Anaesth *58*:779–789, 1986.

37. Modig J, Borg T, Karlstrom G, et al: Thromboembolism after total hip replacement: role of epidural and general anesthesia. Anesth Analg *63*:174–180, 1983.

38. Francis CW, Marder VJ, Evarts CM, et al: Two-step warfarin therapy: prevention of postoperative venous thrombosis without excessive bleeding. JAMA *249*:374–378, 1983.

39. Leyvraz PF, Richard J, Bachmann F, et al: Adjusted versus fixed-dose subcutaneous heparin in the prevention of deep-vein thrombosis after total hip replacement. N Engl J Med *309*:954–958, 1983.

40. Harris WH, Athanasoulis CA, Waltman AC, Salzman EW: Prophylaxis of deep-vein thrombosis after total hip replacement: dextran and external pneumatic compression compared with 1.2 or 0.3 gram of aspirin daily. J Bone Joint Surg [Am] *67*:57–62, 1985.

41. Fredin HO, Nillius AS: Fatal pulmonary embolism after total hip replacement. Acta Orthop Scand *53*:407, 1982.

42. Ohlund C, Fransson SG, Stark SA: Calf compression for prevention of thromboembolism following hip surgery. Acta Orthop Scand *54*:896–899, 1983.

43. Ishak MA, Morley KD: Deep venous thrombosis after total hip arthroplasty: a prospective controlled study to determine the prophylactic effect of gradual pressure stockings. Br J Surg *68*:429–432, 1981.

44. Consensus Conference: Prevention of venous thrombosis and pulmonary embolism. JAMA *256*:744–749, 1986.

45. Rosenow EC III, Osmundson PJ, Brown ML: Pulmonary embolism. Mayo Clin Proc *56*:161–178, 1981.

46. Dehring DJ, Areus JF: Pulmonary thromboembolism: disease recognition and patient management. Anesthesiology *73*:146–164, 1990.

47. Oxorn DC, Skurdal D, Belzberg H, Rosenbaum RC: Pneumothorax and pulmonary embolism complicity post-traumatic hip surgery. Can J Anaesth *34*:174–177, 1987.

48. Enright AC, Quartey GR, McQueen JD: Pulmonary embolism during operation. Can Anaesth Soc J *27*:65–67, 1980.

49. International Multicentre Trial: Prevention of fatal postoperative pulmonary embolism by low doses of heparin. Lancet *2*:45–51, 1975.

50. Bell WR, Simon TL, DeMets DL: The clinical features of submassive and massive pulmonary emboli. Am J Med *62*:355–360, 1977.

51. Bynum LJ, Wilson JE III: Radiographic features of pleural effusions in pulmonary embolism. Am Rev Respir Dis *117*:829–834, 1978.

52. Dautzker DR, Bower JS: Alterations in gas exchange following pulmonary thromboembolism. Chest *81*:495, 1982.

53. Stein PD, Dalen JE, McIntyre KM, et al: The electrocardiogram in acute pulmonary embolism. Prog Cardiovasc Dis *17*:247–257, 1975.

54. Kipper MS, Moser KM, Kortman KE, Ashburn WL: Long-term followup of patients with suspected pulmonary embolism and a normal lung scan: perfusion scan in embolic suspects. Chest *82*:411–415, 1982.

55. Hull RD, Hirsch J, Carter CJ, et al: Diagnostic value of ventilation-perfusion lung scanning in patients with suspected pulmonary embolism. Chest *88*:819–828, 1985.

56. Lund O, Nielson TT, Schifter S, Roenne K: Treatment of pulmonary embolism with full dose heparin,

streptokinase or embolectomy: results and indications. Thorac Cardiovasc Surg *34*:240–246, 1986.

57. National Cooperative Study: The urokinase pulmonary embolism trial. Circulation *47*(suppl):1–108, 1973.

58. National Institutes of Health Consensus Development Conference: thrombolytic therapy in thrombosis. Ann Intern Med *93*:141–144, 1980.

59. Verstraete M, Miller GAH, Bounameaux H, et al: Intravenous and intrapulmonary recombinant tissue-type plasminogen activator in the treatment of acute massive pulmonary embolism. Circulation *77*:353–360, 1988.

60. Molloy WD, Lee KY, Girling L, et al: Treatment of shock in a canine model of pulmonary embolism. Am Rev Respir Dis *130*:870–874, 1984.

61. Spotnitz HM, Berman MA, Epstein SE: Pathophysiology and experimental treatment of acute pulmonary embolism. Am Heart J *82*:511–520, 1971.

62. Bates ER, Crevey BJ, Sprague FR, Pitt B: Oral hydralazine therapy for acute pulmonary embolism and low output state. Arch Intern Med *141*:1537–1538, 1981.

63. Woolson ST, Harris WH: Greenfield vena caval filter for management of selected cases of venous thromboembolic disease following hip surgery. Clin Orthop *204*:201–206, 1986.

64. Hopkins NFG, Vauhegan JAD, Jamieson CW: Iliac aneurysm after total hip arthroplasty. J Bone Joint Surg [Br] *65*:359, 1983.

65. Berquist D, Carlsson AS, Ericsson BF: Vascular complications after total hip arthroplasty. Acta Orthop Scand *54*:157, 1983.

66. Hattrup SJ, Bryan RS, Gaffey TA, Stanhope CR: Pelvic mass causing vesical compression after total hip arthroplasty. Clin Orthop *227*:184–189, 1988.

67. Ray B, Baron TE, Bombeck CT: Bladder and urethral displacement: complication of replacement hip arthroplasty. Urology *5*:554–556, 1979.

68. Stulberg BN, Insall JN, Williams GW, Ghelman B: Deep-vein thrombosis following total knee arthroplasty. J Bone Joint Surg [Am] *66*:194–201, 1984.

69. Morrey BF, Adams RA, Ilstrup DM, Bryan RS: Complications and mortality associated with bilateral or unilateral total knee anthroplasty. J Bone Joint Surg [Am] *69*:484–488, 1987.

70. Dorr LD, Merkel C, Mellman MF, Klein I: Fat emboli in bilateral total knee arthroplasty. Clin Orthop *248*:112–119, 1989.

71. Gibbons PA, Lee IS: Scoliosis and anesthesia. Int Anesthesiol Clin *23*(4):149–161, 1985.

72. Kafer ER: Respiratory and cardiovascular functions in scoliosis and the principles of anesthetic management. Anesthesiology *52*:339, 1980.

73. Anderson PR, Puno MR, Lovell SL, Swayze CR: Postoperative respiratory complications in non-idiopathic scoliosis. Acta Anaesthesiol Scand *29*:186–192, 1985.

74. Diaz JH, Lockhart CH: Postoperative quadriplegia after spinal fusion for scoliosis with intraoperative awakening. Anesth Analg *66*:1039–1042, 1987.

75. Ginsberg HH, Shetter AG, Raudzens PA: Postoperative paraplegia with preserved intraoperative somatosensory evoked potentials. J Neurosurg *63*:296, 1985.

76. Johnston CE, Happel LT, Norris R, et al: Delayed paraplegia complicating sublaminar segmental spinal instrumentation. J Bone Joint Surg [Am] *68*:556–563, 1986.

77. Nakai S, Zielke K: Chylothorax—a rare complication after anterior and posterior spinal correction. Spine *11*:830–833, 1986.

78. Gurman AW, Seimon LP: Iliofemoral thrombosis following Harrington spinal instrumentation. J Bone Joint Surg [Am] 67:1273–1274, 1985.

79. Sherman O, Fox J, Snyder S, et al: Arthroscopy—"No problem surgery." J Bone Joint Surg [Am] *8*:256–265, 1986.

80. Swanson AJ: The incidence of prepatellar neuropathy following medial meniscectomy. Clin Orthop *181*:151–153, 1983.

81. Parnass SM, McCarthy RJ, Bach B, et al: A prospective evaluation of epidural versus general anesthesia for outpatient arthroscopy. Anesthestiology *73*:A23, 1990.

82. Bowe EA, Baysinger CL, Sykesh A, Bowe LS: Subarachnoid blockade versus general anesthesia for knee arthroscopy in outpatients. Anesthesiology *73*:A45, 1990.

83. Kang SB, Goodnough DE, Lee YK, et al: Spinal anesthesia with 27-gauge needles for ambulatory surgery patients. Anesthesiology *73*:A2, 1990.

18 PROBLEMS AFTER HEAD, NECK, AND MAXILLOFACIAL SURGERY

KEITH H. BERGE and WILLIAM L. LANIER

Otolaryngologic surgery presents unique postoperative challenges to the anesthesiologist. Added to the routine post anesthetic considerations are the potential problems created by surgery within the airway or upon tissues surrounding the airway. In this chapter we concentrate primarily on postoperative problems related to the airway with brief consideration of several nonairway problems.

TRACHEAL EXTUBATION

Extubation of the trachea following otolaryngologic surgery is often performed in the operating room. Many operations cause derangement of airway anatomy, bleeding, or edema that may result in postextubation airway compromise. The operating room, with trained personnel, monitoring, supplies, good lighting, suction, and a surgeon immediately available, is the safest location for even routine extubation.

Surgical procedures resulting in the greatest anatomic derangement (i.e., laryngectomy, neck dissection) are typically performed following a tracheostomy. In this setting extubation is not a consideration, and the patient can be moved to the recovery room with a secure airway.

"Minor" operations such as tonsillectomy or thyroidectomy occasionally result in serious airway compromise and require careful evaluation prior to extubation. The patient should either be awake or deeply enough anesthetized that laryngeal reflexes are obtunded. With "deep" extubation the patient is at a decreased risk for laryngospasm and bronchospasm but is placed at an increased risk of tracheal aspiration of blood or regurgitated gastric contents. Should extubation be postponed until the patient is awake, the irritating stimulation of the endotracheal tube may result in hypertension and coughing or "bucking." The resulting rise in systemic and venous blood pressure may increase bleeding in the wound. The least desirable anesthetic state for extubation is that of light anesthesia (i.e., between "deep" and awake) because it increases the risk of laryngospasm.[1]

Prior to extubation all loose packs should be removed from the pharynx and gentle suctioning performed. After a surgical procedure in the airway, the posterior pharynx should be visually inspected using a laryngoscope to rule out continued bleeding or the presence of residual packing material. The nasopharynx should be free of residual debris (e.g., adenoid remnants following adenoidectomy). The endotracheal tube can then be withdrawn with gentle positive pressure applied to the rebreathing bag to expel any secretions from the vocal cords and supraglottic region into the pharynx. Once airway patency is established, the patient may be moved to the recovery area and given supplemental oxygen. Following airway procedures in which continued bleeding into the pharynx is likely, there is a risk of aspiration of blood. It is therefore common to transport such patients slightly head-down in the lateral position, the "tonsil position," which allows blood and secretions to passively drain away from the larynx.[2]

It is sometimes best to defer extubation until the patient is fully cooperative. One setting in which this procedure is desirable is following nasal surgery, where nasal packing precludes nasal breathing. Unless fully awake prior to extubation, these patients may become agitated and combative owing to their perceived inability to breathe. Once awake and cooperative, they can respond to instructions to breathe through the mouth. It is also preferable to delay extubation in the patient with dental wiring that limits or precludes jaw opening until the patient is awake and comfortable. These patients should always have wire cutters attached to their gowns to provide access to the airway should difficulty develop.

The recovery room should be equipped with a full array of airway management and resuscitation supplies, including suction. Arterial oxygen saturation should be monitored with a pulse oximeter in any patient with the potential for airway compromise. The anesthesiologist and, if needed, the surgeon should be in attendance for recovery room extubations following airway surgery.

PROBLEMS FOLLOWING EXTUBATION

The most common life-threatening problems that occur during the postoperative period following otolaryngologic surgery are complete or partial airway obstruction (Fig. 18–1) and bleeding into the airway.

COMPLETE AIRWAY OBSTRUCTION

Airway obstruction may range in degree from minimal to complete. Complete airway obstruction is a true emergency. It is typically manifested by absence of breath sounds over the chest or trachea despite obvious efforts by the patient to breathe. The patient develops a paradoxical breathing pattern in which negative intrathoracic pressure generated by contraction and descent of the diaphragm during attempts at inspiration cause the thoracic cage to collapse inward. The diaphragm simultaneously displaces the abdominal contents downward, and the abdominal wall moves outward. With relaxation of the diaphragm, the abdominal wall falls while the chest expands. The net effect is a "rocking" alternation between chest and abdominal rise and fall. Immediate complications from airway obstruction may include hypoxemia, hypercarbia, and pulmonary edema.

A large number of potential causes of airway obstruction exist. They include laryngospasm, airway edema, foreign bodies, and

hypopharyngeal obstruction by posterior displacement of the tongue. Most of the causes of complete airway obstruction represent extreme forms of entities that have developed from less critical obstruction. These problems are addressed in more detail in the discussion of partial airway obstruction. Laryngospasm, an all-or-nothing phenomenon, can result in an immediate onset of complete airway obstruction. Laryngospasm is therefore discussed here in detail, along with initial therapy for all forms of complete airway obstruction.

Laryngospasm is a common cause of postextubation complete airway obstruction following otolaryngologic surgery. It may occur as a result of stimulation of glottic or supraglottic mucosa by irritants such as blood, mucus, vomitus, or irritant inhalational anesthetics.[3] This irritation results in forceful closure of the glottis at the vocal cords, as well as a ball valve retraction of the supraglottic tissues and an approximation of the false vocal cords.[4] Fink differentiated this intense ball valve "laryngospasm" from stridor, which he defined as intermittent laryngeal obstruction arising only at the level of the glottis.[4] In contrast to stridor, true laryngospasm results in complete occlusion of the airway, preventing positive pressure ventilation by mask.[4] Although hypoxia may ultimately abolish laryngospasm,[1] emergency intervention is required.

Initial therapy for laryngospasm, as well as for other forms of complete airway obstruction, consists in anterior dislocation of the mandible during attempts to provide positive pressure ventilation by mask. This mandibular displacement maneuver results in anterior motion of the hyoid bone, which in turn, via the hyoepiglottic ligaments, elevates the epiglottis from the false cords, relieving the ball valve obstruction. Fink observed that whereas this maneuver often succeeds in infants and children, the adult jaw muscles may be too strong to overpower.[4] If these attempts fail to restore a patent airway rapidly, succinylcholine 0.15 to 0.30 mg/kg IV should quickly resolve the obstruction and allow assisted ventilation.[5] If the intravenous route is not readily available, succinylcholine 4.0 mg/kg IM may be given. Intramuscular succinylcholine requires 3 to 4 minutes for maximum effect,[6] although initial relaxation of the laryngeal muscles begins much earlier. The small intravenous dose of succinylcholine has a brief duration of action, whereas the larger intramuscular dose requires approximately 20 minutes for recovery in most patients.[6] After succinylcholine ad-

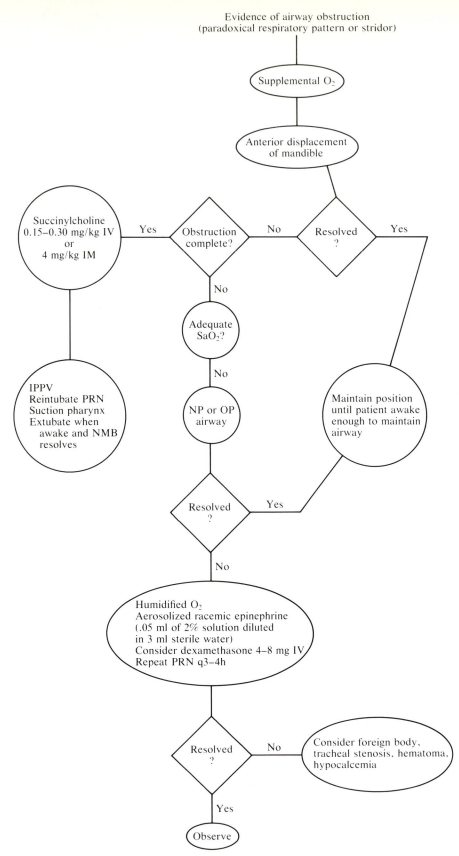

FIGURE 18–1. Management of airway obstruction. SaO₂ = arterial oxygen saturation; IPPV = intermittent positive pressure ventilation; NMB = NP = nasopharyngeal; OP = oropharyngeal.

ministration, regardless of the dose, positive pressure ventilation must be maintained until neuromuscular blockade resolves. In addition, when using the larger dose of succinylcholine or in any case of prolonged neuromuscular blockade, reintubation of the trachea may be desirable to facilitate prolonged ventilation. Pharyngeal suctioning also should be performed prior to full recovery from neuromuscular blockade to decrease the likelihood of laryngospasm recurrence.

Laryngospasm may be more common after otolaryngologic surgery than after other types of surgery. In a retrospective study, Olsson and Hallen[7] reported 1197 cases of laryngospasm in a series of 136,929 patients (0.9 per cent). After otolaryngologic surgery this incidence was 1.0 per cent, and after tonsillectomy it was 1.4 per cent. A much higher incidence of laryngospasm following tonsillectomy has been reported in the prospective studies of Leicht et al.[8] and Baraka[9] in which incidences of 22 and 20 per cent were reported, respectively. It should be noted that the definition of laryngospasm in all these studies included partial or complete obstruction of the laryngeal airway. This definition results in a much higher incidence of laryngospasm than would be expected if Fink's definition were used.[4] Indeed, in prospective studies of tonsillectomy that segregated patients with complete airway obstruction from those with incomplete obstruction,[8,10] the incidence of complete airway obstruction has been 6 to 8 per cent. The increased incidence of laryngospasm following otolaryngologic surgery is likely to be associated with the presence of blood in the airway, particularly following tonsillectomy. Other factors associated with an increased risk of laryngospasm include age less than 9 years, presence of a nasogastric tube, and current upper respiratory tract infection.[7]

Laryngospasm is a potentially serious complication of general anesthesia and is associated with other severe complications. Vomiting (7 per cent), bronchospasm (4 per cent), aspiration (1 per cent), and cardiac arrest (0.5 per cent) were seen in a series of 1197 cases of laryngospasm.[7] Another potential complication of laryngospasm in both children and adults is the development of pulmonary edema. Onset may be sudden[11,12] or delayed by up to 80 minutes.[13] The probable cause is a transient transudation of extraalveolar fluid into the pulmonary interstitium and alveoli as a result of the large transpulmonary pressure gradient created by vigorous attempts to breathe against a closed glottis.[11,12] Therapy is similar to that for other forms of noncardiogenic pulmonary edema, consisting in supplemental oxygen with close monitoring of serial chest roentgenograms and arterial blood gases. Intubation and mechanical ventilation with positive end-expiratory pressure (PEEP) may be necessary to maintain arterial oxygen saturation. The pulmonary edema usually resolves rapidly and completely within 24 to 48 hours.[11-13]

To minimize the risk of laryngospasm, the patient should be extubated when awake enough to respond to commands after careful pharyngeal inspection and suctioning to remove blood and secretions. Early reports showed a decrease incidence of laryngospasm if lidocaine 1 to 2 mg/kg IV was administered 1 to 2 minutes prior to extubation.[9,10] It was unclear whether this effect was due to direct suppression of the laryngeal reflexes by lidocaine or was merely a result of lidocaine's ability to transiently deepen the level of anesthesia just prior to extubation. A more recent study of 100 children extubated with prophylactic lidocaine 1.5 mg/kg following tonsillectomy failed to demonstrate a difference in the incidence of laryngospasm.[8] These investigators waited a mean 4.5 minutes between the lidocaine bolus and extubation, attempting to extubate both the control and test groups at a similar depth of anesthesia as judged by clinical criteria. They attributed the success of previous reports to lidocaine's ability to deepen the anesthetic level and not to any direct effects of lidocaine on the airway.[8]

PARTIAL AIRWAY OBSTRUCTION

Stridor is pathognomonic for partial airway obstruction and is a result of turbulent airflow past an airway constriction. It has been defined as a loud musical sound of constant pitch that connotes tracheal or laryngeal obstruction.[14] Others define stridor as originating only at the glottic level.[4] Our discussion uses the broader definition.

Stridor during inspiration usually indicates partial glottic or supraglottic obstruction, whereas biphasic or expiratory stridor is often a result of partial subglottic obstruction.[15] There are many possible causes of stridor, particularly in children.[15] This discussion is limited to those causes of partial airway obstruction that are frequently seen after otolaryngologic surgery and classifies them based on source: subglottic, glottic, or supraglottic.

Partial airway obstruction may manifest in varying degrees from trivial to near complete. It may occur immediately after tracheal extubation or be delayed and gradual in onset. When initially assessing the patient with partial airway obstruction, the immediate concern is establishment of a patent airway capable of supporting gas exchange. In addition, the inspired oxygen concentration should be enriched to delay the onset of hypoxemia in the face of compromised ventilation. Inability to maintain adequate ventilation and oxygenation constitutes an emergency and requires aggressive intervention, initially with attempts at positive pressure ventilation by mask or, failing that, reintubation. Less severe degrees of partial airway obstruction allow more time to assess, diagnose, and treat the problem.

It may be difficult to quickly and reliably ascertain the level of partial airway obstruction. The approach therefore becomes one of a logical series of therapeutic maneuvers that define the level by virtue of their success or failure in resolving the obstruction. The following should be considered a general approach to any patient with postextubation partial airway obstruction.

Supraglottic Obstruction

Recently extubated patients may not have fully regained pharyngeal tone owing to the residual effects of anesthetics, narcotics, and sedatives. When aroused, the patients may spontaneously breathe with a patent airway; but when left unstimulated, they may develop pharyngeal obstruction due to relaxation of the tongue and soft palate against the posterior pharyngeal wall. This degree of obstruction is frequently temporary and resolves with further emergence. An initial temporizing maneuver is anterior displacement of the mandible ("jaw thrust") with head extension. This simple step has been shown radiographically to increase clearance between the tongue and the posterior pharyngeal wall from an average 2 mm to an average 16 mm in anesthetized, paralyzed patients.[16] If this step resolves the obstruction, the level of the obstruction is most likely the hypopharynx. It may be possible to resolve the obstruction by repositioning the head with pillows, thus obviating the need for recovery room staff to hold the jaw thrust position. If an obstructed airway persists or recurs, an oropharyngeal or nasopharyngeal airway should be inserted. These devices function to elevate the tongue, and in the case of the nasopharyngeal airway the soft palate, away from the posterior wall of the pharynx. In patients with an intact gag reflex, oropharyngeal airways are often poorly tolerated and may elicit vomiting. Nasopharyngeal airways are better tolerated but carry the risk of epistaxis with placement.

A potential cause of supraglottic obstruction that may not be relieved by any of the above measures is generalized mucosal or lingual edema, which may follow surgical trauma or positioning that causes occlusion of venous or lymphatic drainage. Ideally, these patients have not been extubated prior to the resolution of the edema, as reintubation may be both essential and difficult. Another potential cause of obstruction at any level would be a pharyngeal pack that had not been removed prior to extubation.

Glottic Obstruction

Inspiratory stridor (crowing) is pathognomonic for partial obstruction at the glottic level. Fink differentiated stridor from laryngospasm by the mechanism of obstruction.[4] True spasm causes a "ball valve" laryngeal closure involving the true vocal cords, false vocal cords, and epiglottis. Stridor occurs purely at the glottic or true vocal cord level. Inspiratory stridor can occur as a result of any mechanism that interferes with normal abduction of the vocal cords during inspiration, e.g., recurrent laryngeal nerve dysfunction following thyroid surgery,[17] vocal cord edema, or cricoarytenoid joint arthritis.[18]

The partial glottic obstruction that is occasionally seen during emergence from anesthesia is distinct from true laryngospasm and occurs as a result of recovery of diaphragmatic function prior to recovery of skeletal (laryngeal) muscle tone.[4] With spontaneous inspiration, the Bernoulli effect (the pressure of a fluid flowing through a narrowing passage is lowest in the region of highest velocity) generates a low pressure area at the glottic level resulting in the vocal cords being drawn together. The partially anesthetized patient may lack adequate vocal cord abduction to counteract this effect, and the net effect is one of glottic obstruction. The stronger the inspiratory effort generated by the patient, the greater is the degree of obstruction. Expiration is unobstructed as positive intrathoracic pressure "blows" the glottis open.

Treatment consists in oxygen by mask with gentle continuous positive airway pressure (CPAP). With attempts at spontaneous breaths, CPAP counteracts the force that is drawing the glottis closed and results in free gas exchange.[4] The airway can continue to be further supported with CPAP, or the level of obstruction can be bypassed by reintubating the trachea until the patient is sufficiently awake to support his or her own airway.

Edema of the vocal cords may result from even short periods of tracheal intubation and may cause partial obstruction to airflow at the glottic level.[19] This problem can sometimes be differentiated from more distal airway obstruction resulting from edema (croup) in that the obstruction usually occurs during inspiration, whereas croup is characterized by expiratory or biphasic stridor.[15] Postextubation croup is more common in children, whose already anatomically small airways can be compromised by what would be a trivial degree of swelling in an adult. Postextubation croup is generally defined as hoarseness, stridor, or retraction with inspiration. Its reported incidence in children ranges from 1.0 to 3.3 per cent.[20,21]

The therapy for edema-generated partial airway obstruction at the glottic of subglottic level is the same and consists in humidified oxygen-enriched inspiratory gases and adequate hydration. Corticosteroids alone[22] or in combination with nebulized racemic epinephrine[20] are reported to effectively reverse established laryngeal or tracheal edema in children. This medical therapy often obviates the need for reintubation or tracheostomy. Koka et al.[21] reported that only two reintubations were required in 80 cases of postextubation croup using a therapeutic regimen consisting of dexamethasone 4 to 8 mg IV and humidified oxygen at an F_IO_2 of 0.6. The dexamethasone was repeated at 3 hours if no improvement was noted. Only three of these children were treated with racemic epinephrine (0.5 ml of 2 per cent racemic epinephrine mixed with 3 ml sterile water delivered by aerosol). In another series of 110 cases of postextubation croup, Jordan et al.[20] reported that no reintubations were required in patients treated with humidified oxygen and the previously mentioned dose of aerosolized racemic epinephrine. In four children in whom the obstruction persisted, the aerosol was repeated after 4 hours. No child required a third treatment. No corticosteroids were used in this study, although the authors stated that they believe steroids are helpful for arresting the progression of symptoms. No benefit has been shown from the routine prophylactic use of steroids to prevent postextubation airway inflammation.[23]

There are other potential sources of pre- and postoperative inspiratory stridor. Neoplasia (e.g., carcinoma, papillomas) at the glottic level may result in obstruction to airflow. The nature of such an obstruction should be well documented prior to anesthetic induction, and optimal airway management during the perioperative period involves close cooperation between the anesthesiologist and the surgeon. Acute hypocalcemia can cause inspiratory stridor by increasing irritability of the intrinsic muscles of the larynx. This situation may arise after surgery that damages the parathyroid glands, e.g., parathyroid or thyroid gland resection. Treatment requires placement of calcium intravenously until evidence of neuromuscular irritability resolves.

Subglottic Obstruction

If partial airway obstruction persists despite all of the above interventions, one must consider several relatively uncommon causes. Airflow through a congenital or acquired tracheal stenosis can change from adequate to inadequate owing to a seemingly trivial degree of edema. Fiberoptic bronchoscopy may be diagnostic and should be performed prior to reintubation if possible. The obstruction may be bypassed by an endotracheal tube and therefore not be diagnosed if bronchoscopy is performed after reintubation. If reintubation is required prior to definitive diagnosis, the patient can be treated with corticosteroids for 48 hours and extubation attempted again over a flexible fiberoptic bronchoscope. This technique allows rapid reestablishment of the airway if necessary. This technique also allows evaluation of the trachea and larynx during withdrawal of the bronchoscope.

The possibility of aspiration of a foreign body such as a dislodged tumor fragment, a tooth, or a pack should also be considered. With suspected foreign body aspiration, a chest roentgenogram may be diagnostic, but only if the occlusion is caused by a radiopaque object. Fiberoptic bronchoscopy may facilitate diagnosis and removal of the foreign body.

Tracheomalacia may result from long-standing extrinsic compression of the trachea by a large mass, most commonly a thyroid mass. It may result in tracheal collapse and obstruction following extubation.[24] Should tracheomalacia be noted intraoperatively, tracheostomy should be considered at that time.

After neck surgery, particularly thyroid or carotid artery procedures, the airway may be compromised by an expanding wound hematoma. The wound dressing should be removed and the neck observed. An expanding hematoma may cause tracheal shift and kinking. It may also dissect behind the trachea and compress its membranous portion into the tracheal lumen. Further obstruction may be caused by venous congestion and swelling of the tracheal mucosa as a result of impaired venous drainage.[24]

Airway compromise resulting from an expanding hematoma is a potential emergency. The surgeon must be notified immediately. If no airway compromise is present, anesthetic induction and tracheal intubation may be initiated prior to surgical exploration. In this situation, anesthetic induction is best performed with the patient breathing spontaneously to prevent the loss of respiratory muscle tone from causing further collapse of the tracheal lumen. The surgeon should be present at anesthetic induction to assist with airway management should expansion of the hematoma lead to rapid deterioration of airway patency. In contrast, if moderate or severe airway compromise is suspected upon identifying the formation of a hematoma in the awake patient, the trachea should be reintubated with the patient awake, using either direct or fiberoptic laryngoscopy. The exception to this rule occurs in the setting of moderate airway obstruction in the uncooperative patient or in the patient in whom the hemodynamic responses elicited by awake intubation are poorly tolerated (e.g., the patient with unstable angina). In this setting, the patient may require sedation or general anesthesia prior to tracheal intubation. If airway patency worsens prior to or during anesthesia induction, but ventilation is still possible, the surgeon may facilitate ventilation and subsequent tracheal intubation by partially reopening the wound.[24] This maneuver decompresses the hematoma and may subsequently improve airway patency. The maneuver, however, increases the likelihood of brisk blood loss from arterial sources. Should anesthesia personnel be unable to maintain adequate ventilation despite the above interventions or be unable to reintubate the trachea in the presence of a severely compromised airway, the surgeon should proceed immediately with a cricothyrotomy. Failure to proceed promptly will likely result in disastrous consequences.

POSTOPERATIVE BLEEDING INTO THE AIRWAY

Continued bleeding following tonsillectomy or other upper airway surgery may go unnoticed in the recovery room. As has been previously discussed, blood on the vocal cords is a potent stimulant for laryngospasm.[3] Although aspiration of small amounts of blood does not lead to major derangements in lung anatomy and physiology (in contrast to the pulmonary derangements seen with gastric acid aspiration syndromes), aspiration of large amounts of blood can result in intrapulmonary shunting and hypoxemia.[25] Hemodynamic compromise and decreased peripheral delivery of oxygen may result from hypovolemia and anemia. The anesthesiologist and recovery room nurse must have a high index of suspicion in order to diagnose continued bleeding promptly. Patients tend to swallow the blood, and therefore the hemorrhage may not become apparent until the patient vomits. Earlier indications of ongoing bleeding are subtle; they include frequent swallowing and changes in hemodynamics consistent with hypovolemia, i.e., tachycardia and hypotension.[26]

Once bleeding is recognized, the surgeon should be notified and the patient carefully evaluated to determine the degree of anemia and hypovolemia. A blood sample should be obtained for crossmatch and hemoglobin determination. Hemodynamic status should be stabilized with blood and volume replacement as indicated. After correction of hypovolemia, the patient should be returned to the operating room for optimal control of the bleeding.

In the cooperative adult patient the surgeon may be able to control the bleeding while the patient is awake using a ligature or by pressure held with a gauze sponge soaked with a vasoconstrictor such as epinephrine or phenylephrine.[26] Uncooperative adult patients and pediatric patients may require anesthesia induction before bleeding can be controlled.

To prevent ongoing aspiration of blood under anesthesia, the airway must be protected with an endotracheal tube, preferably cuffed, until the bleeding is controlled. Reintubation of these patients carries several risks. In the presence of brisk bleeding, intubation may be difficult as blood may obscure the landmarks. If the patient is anesthetized prior to attempts at intubation, the protective laryngeal reflexes are blunted and aspiration may occur. In a cooperative patient, the best options would therefore be to place the endotracheal tube with the patient awake using either the oral route following adequate supraglottic topical anesthesia or the blind nasal route. Although a fiberoptic intubation may be attempted, the bleeding would likely preclude adequate visualization of the airway landmarks. In the child or uncooperative patient, the only option may be a rapid sequence induction and intubation using cricoid pressure and preoxygenation. Whatever approach is selected, adequate suction and experienced help must be available. The surgeon should also be available in the operating room with equipment ready to perform an emergency cricothyrotomy should attempts at intubation be unsuccessful.

MISCELLANEOUS PROBLEMS

VERTIGO, NAUSEA AND VOMITING

Nausea–vomiting following anesthesia and surgery is probably multifactorial in origin. Perioperative narcotics, female gender, young age, and a history of postoperative nausea and vomiting are associated with an increased risk.[27] Ear surgery is also associated with a high incidence of postoperative nausea and vertigo.[28] Stapedectomy, where perilymph may actually extrude from the vestibular apparatus, is routinely associated with mild nausea and vertigo that is exacerbated by patient movement.[29] Prophylactic administration of an antiemetic such as droperidol 10 to 40 μg/kg IV intraoperatively may reduce the nausea.[28] The antiemetic effect of droperidol results from inhibition of dopaminergic receptors in the chemoreceptor trigger zone of the medulla. It has no effect on labyrinthine-induced motion sickness.[30] The labyrinthine component of the nausea is usually self-limiting and should resolve within 24 hours.[29] Therapy consists in hydration, sedation, bed rest, and nursing the patient in the slightly head-up position to reduce the leakage of perilymph.[29]

COMPLICATIONS FOLLOWING TRACHEOSTOMY

There are many potential complications following tracheostomy.[31] With an experienced surgeon, however, the complications are un-

likely during the immediate postoperative period. We consider here only dislodgement, hemorrhage, and pneumothorax.

Care should be taken to prevent dislodgment of the newly placed tracheostomy tube. Until the stoma tract has begun to mature around the tube, a process requiring 7 to 10 days, the trachea may be difficult or impossible to recannulate.[32] To prevent dislodgment, the tube should be sutured securely in place. The tracheostomy tube obturator should be available at all times, preferably attached to the patient's gown. Should dislodgment occur, the surgeon must be notified immediately. The obturator should be inserted into the tracheostomy tube and an attempt made to reinsert the tube. If the tube does not readily reenter the tracheal lumen, the patient should be reintubated by the oral or nasal route. If the tracheostomy tube is replaced, great care must be taken to ensure that it is in the tracheal lumen and has not dissected into a tract in the pretracheal soft tissues. Undiagnosed, this situation quickly results in respiratory and cardiac arrest.

Occasionally there is minor bleeding from the tracheostomy wound site. It is generally of little consequence and resolves with cautery or packing.[32] Occasionally, more significant bleeding results from the thyroid isthmus and requires surgical reexploration. A potentially catastrophic late complication of tracheostomy is tracheoarterial fistula formation resulting from erosion of the tube cuff through the tracheal wall and into the innominate artery.[26,31,32] Arterial pulsations reflected in the tracheostomy tube warn of the potential for this occurrence. Should a fistula occur, immediate management consists in inflating the cuff of the tracheostomy in an attempt to tamponade the bleeding. If this measure fails to control bleeding into the bronchial tree, an attempt should be made to compress the innominate artery against the posterior aspect of the sternal manubrium by inserting a finger into the tracheal stoma. Pressure must be held until the bleeding artery can be ligated or repaired in the operating room.

Tracheostomy placement may result in pneumothorax, pneumomediastinum, or subcutaneous emphysema. A routine posttracheostomy chest roentgenogram can rule out these complications. Whereas a pneumothorax would likely necessitate chest tube thoracostomy drainage, subcutaneous emphysema or pneumomediastinum should resolve spontaneously.

NERVE TRAUMA

Surgery on the head and neck may result in unintentional damage to, or intentional sacrifice of, cranial or sympathetic nerve pathways. It may influence post anesthetic management and should be discussed with the surgeon prior to the patient's emergence and extubation. Radical neck dissections involve sacrifice of multiple structures including a portion of the sympathetic fibers innervating the heart. Head and neck cancer resections frequently result in anatomic derangement of the airway or in cranial nerve damage, either of which may result in glottic incompetence and acute or chronic aspiration.

Potentially fatal cardiac dysrhythmias have been noted following right radical neck dissection.[33] The Q-T interval is prolonged, which is believed to reflect a complex state of greater than normal disparity of repolarization times within the ventricle,[34] rendering the patient susceptible to ventricular tachydysrhythmias of the torsade de pointes morphology. Although this dysrhythmia typically resolves spontaneously within 1 minute, the rhythm may deteriorate further to ventricular fibrillation. The Q-T interval is not prolonged following either left radical neck dissection or right neck dissection that spares the sternocleidomastoid muscle, internal jugular vein, and accessory nerve.[33]

CONSEQUENCES OF BILATERAL INTERNAL JUGULAR VEIN LIGATION

Bilateral radical neck dissection involves sacrifice of both internal jugular veins. Reported complications of bilateral internal jugular vein ligation include intracranial hypertension, facial edema and cyanosis, retinal edema and hemorrhage, and generalized lethargy.[35] These complications appear to result from venous congestion. The intracranial hypertension is exacerbated by a decreased rate of cerebrospinal fluid resorption.[36] Anecdotal reports of deaths resulting from bilateral internal jugular vein ligation exist.[37,38]

VASOCONSTRICTOR-INDUCED PULMONARY EDEMA

Vasoconstrictors such as cocaine, epinephrine, and phenylephrine are used in otolaryngologic surgery to diminish blood loss and improve exposure while operating on the highly vascular mucosa of the nose. They are also commonly used prior to nasotracheal intubation to reduce the risk of epistaxis. Warner et al.[39] reported three cases of pulmonary edema in otherwise healthy young patients undergoing oral cavity and pharyngeal procedures. All had enzyme elevations suggestive of myocardial damage. The authors believed the cause was 0.5 per cent phenylephrine nasal decongestant delivered by a commercially available spray bottle. These spray bottles were designed for use in the upright position, and their use in a supine patient resulted in an apparent overdosage.

OTHER CONSIDERATIONS: COEXISTING DISEASES

Many head and neck cancers occur in patients with histories of chronic tobacco and alcohol abuse. Frequently, a patient presenting with such a history has associated health problems such as emphysema, bronchitis, liver disease, and malnutrition, as well as the potential to develop symptoms of acute alcohol withdrawal.

SUMMARY

Many immediate post anesthetic problems following otolaryngologic surgery involve maintaining the patency and integrity of the airway. These problems include laryngospasm, partial airway obstruction, and bleeding within the airway. Other less common problems associated with the recovery from otolaryngologic surgery include vertigo, nausea, tracheostomy complications, chronic aspiration, cardiac dysrhythmias, and vasoconstrictor-induced pulmonary edema.

References

1. Roy WL, Lerman J: Laryngospasm in paediatric anaesthesia. Can J Anaesth 35:93–98, 1988.
2. Donlon JV Jr: Anesthesia for eye, ear, nose, and throat. *In* Miller RD (ed): Anesthesia, 2nd ed. New York, Churchill Livingstone, 1986, pp. 1872–1874.
3. Rex MAE: A review of the structural and functional basis of laryngospasm and a discussion of the nerve pathways involved in the reflex and its clinical significance in man and animals. Br J Anaesth 42:891–899, 1970.
4. Fink BR: The etiology and treatment of laryngeal spasm. Anesthesiology 17:569–577, 1956.

5. Stoelting RK, Miller RD: Recovery room. *In* Basics of Anesthesia. New York, Churchill Livingstone, 1984, p. 422.

6. Liu LMP, DeCook TH, Goudsouzian NG, et al: Dose response to intramuscular succinylcholine in children. Anesthesiology 55:599–602, 1981.

7. Olsson GL, Hallen B: Laryngospasm during anesthesia: a computer-aided incidence study in 136,929 patients. Acta Anaesthesiol Scand 28:567–575, 1984.

8. Leicht P, Wisborg T, Chraemmer-Jorgensen B: Does intravenous lidocaine prevent laryngospasm after extubation in children? Anesth Analg 64:1193–1196, 1985.

9. Baraka A: Intravenous lidocaine controls extubation laryngospasm in children. Anesth Analg 57:506–507, 1978.

10. Bidwai AV, Rogers C, Stanley TH: Prevention of post-extubation laryngospasm after tonsillectomy. Anesthesiology 51:S50, 1979 (abstract).

11. Lee KWT, Downes JJ: Pulmonary edema secondary to laryngospasm in children. Anesthesiology 59:347–349, 1983.

12. Lorch DG, Sahn SA: Post-extubation pulmonary edema following anesthesia induced by upper airway obstruction: are certain patients at increased risk? Chest 90:802–805, 1986.

13. Glasser SA, Siler JN: Delayed onset of laryngospasm-induced pulmonary edema in an adult outpatient. Anesthesiology 62:370–371, 1985 (letter to the editor).

14. Hollingsworth HM: Wheezing and stridor. Clin Chest Med 8:231–240, 1987.

15. Maze A, Bloch E: Stridor in pediatric patients. Anesthesiology 50:132–145, 1979.

16. Ruben HM, Elam JO, Ruben AM, Greene DG: Investigation of upper airway problems in resuscitation. 1. Studies of pharyngeal x-rays and performance by laymen. Anesthesiology 22:271–279, 1961.

17. Caldarelli DD, Holinger LD: Complication and sequelae of thyroid surgery. Otolaryngol Clin North Am 13:85–97, 1980.

18. Funk D, Raymon F: Rheumatoid arthritis of the cricoarytenoid joints: an airway hazard. Anesth Analg 54:742–745, 1975.

19. Colice GL: Prolonged intubation versus tracheostomy in the adult. J Intens Care Med 2:85–102, 1987.

20. Jordan WS, Graves CL, Elwyn RA: New therapy for postintubation laryngeal edema and tracheitis in children. JAMA 212:585–588, 1970.

21. Koka BV, Jeon IS, Andre JM, et al: Postintubation croup in children. Anesth Analg 56:501–505, 1977.

22. Deming MV, Oech SR: Steroid and antihistaminic therapy for post intubation subglottic edema in infants and children. Anesthesiology 22:933–936, 1961.

23. Goddard JE Jr, Phillips OC, Marcy JH: Betamethasone for prophylaxis of postintubation inflammation—a double-blind study. Anesth Analg 46:348–353, 1967.

24. Wade JSH: Respiratory obstruction in thyroid surgery. Ann R Coll Surg Engl 62:15–24, 1980.

25. Goodwin SR: Aspiration syndromes. *In* Civetta JM, Taylor RW, Kirby RR (eds): Critical Care. Philadelphia, Lippincott, 1988, p. 1082.

26. Walike JW, Chinn J: Evaluation and treatment of acute bleeding from the head and neck. Otolaryngol Clin North Am 12:455–464, 1979.

27. Muir JJ, Warner MA, Offord KP, et al: Role of nitrous oxide and other factors in postoperative nausea and vomiting: randomized and blinded prospective study. Anesthesiology 66:513–518, 1987.

28. Feinstein R, Owens WD: Anesthesia for ENT. *In* Barash PG, Cullen BF, Stoelting RK (eds): Clinical Anesthesia. Philadelphia, Lippincott, 1988, p. 1076.

29. Willis R: Stapedectomy complications. J Laryngol Otol 90:31–40, 1976.

30. Stoelting RK: Pharmacology and Physiology in Anesthetic Practice. Philadelphia, Lippincott, 1987, p. 351.

31. Stauffer JL, Silvestri RC: Complications of endotracheal intubation, tracheostomy, and artifical airways. Respir Care 82:417–434, 1982.

32. Hughes J: Tracheostomy. *In* Rippe JM, Irwin RS, Alpert JS, Dalen JE (eds): Intensive Care Medicine. Boston, Little, Brown, 1985, pp. 148–149.

33. Otteni JC, Pottecher T, Bronner G, et al: Prolongation of the Q-T interval and sudden cardiac arrest following right radical neck dissection. Anesthesiology 59:358–361, 1983.

34. Ruskin JN: Ventricular arrhythmias. *In* Johnson RA, Haber E, Austen WG (eds): The Practice of Cardiology. Boston, Little, Brown, 1980, p. 171.

35. Comerota AJ, Harwick RD, White JV: Jugular venous reconstruction: a technique to minimize morbidity of bilateral radical neck dissection. J Vasc Surg 3:322–329, 1986.

36. Kawajiri H, Furuse M, Namba R, et al: Effect of internal jugular vein ligation on resorption of cerebrospinal fluid. J Maxillofac Surg 11:42–45, 1983.

37. Sugarbaker ED, Wiley HM: Intracranial-pressure studies incident to resection of the internal jugular veins. Cancer 4:242–250, 1951.

38. Royster HP: The relation between internal jugular vein pressure and cerebrospinal fluid pressure in the operation of radical neck dissection. Ann Surg 137:826–832, 1953.

39. Warner MA, Warner ME, Narr BJ: Major perioperative morbidities: analysis for sentinel events. Anesthesiology 69:A904, 1988 (abstract).

19 POSTOPERATIVE PAIN MANAGEMENT

HUGH C. GILBERT

Every physician and nurse involved in the care of postoperative patients recognizes that pain control plays an important role in facilitating the recovery process. Although it may be difficult to quantify, postoperative pain is easily diagnosed after emergence from anesthesia by the changes in heart rate, blood pressure, and emergence behavior. When mental faculties return, patients often verbalize their feelings regarding the need for analgesics. The degree of pain reported is highly variable.[1,2]

In the post anesthesia care unit (PACU), physicians and nurses interpret the extent of pain by observing a patient's emergence behavior. Unfortunately, there are no specific signs that consistently indicate the extent of pain. Clinical signs commonly associated with the development of postsurgical pain after emergence from anesthesia are as follows.

Verbalized responses
Agitation (rule out hypoxia)
Tearing or crying
Splinting
Changes in vital signs
    Hypertension
    Tachycardia
Changes in posturing
    Writhing
    Sitting up
    Moving from side to side

Many factors can influence the severity of pain symptoms. Thoracic and abdominal incisions have consistently been found to be associated with severe pain. Less consistent factors include the type of anesthesia, premedication, preoperative anxiety and teaching, and the cultural and social background of the patient.[3]

It is apparent that in many instances postoperative analgesia often falls short of both patient expectations and objective needs. The widespread dissatisfaction with present methods of prescribing analgesic drugs for postoperative pain is well documented.[4] There is an enormous literature on the subject of analgesia and the means and methods necessary for effective pain control. This chapter focuses attention on the practical application of principles necessary for effective control of pain during the early postoperative period.

ASSESSMENT OF POSTOPERATIVE PAIN

Analgesia, like any other medical therapy, must adhere to the stringent tests of a scientific methodology. Unfortunately, the search for subjective relief of the *hurt* has dominated both analgesic practice and investigational design. Littlejohns and Vere have enumerated the complexity of the clinical assessment of pain.[5] Beecher, in his classic monograph, emphasized that perception of pain has two components: the original injury (nociception) and the reaction or processed response following the pain stimulus.[6] It is easy for physicians and nurses to link the unpleasant sensory and emotional experiences associated with surgery. Yet when assessing postsurgical pain and its treatment, we must still depend on the willingness and ability of the patient to communicate how our interventions have met their expectations.[7]

Presumably, pain following surgery results from nociceptive input of variable intensity that is derived from the consequence of surgical wounding or preexisting painful conditions. Postsurgical pain has been difficult to quantify. Verbal responses, patient behavior, and changes in vital signs may reflect the severity of the pain and the effect of analgesic medications. In fact, many physicians and nurses individualize analgesic therapy based on their expectations of "normal" postoperative pain behavior.

Analgesic studies require an assessment tool. Many investigators have relied on either ordinal pain scales or visual analogue scales (VAS) for pain quantification. Although the validity of pain measurement is impossible to quantify, ordinal scales, or VAS, are helpful for tracking spontaneous pain changes and the effect of analgesics. Pain scales and questionnaires are useful for assessing analgesic effects in most adult patients. VAS, pain drawings, and color scales have helped investigators track the effect of analgesia in patients who cannot effectively express their feelings. All of the above techniques for assessing postoperative pain are introspective in that each uses the patient to describe the changes produced by the analgesic medication administered. Papper et al. simply counted the number of standard doses of analgesics used for treating postoperative pain. In this way, they thought that they could establish equipotency of narcotic analgesics.[8]

Many investigators have relied on spirometric measurements for quantification of the effectiveness of analgesic therapy. It is well known that reductions in vital capacity and peak expiratory flow rates result when thoracic or abdominal surgery has been performed. Pain has been considered to be a predominant factor in the reduction of effort-dependent measurements of pulmonary function during the postoperative period (splinting). It has been suggested that improvement in these measurements represents a quantifiable salutary effect of analgesia.[9] The value of spirometric measurements as a means of assessing analgesia is often questioned; yet one of the most compelling clinical needs has been the search for analgesic techniques that allow patients at risk to improve coughing and thus mobilize secretions.[1]

There has been interest in assessing the influence of analgesia on the outcome in surgical patients known to be at risk for postoperative complications. Good analgesia, by definition, advances postoperative care by promoting effective ventilation, early ambulation, and reducing postoperative complications that result when patients are restricted to bed and remain immobile.

OPIOID ANALGESICS AND OPIOID RECEPTOR MECHANISMS

Opioid analgesics act by interaction with specific opioid receptors. The major effects of opioids (analgesia, cough suppression, altered mood) and their side effects (nausea, vomiting, decreased gastric motility) result from opioid–receptor interactions. Studies of opioid mechanisms and their distribution have advanced our concept of how nociception is influenced by both endogenous opioids and the narcotic analgesics. Although there are some indications that opioids may act directly on the nerve endings of primary afferent nerves, attention has been directed to modulation of primary afferents at the spinal cord level.[10] The effects of opioids on primary afferent transmission and supraspinal control have been reviewed by Fields and Basbaum.[11] The distribution of opioid receptors in the spinal cord coincides with the transmission areas of the C fibers. The action of opioids on neuronal transmission has been characterized as inhibitory.

Analgesia results when the narcotic agonists bind to opioid receptors located in both the brain and spinal cord. Each of these sites requires narcotic analgesics to have the pharmacologic capability to cross the blood-brain barrier (BBB). The diversity of the distribution of endogenous opioids and opioid receptors and their interaction with other neurotransmitters account for the wide variability of effects that can be demonstrated in the laboratory and when opioid analgesics are used clinically.[12]

Many of the complications attributed to narcotic analgesics are the result of opioid–receptor interactions. Of greatest concern has been the interactions of opioids with respiratory and circulatory control systems of the brainstem. The physiologic role of opioid peptides on these control systems is not fully understood. However, there are data suggesting that endogenous opioid peptides do not play an important role in normal respiratory and cardiovascular control in humans. This situation changes during stressful conditions such as anesthesia, surgery, pain, hypoxia, and shock.[13] Therefore conditions that frequently occur postoperatively may be associated with significant opioid interactions that affect respiratory and cardiovascular homeostasis.

It has been proposed that narcotic analgesics interact with specific opioid receptors that normally are the site of action of endogenous polypeptide opioids termed endorphins.[14] A pure mu agonist (e.g., morphine) binds to mu receptors and activates the mu opioid effector mechanism. By definition, a pure antagonist (e.g., naloxone) has affinity but no efficacy. For the purposes of this discussion, narcotic analgesics are classified as either mu agonists, antagonists, or agonist-antagonists. Although it is clear that there are clinically useful narcotic analgesics with kappa and delta receptor affinity, their use in analgesic strategies needs further evaluation.

Opioid receptor physiology has given us a unifying concept.[15] All mu agonists should have similar effects after crossing the BBB. Differences in potency and effect are related to the structure–activity relations and physiochemical properties of the individual narcotic analgesics. Unfortunately, other clinically important differences have been demonstrated. For example, intravenous morphine releases histamine, which may result in clinically significant vasodilation.[16] Meperidine and codeine also increase plasma histamine. Increases in plasma histamine have not been associated with the use of methadone or fentanyl.

The hemodynamic effects of mu agonists are difficult to quantify. Mu agonists decrease heart rate, a response thought to be vagal secondary to the activation of receptors at the nucleus ambiguous. Following the administration of mu agonists, vasomotor tone often decreases, most likely resulting from a reduction in sympathetic output.[17] Increases in myocardial work have been demonstrated to occur when postoperative patients experience pain.[18] Therefore the cardiovascular effects of mu agonists can be beneficial when they are administered to postoperative patients having pain. Likewise, administration of opioid analgesics in unstable patients may be associated with serious hypotension.

The respiratory consequences of mu agonists are not as forgiving. Administration of narcotic analgesics in awake subjects results in rightward displacement of the carbon dioxide response curve.[19] Sleep increases the effect of narcotic analgesics by changing the slope of the ventilatory responses to carbon dioxide.[20]

Jordan has reviewed the methods used to assess the respiratory effects of analgesics,[21] and Catley has underscored the deficiencies of the clinical assessment of the respiratory effects of analgesics using respiratory rate alone.[22] Furthermore, the effective use of mu agonist analgesics has been hampered because nurses and physicians recognize the risk of respiratory depression and may limit the availability of narcotic analgesics. Sensitivity to hypoxia and hypercarbia is reduced when narcotic analgesics are used clinically. The extent and potential for clinically important changes in ventilatory effects depend on the age of the patient, preexisting respiratory function, dose and route of narcotic administration, site of operation, and the interplay of other drugs that may interact with ventilatory function. Increases in intracranial pressure result when narcotic analgesics reduce minute ventilation. Therefore narcotic analgesics must be used with caution in any patient in whom increases in intracranial pressure might be harmful. Effective pain control using mu agonists can be achieved with a low incidence of clinically significant respiratory depression. Although it does not seem possible to distinguish respiratory depression from opioid analgesia, there are several therapeutic strategies that minimize or reverse the ventilatory effects. These strategies are described in the following sections.

EFFECTIVE PAIN RELIEF

Inadequate pain relief is common following surgery.[23] The current practice of administering narcotic analgesics intramuscularly or subcutaneously pro re nata (PRN) has not provided consistent postoperative analgesia. Many reasons have been offered to explain the deficiencies of current analgesic practice. Inadequate analgesia results when the responsibility for postoperative comfort rests on a system wherein a patient must be in pain and call for help, and a nurse must then assess the degree of pain and the need for treatment, review the physician's orders, decide on the drug dose that matches the need, find the key to the locked narcotics cabinet, and administer the drug, finally initiating therapy. This inefficient drug delivery system cannot possibly provide a steady-state plasma concentration, nor can it hope to provide relief for the changing pain intensity that occurs during convalescence. Analgesia fails when physician orders are vague and the drug doses prescribed are inadequate. PRN dosing regimens compound the problem because nurses often make illogical choices regarding the timing and dosage of the narcotic to be administered. The logistics of getting a bolus of narcotic administered to a postoperative patient can be cumbersome. Intramuscular PRN dosing regimens fail when they are ordered and administered without regard to the pharmacokinetic and pharmocodynamic factors that determine the effectiveness of opioid analgesia.

Conventional narcotic analgesic dosing

does not provide for widely differing individual drug requirements of postsurgical patients.[24] Studies by Austin and colleagues have established that for each postoperative patient there is a minimum effective analgesic concentration necessary for pain relief that is independent of the method of drug delivery. Analgesia does not result unless a critical blood concentration of opioid is achieved. This point on the concentration–effect curve is termed the minimal effective analgesic concentration (MEAC). In the standard normal population, MEAC can vary by fourfold.

Analgesic responses following injection of intramuscular narcotics are variable because it is difficult to maintain plasma concentrations of narcotics at or above the MEAC. Furthermore, studies of intramuscular drug delivery in both patients and volunteers have demonstrated that not only are peak concentrations diverse but so is the time of their occurrence. These two features make intramuscular dosing unpredictable.

Individual characteristics such as age, body weight, and gender have been used by physicians to adjust narcotic analgesic dosing. Studies in adult patients have found no correlation between body size, gender, and analgesic demand. However, an increased sensitivity to narcotic analgesics has been demonstrated to occur with advancing age. Elderly patients have higher peak concentrations of narcotics than young adults receiving the same bolus of narcotic. Age-related differences in opioid pharmacokinetics have been described. Many older patients report better pain relief than young patients. However, age by itself should not be considered an important predictor of analgesic need. Although patients' physical characteristics do not predictably influence analgesic drug needs, their individual pain tolerance plays an important role in determining the drug dosages necessary for effective analgesia. Individual variability in analgesic requirements has been demonstrated to occur irrespective of drug delivery. Individual variability of analgesic need is a clinical manifestation of the relation between opioid drug concentration at the receptor level (biophase) and the intensity of effect.

Effective narcotic pain relief, by definition, requires a capability to fine-tune the state of analgesia as indicated by the patient's response to therapy. The treatment of severe postoperative pain by repeated intramuscular injections results in variable analgesic responses. Often the first dose of intramuscular narcotic fails to approach the MEAC, resulting in undertreatment of pain. With subsequent injections a waxing and waning of plasma concentration occurs that is associated with periods of sedation followed by periods of pain. Figure 19–1 depicts the plasma–time relation for intramuscular narcotics.

Intramuscular narcotic injection has become the most popular analgesic delivery system because of its simplicity and low cost. As currently practiced, patients often receive an insufficient amount of narcotic administered at inflexible intervals that often results in inadequate analgesia.[24] The variability of the rate of narcotic absorption even when dosing occurs at predefined intervals makes intramuscular narcotic administration an unpredictable method of analgesic delivery. PRN intramuscular injections have been considered to be a safe method of narcotic administration because the timing of each dose is supervised by a registered nurse. However, physicians and nurses tend to restrict the availability of narcotics when they are concerned that the potential for narcotic-induced respiratory depression exists.[25]

The diversity of subjective responses in pa-

FIGURE 19–1. Plasma concentration required for bolus intramuscular narcotic injections. ● = intramuscular injection of narcotic analgesic. (Adapted from White PF: Patient controlled analgesia: a new approach to the management of postoperative pain. Semin Anesth 4:255, 1985. With permission.)

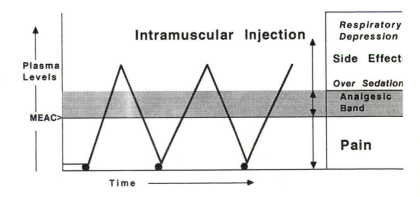

tients administered standard doses of narcotics suggests that there are fundamental differences in pain perception. Almay and co-workers have postulated that increases in pain sensitivity represent a deficiency in the production of endogenous opioid peptides.[26] Tamsen and associates[27] have determined the relation between preoperative cerebrospinal fluid (CSF) endorphin levels and postoperative meperidine usage following laparotomy. They observed that there was an inverse relation between CSF meperidine levels and the preoperative endorphin levels. These observations support the concept that the diversity of narcotic needs has a physiologic basis. Similar relations have been described for morphine and plasma β-endorphin during postoperative pain and in children with burns.[28]

Effective pain relief with opioid analgesics requires a capability to individualize therapy based on periodic assessment of the patient's response to therapy.

PHARMACOKINETICS AND PHARMACODYNAMICS

Many factors influence the relation between the degree of pain relief and the dose of analgesic administered. In the previous section, it was suggested that effective analgesia results when opioid plasma concentrations exceed the MEAC. The dosage of opioid necessary to achieve analgesia depends on a number of factors. Opioid dosing depends on the site of administration and the physiochemical characteristics and pharmacokinetic profile of the opioid administered. Unfortunately, the relation between dose and analgesic effect is complex.

After distribution into the plasma, only the un-ionized fraction that is unbound to plasma proteins can penetrate lipid membranes and cross the BBB. Once the opioid penetrates the BBB, there is diffusion of drug to receptor sites. The concentration of opioid at the receptor depends on the ability of the opioid to penetrate the lipid-rich biophase. Each opioid analgesic has a physiochemical profile that determines its ability to penetrate the BBB and interact with opioid receptors. The diffusion characteristics and lipid solubility of opioids influence their latency and duration of action. Morphine has the least lipid diffusion potential of all clinically useful opioids. After an intravenous bolus, there is a delay in achieving the onset of maximal effect. However, once in the biophase, there is little diffusion away from receptors. Although highly lipid-soluble narcotic analgesics have the advantage of being able to penetrate the BBB, the lipid-rich central nervous system (CNS) buffers the lipid-soluble opioids, reducing the effective concentration at receptors. The duration of action of a bolus of opioid depends on receptor affinities, lipid diffusion in the CNS, and the changing plasma concentration.

Pharmacokinetics are helpful for predicting differences in the plasma profiles of various opioid narcotics. Unfortunately, monitoring of opioid plasma concentrations is not currently available for determining the therapeutic level of opioid analgesics. Effective postoperative analgesia, then, remains an art based on the scientific foundations of pharmacokinetics.

PAIN CONTROL IN THE PACU

The need for pain control often first appears in the PACU. With emergence from general anesthesia or the return of sensation following regional anesthesia, nociceptive function becomes operational. As wakefulness and the ability to speak reappear, subjective assessment of the state of pain is possible. The technique of anesthesia, its duration, and the site of surgery can influence not only the degree of pain but also its onset. McQuay et al. have reported striking variations in the first request for pain medications following orthopedic surgery, suggesting that premedication and type of anesthesia influence to a great degree the onset of postoperative pain.[29] Recovery times after general anesthesia vary depending on the duration of anesthesia, type of drugs administered preoperatively and intraoperatively, and the age and state of health of the patient. Modern anesthetic techniques have reduced recovery time. After general anesthesia, it is likely that the capability of pain perception is present following the return of orientation to time and place. Korttile and Valanne have evaluated recovery following the commonly used potent inhalation agents isoflurane and enflurane.[30] Following the cessation of inhalational anesthetics, orientation to time and place returns within 20 minutes. Frequently, anesthesiologists include an intravenous narcotic administered intraoperatively as a means to provide a smooth early transition between anesthetic emergence and the initiation of postoperative pain control in the PACU. Clearly, the drugs and techniques used pre-

and intraoperatively can influence analgesic requirements during the early postoperative period.

A good example of this interplay is demonstrated by the studies of Gourlay and colleagues comparing the efficacy of intraoperatively administered methadone and morphine.[31] Using a loading dose of 20 mg of methadone intraoperatively, it was possible to afford pain relief for as long as 22.6 hours postoperatively. Morphine administered in the same fashion resulted in effective pain relief for only 7.8 hours.

Preoperative preparation of the patient can also be helpful for minimizing the responses to surgical wounding, as the pharmacodynamic responses that determine analgesic effectiveness are influenced by the patient's personality characteristics, previous pain experiences, and expectations.

Narcotic analgesics are an important component of modern anesthetic technique. The philosophy of the anesthesia care team influences the need for pain control during the early postoperative period to the same extent as the constraints of the clinical situation presented. Modern general anesthesia often consists of the smallest doses of anesthetic agents necessary to ensure the patient's comfort and safety. Trends promoting day surgery have increased interest in anesthetic techniques that result in a prompt return of cognitive function.

The PACU has the most diverse collection of postoperative patients, ranging from infants and children to the severely compromised elderly. The diversity of the patient mix requires a pain management program that is adaptable. Most adult surgical patients expect a certain degree of discomfort following their operation. Often the most distressing pain occurs during the early postoperative period. Studies of narcotic analgesic requirements demonstrate that narcotic utilization is greatest during the first day after surgery.

In many hospitals postoperative pain control is a shared responsibility. PACU pain management is often under the direct supervision of an anesthesiologist, whereas the postoperative orders for analgesic administration on the surgical floors are under the direction of the surgeon. In many centers PACU pain is treated with incremental intravenous injections of narcotics, whereas on the wards postoperative pain is managed with intermittent intramuscular narcotics. Unfortunately, information gained by the anesthesiologist in the PACU regarding an individual's specific nar-

cotic requirement does not influence the postoperative orders written by the surgical service.

Many institutions have established acute pain services (APSs). APSs develop management strategies for the treatment of postoperative pain from admission to the PACU through the first several days when postoperative pain is most distressing and traditionally undertreated. APSs can improve the scope of pain management. The APS is designed to increase patient comfort, reduce or prevent pain-related postoperative complications, and promote research and teaching. APSs provide comprehensive pain management strategies that offer postoperative patients powerful alternatives to conventional analgesia.

Pain strategies in the PACU are often influenced by the philosophy of the anesthestiologist as well as the clinical situation. The use of intramuscular narcotics for treatment of PACU pain can be condemned based on the wide variation in absorption noted following surgery and anesthesia. Intramuscular administration has a slow, unpredictable onset. All PACU patients have intravenous access, which represents the preferred route of administration for narcotic analgesics. Most PACUs use intermittent intravenous injections of narcotic analgesics for the treatment of postoperative pain. The frequency of repeated bolus injections depends on the size of the initial dose and the duration of action of the drug administered. Once a desired analgesic effect is achieved, its effect over time can be observed by the nursing staff. Effective analgesia in the PACU provides for a level of pain control that allows timely transfer to the postsurgical floor or, in the case of day surgery, a timely discharge home. Typically, the anesthesiologist orders a narcotic analgesic, determines a dosage to be administered, and prescribes an interval for observation before a second bolus of the narcotic analgesic is administered. The effectiveness of this "nurse-controlled analgesia (NCA) regimen" depends on the response time of the staff nurses to medicate and evaluate the resulting changes in pain as well as the attitudes of the doctor, patient, and nurses regarding "normal" postoperative pain.

When narcotic analgesics are administered intravenously at regular intervals, the plasma concentration tends to sawtooth around a steady-state plasma concentration. If NCA permits the patient to maintain a plasma concentration above their MEAC, effective anal-

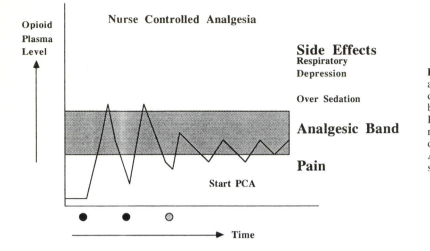

FIGURE 19–2. Nurse-controlled analgesia. ● =intravenous bolus of narcotic; ◯ = 1/2 intravenous bolus. (Adapted from White PF: Patient controlled analgesia: a new approach to the management of postoperative pain. Semin Anesth *4*:255, 1985. With permission.)

gesia is possible. The drug dose required for effective analgesia depends on the physiochemical profile of the drug prescribed, the patient's MEAC, and the patient's capacity to eliminate the drug prescribed. Figure 19–2 depicts the plasma–time relations of NCA.

NARCOTIC ANALGESICS IN THE PACU

Lasagna and Beecher have defined the optimal dose of a narcotic analgesic as the dose that provides the desired therapeutic effect with a minimum of undesirable side effects.[34] There have been numerous publications that have attempted to define the optimal dose of morphine for the standard surgical population. Many more espouse the attributes of other narcotics. This presentation has focused attention on the concept that the optimal dose of a narcotic is related not only to the characteristics of the drug administered but also to the pharmacodynamic variability of the patient in whom the drug has been administered. Many narcotic analgesics are used for the treatment of postoperative pain in the PACU. Generally, small incremental intravenous doses of a mu agonist can be titrated to the individual's needs. It is helpful for the PACU staff to establish analgesic protocols that clearly define the procedure for the titration of narcotic analgesics. Generally, this analgesic regimen specifies the loading dose of the analgesic (bolus), the period for observation (lock-out), and the incremental doses to be given when further therapy is indicated. Initially, a patient is "empty" of narcotic analgesic. Each de-

mand dose leads to a rapid rise in plasma drug concentration followed by a rapid decline. The lock-out period is adjusted for the latency of the narcotic administered. Thus morphine requires a longer lock-out period than fentanyl. As more narcotic is administered, redistribution occurs, the tissues become saturated, and the ability to maintain a plasma concentration is increased. As the plasma concentration reaches MEAC and passes into the therapeutic band, patients experience comfort, and the need for further narcotic depends on incidental changes in pain threshold or reductions in opioid concentrations at the biophase. As CNS concentrations of narcotics increase, undesired side effects (e.g., nausea or vomiting) can be expected. Unwanted side effects may require additional drug management or even a change in the analgesic management plan.

Morphine has become the opioid standard against which all narcotic analgesics are compared. With the development of pain in the PACU, 1 to 4 mg of morphine administered intravenously represents a reasonable starting point for the initiation of NCA in an adult patient. After its administration, the PACU staff evaluate changes in vital signs, comfort, and level of consciousness. After a lock-out period of 6 to 10 minutes, the PACU nurse assesses the need for additional analgesia. Typically, several injections eventually establish a level of analgesia commensurate with the goals of the PACU unit. NCA is rarely associated with clinically significant hypoventilation. However, one must always remember that the effect of narcotic analgesics on ventilatory control mechanisms is potentiated by sleep and the residual of even well conducted general anesthesia. Likewise, pain and stress may act as respiratory stimulants during the early postoperative period. Therefore it is prudent to pay particular attention to the rate, depth, and pattern of breathing during analgesic dosing. Many physicians restrict the dosing of narcotics when the respiratory rate falls below 10 to 12 breaths/min. The PACU staff must learn to recognize impending ventilatory failure and initiate supportive measures, starting with "wake-up reminders" and advancing as needed to bag-and-mask ventilation, administration of narcotic antagonists, or even endotracheal intubation and mechanical ventilation.

Attention to the character and location of pain symptoms is necessary to prevent NCA overtreatment. Narcotics are not appropriate treatment for the pain of an unrecognized distended bladder or a wound hematoma. It is important for the PACU staff to assess all painful symptoms and consult with the anesthesiologist and surgeon if any unusual symptoms or signs are noted. Pain may occur for many reasons during the early postoperative period. Unexpected painful symptoms, e.g., chest pain or back pain, require careful evaluation. Their occurrence may be insignificant (e.g., pain related to positioning) or can require further diagnosis and therapy, as in the case of pain associated with myocardial ischemia.

Nurse-controlled analgesia is effective when administered to PACU patients who are communicative and have pharmacodynamic profiles that fit the anticipated expectations of the PACU staff. The use of pulsed intravenous narcotics may be associated with periods of sedation. Somnolence represents the top of the plasma analgesic concentration band. Frequently, NCA produces a sedated patient who is arousable. As sleep develops it is imperative to ensure a patent airway. Narcotic sedation is associated with a reduced response to hypoxia. The need for supplemental oxygen must be evaluated in all postoperative patients receiving NCA. It is difficult to assess hypoxemia clinically. Pulse oximetry can be helpful when evaluating changes in oxygen needs that can occur with NCA. Occasionally, the NCA program does not meet the expectations of the patient or staff. This situation does not represent a failure of narcotic analgesics but, rather, underscores the wide range of analgesic needs following surgery. When faced with a patient whose analgesic demands exceed protocol drug dosing, it is important that the supervising physician evaluate the clinical situation at the patient's bedside. Occasionally, an alternative analgesic management plan proves beneficial. For example, it may be appropriate to increase the usual standard titration of intravenous opioid or administer an adjunctive medication. NCA is based on maintaining MEAC plasma levels using a reasonable demand dose of narcotic that is titrated to effect.

Many narcotic analgesic drugs are suitable for administration in the PACU. Short-acting narcotics such as alfentanil do not lend themselves to NCA because they require a continuous background infusion; likewise, long-acting narcotic analgesics have effects that extend beyond the stay in the PACU. Fentanyl is an effective drug for intermittent administration in the PACU. After a single intravenous bolus, its duration of action can be expected to be limited by redistribution. Fentanyl is an ideal analgesic for administration in situations where a quick clinical effect is needed. Hug and Murphy demonstrated that after an intravenous bolus injection peak concentrations of fentanyl occurred within 2 to 10 minutes in the CSF of canines.[32] As fentanyl redistributes to other tissues, its analgesic effect can be expected to wean. Multiple intravenous injections cause accumulation of fentanyl in plasma and decrease the redistribution gradient from brain to the tissues. Secondary increases in fentanyl plasma concentration have been observed in patients and volunteers and have been attributed to mobilization of fentanyl from tissue depots. Secondary peaks have been identified as a possible concern for the development of late-onset respiratory depression. Fentanyl is a good analgesic choice in situations where a quick, transient step-up in analgesia is needed. Fentanyl is useful for postoperative pain in day surgery patients who are expected to have a short PACU stay.

Many believe that there are objective differences in the analgesia that results from the administration of the various mu agonists. Few data exist comparing the dose-response curves for the mu agonists in management of postoperative pain in the PACU. Dose relations for narcotic analgesics have been determined in both the laboratory and clinical settings. At issue is the possibility that, at equianalgesic doses, a particular narcotic analgesic offers an advantage over other opioid analgesics. The effectiveness of opioids used for NCA depends on several independent variables: the pharmacokinetic profile of the

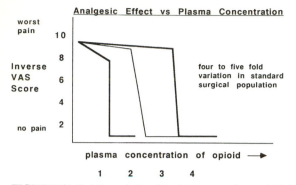

FIGURE 19–3. The relationship between pain control (depicted as an inverse VAS scale) and the plasma concentration achieved is very steep. Typically, a 4 to 5 fold variance is found in the standard normal surgical population. (Modified from Austin KL, Stapleton JV, Mather LK: Relationship between blood meperidine concentrations and analgesic response: a preliminary report. Anesthesiology *53*: 460–466, 1980.)

drug administered, the pharmacodynamic profile of the patient, and the willingness of PACU staff to administer appropriate doses of the opioid. The effectiveness of any narcotic analgesic depends on the size of the initial dose and the interval and size of subsequent doses. Accumulation in the plasma can be expected when the frequency of the narcotic administration exceeds either the redistribution

or the elimination of the drug. The slope of the relation of opioid plasma levels and analgesic effect (VAS) is steep (Fig. 19–3).

When MEAC concentrations are achieved, the interval between further doses depends on the pharmacokinetic profile of the drug administered and any alteration in incidental pain. The characteristics for dosing are identical to those for patient-controlled analgesia (PCA) except the patient's needs and delivery are dependent on the assessment of the PACU staff nurse.

At our institution, most PACU patients are started on NCA using hydromorphone (Dilaudid), a semisynthetic derivative of morphine. The hydroxyl substitutions markedly improve lipid solubility and potency. Clinical studies suggest that hydromorphone is 7- to 10-fold more potent than morphine.[33] Typically, 0.25 to 0.50 mg of hydromorphone is administered intravenously with a lock-out of 5 to 10 minutes. Effective analgesia results within 10 to 20 minutes. Hydromorphone shares features with morphine. However, our staff believes it to be superior to morphine in two respects: At equipotent doses morphine has been associated with greater changes in hemodynamic stability. Recognizing the potential for hypotension, our PACU nurses are reluctant to bolus morphine in doses comparable to hydromorphone doses.

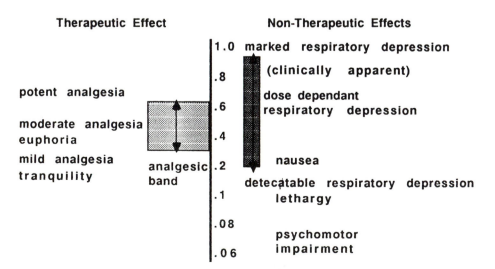

FIGURE 19–4. Relation between meperidine plasma levels and pharmacologic effects and side effects. The numbers (1.0 to .06) indicate the plasma meperidine levels in micrograms per deciliter. (Modified from Kitz RJ, Laver MB: Scientific basis of clinical anesthesia. *In* Stanski DR, Watkins WD, eds. Drug disposition in Anesthesia. Orlando: Grune & Stratton, 1982, p. 150. With permission.)

Meperidine (Demerol) has been considered by many to be a good analgesic for the treatment of postoperative pain. Its ability to diminish postoperative shivering when administered intravenously in small doses has been useful in the PACU. Austin and associates[24] measured whole blood meperidine concentrations in patients receiving the drug intramuscularly, by intravenous infusion, or by on-demand intravenous analgesia. They established the relation between blood concentration and analgesic effect. The studies substantiated that an individual's narcotic requirement appears constant during the postoperative recovery period. Their research suggested that drug delivery is an important consideration when achieving effective pain control. When the administration technique allowed meperidine to achieve and maintain MEAC, effective analgesia resulted. Figure 19–4 depicts the relation of therapeutic and nontherapeutic effects as a function of increasing plasma meperidine levels. The scale shifts upward or downward depending on the individual's "pain thermostat."

CONTINUOUS INTRAVENOUS ANALGESIA

Demand analgesia using a nurse observer is effective in any intensive care setting. However, it is impractical to implement NCA on a busy postsurgical ward. The postsurgical ward requires a drug delivery system that can be individualized to each patient's needs without serious constraints on nursing personnel.

Continuous intravenous infusions of narcotic analgesics have been recommended as offering advantages over intermittent intramuscular injections. When a narcotic is administered intravenously at regular intervals, the plasma concentration eventually oscillates around a steady-state concentration. Pharmacokinetic theory predicts that continuous intravenous analgesia (CIV) produces a steady state in about six half-lives. The half-life for meperidine has been estimated at 3 to 7 hours. Therefore if meperidine were administered by CIV at a constant infusion rate, it would take around 24 hours to achieve a steady-state blood concentration. Increasing the amount of meperidine infused per unit time decreases the time it takes to achieve MEAC. As the infusion continues, overdosing could occur.

Continuous intravenous analgesia has, for the most part, been replaced by PCA. How-

ever, the pharmacologic concepts that have evolved from the study of CIV are the foundation on which PCA is based. These regimens have been reviewed by Tamsen.[35] CIV requires close supervision. It can be effective in patients who cannot cope with interacting with a computer for the titration of analgesia. Such patients include the debilitated and the very young who are recovering in an intensive care setting. The precision of CIV has improved dramatically with the advent of intravenous pump controllers on postoperative wards. However, the potential for developing life-threatening respiratory depression during the unwavering administration of analgesic narcotics has diminished its application. A CIV analgesic program needs fine-tuning if incidental changes in pain that normally occur in recovering postsurgical patients are to be treated. The combination of CIV and PCA has been found to dramatically improve analgesia when mechanisms for monitoring and supervising the analgesic program are in place.

PATIENT-CONTROLLED ANALGESIA

Demand dosing by nursing personnel, however effective, is impractical because it requires a level of nursing supervision found only in specialized care units. Since the 1970s instruments that permit patients to self-administer small boluses of narcotic analgesics intravenously have been designed and tested. Early systems incorporated a timing device linked electronically to valves that permitted the infusion of a predetermined amount of narcotic analgesic into the patient's intravenous line when the patient depressed a button. The analgesic delivery system was designed to remain refractory for a present period, minimizing the possibility that patients would deliver excessive narcotic doses.[36] Early experience with PCA was encouraging. Comparisons with conventional intramuscular regimens demonstrated that PCA enhanced postoperative pain management and reduced the incidence of inadequate pain relief.[37] Experience with the first commercially available PCA device (Cardiff Palliator) was reported in 1976.[38] During the ensuing years, many new devices have been marketed for the administration of PCA.

Most PCA devices use digital electronics to control the dose of analgesic delivered by a syringe pump. The size of each incremental bolus and the minimum time interval between doses is programmable. Many of these devices are able to maintain a continuous background infusion that is also programmable. These devices are pole-mounted to facilitate their use in ambulatory patients. They are small and compact, and they operate on internal battery power for extended periods. Programming is easily adjusted using keyboards or wheeled switches that are tamperproof. Security locks and alarms are standard features. These "intelligent" infusion pumps can be interfaced with printers that provide hard copy of the current settings, profiles of usage, and number of demands requested by the patient. Computer-controlled PCA devices have been available in the United States since 1984.

Conventional intramuscular narcotics have been demonstrated to produce inadequate analgesia when the dosing interval or the prescribed dose fails to provide sustained MEAC levels. PCA, by design, can accommodate the wide variability in pharmacodynamics observed in the standard surgical population. Sechzer, using small intravenous boluses of morphine and meperidine, studied the behavior of patients using a demand system for analgesia.[39] He found that analgesic demand was a measure of the individual's pain experience, and he compared demand analgesia to operant conditioning.

Patients pressed the analgesic demand button until their personal target of pain relief was satisfied. As a direct result of PCA research, a number of important concepts regarding postoperative pain management have been identified. Tamsen and associates, in a series of publications, demonstrated that analgesic demand after PCA is not related to age, sex, or body weight.[40,41] Furthermore, these investigators demonstrated fairly constant plasma concentrations of narcotic analgesics when patients use PCA. With PCA, it has been possible to quantify dosage requirements and mean consumption rates of various narcotic analgesics.[42] Individual variability of these "pseudo-steady-state" blood levels reinforce the concept of MEAC. The practicality, efficacy, and side effects of PCA have been studied in many clinical situations. Despite the difficulty of quantifying adequacy of analgesia, it is apparent that nurses appreciate the improved responsiveness of PCA and patients delight in having more control over the treatment of their pain symptoms. Despite its popularity, there are no large-scale clinical studies that demonstrate superiority to other *effective* methods of managing postoperative pain. Furthermore, there are no studies that compare the safety or efficacy of the various delivery options that are currently available.

Many PCA devices can be programmed to provide a background infusion of the narcotic analgesic. Using this mode, bolus injections administered on demand fine-tune the analgesic delivery for incidental pain. PCA allows titration of an individual's analgesic needs. As with NCA, as the patient emerges from anesthesia, intravenous boluses of an opioid analgesic are titrated to achieve an adequate level of pain relief. Typically, loading doses are administered in the PACU using the same drug that is to be administered by PCA. After loading, the PCA device is placed in line with the intravenous infusion, and the device is programmed according to the physician's prescription. Typically, this prescription specifies the loading dose, the incremental bolus dose, and the lock-out interval. A maximum 4-hour administration limit is usually specified. Inherent to the PCA prescription are instructions for the titration of bolus doses based on specific observations. Thus the amount of opioid to be administered might be increased or decreased by a specific amount when pain ratings or levels of consciousness change. PCA prescriptions include orders regarding the administration of narcotic antagonists should evidence for serious narcotic depression occur. Many PCA devices record the number of attempts for narcotic administration. When a patient depresses the administration button during a lock-out, no medication is administered. Once the PCA device is programmed, it is recommended that the instrument's instructions be double-checked by a second staff member, thereby avoiding setup errors.

Inherent to PCA, the frequency of narcotic administration is controlled by the patient. Some early PCA devices required patients to depress the demand switch twice within a 1-second interval in order to reduce erroneous demand requests. Current devices limit demand by lock-out alone. To date, PCA has a good safety record. PCA devices are engineered for the safe, autonomous administration of medications that have inherent risks. With PCA therapy, analgesia can be sustained at a level that produces few side effects. Each patient using PCA needs to be assured that their analgesic therapy is being monitored by the nursing staff so as to ensure that the analgesic prescription is not only effective but safe. The potential for overdose is minimized when small bolus doses are used with a mandatory lock-out interval that is matched to the pharmacokinetic profile of the narcotic analgesic prescribed. Should excessive sedation result, the patient can reduce demand and the plasma levels will fall, minimizing the risk of overdose. This feedback loop represents an important safety feature that is unique to patient dosing systems.

Disruption of sleep occurs with all intermittent techniques for analgesia. Nocturnal disruptions because of pain can be reduced if the evening dosing increment is increased.

SPINAL OPIOIDS

Following the identification of opioid receptors in the brain and spinal cord, many investigators have studied the activity of spinally administered opioids. In 1976 Yaksh and Rudy determined that morphine administered intrathecally produced analgesia in rats.[43] Three years later, Wang et al. reported that profound analgesia resulted from intrathecal morphine in patients with intractable cancer pain.[44] Since these pioneering studies, it has become apparent that epidural and spinal administration of opioids are powerful techniques that can improve analgesia for a wide range of acute and chronic pain problems.

When narcotic analgesics are administered epidurally, they diffuse into the CSF. The rate of absorption into the CSF depends on the physiochemical properties of the drug administered. When opioids are administered spinally or epidurally, their site of action resides at the pre- and postsynaptic opioid receptors located in the substantia gelatinosa of the dorsal horn of the spinal cord. Spinally administered opioids offer a major advantage over epidural or spinal local anesthetics because they produce a *selective blockade* of the pain pathways. Local anesthetics, on the other hand, block sodium conductance of axonal membranes. They do not discriminate between pain and nonpain pathways.

Theoretically, spinally administered opioids produce a selective *segmental* analgesia if opioid receptor sites corresponding to the nociceptive pathways transmitting the surgical pain messages are activated. At the spinal cord, local anesthetics produce analgesia by virtue of the loss of sensation, which is always associated with sympathetic blockade and frequently associated with impaired motor function.

The degree of sensory and motor impair-

ment depends on the concentration, volume, and local anesthetic administered. As clinical experience with epidural and intrathecal narcotics grew, it became clear that both techniques produce profound analgesia with greatly reduced dosages of narcotic compared to other methods of narcotic delivery. This increased efficacy of spinally administered narcotics results from the ability of narcotic analgesics to distribute to the opioid receptor sites. Conventional methods of analgesic administration require sustained plasma levels to drive the narcotic analgesic across the BBB to the active sites in the CNS. After intrathecal administration, narcotic analgesics distribute into the CSF and then penetrate the spinal cord. Epidurally administered narcotics are separated from the subarachnoid space by the dura mater and the arachnoidea. These tissues, along with the capillary endothelium, constitute the BBB. The analgesia produced by the epidural administration of narcotic analgesics is thought to be related to the dramatic levels of narcotic that result in the CSF owing to dural diffusion and subsequent penetration of the spinal cord.

Early experience with epidural and intrathecal morphine demonstrated prolongation of the duration of action of morphine when compared to its intravenous or intramuscular administration. Weddel and Ritter reported that clinical analgesia using morphine can last 18 to 36 hours.[45] After epidural administration, serum levels of narcotic analgesics were found to vary from patient to patient. Unlike all other forms of narcotic analgesic administration, analgesia resulting from epidural or intrathecal opioids is not related to sustaining plasma opioid levels at MEAC. However, pharmacokinetic studies of various opioid narcotics have demonstrated plasma concentrations of narcotic analgesics that cannot be ignored, especially when lipid-soluble narcotic analgesics are administered epidurally.

Equipotent doses of mu agonists produce similar effects when administered intraspinally. The speed of onset and duration of effect are related to the lipid solubility of the narcotic analgesic. Morphine, a highly water-soluble opioid, has the greatest latency and duration of action. Its half-life after epidural administration has been reported to be 18.1 ± 6.8 hours.

Lipophilicity plays a key role in the dural transfer of opioids. Sjöstrom and colleagues have studied the pharmacokinetics of both epidural and intrathecal morphine and meperidine in postoperative patients.[46,47] For both opioids, the measured plasma concentrations fell below MEAC well before the disappearance of analgesia. In contrast to morphine, meperidine CSF concentrations declined rapidly, suggesting that meperidine was unlikely to migrate cephalad in the CSF to the brainstem. Complications can be expected when analgesic delivery systems distribute water-soluble (ionized) opioid molecules to brainstem opioid receptors. Ideally, spinally administered narcotics bind with opioid receptors at the spinal segments that transmit and modulate the pain messages, leaving few molecules available for transport in the CSF to the opioid receptors of the midbrain.

A necessary condition for using spinally administered narcotics is either placement of an epidural catheter or performance of a spinal tap. Therefore unlike other methods of narcotic administration, spinally administered narcotics require the expertise of anesthesiologists. Typically, the decision to use spinally administered narcotics is made preoperatively.

Since 1979 intraspinal analgesia has been widely studied in many clinical situations. Comparisons with other regional anesthetic techniques and the more traditional forms of narcotic administration have been described. Spinally administered opioids have been shown to be effective in relieving both visceral and somatic pain. Using VAS scales, effort-dependent pulmonary function studies, blood gas assays, and patient or nursing satisfaction scales, intraspinal narcotics have been found to provide enhancements that compared favorably to both PCA and local anesthetic techniques. Furthermore, the analgesic effect of a small bolus of morphine (3 to 8 mg epidurally) produces long-lasting, effective analgesia that could not be duplicated by other narcotic delivery systems.

However, despite the theoretic benefits of "selective segmental analgesia" and the growing number of clinical reports extolling its clinical superiority, it is difficult to define precisely the clinical indications where spinally administered narcotics demonstrate clear-cut advantages to other *well-managed* analgesic techniques. The decision to use a spinally administered narcotic can be controversial. Every anesthesiologist must choose not only the method of drug delivery (spinal or epidural) but also the spinal level, the analgesic, and whether the opioid analgesic is to be administered as a bolus or by continuous infusion.

These choices may have an impact on manpower requirements and the need for additional surveillance during the early postoperative period. Analgesic choices can influence hospital expenditures. Intraspinal analgesic regimens have differing levels of manpower requirements. A single instillation of morphine subarachnoidally does not require the same personal attention from the anesthesia care team as does bolus or infusion epidural narcotic analgesia.

Patients receiving spinally administered narcotics require a high level of observation to prevent serious respiratory side effects. Bromage and associates have demonstrated the rostral spread of analgesia in human volunteers following the epidural instillation of 10 mg of morphine.[48] Trigeminal analgesia resulted 5 to 9 hours after the epidural administration of morphine. Alterations in pain sensitivity correlated with profound decreases in the ventilatory response to carbon dioxide.[49] Respiratory depression followed the same time course as the progressive, upward analgesia. The greatest impairment in ventilatory responses were noted when the subjects demonstrated analgesia of the face. Bromage and coworkers reported significant impairment in ventilatory responses to carbon dioxide that peaked 6 to 9 hours after epidural morphine administration. This "late respiratory depression" has been demonstrated to occur in postsurgical patients receiving either epidural or intrathecal morphine.

Clinical and experimental evidence suggests that intraspinal morphine migrates with the CSF flow cephalad to the brainstem. Spinal fluid transport from lumbar levels to the rapid circulation of the intracranial CSF occurs within 3 to 6 hours. This "narcotic elevator" has important clinical ramifications. Certainly, the potential for developing unwanted opioid receptor-mediated side effects depends on the availability of the opioids to interface at these higher centers. Therefore techniques that target segmental mu receptors may substantially reduce the potential for unwanted side effects. On the other hand, many anesthesiologists deliberately use CSF transport to deliver narcotic to thoracic spinal segments, thus avoiding the hazards of thoracic epidural catheter placement. Although the incidence of life-threatening respiratory depression is low, every patient, including many receiving lipid-soluble opioids, demonstrate an impaired ventilatory response to carbon dioxide. In many instances this depression in ventilation is *not* clinically apparent and is no different from the depression found after conventional narcotic delivery. Respiratory depression within several hours of epidural injection has been described.[50] Unlike late respiratory depression, early respiratory effects probably are related to vascular absorption and transport via the basivertebral venous plexus to the centers of respiratory control. Complications resulting from vascular uptake can occur with any opioid. During catheter placement or during epidural bolus injections, it is valuable to ascertain the possibility of catheter migration with an aspiration test. After proper placement, epidural catheters can, over time, penetrate either the dura or the thin walls of epidural veins. Both circumstances have been associated with serious complications.

Although the potential for life-threatening respiratory depression always exists when intraspinal narcotics are used, the incidence of serious sequelae appears to be small. Many thousands of patients have had effective analgesia using epidural or intrathecal narcotics. The percentage of patients requiring a "naloxone rescue" or who have had documented respiratory arrest as the result of their analgesic management is unclear.

Gustafsson et al. summarized the Swedish anesthesiologists' experience using intraspinal morphine and meperidine from 1979 to 1981. Ventilatory depression requiring "naloxone rescue" occurred in 22 patients receiving epidural morphine (0.33 per cent) and in six patients treated with intrathecal morphine (5.5 per cent).[51] Many investigators have attempted to determine not only factors that identify patients at risk for developing respiratory depression but also strategies that would improve on the safety of intraspinal administration of morphine. Rawal et al. have reported on the present state of epidural and intrathecal opioid analgesia in Sweden.[52] The statistics from Sweden suggest that the incidence of delayed respiratory depression following epidural opioid analgesia has been reduced to 0.09 per cent. Respiratory depression following intrathecal opioid analgesia has fallen to 0.36 per cent. Factors that have been associated with increasing the risk for developing delayed respiratory depression are as follows.

Preexisting pulmonary impairment
Extremes of age
Additive effect of CNS depressants
Excessive opioid administration
Water solubility of drug administered (morphine)
Inadvertent dural puncture
Increased intraabdominal or intrathoracic pressure

Epidural morphine has not fulfilled the promise of selective, segmental analgesia. Its clinical use has been associated with troublesome side effects. Nausea, vomiting, and respiratory depression are side effects that result from the rostral spread of morphine. Their incidence is related to the dose of morphine administered and the time required for the opioid to be transported to the midbrain. Nausea and vomiting were observed in 50 per cent of the human volunteers after administration of 10 mg morphine epidurally. Reiz and Westberg reported that 17 per cent of postoperative patients receiving epidural morphine complained of nausea and vomiting.[53] Although the incidence of nausea and vomiting is high, comparison studies suggest that it is similar when sufficient morphine is administered intramuscularly.[54] Nausea and vomiting can be effectively treated with small doses of intravenous naloxone without diminishing the analgesic effects of epidural morphine. Likewise, the respiratory effects following epidural morphine can be treated with the intravenous infusion of either naloxone or the kappa agonist nalbuphine.[55]

The potential for serious respiratory depression and the difficulty of predicting its occurrence has challenged clinicians. Many have restricted the use of epidural narcotics to the intensive care setting, where constant vigilance diminishes the potential for serious sequelae. Electronic devices that monitor ventilatory motion are commercially available. These apnea monitors continuously track the respiratory rate. They are equipped with auditory alarms that warn the nursing station when apnea or bradypnea occurs. Many believe that these devices permit the safe use of epidural morphine outside an intensive care setting.

Urinary retention has been reported to occur after intraspinal administration of morphine. This effect is not dose-related and is purported to be mediated at the sacral spinal cord. Inhibition of the micturation reflex is sensitive to naloxone reversal. Although urinary retention is a common postoperative occurrence, systemic morphine does not routinely inhibit the micturation reflex. Intraspinal techniques for pain control are most commonly utilized in patients having operations for which bladder catheterization is routine.

Itching commonly follows the administration of epidural morphine. Pruritus occurs more often after intrathecal morphine. It can be localized to the face and trunk or manifest as a generalized phenomenon. Its mechanism is unknown. Antihistamines or naloxone can be helpful when pruritus becomes troublesome. The concurrent administration of epidural bupivacaine (0.100 to 0.125 per cent) appears to reduce the incidence of itching.

The goal of selective segmental analgesia has been difficult to achieve. El-Baz and associates found that additional intravenous morphine was needed when 5 mg of epidural morphine was injected via a "targeted" thoracic catheter in patients recovering from thoracotomy. Several patients developed serious respiratory depression requiring not only "naloxone rescue" but also mechanical assisted ventilation.[56] These investigators were able to achieve a more effective and selective analgesia by infusing targeted thoracic catheters with morphone 0.1 to 0.5 mg/hr. Incidental pain was treated with incremental, on-demand intravenous morphine 2 mg. Despite the need for systemic narcotics, serum morphine levels were found to be below the MEAC. The continuous epidural infusion of morphine enhanced safety and reduced the need for intensive care surveillance, and it reduced the demands on the anesthesia staff.

More recently, Fischer and colleagues[57] have reported on further refinements in the management of postoperative pain using continuous epidural infusions. Both morphine and fentanyl were administered in a 0.1 per cent bupivacaine solution. In this study, fentanyl and morphine were administered at a fixed rate of infusion. The infusion rates (fentanyl 60 μg/hr, morphine 0.5 mg/hr) were chosen to fall below the threshold levels that have been determined in human volunteers to produce clinically significant respiratory depression. Supplemental pain needs were treated with intramuscular meperidine. This combined method of analgesia was found to be effective and safe. Patients were managed in a standard hospital setting without special apnea monitors. Patients receiving the fentanyl–bupivacaine infusion had significantly less pruritus and nausea than the morphine–bupivacaine group.

Methods of analgesia must be assessed based not only on their ability to improve analgesia but also on their associated risk/benefit ratio. Intraspinal opioid administration has been found to be efficacious in a number of prospectively controlled studies of postoperative pain. Its use in patients at high risk for developing complications postoperatively has been advocated.[58] It is still impossible to determine with certainty if intraspinal opioid administration offers measurable enhancements compared to other well managed forms of opioid administration. Several concepts need further clarification. Currently, the dose of morphine has been reduced compared to the doses of early reports. However, the margin of safety between the analgesic dose and a dose that is associated with significant rostral migration is small. The alternative—using a lipid-soluble opioid such as fentanyl—has been shown to reduce unwanted side effects. However, fentanyl's duration of action is sufficiently short to place unrealistic demands on the analgesic management team. Epidural fentanyl infusions have been proposed to fulfill these limitations.

The following questions still need clarification.

1. How important is the concept of targeting a catheter to the surgical field?
2. When using epidural fentanyl infusions, to what degree does systemic absorption play in the overall analgesic effect?
3. Is it safe to use epidural fentanyl infusions outside the intensive care or intermediate care setting?
4. Should incidental pain be managed using "patient-controlled" epidural analgesia?

LOCAL ANESTHETIC TECHNIQUES

Local anesthetic blocks can be beneficial in the management of postoperative pain. Unfortunately, a local anesthetic with an extended duration of action is not currently available. When compared to the other methods for achieving postoperative analgesia, local anesthetic techniques have not received the enthusiastic support of anesthesiologists. Misconceptions regarding their efficacy, safety, and side effects have limited their use. Local anesthetic techniques require a high degree of personal involvement by anesthesiologists. The potential for patient dissatisfaction, complications, and side effects and an unpredictable legal climate have dissuaded many to not even gain proficiency in their administration.

Local anesthetic blockade can, in many surgical populations, provide a truly regional approach to nociception that avoids many of the problems associated with conventional analgesia. Local infiltration of wound surfaces and peripheral neural blockade are two examples where local anesthetic techniques can effectively improve postoperative pain management. Infiltration blocks can substantially reduce postoperative pain in children undergoing inguinal hernia repair, orchiopexy, and penile surgery. Broadman and associates have demonstrated that a subcutaneous ring block reduces the need for narcotic analgesia and shortens the time required to meet PACU discharge requirements.[59] The ring block of the penis requires no special skills and is an excellent adjunct to operative anesthesia. Similarly, postoperative pain of inguinal incisions can be substantially reduced when ilioinguinal and iliohypogastric nerve blocks are performed.[60] Even in healthy adults, the advantages of intraoperative infiltration and peripheral nerve block can far outweigh the risks and time required for their performance. Their use requires collaboration with anesthesiologists and surgeons. With presently available local anesthetic drugs (e.g., 0.5 per cent bupivacaine) 10 to 12 hours of analgesia can be achieved.

The risks following local infiltration are associated with the anatomic location of the block and the toxicity characteristics of the local anesthetic employed. All local anesthetic drugs have low therapeutic ratios that mandate care when they are administered. Most of the serious problems occur during the period of observation immediately after their administration. With the advent of continuous infusion techniques, it is imperative that the nursing team be familiar with the basic concepts of the recognition and treatment of local anesthetic toxicity.

Local anesthetics are absorbed from the site of instillation. Accidental intravascular injection can result in toxic plasma levels. Local anesthetic toxicity can result from an imbalance between absorption and the ability of the patient to distribute and metabolize the drug. The site of instillation, the dosage and drug administered, and the size of the patient are important factors that determine the potential of developing high plasma concentrations of local anesthetics. As plasma concentrations of local anesthetics increase to toxic levels, patients experience circumoral numbness and lightheadedness, and they begin to have visual disturbances. If the plasma levels continue to rise, these premonitory signs are then followed by muscular twitching, convulsions, and finally coma or respiratory arrest. With an overwhelming overdose, a patient may present with cardiovascular collapse and cardiac arrest. It is imperative that the PACU and postsurgical ward staff understand the importance of the signs and symptoms of local anesthetic toxicity. Early recognition of local anesthetic toxicity can reduce the potential for serious sequelae. Treatment of local anesthetic toxicity includes the following steps.

1. Establish a clear airway.
2. Give oxygen by face mask.
3. Ensure adequate ventilation.
4. Determine circulatory status.
5. Evaluate the patient.
   a. Assess need for artificial ventilation.
   b. Assess need for cardiovascular support.
   c. Assess need for anticonvulsants.

It is unlikely that local anesthetic toxicity will result from peripheral nerve blocks or wound infiltration. However, many local anesthetic techniques, whether intermittent or continuous, have been demonstrated to produce plasma levels that are associated with the development of local anesthetic toxicity.

In many institutions, intercostal nerve blocks (ICBs) play an important role in enhancing analgesia after pulmonary resection. Performed intraoperatively while the thorax is open, the potential for lung injury is nil. However, paravertebral, epidural, and even intrathecal spread has been described with its associated adverse effects on circulation and ventilation.[61] Pain relief following an ICB results from sensory block of the chest wall and upper abdomen. Splinting, the restriction of breathing that occurs after thoracic or abdominal wounds, can be effectively reduced or abolished following sensory blockade. Midline incisions require bilateral ICBs. Because of the close proximity of the intercostal nerves with the intercostal artery and vein, systemic absorption of local anesthetic is great. Excessive systemic blood concentrations can be minimized by using epinephrine-containing solutions of local anesthetic.

Blockade of intercostal nerves should produce no cardiovascular effects. However, there is ample clinical and experimental evidence supporting the capability of large volumes of local anesthetics to distribute several levels above and below the level of injection.[62] Sympathetic nervous system blockade, systemic toxicity, or tension pneumothorax may follow an ICB. Each of these potential complications is associated with alteration in cardiovascular stability. In most cases their occurrence can be ruled out by physical examination.

Pneumothorax is a rare complication of ICB. Based on follow-up chest films, a 1 to 2 per cent incidence can be expected. Pneumothorax following ICB is most often asymptomatic. Resorption of the pneumothorax can be facilitated by administration of high flow oxygen. However, the potential for puncturing the visceral pleura and having a persistent air leak exists. As air accumulates in the pleural space, ventilatory embarrassment may necessitate placement of a chest tube.

Enthusiasm for ICB for the management of postoperative pain is based on the ability of ICB to reduce splinting and improve pulmonary function. Many patients undergoing thoracic and upper abdominal surgery have measurable changes in their ability to perform effort-dependent pulmonary function tests. Conventional narcotic analgesia with its inherent effect on ventilatory control can compound the problem. When compared to conventional narcotic analgesia, ICB produces segmental analgesia that reduces "splinting," which results in improvement of peak expiratory flow, mobilization of secretions, and arterial oxygenation.[63] After surgery ICB can be an effective technique for the treatment of somatic pain. The quality and duration of the analgesia and the improvement in ventilatory function compare favorably with intraspinal narcotics.[64] However, patients and nurses often prefer spinally administered narcotic analgesia over ICB because ICB requires repeated needle insertions, and often its analgesia is spotty. ICB is an effective adjunct to other forms of analgesia. The potential for local anesthetic toxicity, pneumothorax, and short duration of action have limited its use by both surgeons and anesthesiologists.

Many have recommended that ICB can be enhanced by placing a catheter in the region of the intercostal neurovascular bundle. Large volumes (20 ml) of local anesthetic solution were found to spread and block several dermatomes. Continuous ICB might enhance the quality and duration of analgesia.[65] Reistad and Stromskag, investigating catheter ICB, found that the intrapleural administration of bupivacaine relieved ipsilateral incisional pain following mastectomy, cholecystectomy, and renal surgery.[66] Since this enthusiastic report,

many have begun investigating the efficacy and risk associated with intrapleural infusion administration (IPA). Currently, the experience has been mixed. Seltzer and coworkers demonstrated that significant amounts of bupivacaine are absorbed from the pleural space.[67] The potential for toxic bupivacaine levels has been substantiated in children and adults. The effectiveness of IPA is currently undergoing careful scrutiny. IPA could offer advantages if effective analgesia could be achieved without local anesthetic toxicity, urinary retention, or the cardiovascular changes associated with sympatholysis. Some preliminary reports have suggested that IPA does not offer enhancements over other regional anesthetic techniques; on the other hand, McIlvane and associates enthusiastically endorsed IPA as effective for treating postthoracotomy pain in children.[68] Although local anesthetic toxicity was not demonstrated, the measured bupivacaine levels underscored the potential for toxicity. The observations of McIlvane et al. suggested that IPA can produce sympathetic blockade involving not only the thoracic chain but also the cervical sympathetics. Splinting and its ventilatory consequences were effectively reduced.

More studies are needed to determine the usefulness of IPA. Current questions include the following.

1. Where should infusion catheters be placed for optimal analgesia?
2. What is the effective infusion dose?
3. Is IPA compatible with early ambulation?
4. What are the benefits compared to the potential risks?

EPIDURAL BLOCK

Epidural catheter techniques (epidural block, or EDB) can be adapted to provide analgesia and sympathetic blockade for the management of postoperative pain. As originally conceived, EDB could replace or reduce the need for centrally depressing narcotics by producing peripheral deafferentation at the spinal cord level. Ideally, the block would ensure adequate comfort, improve breathing and coughing, and allow early ambulation.[69] Epidural analgesia can be associated with significant physiologic effects that demand careful observation. The extent of the physiologic trespass depends on many factors. Features that can be controlled include the following.

1. Volume and concentration of local anesthetic
2. Use of vasoconstrictors and vasopressors
3. Level of catheter placement
4. Intravascular volume state of the patient
5. Position of the patient

Physiologic effects following epidural local anesthetic administration result from either direct, segmental blockade of the spinal roots and spinal cord or the effects of absorption of the local anesthetic. Therefore the success of EDB in a comprehensive pain program depends in large measure on patient selection, the austerity and vigilance of the anesthesiologist, and the overall competence of the postoperative care givers.

Cardiovascular changes following EDB can vary in significance. In general, these effects result from blockade of the sympathetic nerves, which are sensitive to local anesthetic blockade. Circulatory changes result from alterations in vasomotor tone, decreased heart rate, and contractility. The overall effects vary with the clinical situation. The effects of sympatholysis following EDB can be dangerous in hypovolemic patients in whom cardiovascular function is maintained by virtue of the sympathetic nervous system and its effects on the heart, vasculature, and adrenal glands. On the other hand, major vascular surgery is often associated with postoperative hypertension resulting from the release of endogenous catecholamines and activation of the sympathetic nervous system. Kumar and Hibbert have suggested that EDB can effectively treat the postoperative hypertension that may follow major vascular surgery.[70]

Epidural block offers real advantages to postoperative patients despite the potential for adverse circulatory changes. After upper abdominal and thoracic surgery, there is consistent impairment of pulmonary function characterized by a reduced inspiratory capacity, vital capacity, and reduction in functional residual capacity. These changes diminish coughing and deep breathing and can lead to the retention of secretions, atelectasis, and pneumonia. EDB can alter the impaired mechanical ventilatory effects that follow surgery. However, measurements of peak expiratory flow rate, vital capacity, and functional residual capacity do not return to preoperative values. Several studies have suggested that EDB improves pulmonary function tests to a greater degree than conventional narcotic administration.[71] The improvement in effort-dependent pulmonary function following EDB have been reported to enhance coughing and reduce the need for mechanical ventilation in postthoracotomy patients at risk for pulmonary failure.[72] However, both PCA and intraspinal opioids also improve postoperative breathing to a similar extent. EDB can modify the endocrine and metabolic responses that are associated with surgical wounding. Amelioration of the stress response results from the reduction in catecholamines, cortisol, and insulin levels.[73] Local anesthetic blockade can modify the stress responses by either sympatholysis or a reduction in reflex activation. EDB has a profound effect on the neurohumeral responses following surgical wounding. Unfortunately, it is difficult to determine if the benefits described influence surgical morbidity or mortality.

Epidural block has been used for postoperative pain control following thoracoabdominal and thoracic surgery,[74] vascular surgery,[75] abdominal and gynecologic surgery,[76] and total hip replacement.[77] Further data are needed to confirm the clinical impression that espouses derived benefits compared to traditional narcotic analgesic regimens. Many believe that EDB improves alimentary function, promotes early ambulation, improves arterial oxygen tension, and reduces the risk of pulmonary infection.

Most commonly, EDB is initiated intraoperatively by the anesthesiologist who incorporates it in the anesthetic management plan. Following surgery, EDB options include intermittent top-up local anesthetic administration, continuous infusion local anesthetic block, intermittent or continuous infusion of local anesthetic-epidural narcotic mixtures. The training, staffing, and attitudes of the medical and nursing personnel determine the extent to which EDB is utilized. Local anesthetics, by virtue of their mechanism of action, have the potential to provide a quality of analgesia that is unparalleled. Several limitations must be considered when contemplating EDB as a postoperative pain strategy. All catheter techniques should be used with caution in patients with a septic focus. Local injection, circulatory instability, and head injury are patient factors that contraindicate EDB analgesia. The milieu of the postoperative ward and staffing may also place limits on the ability of the anesthesiologist to ensure patient safety. The use of epidural catheter techniques in patients who either are anticoagulated during vascular surgery or receive anticoagulant therapy postoperatively is controversial. Many believe that with scrupulous technique the potential for epidural hematoma can be minimized.[75,78] Certainly, clinical circumstances can warrant EDB or epidural opioid administration in patients in whom anticoagulation is anticipated. Catheter insertion should be atraumatic and timed to be performed before anticoagulation. Likewise, removal of the epidural catheter should follow documentation of heparin reversal. The onset of back pain and the development of a neurologic deficit that cannot be ascribed to a local anesthetic effect requires prompt evaluation. Surgical decompression of an epidural hematoma may prevent permanent paralysis.

Unlike other analgesic techniques, EDB often influences motor function, making early ambulation hazardous. The cardiovascular effects of EDB can produce orthostatic hypotension or diminish a patient's ability to adjust to fluid shifts that frequently occur during the early postoperative period. Ideally, the epidural technique is planned to limit the potential for these sequelae. Several options have been described to "tame" EDB, including the infusion of dilute local anesthetic solutions of low concentration. As with any analgesic technique, the effect over time must be monitored not only for complications but also to determine effectiveness. However, the potential for extension of the sensory blockade, due to either unintentioned (intrathecal) catheter migration or overinfusion, needs to be assessed at regular intervals. Although pharmacokinetic studies suggest that continued infusion of epidural bupivacaine is not associated with plasma accumulation, the potential for local anesthetic toxicity is ever present, particularly in patients with abnormal hepatic or renal function.[79]

Somatic blockade can have profound effects on nursing care. Urinary retention can be expected when sacral nerves are blocked. Patients with sensory deficits require frequent changes in position to prevent pressure sores. Heat loss is exacerbated during EDB, and EDB may influence postoperative fluid management. Vital signs and the extent of analgesia must be monitored. Like other effective analgesic techniques, EDB is labor-intensive. The safe use of EDB requires not only the skill and expertise of anesthesiologists but also a commitment from surgeons and nurses that the benefits of neural blockade outweigh the burdens that ensure patient safety.

Unlike narcotic techniques that provide central sedative and euphoric effects, local anesthetic techniques fix the hurt with little influence on emotional distress or anxiety. In many instances, tranquilizers are helpful for reducing anxiety or emotional distress.

SYMPTOM CONTROL

The side effects of analgesic regimens often require additional medications to promote safety and a general feeling of well-being. Historically, physicians have used many combinations of drugs and medications, trying to improve on the potency and duration or to reduce the side effects associated with the use of narcotic analgesics. Many of these combinations are still useful, e.g., the addition of antihistamines for their antiemetic and ataractic effects. Hydroxyzine has been found to improve pain scores following its administration with intramuscular narcotics.[80] Other examples include efforts to couple respiratory stimulant drugs such as dextroamphetamine or doxapram with narcotic analgesics.[81] These adaptations have not been enthusiastically supported.

Pharmacologic remedies that reduce the potential for respiratory depression after administration of epidural narcotics have also been suggested. The simultaneous infusion of low dose naloxone 5 to 10 μg/kg/hr[83] or the administration of the narcotic agonist-antagonist nalbuphine 0.05 mg/kg/hr[84] has been suggested to reduce the need for an intensive care admission following ISN.

Narcotic analgesia is frequently associated with nausea irrespective of the route of drug delivery. Nausea results from stimulation of the medullary chemoreceptor trigger zone. Droperidol, a butyrophenone tranquilizer, has been found to be an effective antiemetic when administered at 10 μg/kg IV.[85] Although it has no inherent analgesic effect, droperidol prolongs the duration of action of parentrally administered narcotics without affecting potency.[86] Narcotic analgesia and regional anesthetic techniques have not been perfected to a degree that ensures satisfactory pain relief without unwanted side effects and risks. The search for a more effective drug delivery system, a longer-acting local anesthetic, or a better, safer narcotic is ongoing. Historical references to the use of electricity as a treatment for pain have stimulated interest in applying electrical currents to surgical wounds. Transcutaneous electrical stimulation (TENS) has been demonstrated to reduce narcotic requirements after surgery.[87] Unfortunately, the lack of uniformity regarding stimulation parameters, duration of treatment, and lead placement have made it difficult to evaluate the importance of TENS in a comprehensive postoperative pain program. It is possible that the various stimulation modes have differing physiologic effects by virtue of several mechanisms of action. Stimulation modes that produce muscular contractions have been shown to promote the release of endorphins.[88] Conventional TENS has been suggested to stimulate large low threshold afferents that inhibit T cell transmission of nociception (Gate theory of pain).[89] Brief, intense TENS may produce anodal conduction block of peripheral nerves.[90] The importance of TENS as an adjuvant to other analgesic regimens needs further evaluation.

PHARMACOLOGIC APPROACHES TO POSTOPERATIVE PAIN CONTROL

Drug therapy for pain management has been a major area of investigation. Analgesic drugs can be divided into three major groups.

Group I includes the nonsteroidal antiinflammatory drugs (NSAIDs). These drugs act peripherally and produce analgesia through their ability to inhibit prostaglandin synthesis. The analgesic effects of group I drugs demonstrate a ceiling effect. When combined with narcotic analgesics, NSAIDs have additive effects. Their use for postoperative pain control has been limited by gastrointestinal and hematologic side effects and uncertain uptake. Currently available oral NSAIDs have an effect equivalent to that of 6 to 10 mg of morphine.[91] NSAIDs are most effective in circumstances where inflammatory responses are ongoing. It is expected that future developments in NSAID pharmacology will improve potency and reduce side effects, yielding analgesia that is truly peripheral in effect. Several promising prototype drugs are being tested for clinical efficacy. The introduction of ketorolac tromethamine (KT) for intramuscular administration offers clinicians nonnarcotic alternatives for treating postoperative pain. Comparison studies suggest that 30 mg of KT provides similar analgesia to 12 mg morphine sulfate.[92]

Group II analgesics are opioid receptor agonists. This chapter has focused attention on their importance in effective postoperative pain management. Currently, the effective use of these drugs requires balancing the desired analgesic effect against undesirable side effects. Much of the difficulty in achieving effective postoperative analgesia arises from individual variations in response to standard doses of narcotic analgesics. Over the last several decades, drug delivery systems based on pharmacokinetic and pharmacodynamic principles have enhanced the capability of achieving postoperative pain control.

Group III drugs represent a diverse collection of pharmacologic agents that may be helpful in augmenting narcotic analgesia or treating unpleasant side effects that result from opioid–receptor interaction. Group III drugs are adjuvants that play an important role in the management of cancer pain and deafferentation pain. Many of these drugs are useful in special circumstances that occur postoperatively. Phenothiazines, for example, enhance narcotic analgesia and are antiemetic. Butyrophenones can be useful when confronted with postoperative delirium or psychosis. Tricyclic antidepressants may augment analgesia by increasing central serotonin stores. These examples underscore how many different pharmacologic actions can alter a postoperative patient's attitude toward their surgical wound pain. It is possible that the next important advance in analgesia will be found in the area of group III pharmacology.

ADVANCES IN METHODS OF DRUG DELIVERY

Advances in "controlled release technology" offer hope that new routes of administration will sustain analgesic plasma levels near MEAC without peaks and valleys. Improvements, particularly in the areas of convenience and safety, are expected to be introduced into clinical practice. Three narcotic delivery systems are currently undergoing investigation. Iontophoresis of ionized drugs such as morphine can produce plasma levels that vary in proportion to the electrical field applied. Preliminary investigations have demonstrated that MEAC plasma levels can be achieved. However, it is not clear as to the risk/benefit ratio for iontophoresis. Transdermal patches (TPF) that sustain the controlled bioavailability of fentanyl are currently being evaluated for treating postoperative pain. Clinical data suggest that a constant effective level of analgesia can be demonstrated in the treatment of somatic pain following orthopedic surgery.[93] Transdermal fentanyl delivery (75 µg/hr) resulted in stable plasma fentanyl levels that often exceed MEAC.[94] TPF offers postoperative patients a simple, effective method of opioid drug delivery. More experience is needed to determine how to utilize TPF when treating complex pain problems. TPF may be an important tool for the treatment of "background" pain particularly in cancer patients. Plasma decay following removal of the TPF system declines slowly. Like other narcotic delivery systems, side effects are related to the peak plasma levels achieved. TPF (Duragesic) has been approved for clinical usage and is marketed in patches that release 25 to 100 µg/hr. The effective duration of action for TPF is approximately 72 hours.

Transmucosal and nasal aerosol narcotic delivery systems have been tested in children and adults as an alternative to intravenous narcotic administration. In general, lipid-soluble drugs, e.g., fentanyl, sufentanil, and buprenorphine, have been studied. Sublingual or buccal buprenorphine 0.4 mg produces analgesia that has an onset similar to that with intramuscular administration. It is possible to use mucosal absorption in a patient-demand mode. Further study is needed to determine the feasibility of employing mucosal delivery of potent narcotic analgesics for the treatment of postoperative pain.

CONCLUSION

The adverse effects of poorly controlled postoperative pain are well known to the patient, physician, and nursing staff. In most circumstances, current techniques in pain control not only can substantially improve a patient's feeling of well-being, they also help reduce postoperative complications and ultimately postoperative mortality. These goals can be achieved by developing protocols for analgesia that are formulated on principles herein described. Unfortunately, many factors interplay in the implementation of effective analgesia. The ability to provide PCA, regional administration of local anesthetics, or intraspinal narcotics demands more than the knowledge and commitment of physicians. These techniques, although enhancing analgesia, substantially change the level of observation required during the early postoperative period. They require extensive training of nursing staffs as to their pharmacologic and physiologic effects. Evidence is mounting that effective analgesia can, in many situations, improve patient ambulation and pulmonary function and can shorten the hospital stay and costs. The issue of weighing the benefits of specific analgesic programs with the costs of implementation must be addressed in all hospitals. Conventional intramuscular narcotics have been the mainstay of postoperative pain management because of their long history and ease of administration. Dissatisfaction with the quality of the analgesia is related not so much to the obvious problems with bioavailability but in large measure to the hospital ward system of drug delivery that has evolved. Effective use of opioid analgesics requires drug delivery that is based on pharmacokinetic and pharmacodynamic principles. Unfortunately, the therapeutic window for analgesic techniques is narrow. Without adequate medical and nursing supervision, it is impossible to implement any comprehensive program of analgesia.

References

1. Loan WB, Dundee JW: The value of postoperative pain in the assessment of analgesics. Br J Anaesth *39*:743–749, 1967.
2. Pflug AE, Bonica JJ: Physiopathology and control of postoperative pain. Arch Surg *112*:733, 1977.
3. Bullingham RES: Postoperative pain. Postgrad Med *60*:847–851, 1984.
4. Utting JE, Smith JM: Postoperative analgesia. Anesthesia *34*:320, 1979.
5. Littlejohns DW, Vere DW: The clinical assessment of analgesic drugs. Br J Clin Pharmacol *11*:319–332, 1981.
6. Beecher HK: Measurement of Subjective Responses: Quantitative Effects of Drugs. New York, Oxford University Press, 1959.
7. Turk DC, Flor H: Pain & pain behaviors: the utility and limitations of the pain behaviour construct. Pain *31*:277–295, 1987.
8. Papper EM, Brodie BB, Rovenstine EA: Postoperative pain: its use in the comparative evaluation of analgesics. Surgery *32*:107–109, 1952.
9. Bromage PR: Spirometry in assessment of analgesia after abdominal surgery. Br Med J *2*:589–593, 1955.
10. Nincovic M, Hunt SP, Gleave RJW: Localization of opiate and histamine H_1-receptors in the primate sensory ganglia and spinal cord. Brain Res *241*:197, 1982.
11. Fields HL, Basbaum AI: Brainstem control of spinal pain transmission neurons. Annu Rev Physiol *40*:217, 1978.
12. Tyers MB: A classification of opiate receptors that mediate antinociception in animals. Br J Pharmacol *69*:503, 1980.
13. McQueen DS: Opioid peptide interactions with respi-

ratory and circulatory systems. Br Med Bull *1*:77–82, 1983.

14. Terenius L, Tamsen A: Endorphins and the modulation of acute pain. Acta Anaesthesiol Scand [Suppl] *74*:21, 1982.
15. Neil A, Terenius L: Receptor mechanisms for nociception. Int Anesthesiol Clin *24*:1–15, 1986.
16. Rosnow CE, Moss J, Philibin DM, Savarese JJ: Histamine release during morphine and fentanyl anesthesia. Anesthesiology *56*:93–96, 1982.
17. Lowenstein E, Whitting RB, Bittar DA, et al: Local and neurally mediated effects of morphine on skeletal muscle vascular resistance. J Pharmacol Exp Ther *180*:359–367, 1972.
18. Sjogren S, Wright B: Circulatory changes during continous epidural blockade. Acta Anaesthesiol Scand *46*:5–25, 1972.
19. Bellville W, Fleischli G: The interaction of morphine and nalorphine on respiration. Clin Pharmacol Ther *9*:152–161, 1968.
20. Forrest W, Bellville J: The effect of sleep plus morphine on the respiratory response to carbon dioxide. Anesthesiology *25*:137–141, 1964.
21. Jordan C: Assessment of the effects of drugs on respiration. Br J Anaesth *54*:763, 1982.
22. Catley DM: Postoperative analgesia and respiratory control. Int Anesthesiol Clin *22*:95–111, 1984.
23. Cohen FL: Postsurgical pain relief: patient's status and nurses' medication choices. Pain *9*:265–274, 1980.
24. Austin KL, Stapleton JV, Mather LE: Multiple intramuscular injections a major source of variability in analgesic response to meperidine. Pain *8*:47–62, 1980.
25. Sriwatanakul K, Weiss OF, Alloza JL, et al: Analysis of narcotic analgesic usage in the treatment of postoperative pain. JAMA *250*:926–929, 1983.
26. Almay BG, Johansson F, von Knorring L, et al: Endorphins in chronic pain. 1. Differences in CSF endorphin levels between organic and psychogenic pain syndromes. Pain *5*:153–162, 1978.
27. Tamsen A, Sakurada T, Wahlström, A, et al: Postoperative demand for analgesics in relation to individual levels of endorphins and substance P in cerebrospinal fluid. Pain *13*:171–183, 1982.
28. Szyfelbein SK, Osgood PF, Carr DB: Pain assessment and beta-endorphin plasma levels in burned children. Anesthesiology *50*:A198, 1983.
29. McQuay HJ, Carroll D, Moore RA: Postoperative orthopedic pain—the effect of opiate premedication and local anesthetic blocks. Pain *33*:291–295, 1988.
30. Korttile K, Valanne J: Recovery after outpatient isoforane and enflurane anesthesia. Anesth Analg *64*:239, 1985.
31. Gourlay GK, Willis JR, Lamberty J: A double-blind comparison of the efficacy of methadone and morphine in postoperative pain control. Anesthesiology *64*:322–327, 1986.
32. Hug CC, Murphy MR: Fentanyl disposition in cerebrospinal fluid and plasma and its relationship to ventilatory depression in the dog. Anesthesiology *50*:642–349, 1979.
33. Mahler DL, Forrest WH: Relative analgesic potencies of morphine and hydromorphone in postoperative pain. Anesthesiology *42*:602–607, 1975.
34. Lasagna L, Beecher HK: The optimal dose of morphine. JAMA *156*:230–234, 1954.
35. Tamsen A: Comparison of patient-controlled analgesia with constant infusion and intermittent intramuscular regimes. *In* Harmer M, Rosen M, Vickers MD

(eds): Patient-Controlled Analgesia. Oxford, Blackwell Scientific Publications, 1985, pp. 111–123.
36. Forrest WH Jr, Smethurst PWR, Kienitz ME: Self-administration of intravenous analgesics. Anesthesiology *33*:363–365, 1970.
37. Keeri-Szanto M, Heaman S: Postoperative demand analgesia. Surg Gynecol Obstet *134*:647–651, 1972.
38. Evans JM, McCarth JP, Rosen M, Hogg MIJ: Apparatus for patient controlled administration of intravenous narcotic during labour. Lancet *1*:17–18, 1976.
39. Sechzer PH: Studies in pain with the analgesic-demand system. Anesth Analg *50*:1–10, 1971.
40. Tamsen A, Hartvig P, Fagerlund C, et al: Patient-controlled analgesic therapy: clinical experience. Acta Anaesthesiol Scand *5*:462–470, 1982.
41. Dahlstrom B, Tamsen A, Paalzow L, et al: Patient controlled analgesic therapy: pharmacokinetics and analgesic plasma concentrations of morphine. Clin Pharmacokinet *7*:266–279, 1982.
42. Behar M, Rosen M, Vickers MD: Self-administered nalbuphine, morphine, and pethidine: comparison by intravenous route following cholecystectomy. Anesthesia *40*:529–532, 1985.
43. Yaksh TL, Rudy TA: Analgesia mediated by a direct spinal action of narcotics. Science *192*:1357, 1976.
44. Wang JK, Nauss LE, Thomas JE: Pain relief by intrathecally applied administration of morphine in man. Anesthesiology *50*:149, 1979.
45. Weddel SJ, Ritter RR: Serum levels following epidural administration of morphine and correlation with relief of postsurgical pain. Anesthesiology *54*:210–214, 1981.
46. Sjostrom S, Hartvig P, Persson P, Tamsen A: Pharmacokinetics of epidural morphine and meperidine in humans. Anesthesiology *67*:877–888, 1987.
47. Sjostrom S, Tamsen A, Persson P, Harvig P: Pharmacokinetics of intrathecal morphine and meperidine in humans. Anesthesiology *67*:889–895, 1987.
48. Bromage PR, Camporresi EM, Durant PAC, et al: Rostral spread of epidural morphine. Anesthesiology *56*:431, 1982.
49. Bromage PR, Camporesi EM, Leslie J: Epidural narcotics in volunteers: sensitivity to pain and to carbon dioxide. Pain *9*:145, 1980.
50. Scott DB, McClure J: Selective epidural analgesia. Lancet *1*:1410, 1979.
51. Gustafsson LL, Schildt B, Jacobsen KF: Adverse effects of extradural and intrathecal opiates: report of a nationwide survey in Sweden. Br J Anaesth *54*:479–486, 1982.
52. Rawal N, Arner S, Gustafsson LL, Allvin R: Present state of extradural and intrathecal opioid analgesia in Sweden. Br J Anaesth *59*:791–799, 1987.
53. Reiz S, Westberg M: Side effects of epidural morphine. Lancet *2*:203–204, 1980.
54. Lanz E, Theiss D, Riess W, Sommer V: Epidural morphine for postoperative analgesia: a double-blind study. Anesth Analg *61*:236–240, 1982.
55. Rawal N, Wattwil M: Respiratory depression following epidural morphine: an experimental and clinical study. Anesth Analg *63*:8–14, 1984.
56. El-Baz NM, Farber P, Jensik RJ: Continuous epidural infusion of morphine for treatment of pain after thoracic surgery: a new technique. Anesth Analg *63*:757–764, 1984.
57. Fischer RL, Lubenow TR, Liceaga A, et al: Comparison of continuous epidural infusion of fentanyl-bupivacaine and morphine-bupivacaine in management

of postoperative pain. Anesth Analg 67:559–563, 1988.

58. Yeager MP, Glass DD, Neff RK, Brinck-Johnse T: Epidural anesthesia and analgesia in high-risk surgical patients. Anesthesiology 66:729–736, 1977.

59. Broadman LM, Hannallah RS, Belman B, et al: Post-circumcision analgesia—a prospective evaluation of subcutaneous ring block of the penis. Anesthesiology 67:399–402, 1987.

50. Hannallah RS, Broadman LM, Belman AB, et al: Comparison of caudal and ileo-inguinal/iliohypogastric nerve blocks for control of post-orchiopexy pain in pediatric ambulatory surgery. Anesthesiology 66: 832–834, 1987.

61. Benumof JL, Semenza J: Total spinal anesthesia following intrathoracic intercostal nerve blocks. Anesthesiology 43:124, 1975.

62. Murphy DF: Continuous intercostal nerve blockade: an anatomical study to elucidate its mode of action. Br J Anaesth 56:627, 1984.

63. Bridenbaugh PO, DuPen SL, Moore DC, et al: Postoperative intercostal nerve block analgesia versus narcotic analgesia. Anesth Analg 52:81, 1973.

64. Rawal N, Sjostrand UH, Dahlstrom B, et al: Epidural morphine for postoperative pain relief: a comparative study with intramuscular narcotic and intercostal nerve block. Anesth Analg 61:93, 1982.

65. Ablondi MA, Ryan JF, O'Connell CT, et al: Continuous intercostal nerve blocks for postoperative pain relief. Anesth Analg 45:185, 1966.

66. Reistad F, Stromskag KE: Intrapleural catheter in management of postoperative pain. Reg Anesth 11:89–91, 1986.

67. Seltzer JL, Larijani GH, Goldberg ME, Mark AT: Intrapleural bupivacaine—a kinetic and dynamic evaluation. Anesthesiology 67:798–800, 1987.

68. McIlvane WB, Knox RF, Fennessey PV, Goldstein M: Continuous infusion of bupivacaine via intrapleural catheter for analgesia after thoracotomy in children. Anesthesiology 69:261–264, 1988.

69. Bromage PR: Extradural analgesia for pain relief. Br J Anaesth 39:721, 1967.

70. Kumar B, Hibbert GR: Control of hypertension during aortic surgery using lumbar extradural blockade. Br J Anaesth 56:797, 1984.

71. Spence AA, Smith G: Postoperative analgesia and lung function: a comparison of morphine with extradural block. Br J Anaesth 43:144, 1971.

72. Shuman PL, Peters RM: Epidural anesthesia following thoracotomy in patients with chronic obstructive airway disease. J Thorac Cardiovasc Surg 71:82, 1976.

73. Kehlet H: Pain relief and the modification of the stress response. In Cousins MJ, Phillips GD (eds): Acute Pain Management. New York, Churchill Livingstone, 1986, pp. 49–75.

74. Alon E: Postoperative pain relief: epidural versus parenteral analgesia. Acta Anaesthesiol Scand [Suppl] 27:71, 1983.

75. Odoom JA, Sih IL: Epidural analgesia and anti-coagulant therapy: experience with 1000 cases of continuous epidurals. Anaesthesia 38:254, 1983.

76. Scott DB, Schweitzer S, Thorn J: Epidural block in postoperative pain relief. Reg Anesth 7:135, 1982.

77. Modig J, Borg T, Karlstrom G, et al: Thromboembolism after total hip replacement: role of epidural and general anesthesia. Anesth Analg 62:174, 1983.

78. Rao TLF, El-Etr AA: Anticoagulation following placement of epidural and subarachnoid catheters: an evaluation of neurologic sequelae. Anesthesiology 55:618, 1981.

79. Denson DD, Raj PP, Saldahna F, et al: Continuous perineural infusion of bupivacaine for prolonged analgesia: pharmacokinetic considerations. Int J Clin Pharmacol Ther Toxicol 21:591, 1983.

80. Beaver WT, Feise G: Comparison of the analgesic effects of morphine, hydroxyzine and their combinations in patients with post-operative pain. In Bonica JJ, Albe-Fessard D (eds): Advances in Pain Research and Therapy, Vol. 1. New York, Raven Press, 1975, pp. 553–557.

81. Forrest WH, Brown BW, Brown CR: Dextroamphetamine with morphine for the treatment of post-operative pain. N Engl J Med 296:712–715, 1977.

82. Gawley TH, Dundee JW, Gupta RK, Jones CJ: Role of doxapram in reducing pulmonary complication after major surgery. Br Med J 1:122–124, 1976.

83. Rawak N, Schott U, Dahlstrom B, et al: Influence of naloxone infusion on analgesia and respiratory depression following morphine. Anesthesiology 64:194–201, 1986.

84. Doran R, Baxter AD, Samson B, et al: Prevention of respiratory depression from epidural morphine in post-thoracotomy patients with nalbuphine hydrochloride. Anesthesiology 67:A248, 1987.

85. Loesser EA, Bennet G, Stanley TH, et al: Comparison of droperidol, haloperidol and prochlorperazine as postoperative anti-emetics. Can Anaesth Soc J 26:125, 1979.

86. Morrison JD, Load WB, Dundee JW: Controlled comparison of the efficacy of fourteen preparations in the relief of postoperative pain. Br Med J 3:287, 1971.

87. Rosenberg M, Curtis L, Bourke DL: Transcutaneous electrical nerve stimulation for the relief of postoperative pain. Pain 5:129–133, 1978.

88. Sjolund BH, Terenius L, Eriksson MBE: Increased cerebrospinal fluid levels of endorphin after electroacupuncture. Acta Physiol Scand 100:382–384, 1977.

89. Wall PD, Sweet WH: Temporary abolition of pain in man. Science 155:108–109, 1967.

90. Ignelzi RJ, Nyquist JK: Excitability changes in peripheral nerve fibers after repetitive electrical stimulation: implications in pain modulation. J Neurosurg 51:824, 1979.

91. Tammisto T, Tigerstedt I: Mild analgesics in postoperative pain. Br J Clin Pharmacol 10(suppl):347–350, 1980.

92. Fragen RJ, O'Hara D: A comparison of intramuscularly injected ketorolac and morphine in postoperative pain. Clin Pharmacol Ther 41:212, 1987.

93. Caplan RA, Ready LB, Olsson GL, Neely ML: Transdermal delivery of fentanyl for postoperative pain control. Anesthesiology 65:A210, 1986.

94. Plezia PM, Linford J, Kramer TH, et al: Transdermally administered fentanyl for postoperative pain: a randomized double-blind, placebo controlled trial. Anesthesiology 69:A364, 1988.

Bibliography

Cousins MJ, Phillips CD: Acute Pain Management. New York, Churchill Livingstone, 1986.

Harmer M, Rosen M, Vickers MD: Patient-Controlled Analgesia. Oxford, Blackwell Scientific Publications, 1985.

PROBLEMS OF AMBULATORY SURGERY 20

SAMUEL M. PARNASS

Many changes have taken place in anesthesia and surgery since Ralph Waters opened the Downtown Anesthesia Clinic in Sioux City, Iowa in 1916.[1] Since that time, the field of outpatient anesthesia has grown considerably and now accounts for a major percentage of surgeries performed at many institutions. At Rush-Presbyterian-St. Luke's Medical Center in Chicago the incidence is 30 to 40 per cent. Criteria for patient acceptance and economic demands have fueled the rapid growth of outpatient care. Ambulatory surgery is no longer restricted to only American Society of Anesthesiologists (ASA) physical status I or II patients. Wetchler stated that the ASA physical status III patient is now acceptable if the patient's systemic disease is medically stable.[2] The anesthesiologist must assess each individual's acceptability for ambulatory surgery through preoperative evaluation.

ANESTHESIA FOR AMBULATORY PROCEDURES

PATIENT SELECTION

Surgeons are often responsible for the initial history and physical examinations that must be provided for each patient according to the Joint Commission for the Accreditation of Hospitals (JCAH) requirements. Wilson et al.[3] has shown that simple screening questions correlate with a consensus of fitness for anesthesia. These questions can be easily answered by the patients and serve as a screening device or "red flag" to indicate which patients need further work-up (Table 20–1). Preoperative screening performed by an anesthesiologist through chart reviews, telephone interviews, or direct history and physical examination is beneficial. The practice of seeing patients the day of the surgery is often adequate for ASA class I or II patients; however,

delays may result if problems are found the day of surgery. All class III patients should be reviewed by anesthesia personnel prior to the day of surgery.

Each outpatient center should develop guidelines for minimal preoperative laboratory test requirements. At Rush-Presbyterian-St. Luke's Medical Center separate criteria for each ASA class patient have been established. Table 20–2 lists the current requirements.

Blery et al.[4] selectively orders preoperative tests based on a protocol of suspected diseases. In a series of 3866 patients, they found that only 0.2 per cent of omitted tests would have been useful based on an anesthetists' questionnaire. Roizen[5] has suggested that utilizing this protocol and eliminating unnecessary laboratory tests would result in a 93 to 97 per cent reduction in patient charges and hospital costs.

The individual anesthesiologist must decide what range of laboratory abnormalities are acceptable based on the specific clinical situation. However, prior teaching that the hemoglobin level must be greater than 10 gm/dl or the potassium greater than 3.5 mEq/L are no longer applicable given the current climate regarding transfusion-associated disease and data about the safety of mild hypokalemia and general anesthesia.[6]

ANESTHETIC TECHNIQUES

Regional Anesthesia

Although common complications of general anesthesia, e.g., oversedation, nausea and vomiting, and residual pain, are generally considered benign, they are significant in the outpatient setting. They delay or prevent discharge, disrupt the smooth functioning of ambulatory surgery units, and aggravate patients and their families who are eager to return home. The use of regional anesthesia of-

TABLE 20–1. QUESTIONS TO EVALUATE FITNESS FOR ANESTHESIA

1. Do you feel sick?

2. Have you had any serious illnesses in the past?

3. Do you get more short of breath on exertion than others of your age?

4. Do you have a cough?

5. Do you have a wheeze?

6. Do you have any chest pain or exertion?

7. Do you have any ankle swelling?

8. Have you taken any medications over the past three months?

9. Have you any allergies?

10. Have you had an anesthetic during the past two months?

11. Have you or your relatives had any problems with anesthesia?

From Wetchler BV (ed): Problems in Anesthesia: Outpatient Anesthesia. Philadelphia, Lippincott, 1988, pp. 9–17. With permission.

ten can avoid these problems and improve the outpatient experience. When coupled with light sedation, patient anxiety can be controlled without delaying discharge time. There is also a lower incidence of nausea and vomiting and unanticipated hospital admissions after regional anesthesia than after general anesthesia.[7,8] Postoperative analgesia, from either residual block (i.e., axillary block) or supplementation with local infiltration, can actually help early ambulation and thereby avoid admission for intractable pain.

Successful regional anesthesia depends on a number of important factors. Proper patient selection is important, as is education regarding the technique and performance of the block, potential residual effects, and possible side effects. Similarly, there should be support from the surgeon, who may be the first person to discuss anesthesia possibilities with the patient. It is important for all personnel to realize that although extra time may be required for the performance of certain techniques the payoff in patient care is worth the investment. Designating a preoperative holding area where blocks can be performed facilitates patient flow and avoids delays, keeping rapid turnover of the surgical patients possible.

Patient cooperation is important; the highly anxious patient is not a good candidate for regional anesthesia. In addition, the proper choice of local anesthetic agent is important. For example, short-acting agents are best used for spinal or epidural blocks; long-acting agents can be utilized in the properly selected patient if limb immobilization using slings, casts, or crutches is expected.

The use of regional anesthesia does not eliminate the potential for aspiration, nor does it eliminate the need for adequate preoperative evaluation. Ambulatory patients are at risk for significant pulmonary complications from aspiration of gastric contents and must have had nothing by mouth (NPO). Manchikanti and Marrero have shown that 60 per cent of outpatients have gastric aspirates with a pH of 2.5 or less and a volume of 25 ml or more.[9] Patients receiving minor blocks may actually be the most ill as a group, and therefore all patients must receive similar anesthetic vigilance. Myers has reported that 5.1 per cent of cataract surgery under local anesthesia generated emergency calls for one group of anesthesiologists.[10] Similarly, Kitz et al.[11] documented that 50 to 75 per cent of patients undergoing "local" or "local/sedation" have significant variations of blood pressure and heart rate, and that 50 to 75 per cent of these patients had oxygen saturations of less than 85 per cent at some point during the procedure.

There are disadvantages to regional anesthesia in the outpatient setting that must be taken into account whenever such a regional technique is contemplated. The overly anxious patient is clearly a poor candidate. The extra time required to perform nonroutine blocks can be a realistic drawback in busy outpatient centers. The time required for the local anesthetic to take effect is also a factor but can be hastened by the appropriate use of fast-acting drugs or by modifying them with alkalinization as shown by Defazio et al. for lidocaine[12] and Hilgier for bupivacaine.[13] One milliliter of $NaHCO_3$ added per 10 ml of 2 per cent lidocaine with epinephrine significantly shortened onset time for epidural block.[12] Much less bicarbonate is needed for bupivacaine, where only 0.1 ml of $NaHCO_3$ added per 10 ml of 0.5 per cent bupivacaine significantly shortened the onset time for axillary block (range of 20 to 32 minutes to 7 to 14 minutes), with a much longer duration of action in the alkalinized group.

The problem of residual numbness following regional block of an extremity has raised concern, but there are no documented problems after arm or foot blocks so long as careful instructions are given to the patient and family

TABLE 20–2. RUSH–PRESBYTERIAN–ST. LUKE'S MEDICAL CENTER (CHICAGO), DEPARTMENT OF ANESTHESIOLOGY POLICIES AND PROCEDURES

1. Routine admission for outpatient surgery is limited to those patients classified as class I and class II by the American Society of Anesthesiologists Patient Status Classification. Class III patients may be admitted if they are medically stable and have anesthesia clearance.

2. Minimal requirements for an adult outpatient surgery patient (class I or II) having surgery under general anesthesia are:
   2.1 History and physical examination
   2.2 Hematocrit
   2.3 Sickle cell preparation as indicated
   2.4 Chest roentgenogram for patients over 60 years of age
   2.5 ECG for male patients over 40 years of age and for female patients over 60 years of age
   2.6 Valid consent

3. Minimal requirements for any adult class III ambulatory surgery patient having surgery under general anesthesia, local/general, or major regional blocks are:
   3.1 History and physical examination
   3.2 Complete blood count
   3.3 Urinalysis
   3.4 SMA-6 with glucose
   3.5 Chest roentgenogram
   3.6 ECG
   3.7 Sickle cell preparation as indicated
   3.8 Valid consent

4. For class I or II patients, laboratory data, ECG, and chest film are accepted up to within 6 months of surgery if there has been no intervening illness or change in the clinical status.

5. For class III patients, laboratory data, ECG, and chest film are accepted up to within 4 weeks of surgery if there has been no intervening illness or changes in the clinical status.

to protect the affected limb from external injury.[14] Furthermore, the residual analgesia provided by the local anesthetic often more than compensates for the extra care needed for its use.

Urinary retention following spinal or epidural blockade is not a major problem when long-acting agents such as bupivacaine and tetracaine are avoided. Hypotension resulting from residual sympathectomy has not been found to be a significant problem so long as ambulation is not attempted prior to documentation of full return of perianal sensation and proprioception.[15] Mulroy found fewer unanticipated hospital admissions due to urinary retention and residual sympathectomy than to intractable nausea and vomiting after general anesthesia.[14]

Postdural puncture headache (PDPH) after either spinal or epidural anesthesia can be a significant problem, although the risk does not increase with ambulation,[16] other than hastening the onset.[17] Whereas Burke has documented a low incidence of PDPH (2 per cent) in outpatients,[18] Flaaten and Raeder[19] found a 37 per cent incidence of PDPH in young outpatients even with a 25-gauge spinal needle. Further data are clearly needed for young populations before definitive criteria can be formulated. Epidural anesthesia has been recommended for young patients,[14] and though the risk of dural puncture is still present it is markedly reduced. Patients who cannot be adequately followed up, however, should not have either technique performed.

Should a dural puncture occur, a prophylactic epidural blood patch can be performed. Although controversy exists regarding its efficacy, successful results have been reported, including the performance of a patch through an epidural catheter placed an interspace above the dural puncture site.[20,21] Alternatively, conservative therapy and counsel for bed rest, hydration, and analgesics can be given over the telephone. Caffeine has been suggested as an effective method of therapy by the intravenous route[22,23] and, in our experience, has provided relief in outpatients when prescribed orally in the form of coffee or the caffeine-rich soft drink "Jolt." Clearly, studies are needed in this area. If the headache persists, the patient should be brought back for either intravenous caffeine or an epidural blood patch. One protocol for intravenous caffeine included 2 liters of intravenous fluid: the first with 500 mg of caffeine sodium benzoate given over 1 hour and the second liter over the subsequent hour. A second course of caffeine is given if needed after a 4-hour rest period. This protocol has been successful in 75 per cent of cases.[24] The remainder received an epidural blood patch. Outpatient epidural blood patches can be performed simply and successfully without the need for an intravenous infusion, and patients can be discharged after a short period of observation.[25]

Certain specific regional blocks may be inappropriate for cases where rapid discharge and minimal follow-up are encountered. For example, sciatic-femoral block may prolong recovery time owing to loss of motor strength and coordination in the blocked leg, whereas a supraclavicular brachial plexus block may be contraindicated because of the potential for pneumothorax.[26] However, Patel and colleagues[27] studied the coordination of a "3-in-1 block" as described by Winnie et al.[28] encompassing the femoral, lateral femoral cutaneous, and obturator nerves for outpatient arthroscopy. They compared this technique with general anesthesia and with the 3-in-1 block with an additional lateral femoral cutaneous block. They found the combination of the 3-in-1 block with the additional lateral femoral cutaneous block to be superior to the 3-in-1 block alone and found significantly shortened discharge times for the regional procedures (57 minutes) when compared to those after general anesthesia (95 minutes).

Intravenous regional anesthesia (Bier block) is particularly well suited for orthopedic outpatient procedures because of the ease and simplicity of performing the block, as well as its rapid disappearance following release of the tourniquet.[29] When properly performed, this technique provides excellent analgesia coupled with adequate muscle relaxation. Although most studies on intravenous regional anesthesia deal with surgery of the upper ex-

tremities, satisfactory surgical analgesia can also be obtained for short procedures on the foot.[30] The tourniquet is placed below the knee, avoiding pressure over the superficial peroneal nerve. Lidocaine is most commonly used: 3 mg/kg or 40 ml of 0.5 per cent solution for upper extremity surgery and 75 to 100 ml of a 0.25 to 0.35 per cent solution for lower extremity surgery.[30]

General Anesthesia

The aims of general anesthesia are similar in many respects to those of regional anesthesia: induction and maintenance of a smooth anesthesia, rapid safe recovery, and minimal postoperative side effects. Particular attention must be paid to postoperative psychomotor and cognitive function, pain, nausea, and vomiting when choosing general anesthetic techniques for ambulatory patients.

Premedication. The routine use of premedication in outpatients is often avoided because of concern for prolonged postoperative sedation and recovery times; furthermore, many centers do not have a separate area available where the patient can be monitored once the premedication is given. The use of potent amnestic agents such as midazolam has also been reported to cause patients to fail to remember having seen their surgeon the day of surgery.[31] Unfortunately, patients receiving amnestic agents may also fail to remember postoperative instructions or answers to their questions. Regardless of this possibility, however, there are patients who are anxious for whom the use of some premedication is appropriate. Therefore it is important to use anesthetic agents that are relatively short-acting and to avoid large doses in order to facilitate timely discharge.[32] In general, small intravenous doses of short-acting narcotics such as fentanyl or sedatives such as midazolam are important adjuncts in a balanced anesthetic technique using premedication. Fentanyl, when used as an intravenous premedication or as an adjunct to balanced anesthesia in a dose of 1 to 2 μg/kg, has been shown to decrease recovery time as a result of the narcotic's ability to decrease anesthetic requirements.[33] The presence of postoperative pain has been well established as a contributing factor to postoperative nausea and vomiting. Therefore the use of small doses of intravenous narcotics to reduce postoperative pain may contribute to lowering the incidence of nausea and vomiting, thereby speeding recovery time.[34]

Other agents that have traditionally been used for premedication (e.g., anticholinergics to block vagal reflexes, antacids and histamine-receptor blockers to increase the pH of gastric contents, and gastrokinetic agents to reduce the volume of gastric contents) may be used in outpatients where specifically indicated. Whether all outpatients should receive prophylaxis for aspiration pneumonitis has been the subject of considerable controversy. Manchikanti et al. reported a significant number of outpatients with increased gastric volume and increased acidity.[35] However, many clinicians still believe that routine administration of antacids or histamine blockers is not indicated for all outpatients because the risk of aspiration is small and there are not outcome data to support such a practice.[36]

Intravenous Anesthetics. Intravenous anesthetic agents are most commonly used for induction of general anesthesia, but they can also be used for maintenance of anesthesia, usually as an adjunct to nitrous oxide. Most recent work focuses on the use of propofol.

Propofol is particularly well suited for outpatient anesthesia because of its associated postoperative speed of recovery.[37] Propofol was found to produce slightly more cardiorespiratory depression than methohexital when used as an induction agent, but the speed and quality of recovery were superior with propofol.[37] When compared to thiopental as an induction agent, propofol was found to have a significantly greater number of "excellent inductions," with significantly more rapid recoveries.[38] Other investigators[39] reported that patients using propofol demonstrated a definite sense of well-being after anesthesia when their postoperative mood state was compared with that of a similar group of patients induced with thiopental.

Propofol has also been associated with fewer side effects, e.g., hiccoughing, nausea, and vomiting, both intraoperatively and postoperatively. Doze and colleagues also showed that recovery times for awakening, orientation, and ambulation were consistently shorter with propofol than with methohexital when they were used as adjuvants to nitrous oxide anesthesia for outpatients.[40] Common side effects from propofol include cardiovascular depression similar to that produced by thiopental and pain on injection depending on the site of administration (greatest with dorsal hand veins).[41]

Intravenous Analgesics. The most common intravenous analgesic agents now being used for outpatient anesthesia are fentanyl, alfentanil, and sufentanil. These drugs are relatively short-acting in comparison to morphine and are most frequently administered as part of a balanced anesthetic technique. Narcotic techniques in combination with nitrous oxide have been utilized for outpatient surgery, but an unacceptably high incidence of nausea and vomiting has made these techniques less favored.[42,43]

Although even small preinduction doses of intravenous narcotic agents have been shown to increase the incidence of postoperative nausea and vomiting,[44] they can reduce the anesthetic requirements as well as decrease the need for postoperative pain control,[45] recovery time, and the incidence of nausea due to pain alone.

Inhalational Agents. There is currently insufficient evidence to strongly recommend any one of the currently available inhalational agents over another for outpatient surgery. A number of studies have been performed that compare recovery times for the various anesthetic techniques. Enflurane has been shown to have shorter recovery times than halothane[46]; however, in comparison to isoflurane, Azar et al.[47] found no significant differences. With procedures that were longer than 90 minutes, Korttila and Valanne[48] found significantly slower recovery with enflurane than with isoflurane. These studies suggest that isoflurane may be the inhalational agent of choice for ambulatory anesthesia in procedures lasting longer than 90 minutes. The future use of desflurane (I653) holds great promise for rapid recovery from general anesthesia. However, its clinical use has yet to be established.

Nitrous oxide is the most common adjunctive anesthetic for both inhalational and intravenous anesthesia techniques. Considerable controversy exists regarding the role of nitrous oxide in the production of postoperative nausea and vomiting.[49–53] There are numerous studies to support either side of the issue, which remains unsettled. Despite this controversy, however, nitrous oxide, with its acceptable odor and rapid induction and emergence, is an important tool as an adjunctive agent; and it continues to be the main adjunct for both inhalational and intravenous anesthesia in the ambulatory setting.

Muscle Relaxants. Many outpatient procedures do not require muscle relaxation. Furthermore, many cases can be performed using a face mask without endotracheal intubation.

However, when endotracheal intubation is used for a case, the most common muscle relaxant to facilitate intubation is succinylcholine. Although succinylcholine is an ideal drug in the outpatient setting because of its rapid onset and ultra-short-acting duration, its numerous side effects, particularly myalgia, can be significant in an outpatient setting. Myalgia after succinylcholine can occur up to 4 days postoperatively, and its effects may be more severe than those of the surgical procedure itself. The use of a defasciculant has been shown to decrease the incidence of myalgia; the preferred agents are those with significant prejunctional effects, e.g., gallamine and tubocurarine.[54] Atracurium has been compared to d-tubocurarine for the prevention of postsuccinylcholine myalgia. Although fewer fasciculations were seen with d-tubocurarine, there was significantly less post anesthesia myalgia in the atracurium group (0.025 mg/kg).[55] Myalgia, however, has been reported even in the absence of fasciculations.[56] The incidence of myalgia was found to be no different in patients receiving either succinylcholine or vecuronium.[57]

When muscle relaxation is needed for surgical procedures lasting less than 20 minutes, the only current option is a succinylcholine infusion. The reason is that there are no currently approved short-acting nondepolarizing muscle relaxants in the United States, although mivacurium (BW B109OU) has been under clinical investigation since 1985 and may be useful in outpatients. Structurally, mivacurium is similar to atracurium, and it also undergoes ester hydrolysis though there is no Hofmann elimination. Mivacurium has the same weak histamine-releasing properties as atracurium and may produce hypotension, tachycardia, and skin flush on induction.[58] Intubating doses of 0.20 to 0.25 mg/kg have an onset time of 2.5 minutes, with 95 per cent recovery within only 30 minutes. This factor makes the duration of onset of the intubating doses of mivacurium about twice as long as that of succinylcholine and half as long as those of atracurium and vecuronium.[59] A dose of 0.1 mg/kg has an onset time of 3.8 minutes with a 95 per cent spontaneous recovery time of 25 minutes.[60]

For procedures lasting longer than 30 minutes, atracurium and vecuronium are valuable clinical options. The durations of action for these drugs are similar; but when used in intubating doses, the duration of action is 50 to 70 minutes, which may be too long for short ambulatory cases.[61] A combination of atracurium (0.125 mg/kg) and vecuronium (0.025 mg/kg) has been shown to produce neuromuscular blockade with onset times similar to those of the intubating doses of either drug, yet with faster recovery than either drug. The combination was found to have recovery to 25 per cent in 32 minutes and to 90 per cent in 48 minutes.[62] This combination could have advantages in an outpatient setting until mivacurium becomes available.

PAIN MANAGEMENT IN THE PACU

Adequate management of postoperative pain, whether for prevention or treatment, is one of the most important factors in successful outpatient surgery. In a study of unexpected hospital admissions, Meridy reported that pain was the most common surgically related reason for unexpected hospital admissions.[8] Pain is also a determining factor in the decision as to when patients are ready for discharge. Finally, patients' perception of the quality of their overall ambulatory surgery experience is greatly enhanced by rapid, effective control of postoperative pain.

The cornerstones of pain management in ambulatory surgery include the following: 1) the use of potent intravenous opioid analgesics during the preoperative and intraoperative periods to provide effective postoperative analgesia and perhaps decrease intraoperative anesthetic requirements; 2) the use of local anesthetic agents used as supplements to general anesthesia or alone at the end of surgery for postoperative analgesia, administered as a regional block or via local infiltration; and 3) the use of potent oral opioid analgesics and nonsteroidal antiinflammatory drugs (NSAIDs) for control of pain at home.

The use of intravenous opioid analgesics as premedicants has been shown to decrease patient anxiety, reduce anesthetic requirement, and provide pain relief early in the postoperative period. No prolongation of recovery time or increase in postoperative side effects were reported with fentanyl (1 to 2 μg/kg), sufentanil (0.10 to 0.25 μg/kg), or alfentanil (7.5 to 15.0 μg/kg).[63] Similarly, Hunt et al. premedicated a group of outpatients scheduled for dilatation and curettage with intravenous fentanyl (75 to 125 μg) and found a significantly reduced frequency of postoperative abdominal pain without an increase in nausea or vomiting.[64] When comparing patients who received intraoperative intravenous opioid analgesics to patients who did not, Epstein et al. found that patients who did not receive intravenous opioids had a significantly higher incidence of postoperative pain and a higher incidence of excitement during their recovery period. Patients who received intraoperative opioids recovered sooner, had a shorter time to ambulation without support, and spent less time in the PACU.[65] Alfentanil has been compared to inhalational anesthesia in a number of studies of short outpatient procedures, with faster recoveries being noted in patients receiving opioid analgesia.

There were no differences in late recovery scores or subjective feelings of drowsiness or unsteadiness.[66-68] There are numerous intravenous opioid analgesics that can be used for ambulatory surgery, but no ideal agent has yet been determined. Although it has been suggested that long-acting drugs such as morphine and meperidine may have too long an action for outpatient use,[69] data comparing meperidine (1.0 to 1.5 mg/kg) with fentanyl (2 μg/kg) did not show any differences in recovery or patient discharge times.[70] Nalbuphine is generally thought to be as effective as morphine. Garfield et al., however, reported that nalbuphine, (0.3 to 0.5 mg/kg) was similar to fentanyl (1.5 μg/kg) regarding postoperative analgesia but had increased recovery room stay, and psychological side effects were seen, e.g., anxiety and dreaming.[71] Bone et al. compared nalbuphine (0.25 mg/kg) to fentanyl and found that nalbuphine patients had significantly lower pain scores at 1 hour and required significantly less postoperative analgesia; there were no significant differences regarding nausea or observer assessment of appearance, though there was some evidence of psychomotor impairment at 2 hours.[72] When butorphanol (40 μg/kg) and fentanyl (2.0 μg/kg) were compared as supplements to balanced general anesthesia, butorphanol was not found to be superior. Although patients receiving butorphanol were generally more pain-free than the fentanyl patients, they were also drowsier. The incidence of nausea and vomiting was similar in the two groups.[73]

Local anesthetics have been successful in preventing and treating pain in the PACU. Infiltration of the ilioinguinal and iliohypogastric nerves with bupivacaine has been shown to decrease pain and vomiting during the recovery period[74] while significantly decreasing anesthetic and analgesic requirements and demonstrating a more rapid return to normal activity.[75] After laparoscopic tubal ligations, infiltration of the mesosalpinx with 0.5 per cent bupivacaine in the area of fallopian ring placement has been shown to significantly decrease patients' pain in the PACU.[76,77] A simple subcutaneous ring block of the penis with 0.25 per cent bupivacaine has been shown to significantly decrease PACU analgesic requirements after circumcision in children.[78] Another technique is the application of topical lidocaine jelly, which was found to be as effective as dorsal nerve block and parenteral morphine for outpatient circumcisions.[79] The use of intraarticular bupivacaine after arthroscopic meniscectomy has been shown to reduce significantly both patient assessment of pain and the amount of supplemental postoperative morphine required.[80] Caudal block supplementation has been used to prevent postoperative surgical pain for pediatric circumcision, correction of hypospadias, and orchiopexy.[81,82] Caudal analgesia has also been shown to be superior to systemic opioids with a more tranquil recovery period, superior analgesia, and a lower incidence of vomiting.[83-86] When comparing patients receiving caudal anesthesia to those receiving dorsal nerve block for circumcision, the latter group demonstrated equal pain relief with earlier micturition and ability to stand unaided, as well as a lower incidence of vomiting.[87]

In summary, the control of postoperative pain in the ambulatory surgery setting can be accomplished in a number of ways. Premedication or supplementation of anesthesia with potent intravenous opioid analgesics can significantly decrease postoperative pain and enhance recovery as well as speed up patient discharge times. The smallest doses that are effective should be employed to minimize problems such as nausea, vomiting, and drowsiness. When possible, infiltration with local anesthetics or regional blocks can be employed either alone or in combination with potent intravenous narcotics to allow the greatest patient comfort in the postoperative setting with the least delay in discharge.

NAUSEA AND VOMITING IN THE PACU

Postoperative nausea and vomiting is a long-standing problem that is vexing to both patients and ambulatory surgery personnel involved in their care. In 1914 the first issue of

Anesthesia and Analgesia featured on its front cover an original article entitled "Prophylaxis of Post Anesthetic Vomiting Period."[88] More than 70 years later, that topic remains one of the major concerns faced by health care providers in the PACU. Postoperative nausea and vomiting are the most common complications reported in the PACU at the Phoenix Surgi-Center. At the Methodist Ambulatory Surgery Center in Peoria, they comprise the fourth most common reason for unanticipated hospital admissions, excluding direct surgical causes, and are often accompanied by somnolence following treatment with potent antiemetics.[89]

It is in the outpatient setting that the problem of postoperative nausea and vomiting is most troublesome because the consequences of delayed discharge times and the need for hospitalization are more acutely experienced. Notwithstanding a perfect surgical result and a well delivered anesthetic, the ambulatory surgery experience can be viewed as a complete failure by outpatients who subsequently have uncontrolled postoperative nausea and vomiting or who need to be admitted.

CAUSES OF POST ANESTHETIC NAUSEA AND VOMITING

Numerous factors are associated with postoperative nausea and vomiting, many of which work in concert. There is considerable controversy regarding some of these factors. Those that have been frequently implicated are included in Table 20–3.

Anesthetic Techniques

Anesthetic techniques such as the use of positive pressure ventilation by mask, often

TABLE 20–3. FACTORS ASSOCIATED WITH POSTOPERATIVE NAUSEA AND VOMITING

Anesthetic techniques
Anesthetic agents
Gender
Age
Weight
Surgical procedure
Pain
History of postoperative nausea and vomiting
History of motion sickness

performed during induction of anesthesia to preoxygenate patients, may increase the incidence of nausea and vomiting by forcing air into the stomach. Potential airway problems may be even more significant in obese patients. Also, the length of anesthetic exposure time has been correlated with an increased incidence of subsequent postoperative nausea and vomiting.

Anesthetic Agents

Certain anesthetic agents used for the induction and maintenance of anesthesia have been shown to influence the incidence of postoperative nausea and vomiting. Although there is controversy regarding some of these agents, it is clear that the use of a narcotic-based technique for the induction or maintenance of anesthesia increases the incidence of postoperative nausea and vomiting. Numerous studies have compared fentanyl or alfentanil with the inhalational anesthetics and have shown a significantly increased incidence of postoperative nausea and vomiting with the narcotic techniques.[90–92]

Nitrous oxide has traditionally been implicated as a major cause of postoperative nausea and vomiting; however, this conclusion has been questioned in a number of well controlled, prospective studies and is currently controversial.[52,93–95] Earlier studies that implicated nitrous oxide as a cause of postoperative nausea and vomiting cited the increased sympathetic activity of nitrous oxide, changes in middle ear pressure, and gastrointestinal distension as factors that produce postoperative nausea and vomiting. However, Muir et al. evaluated nitrous oxide in surgery that excluded otologic, neurologic, intraabdominal, and ophthalmic operations and found no association between nitrous oxide and postoperative nausea and vomiting.[52] Kortilla et al. studied abdominal hysterectomies comparing oxygen/nitrous oxide/isoflurane to oxygen/isoflurane and also found no difference in the incidence of nausea or vomiting.[95] In the pediatric setting, Gibbons et al., studying the effect of nitrous oxide on postoperative vomiting after pediatric eye surgery, found no significant difference between the two groups when they were compared for the incidence of vomiting and the severity of vomiting as measured by the need for antiemetics.[96]

No conclusive data have been published demonstrating significant differences between the various inhalational anesthetic agents. Although enflurane has been suggested as the inhalation agent of choice for gynecologic outpatients (as it appears to be associated with less nausea and vomiting), other studies have found no difference among inhalational agents.[90] Regional anesthesia, by avoiding potent inhalational or intravenous anesthetic agents, has been shown to result in significantly less postoperative nausea and vomiting.[97]

Age, Gender, and Weight

A number of studies have shown that the incidence of postoperative nausea and vomiting is correlated with young age groups. In addition, women are two to four times more likely to experience postoperative nausea and vomiting than men.[90]

The issue of weight and obesity is somewhat controversial, but both factors have been implicated. Previously, it was thought that obese patients have an increased incidence of nausea and vomiting because they sequester drugs in fat compartments and have slower metabolism, which prolongs the release of anesthetics. However, Muir et al. found that the body mass index was not associated with increased postoperative nausea and vomiting.[52] They attributed their differing findings to the fact that they did not ventilate their patients by mask prior to the induction of anesthesia. They speculated that, because obese patients are usually more difficult to ventilate by mask, there is a greater likelihood of gastrointestinal distension from air being forced into the stomach, thus increasing the possibility that nausea and vomiting may result.

Type of Surgical Procedure

Whether the type of surgical procedure is an important predictor of the incidence of postoperative nausea and vomiting has been the subject of much debate. In the pediatric population it has been clear that strabismus and orchiopexy surgery have a significant incidence of postoperative nausea and vomiting. Caldamone and Rabinowitz[98] found that up to 5 per cent of their patients undergoing outpatient orchiopexy needed to be admitted to the hospital for either nausea, vomiting, drowsiness, or more extensive surgery. They found that a 4- to 6-hour recovery room stay was the rule rather than the exception. Tonsillectomies and adenoidectomies have been similarly associated with an increased incidence of postoperative nausea and vomiting. The incidence was found to be twice as common in the pediatric population with procedures lasting longer than 20 minutes and was more frequent in patients over 3 years of age, with an increase of 42 to 51 per cent from age 3 until puberty.[89]

In the adult population increased frequencies in postoperative nausea and vomiting have been reported in patients undergoing gastrointestinal, otologic, and ophthalmic procedures.[99,100] In contrast, however, Burtles and Peckett[101] and Knapp and Beecher[102] reported that the site of surgery is unimportant as a factor relating to postoperative nausea and vomiting. Pataky et al.[103] looked at nausea and vomiting following ambulatory surgery and found a significantly increased incidence with laparoscopy and laparoscopic ovum retrieval compared to that with other procedures. This complication extended the recovery room stay by as much as 56 per cent. Because prolonged recovery room stay may disrupt patient flow they suggested that ambulatory surgery administrators could establish ideal daily scheduling principles in which patients scheduled for procedures associated with a high incidence of nausea and vomiting and long recovery room times could be scheduled early in the day. In addition, it might be desirable to have a separate step-down recovery unit available for these patients so their presence would not disrupt the functioning or capacity of the ambulatory surgery unit.

Pain

The role of postoperative pain as an etiologic factor for postoperative nausea and vomiting has been well established. Anderson and Crohg[104] found a relation between postoperative pain and the frequency of nausea and vomiting. They also found that complete pain relief without simultaneous relief of nausea was unusual. Almost one half their patients with inadequate pain relief and postoperative nausea had both symptoms relieved after the first injection of analgesic, and the other half had the two complaints relieved after the second dose. Only 10 per cent of their patients complained of nausea without complaints of pain. These authors concluded that nausea often accompanies pain during the postoperative period and that it can be relieved in most cases when pain relief is achieved by the use of intravenous opiates.

Preoperative History

It is important to obtain a good preoperative history, especially in outpatients who will be traveling home after their procedure. It has been well documented that patients with a history of postoperative nausea and vomiting are more likely to repeat the syndrome with subsequent anesthetics. Similarly, patients with a history of motion sickness have a high incidence of the complication[52]; therefore a good preoperative history is important so these patients can be targeted for aggressive prophylaxis. The drive home from an outpatient unit may itself stimulate post-PACU nausea and vomiting in patients who did not have this problem in the PACU. Muir et al.[52] found a two- to fivefold increase in postoperative nausea and vomiting from PACU discharge to 24 hours postoperatively. The factors involved included pain, use of narcotic analgesics, mental stress and anxiety, delay of eating, and movement. It should be remembered that reports evaluating postoperative nausea and vomiting only in the PACU underestimate the true frequency of postoperative nausea and vomiting.

PROPHYLAXIS AND TREATMENT

The management of postoperative nausea and vomiting ideally stems from a prophylactic rather than a therapeutic approach (particularly in patients identified to be at risk), which would serve to reduce the discomfort experienced by patients going through ambulatory surgery units. As these patients are generally less sedated, they are more likely to remember incidents of nausea and vomiting when compared to their inpatient counterparts. Furthermore, the delay in discharge caused by nausea and vomiting tends to cause a further deterioration of the outpatient experience as well as upset the unit's patient flow. Preventive therapy may minimize morbidity, increase and maintain patient comfort, and decrease the frustration often felt by nurses trying to manage the problem. It is advantageous for those involved in taking care of these patients, specifically PACU nurses, to have standing orders available for the treatment of postoperative nausea and vomiting and pain. This practice avoids delays that are so common when trying to get the anesthesiologist to give specific orders each time. Preprinted order forms with strict guidelines allow prompt treatment of postoperative nausea and vomiting itself and the pain that may be contributing to this postoperative complication.

Many agents have been used to control postoperative nausea and vomiting. There is controversy regarding some of them, which are listed in Table 20–4. The problem with most of these medications is that, although they may be effective in preventing or controlling postoperative nausea and vomiting, increasing dosages also increase the incidence of postoperative sedation. Although it may not be a significant problem in the inpatient population, it is an important problem for outpatients and can adversely affect discharge times.

Droperidol and Metoclopramide

The two most common anesthetic agents used today are metoclopramide and droperidol. Numerous studies have shown droperidol to be effective in a low dose intravenous format without significantly affecting discharge times.[105–108] Dosage recommendations have ranged from 0.625 to 2.500 mg for the average adult (10 to 20 μg/kg). Dosage guidelines for children range from 25 to 75 μ/kg.

Metoclopramide also has been found efficacious for nausea and vomiting.[109,110] Both metoclopramide and droperidol antagonize dopaminergic receptors and block stimulation of the medullary chemoreceptor trigger zones. However, only metoclopramide is a gastro-prokinetic drug that sensitizes the upper gastrointestinal tissues to the action of acetylcholine, thereby stimulating gastric motility. Metoclopramide also increases the resting tone of the lower esophageal sphincter, relaxes the pyloric sphincter and duodenal bulb during gastric contractions, and simultaneously increases peristalsis of the proximal small bowel. The net result is an accelerated

TABLE 20–4. AGENTS USED FOR TREATMENT OF POSTOPERATIVE NAUSEA AND VOMITING

Droperidol (Inapsine)
Metoclopramide (Reglan)
Benzquinamide (Emete-Con)
Prochlorperazine (Compazine)
Trimethobenzamide hydrochloride (Tigan)
Hydroxyzine (Vistaril)
Ephedrine sulfate
Diphenhydramine (Dramamine)

gastric emptying time and shortened small bowel transit time, which can be important during the preinduction period to help eliminate gastric contents and prevent any chance of aspiration while also helping to decrease the incidence of nausea and vomiting. Prior treatment with anticholingeric agents does not inhibit the gastroprokinetic actions of metoclopramide in normal patients[111] but does so in obese patients[112]; the reason for this difference is not clear. Because the duration of action of metoclopramide is approximately 2 hours, if the drug is given preoperatively for a procedure that lasts 1 to 2 hours the drug may no longer be available in sufficient quantity after surgery to be effective. Therefore it is advantageous to give a second dose of metoclopramide at the end of the procedure in order to obtain good postoperative nausea and vomiting prophylaxis. Higher doses than the average 10 mg/70 kg patient may be needed in certain populations, especially women. Of interest is the fact that oncology patients routinely receive 50 mg metoclopramide per dose for nausea prophylaxis to chemotherapeutic agents. One of the major advantages of metoclopramide is that there is little or no sedative effect.

There are side effects to both droperidol and metoclopramide that must be understood. Droperidol may cause sedation and can also potentiate other central nervous system depressants commonly used during the postoperative period. Droperidol, as an α-blocker, may also cause hypotension and peripheral vascular dilatation; therefore caution should be used in patients who are hypovolemic, are dizzy upon standing, or have low blood pressure. Droperidol may also cause an acute dysphoric reaction as well as extrapyramidal symptoms such as dystonia or oculogyric crisis. Metoclopramide is less likely to cause extrapyramidal symptoms, although they have been reported. It must be remembered that metoclopramide with its gastroprokinetic actions is contraindicated with bowel obstruction or partial bowel obstruction. The treatment for extrapyramidal reactions, should they occur, is benztropine 1 to 2 mg (Cogentin) or diphenhydramine 25 to 50 mg (Benadryl).

FUTURE TRENDS

Although the incidence of postoperative nausea and vomiting has been clearly shown to be decreased with droperidol and in many studies with metoclopramide, the incidence has not been completely reduced. Doze et al.[113] combined droperidol with metoclopramide in an attempt to increase the amount of antiemetic drug given without a concomitant increase in the incidence of sedation or side effects. They found that the combination of droperidol and metoclopramide was more effective in preventing nausea and vomiting than droperidol alone. They were able to decrease the incidence of nausea and vomiting (an average of 40 per cent with droperidol) by one half with the combination therapy, with concomitant shortening of ambulation and discharge times.

Other investigators have approached the problem of postoperative nausea and vomiting from the perspective of motion sickness. It has been well documented that a history of motion sickness is a strong predictive factor for postoperative nausea and vomiting.[52] Bidwai et al.[114] studied diphenhydramine (Dramamine), a commonly used anti-motion-sickness drug and found significantly less nausea (8 per cent) when compared to both droperidol (21 per cent) and placebo (34 per cent). Diphenhydramine is an antihistamine and its anti-motion-sickness effect is thought to be a combination of a primary H_1-blocking effect and central anticholinergic action.

Rothenberg et al.[115] have studied the use of ephedrine in the prevention of postoperative nausea and vomiting in outpatients. They found that prophylactic ephedrine (0.5 mg/kg IM after extubation) was as effective as droperidol in reducing the incidence of nausea, with significantly less postoperative sedation in the ephedrine group and a trend toward earlier discharge times. There were no significant differences regarding mean arterial blood pressure among the groups. Ephedrine has been used for the prevention of motion sickness by the National Aeronautics and Space Administration (NASA)[116] and is commonly used to treat nausea and vomiting following hypotension after spinal or epidural anesthesia. Its mechanism for motion sickness is unknown, but after spinal and epidural anesthesia it undoubtedly reverses the hypotension of the induced sympathectomy through its α-agonist properties. Similarly, many patients are volume-depleted after anesthesia and may have residual vasodilation from potent inhalational anesthetics. This situation is typically manifested by dizziness upon standing and is often accompanied by nausea and vomiting.

These patients may particularly benefit from treatment with ephedrine in the PACU.

Persistent postoperative nausea and vomiting may require repeated doses of antiemetics in the PACU. Standing orders should be available for prompt and rapid institution of such therapy. In addition, careful attention must be given to both pain control and the patient's volume status. Intravenous fluids should be increased to account for fluid losses and should be maintained until oral fluids are tolerated. Fluid losses should be replaced with lactated Ringer's solution or normal saline and should not be replaced with 5 per cent dextrose in water (D_5W) alone because it does not remain in the intravascular compartment.

Furthermore, it is essential that good communication exists between the anesthesiologist, patient, and family. Patients should be warned during the preoperative interview that nausea and vomiting are common side effects of anesthesia and surgery. They are then able to tolerate these situations with less anxiety and are less apt to believe that their experience has been a failure. Although rare, there are patients in whom postoperative nausea and vomiting is refractory to all efforts for control, and these patients must be admitted overnight. A review of unanticipated admissions over a 6-month period at the Ambulatory Surgical Unit of Rush–Presbyterian–St. Luke's Medical Center found that 10 per cent were for uncontrolled postoperative nausea and vomiting, with an overall incidence of 4 per cent. Patients with persistent nausea and vomiting should be treated aggressively with maximum doses of antiemetics, as it is preferable to admit a sedated patient with controlled nausea and vomiting than one who is unsedated and whose nausea and vomiting are uncontrolled.

Conclusion

Postoperative nausea and vomiting remain an important and clinically significant problem for health care providers and patients. Although management of the problem must first and foremost be centered around prevention, placing primary responsibility on the anesthesia team with prompt treatment in the PACU requires a cooperative effort among the anesthesiologist, PACU nurse, and patient, all working toward the goal of decreasing or preventing morbidity and improving patient safety and comfort. Numerous agents have been used prophylactically with varying success rates, most likely due to the inherent difficulty of controlling for the numerous differences among patients, anesthetics, and surgical procedures. Nonetheless, agents are available that effectively control postoperative nausea and vomiting; in addition, more knowledge is available about which anesthetic techniques should be avoided. Good communication between the ambulatory surgical staff and patients, when supplemented with rapid pain control in the PACU, can help to minimize the chances for the potentially negative influence of postoperative nausea and vomiting on the ambulatory surgery experience.

DISCHARGE CRITERIA

There are varying stages of recovery through which patients progress after surgery and anesthesia. Sophisticated tests that can measure subtle psychomotor differences have been developed, but they are usually too complex and time-consuming to be used on a daily basis; therefore practical discharge criteria must be devised and implemented by each ambulatory surgery unit. In general, the criteria must define the point at which the patient is "home-ready," with the understanding that these criteria do not mean that the patient is ready to walk on the street or to drive a car (Table 20–5).

Most centers generally follow a sequence that includes a stage I PACU where patients are kept recumbent, followed by a stage II PACU where they are encouraged to sit up and ambulate. When patients are awake, oriented, and able to walk, they may have liquids offered to them by mouth and be encouraged to ambulate to the bathroom and attempt to void. If these activities are easily accomplished and patients have no excessive pain, nausea, or vomiting, they are considered "home-ready" and may be discharged with an escort who ideally stays with the patient overnight. Although the ability to void before discharge is not a strict requirement for patients who have undergone general anesthesia, patients who have had spinal or epidural anesthesia should demonstrate that they can void before they are allowed to go home.

Prior to discharge, patients should have their dressing checked and are given written instructions for their care at home in the presence of the responsible person. They must be reminded not to drive, operate power tools, or

TABLE 20–5. GUIDELINES FOR SAFE
DISCHARGE AFTER DAY SURGERY

1. Patient must have a responsible "vested" adult to:
   a. Escort patient home.
   b. Provide care at home.

2. Patient's vital signs must have been stable for at least 1 hour.

3. Patient must have no evidence of respiratory depression.

4. Patient must be:
   a. Oriented to person, place, time
   b. Able to dress himself/herself.
   c. Able to walk out without assistance.
   d. Able to maintain orally administered fluids.[a]
   e. Able to void.[a]

5. Patient must not have:
   a. More than minimal nausea or vomiting.
   b. Excessive pain.
   c. Bleeding.

6. Patient should stay at least 1 to 2 hours after extubation.[a]

7. Patient must be discharged by the person who gave anesthesia or a designee. Written instructions for the postoperative period at home, including a contact place and person, must be reinforced.

[a] The role of these variables as criteria for discharge remains to be established.
Reproduced with permission from Kortilla K: Practical discharge criteria. *In* Wetchler BV (ed): Problems in Anesthesia: Outpatient Anesthesia. Philadelphia, Lippincott, 1988, pp. 144–151.

be involved in major decisions for up to 24 hours after their anesthetic.

Patients should also be informed about common postoperative side effects that might be expected in order to allay anxiety that might be associated with these symptoms. Patients should be told to expect mild pain, nausea, and vomiting, sore throat, muscle aches, and headache. They should be given the telephone numbers of the surgeon, ambulatory center, and emergency room in case problems arise after discharge.

New and revised standards issued by the Joint Commission on Accreditation of Health Care Organizations (JCAHO) in the 1988 edition of the *Accreditation Manual for Hospitals* do not require a physician to examine the patient just prior to discharge; however, a licensed independent practitioner rigorously applying relevant discharge criteria must determine the readiness of the patient for discharge. When the patient meets these criteria, he or she can be discharged by the staff. These criteria are shown in Figure 20–1. Above all else, however, it must be remembered that when it is unclear if a patient is ready for discharge a physician should examine the patient, as clinical judgment is the most important indicator of readiness for discharge.

Finally, facilities should have a method of follow-up for their patients after discharge: Telephone calls the day after surgery or postcard evaluations are the most common methods used (Fig. 20–2). These follow-ups help ambulatory surgical centers obtain feedback on their performance while allowing patients the opportunity to express concerns regarding their ambulatory surgery experience.

RUSH-PRESBYTERIAN–ST. LUKE'S MEDICAL CENTER
PRESBYTERIAN–ST. LUKE'S HOSPITAL
CHICAGO, ILLINOIS 60612

POSTOPERATIVE FOLLOW-UP

SURGERY DATE: _____   PROCEDURE: _____

_____

ANESTHESIA: _____ Local   _____ Local/Sedation
            _____ Local/IV Valium   _____ General
            _____ Epidural   _____ Spinal
            _____ Regional

_____

CALLS TO PATIENT:

Date: _____ Time: _____ 1st Call _____RN
Date: _____ Time: _____ If unable to contact on 1st call
                                             2nd Call _____RN

	YES	NO	COMMENT
Headache			
Dizziness			
Nausea/vomiting			
Bleeding/draining > expected			
Pain > expected			
Delay in filling prescription			
Pain not relieved by medicine			

Were the written discharge instructions helpful to you?

_____ Very helpful   _____ Somewhat helpful   _____ Not helpful

Did you have **unanswered** questions about your recovery at home after your surgery?

_____ Many questions   _____ Some questions   _____ No questions

Did you feel prepared and comfortable with your return home after ambulatory surgery?

_____ Very comfortable   _____ Somewhat comfortable   _____ Not comfortable

How would you rate your overall experience in Ambulatory Surgery?

_____ Excellent   _____ Good   _____ Poor

Explain: _____

_____

RN Assessment:
Patient exhibits good understanding of care related to recovery.
_____ Yes   _____ No

_____

C:\WP\ASU.POC

FIGURE 20–1. Checklist of discharge criteria. (From Rush–Presbyterian–St. Luke's Medical Center; Chicago. With permission.)

AMBULATORY SURGERY
RECOVERY AND DISCHARGE RECORD

DATE: _____ TIME: _____ A/P

ADMITTING R.N.: _____

VITAL SIGNS						TIME					
	Pre-op										
B/P											
Pulse											
Respirations											
Temperature											
R.N. INITIALS											

RECOVERY STATUS						TIME					
Awake/alert/oriented											
Moves extremities											
Respirations full/ equal/spontaneous											
Up in chair											
Ambulates with assistance											
IV infusing (include site check)											
Tolerates PO fluids											
Tolerates PO foods											
Dressing dry & intact											
R.N. INITIALS											

MEDICATIONS				IV FLUIDS			
Medication	Dose	Time	R.N.	IV Fluid	Time Hung	Rate	RN

RN INITIALS	SIGNATURE & TITLE

DISCHARGE CRITERIA

___ Voided (if applicable)   ___ Minimal nausea/vomiting   ___ Patient give written post-op
___ Able to ambulate   ___ No pain medication for one (1) hour   instructions/prescriptions
___ Alert & oriented   ___ Minimal post-op pain   ___ No excess bleeding/drainage
___ Discharge to a responsible adult

Ready for Discharge: _____ A/P Discharge Time: _____ A/P

Physician: _____ Discharge R.N.: _____
       Signature & Title   Signature & Title
M/R Form #7843 Recv 7/89

FIGURE 20–2. Postdischarge follow-up form.

References

1. Waters RM: The down-town anesthesia clinic. Am J Surg (Anesth Suppl) *33*:71, 1919.
2. Wetchler BV: Patient and procedure selection: problems. Anesthesiology 2:9–17, 1988.
3. Wilson ME, Williams NB, Baskett PJF: Assessment of fitness for surgical procedures and the variability of anaesthetists' judgements. Br Med J *1*:509, 1980.
4. Blery C, Charpak Y, Szantan M, et al: Evaluation of a protocol for selective ordering of preoperative tests. Lancet *1*:139–141, 1986.
5. Roizen MF: Preoperative Patient Evaluation—What's Appropriate. ASA Refresher Course 1986, p. 412.
6. Hirsch IA, Tomlinson DL, Slogoff S, Keats AS: The overstated risk of preoperative hypokalemia. Anesth Analg 67:131–136, 1988.
7. Bridenbaugh LD, Soderstrom RM: Lumbar epidural block anesthesia for outpatient laparoscopy. J Reprod Med *23*:85–86, 1979.
8. Meridy HW: Criteria for selection of ambulatory surgery patients and guidelines for anesthetic management: a retrospective study of 1553 cases. Anesth Analg *61*:921–926, 1982.
9. Manchikanti L, Marrero TC: Effect of cimetidone and metoclopramide on gastric contents in outpatients. Anesthesiol Rev *10*:9–16, 1983.
10. Myers EF: Problems during eye surgery under local anesthesia. Anesthesiol Rev 6:23–25, 1979.
11. Kitz DS, Aukburg SJ, Lecky JH: It's not "only a local": haemodynamic and oxygen saturation changes among patients receiving local anesthesia. Anesthesiology 67:A264, 1987.
12. DiFazio CA, Carron H, Grosslight KR: Comparison of pH-adjusted lidocaine solutions for epidural anesthesia. Anesth Analg 65:760–764, 1986.
13. Hilgier M: Alkalinization of bupivacaine for tracheal plexus block. Reg Anesth *10*:59–61, 1985.
14. Mulroy MF: Regional anesthesia: when, why, why not? *In* Wetchler BV (ed): Problems in Anesthesia: Outpatient Anesthesia, Vol. 2. Philadelphia, Lippincott, 1988, pp. 82–92.
15. Pflug AE, Aasheim GM, Foster C: Sequence of return of neurological function and criteria for safe ambulation following subarachnoid block (spinal anaesthetic). Can Anaesth Soc J 25:133–139, 1978.
16. Jones RJ: Role of recumbency in prevention and treatment of post-spinal headache. Anesth Analg *53*:788–796, 1975.
17. Carbaat PAT, Van Creuel H: Lumbar puncture headache: controlled study on the preventive effect of 24 hours bed rest. Lancet 2:1133–1135, 1981.
18. Burke RK: Spinal anesthesia for laparoscopy: a review of 1263 cases. J Reprod Med *21*:59–62, 1978.
19. Flaaten H, Raeder J: Spinal anaesthesia for outpatient surgery. Anaesthesia *40*:1108–1111, 1985.
20. Quaynor H, Corbey M: Extradural blood patch—why delay? Br J Anaesth 57:538–540, 1985.
21. Ackerman WE, Colclaugh GW: Prophylactic epidural blood patch: the controversy continues. Anesth Analg 66:913–922, 1987.
22. Schzer PH, Abel L: Post-spinal anesthesia headache treated with caffeine. I. Evaluation with demand method. Curr Ther Res 24:307–312, 1978.
23. Harrington TM: An alternative treatment for spinal headache. J Fam Pract *15*:172–177, 1982.
24. Jarvis AP, Greenwalt JW, Fagraeus L: Intravenous caffeine for postdural puncture headache. Anesth Analg 65:316–317, 1986.
25. Cohen SE: Epidural blood patch on outpatients: a simpler approach. Anesth Analg *64*:458, 1985.
26. Wetchler BV: Outpatient anesthesia. *In* Barash P (ed): Clinical Anesthesia. Philadelphia, Lippincott, 1989, pp. 1346–1347.
27. Patel NJ, Flashburg MH, Parkin S, Grossman R: A regional anesthetic technique compared to general anesthesia for outpatient knee surgery. Anesth Analg 65:185–187, 1986.
28. Winnie AP, Ramamurthy DZ, Durrani Z: The inguinal paravascular technique of lumbar plexus anesthesia: the "3-in-1 block." Anesth Analg 52:989–996, 1973.
29. D'Amato H, Wielding S (eds): Intravenous regional anesthesia. Acta Anaesthesiol Scand 36S, 1969.
30. Philip BK, Covino BG: Local and regional anesthesia. *In* Wetchler BV (ed): Anesthesia for Ambulatory Surgery. Philadelphia, Lippincott, 1985, pp. 248–249.
31. Philip BK: Hazards of amnesia after midazolam in ambulatory surgical patients. Anesth Analg 66:97–98, 1987.
32. Levy ML, Weintraub HD: Premedication: yes or no? *In* Wetchler BV (ed): Problems in Anesthesia. Philadelphia, Lippincott, 1988, pp. 23–28.
33. Epstein BS, Levy ML, Thein MH, et al: Evaluation of fentanyl as an adjunct to thiopental nitrous oxide–oxygen anesthesia for short surgical procedures. Anesth Rev 2(3):24, 1975.
34. Anderson R, Crogh K: Pain as a major source of postoperative nausea. Can Anaesth Soc J *23*:366, 1976.
35. Manchikanti L, Caneloa MG, Hohlbein LJ, et al: Assessment of effect of various modes of premedication on acid aspiration risk factors in outpatient surgery. Anesth Analg 66:81, 1987.
36. Korttila K: Choice of drugs. Curr Opin Anaesthesiol *1*:54–59, 1988.
37. O'Toole DP, Milligan KR, Howe JP, et al: A comparison of propofol and methohexitone as induction agents for day case isoflurane anaesthesia. Anaesthesia *42*:373–376, 1987.
38. Edelist G: A comparison of propofol and thiopentone as induction agents in outpatient surgery. Can J Anaesth 34(2):110–116, 1987.
39. McDonald NJ, Mannion D, Lee P, et al: Mood evaluation and outpatient anaesthesia: a comparison between propofol and thiopentone. Anaesthesia *43S*:68–69, 1988.
40. Doze VA, Westphal LM, White PF: Comparison of propofol with methohexital for outpatient anesthesia. Anesth Analg 65:1189–1195, 1986.
41. Wetchler BV: Outpatient anesthesia. *In* Barash P (ed): Clinical Anesthesia. Philadelphia, Lippincott, 1989, pp. 1349–1350.
42. Zuurmond WW, Van Leeuwen L: Alfentanil vs. isoflurane for outpatient arthroscopy. Acta Anaesthesiol Scand 30:329–331, 1986.
43. Zuurmond WW, Van Leeuwen L: Recovery from sufentanil anesthesia for outpatient arthroscopy: a comparison with isoflurane. Acta Anaesthesiol Scand *31*:154–156, 1987.
44. Horrigan RW, Moyers JR, Johnson BH, et al: Etomidate vs. thiopental with and without fentanyl: a comparative study of awakening in man. Anesthesiology 52:362–364, 1980.

45. White PF, Chang T: Effect of narcotic premedication on the intravenous anesthetic requirement. Anesthesiology 61:A389, 1984.
46. Padfield A: Recovery comparison between enflurane and halothane technique: a study of outpatients undergoing cystoscopy. Anaesthesia 35:508, 1980.
47. Azar I, Karombelkar DJ, Lear E: Neurologic state and psychomotor function following anesthesia for ambulatory surgery. Anesthesiology 35:508, 1980.
48. Korttila K, Valanne J: Recovery after outpatient isoflurane and enflurane anesthesia. Anesth Analg 64:239, 1985.
49. Alexander GD, Skupski JN, Brown EM: The role of nitrous oxide in postoperative nausea and vomiting. Anesth Analg 63:175, 1984.
50. Lonie DS, Harper NJN: Nitrous oxide anaesthesia and vomiting. Anaesthesia 41:703, 1986.
51. Korttila K, Hovorka J, Erkola O: Omission of nitrous oxide does not decrease the incidence or severity of emetic symptoms after isoflurane anesthesia. Anesth Analg 66:S98, 1987.
52. Muir JJ, Warner MA, Offord KP, et al: Role of nitrous oxide and other factors in postoperative nausea and vomiting: a randomized and blinded prospective study. Anesthesiology 66:513, 1987.
53. Melnick BM, Johnson LS: Effects of eliminating nitrous oxide in outpatient anesthesia. Anesthesiology 67:982–984, 1987.
54. Lichtiger M, Wetchler BV, Philip BK: The adult and geriatric patient. In Wetchler BV (ed): Anesthesia for Ambulatory Surgery. Philadelphia, Lippincott, 1985, p. 202.
55. Sosis M, Broad T, Larijani GE, et al: Comparison of atracurium and d-tubocurarine for prevention of succinylcholine myalgia. Anesth Analg 66:657, 1987.
56. Brodsky JB, Ehrenwerth J: Postoperative muscle pain with suxamethonium. Br J Anaesth 52:215, 1980.
57. Zahl K, Apfelbaum JL: Muscle pain occurs after outpatient laparoscopy despite the substitution of vecuronium for succinylcholine. Anesthesiology 70:408–411, 1989.
58. Savarese JJ, Basta SJ, Ali HH, et al: Cardiovascular effects of BW 1090U in patients under nitrous oxide-oxygen-thiopental-fentanyl anesthesia. Anesthesiology 63:A319, 1985.
59. Ali HH, Savarese JJ, Embree PB, et al: Clinical pharmacology of BW 1090U continuous infusion. Anesthesiology 65:A282, 1986.
60. Basta SJ, Savarese JJ, Ali HH, et al: The neuromuscular pharmacology of BW 1090U in anesthetized patients. Anesthesiology 63:A318, 1985.
61. Wetchler BV: Outpatient anesthesia. In Barash P (ed): Clinical Anesthesia. Philadelphia, Lippincott, 1989, pp. 1349–1351.
62. Stirt JA: Accelerated recovery from combined atracurium-vecuronium neuromuscular blockade in man. Anesth Analg 66:S167, 1987.
63. Pandit SK, Kothary SP: Should we premedicate ambulatory surgical patients? Anesthesiology 65:A352, 1986.
64. Hunt TM, Plantevin OM, Gilbert JR: Morbidity in gynecological day-case surgery: a comparison of two anaesthetic techniques. Br J Anaesth 51:785, 1979.
65. Epstein BS, Levy ML, Thein MH, et al: Evaluation of fentanyl as an adjunct to thiopental-nitrous oxide-oxygen anesthesia for short surgical procedures. Anesth Rev 2(3):24, 1975.
66. Sanders RS, Sinclair ME, Sear JW: Alfentanil in short procedures. Anaesthesia 39:1202, 1984.
67. Short SM, Rutherford CS, Sebel PS: A comparison between isoflurane and alfentanil supplemented anaesthesia for short procedures. Anaesthesia 40:1160, 1985.
68. Jellicoe JA: A comparison of alfentanil, halothane, and enflurane for day-case gynaecological surgery. Anaesthesia 40:810, 1985.
69. Wetchler BV: The post anesthesia care unit: managing pain, nausea and vomiting. Probl Anesth 2:135–141, 1988.
70. Soni V, Burney R: Anesthetic techniques for laparoscopic tubal ligation. Anesthesiology 55:A145, 1981.
71. Garfield JM, Garfield FB, Phillip BK, et al: A comparison of clinical and psychological effects of fentanyl and nalbuphine in ambulatory gynecologic patients. Anesth Analg 66:1303–1307, 1987.
72. Bone ME, Dowson S, Smith G: A comparison of nalbuphine with fentanyl for postoperative pain relief following termination of pregnancy under day-case anaesthesia. Anaesthesia 43:194–197, 1988.
73. Pandit SK, Kothary ST, Pandit UA, Mathi NK: Comparison of fentanyl and butorphanol for outpatient anaesthesia. Can J Anaesth 34:130–134, 1987.
74. Shandling B, Stewart D: Regional analgesia for postoperative pain in pediatric outpatient surgery. J Pediatr Surg 15:477, 1980.
75. Hinkle HA: Percutaneous inguinal blocks for the outpatient management of post-herniorrhaphy pain in children. Anesthesiology 67:411–412, 1987.
76. Thompson RE, Wetchler BV, Alexander CD: Infiltration of the mesosalpinx for pain relief after laparoscopic tubal sterilization with yoon rings. J Reprod Med 32:537, 1987.
77. Alexander CD, Wetchler BV, Thompson RE: Bupivacaine infiltration of the mesosalpinx in ambulatory surgical laproscopic tubal sterilization. Can J Anaesth 34:362, 1987.
78. Broadman LM, Hannallah RS, Belman AB, et al: Post-circumcision analgesia—a prospective evaluation of subcutaneous ring block of the penis. Anesthesiology 67:399–402, 1987.
79. Tree-Karn T, Pirayavaraporn S, Lertakyamanee J: Topical analgesia for relief of post-circumcision pain. Anesthesiology 67:395–399, 1987.
80. Chirwa SS, MacLeod BA, Day B: Intra articular bupivacaine after arthroscopic meniscectomy: a randomized double blind controlled study. Arthroscopy 5:33–35, 1989.
81. Hannallah RS, Broadman LM, Belman AB, et al: Control of post-orchiopexy pain in pediatric outpatients: comparison of two regional techniques. Anesthesiology 61:A429, 1984.
82. Takasaki M, Dohi S, Kawahata Y, et al: Dosage of lidocaine for caudal anesthesia in infants and children. Anesthesiology 47:527, 1977.
83. Lund JW: Post-operative analgesia after circumcision. Anaesthesia 34:552, 1979.
84. Bramwell RGB, Bullen C, Radford P: Caudal block for post-operative analgesia in children. Anaesthesia 37:1024, 1982.
85. May AE, Wandless J, James RH: Analgesia for circumcision in children. Acta Anaesth Scand 26:331, 1982.
86. Yeoman PM, Cooke R, Hain WR: Penile block for circumcision. Anaesthesia 38:862, 1983.
87. Vater M, Wandless J: Caudal or dorsal nerve block?

A comparison of two local anaesthetics for postoperative analgesia following day-case circumcision. Acta Anaesthesiol Scand 29:175, 1985.

88. Buckler HW: Prophylaxis of post anesthetic vomiting period. Am J Surg Q [Anesth Analg Suppl] October 1914, p. 13.

89. Wetchler BV: Problem solving in the PACU. In Wetchler BV (ed): Anesthesia for Ambulatory Surgery. Philadelphia, Lippincott, 1985, pp. 275–316.

90. Swenson E, Orkin F: Postoperative nausea and vomiting. In Orkin F, Cooperman L (eds): Complications in Anesthesiology. Philadelphia, Lippincott, 1983, pp. 429–435.

91. Rising S, Dodgson MS, Steen PA: Isoflurane versus fentanyl for outpatient laparoscopy. Acta Anaesthesiol Scand 29:251–255, 1985.

92. Melnick BM, Chalasani J, Lim Uy NT: Comparison of enflurane, isoflurane, and continuous fentanyl infusion for outpatient anesthesia. Anesth Rev 11:36–39, 1984.

93. Alexander GD, Skupski JN, Brown EM: The role of nitrous oxide in postoperative nausea and vomiting. Anesth Analg 63:175, 1984.

94. Loni DS, Harper NJN: Nitrous oxide anaesthesia and vomiting. Anaesthesia 41:703, 1986.

95. Korttila K, Hovorka J, Erkola O: Nitrous oxide does not increase the incidence of nausea and vomiting after isoflurane anesthesia. Anesth Analg 66:761–765, 1987.

96. Gibbons P, Davidson P, Adler E: Nitrous oxide does not affect postop vomiting in pediatric eye surgery. Anesthesiology 67:530, 1987.

97. Mulroy MM: Regional anesthesia: when, why, why not? In Wetchler BV (ed): Problems in Anesthesia: Outpatient Anesthesia, Vol. 2. Philadelphia, Lippincott, 1988, pp. 83–91.

98. Caldamone AA, Rabinowitz R: Outpatient orchiopexy. J Urol 127:286, 1982.

99. Bonica JJ, Crepps W, Mark B, et al: Postoperative nausea, wretching and vomiting. Anesthesiology 19:532–540, 1958.

100. Smessaert A, Schehr C, Artusio J: Nausea and vomiting in the immediate post anesthetic period. JAMA 170:2072–2076, 1959.

101. Burtles R, Peckett BW: Postoperative vomiting. Br J Anaesth 29:114–123, 1957.

102. Knapp MR, Beecher HK: Post anaesthetic nausea, vomiting and wretching. JAMA 160:376–385, 1960.

103. Pataky AO, Kitz DS, Andrews RW, Lecky JH: Nausea and vomiting following ambulatory surgery: are all procedures created equal? Anesth Analg 67:S163, 1988.

104. Anderson R, Crohg K: Pain as a major cause of postoperative nausea. Can Anesth Soc J 23:366, 1976.

105. Wetchler BV, Collins IS, Jacob L: Anti-emetic effects of droperidol on the ambulatory surgery patient. Anesth Rev 9(5):23, 1982.

106. Valanne J, Korttila K: Effect of a small dose of droperidol on nausea, vomiting and recovery after outpatient enflurane anesthesia. Acta Anaesthesiol Scand 29:359, 1985.

107. Lerman J, Eustis S, Smith DR: Effect of droperidol pretreatment on post anesthetic vomiting in children undergoing strabismus surgery period. Anesthesiology 65:322, 1986.

108. Eustis S, Lerman J, Smith D: Droperidol pretreatment in children undergoing strabismus repair: the minimal effective dose. Can Anaesth Soc J 33:S115, 1986.

109. Rao TLK, Madhavareddy S, Chinthangada M, et al: Metoclopramide and cimetadine to reduce gastric fluid pH and volume. Anesth Analg 63:1014, 1984.

110. Diamond MJ, Keeri-Szanto M: Reduction of postoperative vomiting by preoperative administration of oral metoclopramide. Can Anesth Soc J 27:36, 1980.

111. Weiss JA, Goldberg ME, Norris MC, et al: Atropine and glycopyrrolate do not inhibit the effectiveness of metoclopramide and cimetidine in the general surgical population. Anesth Analg 68:S304, 1989.

112. Goldberg ME, Norris MC, Larijani GE, et al: Does atropine inhibit the effect of metoclopramide pretreatment on gastric contents in the morbidly obese population. Anesthesiology 67:A289, 1987.

113. Doze VA, Shafer A, White PF: Nausea and vomiting after outpatient anesthesia—effectiveness of droperidol alone and in combination with metoclopramide. Anesth Analg 66:S41, 1987.

114. Bidwai AV, Meuleman T, Thatte MD: Prevention of postoperative nausea with dimenhydrate (Dramamine) and droperidol (Inapsine). Anesth Analg 68:S25, 1989.

115. Rothenberg D, Parnass S, Newman L, et al: Ephedrine minimizes postoperative nausea and vomiting in outpatients. Anesth Analg 72:58–61, 1991.

116. Wood CD, Graybiel A: Evaluation of sixteen antimotion sickness drugs under controlled laboratory conditions. Aerospace Med 39:1341–1344, 1968.

INFECTIOUS DISEASES

JAMES J. GORDON
and GRANT O. WESTENFELDER

21

Postoperative fever continues to be a significant problem in the care of surgical patients. Although the causes are many, an accurate diagnosis can most often be reached through a working awareness of the spectrum of etiologies, special attention to the temporal onset of the fever, and a thoughtful history and physical examination.

Two broad groups can be used to categorize postoperative fevers: those related to the operative procedure itself and those associated with the generalized postoperative state. Complications due to the operation itself include infection present preoperatively at the operative site and postoperative wound infection. Although any surgical procedure may produce a simple wound infection, the location of the procedure may give clues to other potential complications. For example, an intraabdominal operation may be associated with an intraabdominal, subphrenic, or hepatic abscess. After cardiovascular surgery, sternal osteomyelitis or mediastinitis may ensue. A pelvic operation may be complicated by pelvic abscess or septic pelvic thrombophlebitis. Similarly, in neurosurgical, orthopedic, and other surgical subspecialty procedures, the type of infection may be unique to the type of procedure performed.

Although postoperative fevers due to specific surgical procedures are essential considerations, most postoperative fevers are related to the generalized postoperative state. For instance, causes of fever during the procedure or within the first 24 hours postoperatively may include malignant hyperthermia, transfusion reaction, atelectasis, aspiration pneumonia, drug reaction, endocrinopathies (e.g., thyroid storm, acute adrenal insufficiency, or pheochromocytoma), special types of wound infection, and idiopathic fevers related to the surgery itself.[1-4] Causes of fever typically occurring after the initial 24 to 48 hours are most often due to infection of an intravenous site (with or without bacteremia), wound, urinary tract, or lung or to deep venous thrombosis.[5] Infections unrelated to the operation must also be considered, such as acute cholecystitis.[6] Only after an analysis of the timing of the onset of fever and its relation to the particular operation along with evaluation of the patient's complaints, physical examination, and significant laboratory findings may the cause of fever become apparent.

The remainder of our current discussion is confined to the evaluation and therapy of a selected group of infections that may present within the first 48 to 72 hours postoperatively (Table 21–1). These infections include special types of wound infection, intravenous line infections, urinary tract infections, pneumonia, and sepsis. Life-threatening problems such as malignant hyperthermia are discussed elsewhere (see Chapter 16).

WOUND INFECTION

The overall wound infection rate for all types of operative wounds is about 5 per cent. Wound infection is not only a significant source of morbidity and mortality, but as Green and Wenzel have reported, it is a major source of increased hospital costs.[7] In their study, when wound infection complicated operations, the average length of hospital stay was doubled with a proportional increase in costs.

A variety of principles, when closely adhered to, have been shown to decrease the incidence of infection in clean surgical wounds.[8-10] Such principles include a short preoperative hospital stay (which decreases gram-negative colonization), preoperative hexachlorophene shower with minimal shaving at the surgical site, short surgical procedures, meticulous surgical technique, and avoidance of drains exteriorized through the operative wound. Furthermore, it is essential

TABLE 21–1. CAUSES OF FEVER DURING THE EARLY POSTOPERATIVE PERIOD

Physiologic response
Endocrinopathies
    Acute addisonian crisis
    Thyroid storm
    Pheochromocytoma
Transfusion reactions
Atelectasis
Drug-related fever
    Malignant hyperthermia
    Other drug fevers
Infections
    Wound infection
        Streptococci
        Clostridia
    Urinary tract infections
    Vascular catheter infections
    Pneumonia
Deep venous thrombosis and pulmonary emboli

to stress strict handwashing by hospital personnel caring for surgical patients.

Preoperative antimicrobial prophylaxis has been clearly shown to decrease the incidence of postoperative wound infections for certain operations.[11,12] The primary principle guiding the appropriate use of prophylactic systemic antibiotics during surgery is the anticipated risk of bacterial contamination. Prophylaxis has not traditionally been utilized for operations classified as clean, unless a foreign body is implanted.

The basic components of antibiotic prophylaxis include antibiotic selection, timing of delivery, and route and duration of administration. The antibiotics selected should have antimicrobial efficacy against the microorganisms that most often cause infectious complications in each particular clinical setting. Antibiotic serum and tissue levels must be therapeutic at the time of potential surgical contamination to be most effective. Therefore intravenous antibiotics should be given approximately 0.5 to 1.0 hour prior to the operative procedure. When orally administered antibiotics are utilized, as for elective colon surgery, a 24 hour preparative period is adequate. Longer periods of preoperative preparation are not necessary and have been associated with the isolation of resistant organisms in the colonic lumen at the time of surgery.[13] Administration of antibiotics should generally be continued only through the duration of the operation for clean and clean-contaminated procedures. For "dirty" operations therapy

should usually be continued for 5 to 10 days. Continuation of antibiotics beyond these time periods has not been show to decrease the incidence of wound infection. However, it does increase the risk of drug toxicity and emergence of drug-resistant organisms, which may result in superinfection.

When wound infection occurs within the first 24 hours after an operation, it invariably is due to either *Clostridium* or the group A β-hemolytic streptococcus. These infections are heralded by a rapid clinical presentation, frequently within a few hours postoperatively. Manifestations may include profound systemic toxicity associated with rapid local advance of the infection, often with involvement of all layers of the body wall. Primary treatment includes parenteral antibiotics and careful attention to fluid, electrolyte, and hemodynamic status, as well as aggressive early débridement of devitalized tissues in the case of clostridial infection.

A more recently appreciated wound infection that can occur within the first 24 to 72 hours postoperatively is the wound-related toxic shock syndrome (TSS) due to *Staphylococcus aureus*[14,15] (Table 21–2). Postoperative TSS is similar to that seen in tampon-related disease, manifesting as hypotension, fever, diffuse erythroderma, profuse watery diarrhea, thrombocytopenia, hypocalcemia, hypoalbuminemia, and multiorgan involvement. Key to successful therapy is a high index of clinical suspicion with subsequent prompt diagnosis. Although such patients seemingly have clean surgical wounds, the wound must be promptly reopened, cultured, and thoroughly irrigated. Gram stain of the wound can provide a prompt presumptive diagnosis by demonstrating gram-positive cocci in clusters. Antistaphylococcal antibiotics and careful attention to hemodynamic status and end-organ function are essential to recovery and prevention of relapse.

TABLE 21–2. TOXIC SHOCK SYNDROME

Hypotension
Fever
Diffuse erythroderma
Diarrhea
Thrombocytopenia
Hypocalcemia
Hypoalbuminemia
Multiorgan failure

INTRAVENOUS LINE INFECTIONS

Intravenous line infections account for more than 50,000 cases of nosocomial sepsis each year.[16] Although they occur most often after the catheter has been in place for several days, they should be considered in the differential diagnosis of fever during the immediate postoperative period. They are particularly common in patients who have been hospitalized for several days prior to their operation or who have had intravenous lines inserted under suboptimal conditions in the field.

Most factors that increase the risk of vascular infection are related to poor insertion and maintenance techniques. This observation has been confirmed by the decreased incidence of infection observed when a team approach using standardized insertion and maintenance techniques is utilized.[17,18] Other factors known to decrease the risk of infection are preinsertion skin preparation and use of topical antibiotics at the insertion site.[19,20] Ideally, peripheral venous catheter sites are changed every 3 days and central venous catheter sites every 4 days. (Absolute frequency of line changes are presently controversial.) The use of topical antibiotics is especially valuable if a catheter cannot be changed with "ideal" frequency. The value of topical antibiotics when a catheter is in place for shorter periods is less significant. Practices of no proved benefit in decreasing infection risk include use of in-line filters, changing catheters at intervals over guidewires, or changing the infusate tubing any more frequently than every 48 to 72 hours.[16,21–24]

The clinical features of line sepsis may be indistinguishable from bloodstream infection arising from any other site. Therefore a high index of clinical suspicion is essential for accurate diagnosis. Expressible purulence at the cannula insertion site is an important clue, but this sign is present in fewer than one-third of cases. A minimum of two sets of blood cultures should be obtained from separate sites. In those patients already receiving antibiotics, use of cell wall stabilizing solutions (e.g., high sucrose media) and use of resin-containing media (e.g., an antimicrobial removal device) should be considered. The intravenous catheter itself as well as the entire administration set should be removed when possible. Changing a vascular catheter over a guidewire may be used diagnostically if there is no gross evidence of catheter-related infection in a febrile postoperative patient. However, if the culture is positive for an organism other than *Staphylococcus epidermidis,* removal of the replacement catheter should be considered, as discussed below. The catheter tip should be cultured using the semiquantitative method of Maki et al.[25] Any purulent drainage at the cannula site also should be Gram-stained and cultured. Lastly, a sample of the infusate should be obtained if this source is considered possibly responsible for the infection. In the case of suspected blood contamination, specimens should be incubated at several temperatures, as the causative organism may be cryophilic.

The three organisms responsible for most intravascular catheter infections are coagulase-negative staphylococci (especially *S. epidermidis*), *Staphylococcus aureus,* and yeast.[16] Less frequent causes of line infections include *Enterococcus* spp., *Pseudomonas aeruginosa, Klebsiella pneumoniae, Corynebacterium* sp., *Serratia marcescens,* and others.

Coagulase-negative staphylococci are currently responsible for most of the line infections. This phenomenon may be due to increased use of long-term central venous catheters. Although initially it was believed that catheter removal was essential for recovery, more recent studies have demonstrated that it is often not required.[26,27] Forty to eighty per cent of hospital-acquired organisms are resistant to semisynthetic penicillins.[28,29] Furthermore, although in vitro sensitivity to cephalosporins may appear good, the in vivo performance of these agents in treating coagulase-negative staphylococci is poor. Vancomycin is the drug of choice, although the required duration of therapy is not well defined. In the immunocompetent host, simply removing the catheter or treatment with vancomycin for 3 to 7 days is often adequate. More critically ill patients require a longer course of therapy, and it is reasonable to continue therapy until bone marrow recovery in neutropenic patients who have recently had chemotherapy.[27] For those organisms resistant to vancomycin, trimethoprim-sulfamethoxazole and ciprofloxacin are alternative agents. Caution must be exercised when using orally administered agents in the clearly septic patient, as gastrointestinal absorption may be unpredictable.

Vascular infections due to *S. aureus* frequently require prompt removal of the catheter as well as judicious use of antistaphylococcal antibiotics. However, occasionally these infections can be eradicated without catheter removal. Candidates for leaving the line in place include patients who do not have purulence at the catheter site or who do not appear to be clinically septic and those who respond rapidly to antimicrobial therapy. The appropriate duration of treatment of these line infections is somewhat controversial. Data addressing the likelihood of *S. aureus* bacteremia due to a removable focus of infection being responsible for endocarditis or another metastatic focus of infection are somewhat mixed.[30–33] If 1) the infection is recognized promptly and treated, 2) the patient is not at risk for endocarditis because of prior rheumatic fever or valve replacement, 3) there are no permanent prosthetic devices at risk for infection due to bacteremic seeding, and 4) the patient responds quickly to an antistaphylococcal drug with rapid defervescence and sterilization of blood cultures, a short (2 week) course of antibiotics may be considered adequate. In general, in patients who go on to have a difficult course, complications (e.g., a new heart murmur or metastatic focus of infection) become apparent within the first 2 weeks of therapy. In such patients and in those in whom the initial response to therapy is slow, there is underlying cardiac valvular disease or a prosthetic device, or if the patient is diabetic or otherwise immunocompromised a 4- to 6-week course of therapy is recommended.

The cornerstone of therapy of intravascular infections due to *Candida albicans* is prompt removal of the catheter. Although most immunocompetent patients respond rapidly and completely to this intervention alone, some patients develop disseminated disease, including *Candida* endophthalmitis.[34] In that there is no predictable way to prospectively identify the group of patients destined to develop disseminated disease, if antifungal chemotherapy is withheld it is essential that patients be followed closely for evidence of recurrent yeast infection, including frequent funduscopic examinations. Unequivocal indications for amphotericin B include associated positive blood cultures for *Candida,* persistent fever after catheter removal, retinal lesions consistent with *Candida* infection, evidence of *Candida* infection elsewhere, and occurrence in an immunocompromised host.

Bloodstream infections caused by *Enterobacter cloacae, Enterobacter agglomerans, Pseudomonas* sp. other than *Ps. aeruginosa,* *Citrobacter,* or *Candida* species other than *C. albicans* should immediately raise the possibility of infusate contamination.[35,36]

URINARY TRACT INFECTIONS

Infections associated with urinary catheters typically occur several days after catheter placement, as is generally the case with intravascular catheter infections. However, such infections may present with fever during the immediate postoperative period if the patient had been in the hospital with a catheter in place for any length of time prior to operation. Urinary tract infections currently account for 40 to 50 per cent of nosocomial infections: 85 per cent of them are associated with indwelling catheters, and another 5 per cent follow other types of urologic instrumentation.[37]

As noted previously, duration of catheterization is an important risk factor for infection, as the average rate of acquisition of bacteriuria is 5 to 10 per cent for each day of catheterization.[38] After 10 days of catheterization, approximately 50 per cent of patients have bacteriuria. In addition to duration of catheterization, predisposing factors to the acquisition of bacteriuria include female sex, age over 50 years, and the presence of significant underlying disease.

Autoinfection from the patient's own gastrointestinal flora is the source of most catheter-associated infections.[38] *Escherichia coli* accounts for approximately one-third of infections. Other gram-negative bacilli such as *Proteus* sp., *Klebsiella* sp., *Pseudomonas* sp., and *Enterobacter* sp. are responsible for almost half of the infections. The remainder are due to enterococci, *Candida,* and other gram-negative bacilli.

The severity of infection may range from being asymptomatic, to mild temperature elevations without other symptoms, to frank septic shock. It is critical to determine whether the symptoms are secondary to catheter-associated bacteriuria or the source of fever is a different site. A careful physical examination, including inspection of any operative wounds and all intravascular access sites, is essential.

Therapy involves institution of appropriate antimicrobial therapy based on a Gram stain of the urine, with modification of the treatment regimen if bacterial identification and in vitro sensitivity data so indicate. The catheter should be removed, if possible.

NOSOCOMIAL PNEUMONIA

Nosocomial pneumonia is defined as a lower respiratory tract infection that develops in a hospitalized patient in whom the infection was not present or incubating at the time of hospital admission. It is the third most common hospital-acquired infection, behind urinary tract infections (42 per cent) and wound infections (24 per cent), accounting for 10 to 15 per cent of nosocomial infections.[39] However, compared with infections at alternate sites, nosocomial pneumonia has the greatest total impact on hospital costs and is the most frequent lethal hospital-acquired infection.[40]

PATHOPHYSIOLOGY

Organisms generally cause pneumonia by one of four basic mechanisms: aspiration of oropharyngeal contents, inhalation of aerosolized particles, hematogenous spread, and direct extension from contiguous sites. The latter two mechanisms are unusual and are not discussed further.

Inhalation of aerosolized particles had previously been a significant source of nosocomial pneumonia in patients utilizing nebulizer respiratory therapy devices. However, because of routine decontamination procedures currently employed, it is no longer a significant problem. Outbreaks of nosocomial pneumonia still occasionally occur, though, owing to aerosolized pathogens such as *Legionella* sp., *Mycobacterium tuberculosis, Aspergillus* sp., and hospital-associated viral infection.

The principal mode of acquiring nosocomial pneumonia is aspiration of oropharyngeal contents. Small liquid boluses of 0.001 to 0.0001 ml commonly contain 10^4 organisms, a sufficient amount to result in pneumonia in laboratory animals. When an aerosolized route is utilized, at least 10^7 organisms are required to result in clinically significant disease.[41,42]

Aspiration of oropharyngeal contents is a common event, even in healthy individuals. At least 70 per cent of patients with impaired consciousness experience aspiration of oropharyngeal secretions, as do 50 per cent of normal individuals during sleep.[43] Clearly, not all of these individuals develop clinical pneumonia. In patients with significant underlying illness, primary lung defenses may be inadequate to clear microaspiration. In patients with impaired consciousness, the volume of aspirated material and subsequently the pathogenic load may be significantly greater.

In that aspirated organisms are the principal pathogens in nosocomial pneumonia, the host's oropharyngeal flora dictates the etiology of the infection. Normal hosts are typically colonized by a number of gram-positive and anaerobic organisms of relatively low pathogenicity. Fewer than 2 per cent of normal hosts are colonized by gram-negative organisms.[44] However, chronically debilitated and acutely ill patients frequently become colonized with gram-negative pathogens. In the intensive care unit (ICU) setting, more than 50 per cent of patients are commonly colonized, correlating with the degree of illness of the patient.[45]

With *typical nosocomial pneumonia* there is an alteration of the host's normal oropharyngeal flora with emergence of gram-negative organisms. This change is followed by aspiration of oropharyngeal contents, overwhelming of host defenses, and clinical pneumonia.

A subset of nosocomial pneumonias occurs early in patients' hospital course. These infections have been termed *early-onset pneumonia,* by definition occurring within 4 days of presentation to the intensive care area.[46] In contrast to typical nosocomial pneumonia, early-onset pneumonia frequently occurs in patients who were healthy prior to the onset of their acute illness. It is strongly associated with events inducing impairment of normal airway protective reflexes, e.g., depressed consciousness, myocardial infarction, shock, or a therapeutic intervention. This association together with the microbiologic data, which rarely implicate typical nosocomial organisms in the absence of previous hospitalization, suggest that aspiration of oropharyngeal contents at the onset of a severe event may be the pathophysiologic mechanism. Hence these infections are not truly nosocomial in origin. Nevertheless, they are an important cause of pneumonia in hospitalized patients. In one study, early-onset pneumonia was found to account for more than 50 per cent of nosocomial pneumonias occurring in the ICU setting.[46]

The early-onset variation of "nosocomial" pneumonia has important therapeutic and prognostic implications. Empiric antibiotic therapy must cover organisms that are part of the normal oropharyngeal flora. The prognosis in these patients, in that they are frequently without significant underlying pulmonary disease, is somewhat better than that associated with typical nosocomial pneumonia.

MICROBIOLOGY

In that aspiration of oropharyngeal contents is the most important pathophysiologic mechanism for the development of nosocomial pneumonia, organisms present in the oropharynx at the time of aspiration are the most frequent pathogens. With typical nosocomial pneumonia, gram-negative organisms including *Pseudomonas aeruginosa, Klebsiella pneumonia, Enterobacter* sp., *Serratia marcescens, Escherichia coli,* and *Proteus* sp. account for 60 to 80 per cent of cases. *Staphylococcus aureus* is the most frequent gram-positive organism, accounting for 10 to 15 per cent of all cases.[47] Other gram-positive organisms are relatively unusual pathogens in typical nosocomial pneumonia, although they are frequently encountered in early-onset pneumonia. Anaerobic organisms are infrequently documented as pathogens in nosocomial pneumonia, but this finding may be due to inadequate specimen attainment and culture for these organisms.

In that hospitals are being increasingly populated with immunocompromised patients, the spectrum of opportunistic pulmonary infections has broadened. Organisms not infrequently encountered include fungi such as *Candida* sp., *Aspergillus* sp., and *Cryptococcus neoformans;* viruses such as cytomegalovirus, herpes simplex, and herpes zoster; protozoa such as *Pneumocystis carinii* and *Toxoplasmosis gondii;* and bacterial species such as *Legionella* sp., *Nocardia* sp., *Mycobacterium tuberculosis,* and atypical mycobacteria.

DIAGNOSIS AND THERAPY

The accurate diagnosis of nosocomial pneumonia is often an exceedingly difficult task. Physical examination in critically ill patients is frequently misleading and inaccurate. Isolation of organisms from sputum specimens is often indicative only of oropharyngeal colonization. Similarly, the appearance of an infiltrate on chest roentgenogram is sufficiently nonspecific to render it inadequate when used alone. A variety of noninfectious disorders may mimic a pneumonic infiltrate, e.g., pulmonary edema, adult respiratory distress syndrome, atelectasis, pulmonary emboli, hemorrhage, neoplasia, and injury due to oxygen, drugs, or radiation. The clinical findings of dyspnea and hypoxemia may also be due to any of the above.

Therapy of nosocomial pneumonia is based on establishing a specific microbiologic diagnosis and instituting an antibiotic regimen directed toward the pathogen(s) involved. However, it is frequently a difficult task. Sputum specimens isolate the responsible organism in only 40 to 80 per cent of cases. Frequently, it is impossible to distinguish colonizing organisms from those causing an infection. Moreover, polymicrobial infections are present in some cases, further confusing the clinical scenario. Nevertheless, sputum examination must be attempted in each case. A good quality specimen that is judged to be free of oropharyngeal contamination (fewer than 10 epithelial cells and more than 25 polymorphonuclear leukocytes per high power field) can be helpful. One must be careful to correlate culture findings with Gram stain results. An unremarkable Gram stain with a positive culture is most likely representative of oropharyngeal contamination. Likewise, a Gram stain with many gram-negative bacilli followed by a negative culture may be indicative of an anaerobic infection or one due to fastidious organisms.

Other specimens that may be helpful in determining the etiology of pneumonia include blood and pleural fluid, if available. Invasive diagnostic techniques such as fiberoptic bronchoscopy with a protected brush catheter and bronchoalveolar lavage are useful in selected cases. The latter procedures may be particularly helpful in immunocompromised patients or in those failing standard therapy.

In that a precise and accurate microbiologic diagnosis is often not attainable, antimicrobial therapy of nosocomial pneumonia is often empiric. The initial therapeutic spectrum must be broad enough to include all likely pathogens. Consideration must be given to a variety of factors. Patients who develop pneumonia while on antibiotics for some other purpose frequently are infected with organisms resistant to those agents. Those patients with chronic obstructive pulmonary disease are at particular risk for infections due to *Hemophilus influenza* or *Branhamella catarrhalis.* Patients with various disorders of immune function may be at particular risk for infection with certain organisms. Patients who are intubated and are receiving mechanical assistance are frequently infected with highly virulent gram-negative pathogens. Certain hospitals harbor gram-negative organisms with unusual antibiotic resistance patterns or a high percentage of methicillin-resistant *Staphylococcus aureus*. Other institutions have a high incidence of pneumonias due to less common organisms such as *Legionella pneumophila*. Hence when selecting an antimicrobial regimen it is important to take into account both host and environmental factors.

In that aminoglycoside therapy may be difficult in critically ill patients with concomitant renal insufficiency, and that its activity in the anaerobic, acidic milieu typical of pulmonary infection is questionable, some have questioned the use of these agents for pneumonia, favoring a monotherapy β-lactam regimen. Others have argued that the addition of an aminoglycoside to a β-lactam is synergistic against many gram-negative organisms and is associated with improved outcome.[48] In any event, aminoglycosides should not be used alone for the therapy of any nosocomial pneumonia. Agents with a broad spectrum of activity, e.g., third generation cephalosporins or carbapenams, may be reasonable agents in the nonimmunocompromised patient who is not floridly septic. In patients immunocompromised owing to neutropenia, a combination approach with an aminoglycoside plus a third generation cephalosporin or ureidopenicillin is most prudent. For those patients with impaired cell-mediated immunity, tuberculosis and *Pneumocystis carinii* infection must also be considered. In patients who were not on trimethoprim-sulfamethoxazole prophylaxis, addition of this agent should be considered. For patients who have a central venous catheter or are otherwise at risk for staphylococcal infection, coverage for this organism with vancomycin should be considered as well.

As an alternative to initial empiric therapy, especially for those patients who are immunocompromised or severely ill, an invasive diagnostic procedure should be strongly considered. For the immunocompromised patient the spectrum of possible etiologies is too broad to adequately cover with empiric therapy unless a multitude of agents are employed with resultant increased toxicity, possible antimicrobial antagonism, and increased cost. For those patients who are critically ill, if the diagnosis is not reasonably certain, invasive diagnostic procedures can help guide initial therapy and optimize future therapy based on in vitro susceptibility testing. In the stable, nonimmunocompromised patient, it is reasonable to initiate empiric therapy, as outlined above. If the patient's condition deteriorates or there is no improvement after 2 to 3 days of therapy, the use of more invasive diagnostic techniques may be pursued.

PREVENTION

The initial approach to the prevention of any disorder is the modification of risk factors, if possible. A wide variety of risk factors for nosocomial pneumonia have been identified, including endotracheal intubation, illness severe enough to require ICU admission, use of multiple antibiotics, use of H_2-blocking agents or antacids, advanced age, underlying pulmonary disease, immunosuppression, and recent surgery.[49,50] Those surgical patients who are having thoracic, upper abdominal, or thoracoabdominal procedures, and those who undergo prolonged procedures are clearly at increased risk. Patients should be urged to stop smoking preoperatively and be extubated as expeditiously as possible. Antibiotic use should be limited as much as possible. Lastly, some recommend the use of sucralfate rather than H_2-blocking agents or antacids when gastric stress ulcer prophylaxis is indicated.

Use of prophylactic antibiotics has been explored as a possible means of preventing gram-negative colonization. Use of aerosolized polymyxin B or gentamicin had initially been successful with decreasing gram-negative colonization but was later associated with excessive microbial resistance.[51,52] More recently, attempts have been made to "decontaminate" the oropharynx and gastrointestinal tract with a combined-modality approach, utilizing the oropharyngeal antibiotic paste and oral antibiotics via a feeding tube with[53] or without[54] systemic antibiotics. Despite promising results, these modalities await further study before they can be clinically applicable. At present, strict handwashing, monitoring for nosocomial "outbreaks" and respiratory equipment contamination, and modifying risk factors remain our only means of trying to reduce the incidence of nosocomial pneumonia.

POSTOPERATIVE SEPSIS

EARLY DETECTION

Sepsis is the most common cause of death following major surgery.[55] Early recognition of patients who are developing sepsis prior to development of the full-blown syndrome, with prompt institution of aggressive therapeutic interventions, markedly improves the clinical outcome of these patients. Wilson reported a large group of patients with blood-culture-proved sepsis in whom mortality was decreased from 65 per cent to 12 per cent when the diagnosis was made while the patient had only fever and leukocytosis rather than septic shock.[56] In a study reviewing intraabdominal sepsis, the mortality rate for patients with peritonitis developing soon after the primary operative procedure was 60 per cent compared with 27 per cent in those who had peritonitis at a time removed from their operation.[57] This difference was attributed to delays in diagnosis in the group who had recently undergone operation.

However, in patients who have had recent major surgery, prompt and accurate diagnosis of sepsis often is difficult. Many of the features commonly attributed to sepsis, e.g., fever and leukocytosis, are normal phenomena of the postoperative period. Intraabdominal sepsis may be masked by postoperative narcotics and mimicked by pain at the surgical incision site. Chest roentgenographic changes normally associated with pneumonia may be inaccurately interpreted to be postoperative atelectasis, and decreased urine output and hypotension may be incorrectly attributed to third-spacing of fluids.

The *"septic" syndrome* has been defined in an effort to identify a group of patients at particularly high risk for developing sepsis.[58] These patients can be identified by the presence of a collection of easily obtained clinical parameters (Table 21–3). Positive blood or closed-space confirmative cultures are not among the inclusion criteria. In fact, the first and most important criterion is evidence of an infection based on a high index of clinical suspicion. The patient with the septic syndrome should have fever higher than 101°F or hypo-

thermia less than 96°F, a heart rate of more than 90 beats/min, a respiratory rate of more than 20 breaths per minute, and evidence of organ dysfunction or hypoperfusion. The latter may manifest as altered mentation, a PaO_2 of less than 75 mm Hg, elevated plasma lactic acid levels, or a urine output of less than 30 ml/hr. The rationale for utilizing such a broad definition for the septic syndrome is to facilitate early institution of therapeutic intervention in a population at high risk for significant morbidity and mortality. One study utilizing these criteria identified a group of patients, two thirds of whom ultimately developed septic shock, usually within 24 hours, with a subsequent mortality of 30 per cent.[58]

Although the septic syndrome outlines many of the clinical features of early sepsis, these findings also are common in the uninfected postoperative population, rendering their clinical utility in these patients somewhat limited. Recognition of some of the other more salient features of sepsis, e.g., a depressed platelet count, altered liver function tests, and difficulty attaining an alkaline gastric pH despite the use of antacids or H_2-blocking agents,[59] may be helpful. In patients who have a pulmonary artery catheter in place, depressed systemic vascular resistance or increased mixed venous oxygen saturation values may be early signs of sepsis. In fact, a significant fall in oxygen consumption with a resultant increase in mixed venous oxygen saturation may be observed as early as 12 hours prior to the onset of hypotension in septic patients.[60]

Ultimately, timely diagnosis of sepsis relies heavily on the ability of the clinician to correctly interpret a collection of clinical information and to maintain a high index of suspicion when treating a patient at risk. Hence the possibility of septicemia should be entertained in any patient who develops changes in body temperature, altered mentation, hyperventilation, increased heart rate, or depressed blood pressure. Although reasons other than sepsis may be responsible for these changes, one must be particularly concerned about sepsis when these changes develop during the postoperative period.

The onset of shock may occur as early as 1 to 2 hours after a bacteremic event, as has been demonstrated in patients undergoing urologic instrumentation. The early phase of shock has been described as "warm" shock. In this phase, the high cardiac output and decreased peripheral vascular resistance cause

TABLE 21–3. SEPTIC SYNDROME

Clinical suspicion of infection
Fever ≥101°F or hypothermia of < 96°F
Heart rate >90 beats per minute
Respiratory rate >20 breaths per minute
Evidence of organ dysfunction or hyperperfusion
    Altered mentation
    PaO_2 <75 mm Hg
    Elevated plasma lactic acid levels
    Urine output <30 ml per hour

patients to appear warm, with dry skin, hyperdynamic pulses, and a ruddy complexion. The hypotension in these patients is a result of the inability of the heart to maintain adequate cardiac output owing to decreased preload from intravascular volume redistribution, decreased afterload, and decreased cardiac inotropy. The latter effect has been attributed, in part, to a substance referred to as myocardial depressant factor (MDF).[61]

Impaired mentation is a common finding early in the course of septicemia, particularly in the elderly patient.[62] Cerebral hypoperfusion is probably a prime contributor to impaired mentation, although β-endorphins may also play a role.

Dermatologic findings may precede the clinical onset of septic shock and often give clues to the etiologic diagnosis. Ecthyma gangrenosum is a painful urticarial lesion that progresses to skin necrosis.[63] It usually is associated with sepsis due to *Pseudomonas aeruginosa* but has also been described with *Aeromonas* sp., other gram-negative organisms, and *Candida* fungemia. Other skin lesions associated with gram-negative sepsis include deep-seated nodules, abscesses, and erysipelas-like lesions.[64] Petechiae may be seen as the result of thrombocytopenia. Erythematous or purpuric papules may be seen in sepsis due to *Candida* sp. or *Trichosporon* sp.

Gastrointestinal symptoms such as nausea, vomiting, and diarrhea with or without ileus may occur during this stage owing to the action of potent smooth muscle contracting compounds and alimentary tract hypoperfusion. Gastric erosions, occasionally complicated by major gastrointestinal bleeding, are common in septic shock.[65,66] Some patients develop a pattern of cholestatic jaundice that has been reported to precede the clinical onset of sepsis by several days.[67]

A variety of renal abnormalities occur in the septic patient, varying from minimal proteinuria to acute renal failure. Acute renal failure most often is attributed to acute tubular necrosis as a result of hypotension and relative volume depletion. In septic patients without evidence of frank shock, renal insufficiency may also be due to glomerulonephritis or interstitial nephritis. A multitude of extrarenal infections, e.g., endocarditis, ventriculoatrial shunt infections, and visceral abscesses, have been implicated as causes of glomerulonephritis, some secondary to immune mechanisms.[68-70] Tubulointerstitial disease not due to acute tubular necrosis may also occur secondary to drugs such as methicillin[71] or because of microbial antigen accumulation within the renal interstitium.[72]

Among the most devastating complications seen in bacteremic shock is the development of the adult respiratory distress syndrome (ARDS). Although the exact pathophysiology remains unclear, the final pathway appears to be increased microvascular permeability with resultant noncardiogenic pulmonary edema. The most frequent early finding is tachypnea with a normal chest roentgenogram and an arterial blood gas revealing respiratory alkalosis. Over the following 24 to 48 hours, the patient becomes increasingly dyspneic with progressive hypoxemia, decreased pulmonary compliance, and the development of diffuse pulmonary infiltrates. Frank ARDS is defined in a patient with the above clinical scenario who has a PaO_2 less than 60 mm Hg while receiving more than 50 per cent inspired oxygen.

A variety of aberrations of blood elements may herald the onset of septic shock. A new leukocytosis or leukopenia may be seen, often with an increase in immature forms. Dohle bodies, toxic granulations and vacuoles indicate rapid marrow maturation and release of leukocytes, with increased intravascular activation.[73,74] Mild to moderate thrombocytopenia is a common finding, occurring in up to 70 per cent of patients.[75,76]

Disseminated intravascular coagulation (DIC), a syndrome seen in a variety of clinical situations, involves the simultaneous activation of fibrin formation and fibrinolysis.[77-79] Although gram-negative sepsis is one of the most common causes of DIC, it is only apparent in 11 per cent of patients by laboratory testing and 3 per cent clinically.[80] Other laboratory findings include a prolonged prothrombin time, partial thromboplastin time, and thrombin time, thrombocytopenia, decreased levels of fibrinogen, and an elevated level of circulating fibrin degradation products. Clinically, patients develop bleeding from venipuncture sites, within intradermal or subcutaneous tissues, and from mucous membranes of the nose, mouth, or gastrointestinal tract. Thrombotic events of small vessels may occur, but they are rare.

The later stage of septic shock is characterized by increasing peripheral vascular resistance and decreasing cardiac output. This phase has been termed the "cold" phase of septic shock. As cardiac output decreases, a vicious cycle of deteriorating pulmonary, renal, and cardiac function ensues with progressive impairment of organ function. The resulting hypotension activates the sympathetic nervous system and the sympathoadrenal axis, leading to increased endogenous catecholamine activity and ever-increasing total peripheral vascular resistance. Decreased renal blood flow activates the renin-angiotensin-aldosterone axis, contributing further to increased peripheral vascular resistance. Lactic acidosis ensues with resultant depressed myocardial contractility and further depressed cardiac output. When three or more organ systems are involved, mortality associated with this syndrome approaches 100 per cent.[81,82]

THERAPY

Comprehensive therapy of septic shock requires appreciation of the major causes of patient demise and the rapidity of disease progression. The major causes of patient mortality include hypotension (a result of decreased systemic vascular resistance and impaired myocardial contractility) and multiorgan failure (due to toxin-mediated effects and tissue hypoperfusion). Therefore rapid institution of therapy to maintain adequate tissue perfusion and halt the progression of infection and mediator-induced tissue destruction are the mainstays of therapy. The focus here is on antibiotic management.

Several studies have underscored the importance of antibiotics for reducing the mortality rate associated with septic shock.[83] These agents should be initiated empirically and in maximum doses before culture results are available. Antibiotics should be active against gram-positive and gram-negative organisms, with appropriate alterations as determined by the clinical situation. For example, if a pelvic or gastrointestinal source of infection is suspected, anaerobic organisms should be covered as well. Antibiotic selection is discussed in greater detail later in the chapter.

Glucocorticoids theoretically should be useful in the therapy of septic shock. Among other actions, they block TNF and Interleukin-1 formation and release from macrophages. However, two trials have demonstrated that corticosteroids are without benefit and may actually increase eventual mortality in patients with septic shock.[58,58a]

It had been hoped that use of heparin for sepsis could reverse the coagulation factor consumption and kallikrein-kinin system activation. However, its efficacy in accomplishing these feats has not been demonstrated.

Opiate antagonists such as naloxone have been utilized for septic shock based on findings in animal models, which suggested that hypotension may in part be mediated by β-endorphins.[84] Although one early study indicated that naloxone, a narcotic antagonist, could block hypotension due to sepsis, subsequent studies have failed to demonstrate efficacy, and one study reported a high incidence of naloxone-induced complications.[85,86] Based on these findings, routine use of naloxone for septic shock cannot be recommended at this time.

Antiprostaglandin therapy has successfully reduced the mortality of experimental septic shock in various animal models.[87,88] It may be due to inhibition of formation of thromboxane A_2 (TXA_2), which may be partially responsible for the pulmonary hypertension, capillary leakage, and leukocyte activation seen in the lungs of patients with ARDS. Prostacycline (prostaglandin I_2, or PGI_2) counteracts the activities of TXA_2, leading to improved membrane stabilization and inhibition of platelet aggregation. Infusing PGI_2 prior to endotoxin administration increases survival in experimental animals. Nonsteroidal antiinflammatory drugs (NSAIDs) have the same effect through inhibition of thromboxane synthetase and cyclooxygenase. These agents hold a great degree of promise, and studies are currently under way to evaluate their efficacy.

A number of passive immunization protocols are being evaluated currently and will add significantly to the therapy of septic shock. Antibodies obtained from normal subjects against common lipopolysaccharide (LPS) core antigens of J5 *Escherichia coli* have been found to detoxify the LPSs from many gram-negative bacilli and may improve survival of patients with septic shock.[89] Monclonal antibodies from human and mouse hybridomas against J5 *E. coli* have been shown to be of benefit in experimental animals.[90–92] Two recently completed trials utilizing monoclonal IgM antibodies directed against LPS have demonstrated marked reductions in mortality due to gram negative sepsis in humans.[117,118] Studies evaluating the efficacy of monoclonal antibody to tumor necrosis factor (TNF) are currently in progress.

IMMUNOCOMPROMISED PATIENT

An ever-increasing number of immunocompromised patients are being encountered regularly in surgical practice. These patients present difficult management problems to the practitioner involved in their care for a variety of reasons. In addition to common infectious conditions often presenting with unusual features, unusual infections arise. Tissue fragility is increased, and wound healing often is impaired, contributing to an increased incidence of wound infection and sepsis. Immunocompromised patients may be unable to mount an effective inflammatory response, further complicating their care. There may be as much as a 12-fold increase in postoperative sepsis and mortality in these patients.[93]

The goal of this section is to briefly describe the major disease entities associated with immunodeficiency states. In that infectious complications are difficult to manage in the immunocompromised patient, it is hoped that the anticipation of potential infectious complications will help facilitate prompt recognition and treatment.

SPECIFIC DISEASE STATES

Protein-calorie malnutrition is endemic among both medical and surgical patients.[94,95] In general, hospitalized patients suffering from malnutrition frequently are afflicted with malignancy or other chronic diseases or are exposed to cytotoxic drugs, chronic administration of steroids, radiotherapy, extensive surgery, or other factors that independently result in an immunocompromised state. Other specific nutritional deficiencies may further impair host resistance.

Those patients at the extremes of age are at increased risk for the development of infections. Neonates have an immature immune system that manifests as poor production of specific antibodies until several months of age, lower levels of complement factors, and impaired opsonization and chemotactic functioning.[96,97]

The diabetic and renal failure patient suffers from immune compromise of a variety of types.[98,99] Patients undergoing chronic ambulatory peritoneal dialysis frequently develop peritonitis, most often due to gram-positive microbes.[100] Patients receiving hemodialysis experience multiple needle punctures and frequently have prosthetic devices in place for vascular access. These situations are significant risk factors for intravascular infections. Alcoholics also frequently suffer violations of their first line of defense due to repeated aspiration of stomach contents, depressed cough reflex, reduced glottal closure, and trauma.

Patients who undergo splenectomy for a hematologic or malignant illness have a 5 per cent lifelong risk of developing overwhelming septicemia.[101] For those who suffer traumatic damage to the spleen with resultant splenectomy, the risk is much lower. The principal organisms responsible for septicemia in splenectomized patients are *Streptococcus pneumoniae* and *Hemophilus influenzae,* but infections due to meningococcus and staphylococci have also been reported.[102–104] The high incidence of infection is primarily due to an impaired ability to clear particles that have been opsonized by immunoglobulin. Because of the risk of pneumococcal sepsis after splenectomy, immunization with polyvalent pneumococcal vaccine is recommended, and it should be done prior to the procedure, if possible.

Patients with sickle cell anemia are prone to develop disseminated pneumococcal infections as a result of both a functional asplenic state due to repeated splenic infarcts and deficient opsonization due to a defect in the alternate pathway of complement.[105] They experience repeated bony infarcts, which establish a nidus for osteomyelitis, often due to *Salmonella* sp.[106] As with patients undergoing splenectomy, polyvalent pneumococcal vaccine is recommended for these patients.

Various malignancies induce immunosuppression, as a result of the disease and its therapy. Patients with acute leukemia develop various cytopenias, including neutropenia, lymphopenia, and monocytopenia. Other factors important in the development of infection include mucosal damage due to cytotoxic chemotherapy, tissue infiltration by leukemic cells, and leukostasis in the vasculature. Patients with chronic lymphocytic leukemia and multiple myeloma have decreased levels of functional immunoglobulins, predisposing the patients to recurrent infections due to pneumococcus and *Hemophilus influenzae.* Patients with Hodgkin's disease have impairment of both cell-mediated immunity and some B cell activities.[107]

A variety of immunosuppressive agents are capable of inducing an immunodeficient state, placing the patient at risk for opportunistic infections. Such agents include glucocorticoids, a variety of cytotoxic agents, and cyclosporin A.

VIRAL HEPATITIS AND AIDS

Viral hepatitis and the acquired immunodeficiency syndrome (AIDS) pose potential risk to the health care worker because they can be transmitted via the blood-borne route. Appreciation of the etiology, epidemiology, and spectrum of disease is important for treatment of infected patients and protection of health care workers from potentially fatal infection. Clearly, of the diseases to be discussed, hepatitis B and non-A, non-B hepatitis are much more of a threat to the health care worker than the other forms of hepatitis (hepatitis A and delta infection). Although AIDS can be transmitted via a blood "accident," it is much less contagious than hepatitis B. Hence, as is discussed below, a mindset toward preventing hepatitis B can be effective in terms of preventing other blood-borne diseases, including AIDS.

VIRAL HEPATITIS

Viral hepatitis is an infection of the liver that may be due to one of several groups of viruses, including hepatitis A, hepatitis B, hepatitis C, hepatitis E, and delta hepatitis. Other viruses, e.g., cytomegalovirus and Ebstein-Barr virus, also may cause hepatic infection but usually as part of a more generalized process. Although the viral agents that cause hepatitis have distinct epidemiologic features, they share the ability to induce an inflammatory reaction in the liver. The spectrum of disease is broad; viral hepatitis is usually a self-limited process, but in some instances patients develop fulminant liver failure or chronic hepatitis, or they become asymptomatic carriers. Indeed, people may be asymptomatic carriers even when there is no history of clinical illness.

Typical signs and symptoms common to all the hepatitides include weakness, fever, lassitude, nausea, vomiting, abdominal tenderness, and jaundice with dark-colored urine. Laboratory studies reveal evidence of hepatic damage and dysfunction. Serologic studies are essential for establishing the etiology of viral hepatitis.

Acute fulminant hepatitis is characterized by progressive jaundice, coagulopathies, hepatic encephalopathy, development of hepatorenal syndrome, and death. The progression is often complete within a few weeks. Various treatments have been attempted, including use of corticosteroids, hyperimmune globulin, and exchange transfusions, but none of these has had a significant effect on patient outcome. Hence therapy consists in supportive management, including proper nutrition, rest, and avoidance of concomitant hepatotoxins.

Chronic hepatitis, not seen with infections due to hepatitis A virus, is a common sequel to hepatitis B and hepatitis C. These patients have persistently elevated aminotransferase levels and histologic evidence of chronic inflammation. There may be progression to hepatic cirrhosis and chronic liver failure. Other than possible superinfection with the delta agent, the chronic asymptomatic carrier state of hepatitis B poses no risk to the patient. However, these individuals are capable of transmitting the virus to others.

Hepatitis A (HAV), previously referred to as infectious hepatitis, accounts for 20 to 25 per cent of clinical hepatitis in developed nations.[108] Transmission of HAV generally is via the fecal-oral route, although transmission through blood products has been reported rarely.[109] It can also be passed through contaminated water supplies or foodstuffs; hence a multitude of common-source epidemics have been reported.[110,111] Most infections, however, are acquired through sporadic (endemic) transmission.[112,113]

Hepatitis B is caused by a DNA virus of the hepadnavirus group. It is a major cause of liver failure, cirrhosis, and hepatocellular carcinoma worldwide. The virus can be present in high concentrations in blood and virtually all body fluids of infected individuals. Transmission occurs when hepatitis B virus is spread through mucosal surfaces or through accidental or deliberate breaks in the skin. The virus can be introduced by contaminated needles, sexual contact, or perinatally. Infection also can occur in the setting of close personal contact with an infected individual, presumably through unappreciated exposure to infectious secretions. However, the virus is not transmitted via the fecal-oral route or by food or water contamination.

Each year, in the United States several thousand health care personnel contract hepatitis B through occupational exposure, with more than 1000 hospitalizations and 200 deaths.[114] Between 6 and 30 per cent of unvaccinated individuals who suffer an accidental needlestick from a patient with hepatitis B eventually contract the disease if there is no intervention.[115] Although only approximately 0.001 ml of blood may be passed with an accidental needlestick, this high transmission rate is understandable if one appreciates that the viremia seen in hepatitis B approximates 100 million virion per milliliter of blood.

Hepatitis C has traditionally accounted for 85 to 95 per cent of postransfusion hepatitis in regions where screening of blood products for hepatitis B is practiced routinely.[116] Now that all blood products are routinely screened for hepatitis C, the incidence of transfusion-related hepatitis has markedly decreased.

Although long considered a transfusion-associated disease, in the United States hepatitis C is actually more commonly a result of nontransfusion-related exposure.[119–121] The incubation period of hepatitis C may be as short as that observed for hepatitis A infection or as long as that with infection due to hepatitis B virus.[116] Approximately 50 per cent of patients who develop transfusion-related hepatitis C have persistently elevated transaminase levels.[122] A significant proportion of these people are asymptomatic; but among those who go on to liver biopsy, chronic active hepatitis is found in 60 per cent and cirrhosis in 10 to 20 per cent.[122]

AIDS

Acquired immunodeficiency syndrome is characterized by the occurrence of severe immune derangements without a known cause for immune dysfunction, such as the use of corticosteroids or other immunosuppressive or cytotoxic therapy, a congenital or genetic immunodeficiency atypical of AIDS, Hodgkin's or non-Hodgkin's lymphoma (except for primary brain lymphoma or a high-grade B cell malignancy), lymphocytic leukemia, multiple myeloma, angioimmunoblastic lymphadenopathy, or any other cancer of lymphoreticular or histiocytic tissue.[123] This immunodeficiency of AIDS primarily involves depletion of the T-helper lymphocyte population, with resultant opportunistic infections and malignancies indicative of ineffective function of this cell line.

There are several major at-risk populations,

and they account for most of the cases of AIDS in the United States.[124–126] Homosexual and bisexual men are the most commonly affected and currently represent almost three fourths of all cases. Intravenous drug abusers comprise the next most common risk group, accounting for 15 to 20 per cent of patients. Heterosexual transmission accounts for approximately 4 per cent of cases, generally occurring in individuals with a history of heterosexual contact with someone in a high risk group. Those who received multiple blood transfusions prior to widespread testing for human immunodeficiency virus (HIV) represent approximately 2 per cent of cases, and hemophiliacs account for 1 per cent of patients with AIDS. Children are also susceptible to HIV infections, particularly through perinatal transmission of the virus.[125]

An important issue, which is also laced with intense emotional overtones, is the concern about risk of transmission of HIV to health care workers. Longitudinal studies have shown that the risk of transmission is low, with the most significant risk being imposed by accidental needle sticks.[127] Based on cumulative data from three large cohort studies, the rate of infection after an accidental needlestick injury (from a needle that has come in contact with an HIV-infected individual) is estimated to be 0.37 per cent. This figure is based on the findings of combined data from 10 prospective studies.[127] These data support the contention that the occupational risk of acquiring HIV infection in health care settings is low, and that it is most often associated with percutaneous inoculation of blood from an infected patient. However, despite the low risk of transmission of HIV to health care workers, it is a possibility given the appropriate circumstances. Recommendations for prevention of transmission, and management of needlestick injuries or other exposures are discussed later in this chapter.

Prevention of Infection

Universal Precautions

It is estimated that there are currently 1.0 to 1.5 million persons in the United States who asymptomatically harbor the HIV.[128] There are undoubtedly countless others who are asymptomatic carriers of other blood-borne pathogens. Because a medical history and physical examination cannot reliably identify all patients infected with these agents, blood and body fluid precautions should be consistently used for *all* patients, especially those in emergency-care settings in which the risk of blood exposure in increased and the infection status of the patient is less likely to be known. The following represent recommendations established by the Centers for Disease Control to help prevent transmission of blood-borne pathogens in the health care setting.[129]

The health care provider should use appropriate barrier precautions to prevent skin and mucous membrane exposure when exposure to blood, body fluids containing blood, or other body fluids to which universal precautions apply (see below) is anticipated. One should wear gloves when touching blood or body fluids, mucous membranes, or nonintact skin of all patients; when handling items or surfaces soiled with blood or body fluids; and when performing venipuncture and other vascular access procedures. Change gloves after contact with each patient; do not wash or disinfect gloves for reuse. Wear masks and protective eye wear or face shields during procedures that are likely to generate droplets of blood or other body fluids to prevent exposure of mucous membranes of the mouth, nose, and eyes. Wear gowns or aprons during procedures that are likely to generate splashes of blood or other body fluids.

The health care worker should wash their hands and other skin surfaces immediately and thoroughly following contaminations with blood, body fluids containing blood, or other body fluids to which universal precautions apply. Wash hands immediately after gloves are removed.

One must take care to prevent injuries when using needles, scalpels, and other sharp instruments or devices; when handling sharp instruments after procedures; when cleaning used instruments; and when disposing of used needles. Do not recap used needles by hand, do not remove used needles from disposable syringes by hand; and do not bend, break, or otherwise manipulate used needles by hand. Place used disposable syringes and needles, scalpel blades, and other sharp items in puncture-resistant disposal containers, which should be located as close to the use area as is practical.

Although saliva has not been definitely implicated in HIV transmission, the need for emergency mouth-to-mouth resuscitation should be minimized by making mouthpieces, resuscitation bags, or other ventilation devices available for use in areas in which the need for resuscitation is predictable.

Health care workers with exudative lesions or weeping dermatitis should refrain from all direct patient care and from handling patient-care equipment until the condition resolves.

Universal precautions are intended to supplement rather than replace recommendations for routine infection control, such as hand washing and use of gloves to prevent gross microbial contamination of hands. In addition, implementation of universal precautions does not eliminate the need for other category- or disease-specific isolation precautions, such as enteric precautions for infectious diarrhea or respiratory isolation for pulmonary tuberculosis. Universal precautions are not intended to change waste management programs undertaken in accordance with state and local regulations.

Universal precautions apply to blood and other body fluids containing visible blood. Blood is the single most important source of HIV, hepatitis B virus, and other blood-borne pathogens in the occupational setting. Universal precautions also apply to tissues, semen, vaginal secretions, and the following fluids: cerebrospinal, synovial, pleural, peritoneal, pericardial, and amniotic.

Universal precautions do not apply to feces, nasal secretions, sputum, sweat, tears, urine, and vomitus unless they contain visible blood. Universal precautions also do not apply to human breast milk, although gloves may be worn by health care workers in situations in which exposure to breast milk might be frequent. In addition, universal precautions do not apply to saliva. Gloves need not be worn when feeding patients or wiping saliva from skin, although special precautions are recommended for dentistry, in which contamination of saliva with blood is predictable. The risk of transmission of HIV, as well as hepatitis B virus, from these fluids and materials is extremely low or nonexistent.

An important point with regard to universal precautions, as listed above, requires reiteration. They were designed in an effort to help prevent the transmission of blood-borne illnesses *only*. That is why secretions such as feces and sputum, unless contaminated with visible blood, are not considered to be "universal precaution" substances. However, a variety of illnesses can be transmitted by these substances, especially in the intensive care setting. For instance, hepatitis A and infectious diarrhea are readily transmitted by infected stool. The agents of tuberculosis and viral pneumonia are transmitted through aerosolized particles. Outbreaks of staphylococcal infection frequently occur owing to person-to-person transmission of these organisms. Universal precautions, when closely adhered to, can certainly help decrease the transmission of blood-borne infections in the health care setting. However, they are incomplete and must be regarded as only a single component of an effective infection control program.

Safety of Blood Products

Since 1982, when the first case of blood transfusion-induced AIDS was reported,[130] a significant number of hemophiliacs and transfusion recipients have developed the disease. As a result, a great deal of concern has been generated regarding the safety of the nation's blood supply. With the development of serologic screening tests for HIV in 1984 and their subsequent approval in 1985, all blood and blood products have been screened with an ELISA assay to identify HIV-infected blood.[131]

Currently available ELISA tests for HIV appear to have a false-positive rate of less than 1 per cent and a false-negative rate of less than 3 per cent.[132-134] Conventional ELISA tests measure antibody directed against antigens grown in human cell lines, resulting in contamination with variable amounts of human histocompatibility antigens. Therefore multiparous women, and recipients of transfusions and organ transplants may have false-positive results if their blood has antibodies to the histocompatibility antigens present in the cell line in which the virus was grown. False positive tests have also been noted in patients with liver disease, renal failure, and connective tissue diseases, such as systemic lupus erythematosus. For this reason, confirmatory tests such as the Western Blot are necessary to confirm any positive ELISA test. ELISA assays utilizing recombinant antigens should exhibit improved specificity.[135,136]

ELISA antibody tests typically become positive 4 to 12 weeks after exposure. This "window" period may also be a source of false-negative ELISA results, in that the ELISA assay may be negative despite the infectivity of the patient and his or her blood products. Furthermore, it is now clear that the typical pattern of seroconversion is not universal, and prolonged periods of viral infection may rarely occur in the presence of a negative ELISA test and negative Western Blot analysis.[137,138] Therefore although routine screening of blood for HIV has markedly decreased the chances for transmission of the agent through blood products, this possibility still exists. At its upper limit, this risk has been estimated to be between 1 in 100,000 and 1 in 1,000,000 units of blood. However, although AIDS has been transmitted via whole blood and cellular components, plasma, and clotting factors that have not been heat-treated, there have been no reported cases due to immunoglobulin, albumin, or plasma protein factor.

IMMUNIZATION

Of the diseases discussed above, hepatitis B is the only infection for which active immunization with a vaccine is currently available.

The hepatitis B vaccine is remarkably safe and effective.[139] In those patients who develop protective levels of antibody, protection against symptomatic hepatitis B virus infection appears to last at least 5 years.[140]

Immunization with hepatitis B vaccine is recommended for adults at increased risk of occupational, social, family, environmental, or illness-related exposure to hepatitis B virus.[139] These high risk groups include workers in health-related occupations with frequent exposures to blood, homosexual men, intravenous drug abusers, household and sexual contacts of hepatitis B virus carriers, residents and staff of institutions for the mentally retarded, hemodialysis patients, recipients of coagulation factors, morticians, prison inmates, and travelers likely to have close contact with members of a population where hepatitis B is endemic.

Development of a safe and effective vaccine for infection with HIV would obviously be a major public health breakthrough. Unfortunately, development of such a vaccine is complicated by several unique scientific, logistic, and ethical issues.[141] These include the failure to thus far clearly delineate the viral components, or epitopes, that induce effective immunity in the host, lack of adequate and convenient animal models for the disease, and lack of indicators of protective immunity that can be serially evaluated. Furthermore, evaluation of such a vaccine is made difficult by the prolonged period between a person's initial infection with HIV and the development of disease symptoms, as well as by the nature of spread of HIV infection. In that transmission depends on behavioral factors, with an incubation period lasting many years, assessment of a vaccine's efficacy and safety similarly will take several years. Hence, although much work is currently under way, a clinically useful immunization for HIV infection is still far away.

Sterilization and Care of Anesthesia Equipment

Viruses are able to survive for long periods on dry surfaces. For instance, hepatitis B virus can be recovered after 1 week at 25°C and 42 per cent humidity.[142] HIV can be recovered from dried material after 3 days at room temperature, and it can survive for more than 2 weeks in an aqueous environment at room temperature. Fortunately, HIV happens to be sensitive to a variety of disinfectant chemicals and to relatively low levels of heat.[143–146] Household bleach also provides excellent sterilizing activity at a dilution of 1:10 to 1:1000, depending on the amount of organic soilage present. For linens, the common hospital sterilization techniques using ethylene oxide, steam, and boiling water typically kill all viruses except Creutzfeldt-Jakob disease virus.[147] However, it is critical to point out that proper cleaning of items prior to sterilization is essential. Excessive residual blood or other organic material may negate the effects of disinfectants or heat due to sheer mass effect.

Various bacteria are able to survive and proliferate within the circuitry of anesthetic machinery. Therefore disposable airway circuits, filters, and carbon dioxide absorbers have been used to prevent bacterial spread via air circuitry. In contrast to bacteria, viruses are unable to proliferate independent of the host organism. Therefore any surviving virus that contaminates anesthetic circuitry remains stagnant, with no increase in inoculum size. Given the probable decreased risk of viral spread compared with bacterial spread in airway circuitry, the scientific data to justify the use of disposable anesthesia equipment to prevent the spread of viruses is speculative at best. Nevertheless, some anesthesia departments in the United States that deal with large numbers of HIV-infected patients or patients in high-risk groups are using disposable breathing circuits and occasionally carbon dioxide absorbers.

Only those portions of the breathing circuitry that potentially can come in contact with sputum or other organic materials containing viruses provide sources for viral spread. These items require cleaning, sterilizing, or disinfection where appropriate, although disposable breathing circuits are most commonly used. Except in unusual situations where sputum and other virus-containing organic materials may extend beyond the expiratory limb, use of disposable carbon dioxide absorbers is probably unnecessary.

Laryngoscopes and other nondisposable items that have touched mucosal membranes or contacted blood or secretions from patients should be thoroughly washed with a detergent and water and either gas- or steam-sterilized or subjected to appropriate disinfection. Persons cleaning this equipment should wear disposable gloves. Environmental surfaces, such as those of the anesthesia machine, that are contaminated should be disinfected with an EPA-registered "hospital disinfectant" having a label claim for mycobactericidal activity. Alternatively, a 1:10 to 1:1000 solution of sodium hypochlorite (household bleach) may be used depending on the amount of residual organic material. As with the anesthesia circuitry, disposable laryngoscopes, esophageal stethoscopes, and other equipment that could be contaminated are being used by some anesthesia departments.

Management of Exposure

Despite even the most meticulous care, on occasion the health care worker may become exposed to potentially infectious materials. If so, the patient who is the source of the exposure should immediately be assessed for likelihood of disease. If the patient is likely to harbor either hepatitis or HIV infection and their status is unknown, serologic status should be determined. If the source is HIV-positive, the worker should receive baseline HIV testing and follow-up every 3 months for 1 year. Counseling should be provided regarding the risk of infection and the potential ramifications of seroconversion. If the suspected high risk patient is hepatitis B surface antigen (HBsAg) positive (we suggest rapid screening using the Auscell technique), the exposed person should receive hepatitis B immune globulin (HBIG) as soon as possible; the adult dose is a single intramuscular dose of 0.06 ml/kg or 5 ml. The value of giving HBIG more than 7 days after exposure is unclear. A series of three doses of hepatitis B virus vaccine should also be initiated simultaneously. For those who choose not to take the vaccination, a second identical dose of hepatitis B immune globulin should be given 1 month later. If the exposed person is known to be HBsAb positive because of prior exposure or vaccination, neither HBIG nor hepatitis B vaccine is necessary. In addition to the above, we recommend that an exposed person receive pooled immune globulin (0.06 ml/kg IM) if the patient has active liver disease and is Auscell-negative or if the source of the needlestick is unknown.

There are currently no postexposure prophylactic measures known to be effective for preventing infection in those exposed to HIV-infected blood. However, based on promising results obtained in animal models,[148,149] some centers are investigating the use of a short course of zidovudine (previously referred to as azidothymidine, or AZT).[150] In general, the decision to administer zidovudine is based on the extent of parenteral exposure and the preference of the patient. Although the risk of HIV seroconversion after a trivial needlestick has been estimated to be approximately 0.37 per cent,[150] this rate is higher when infected blood is actually injected into an individual.

Although zidovudine is generally well tolerated, severe anemia, neutropenia, and thrombocytopenia may occur. However, these toxicities rarely appear within the first 4 weeks of therapy.[151] Other adverse effects include headache, fatigue, nausea, insomnia, myositis, paresthesias, and hepatitis. Preexisting hepatic or renal dysfunction represent a relative contraindication to administration of zidovudine. If the drug is utilized in these patients, one must monitor closely for drug toxicity.

The major concern regarding use of zidovudine in postexposure HIV prophylaxis relates to its use in women of childbearing age. Because of its action at the level of DNA polymerase, the possibility of both mutagenesis and teratogenesis exists. Therefore if it is elected to utilize zidovudine in this population of patients, the individual must be made aware of these potential adverse effects.

In animal models, use of zidovudine for postexposure prophylaxis appears to be most effective if initiated *immediately* after exposure. Hence in those individuals who are uncertain if they want a full course of therapy, it may be prudent to initiate therapy immediately on an interim basis pending their final decision. A typical treatment regimen for this indication would be 200 mg PO q4h for 4 to 6 weeks, although the preferred dosage, frequency, and duration have yet to be defined.

Hospitals should develop ways in which exposures can promptly be evaluated and recommendations given regarding zidovudine "prophylaxis" for the potentially at-risk employee.

ANTIMICROBIAL THERAPY DURING THE POSTOPERATIVE PERIOD

Use of antimicrobial agents is widespread in surgical practice. Despite their frequency of use, they are among the most often misused therapeutic agents in medicine. When used appropriately and intelligently, they are effective adjuncts to our own immune system for the treatment of infectious diseases. However, when used inappropriately, therapeutic failures, bacterial or fungal superinfection, or other antibiotic-induced complications may ensue unnecessarily.

Our current discussion is limited to a basic overview of the principles of antibiotic therapy as they apply to empiric antibiotic therapy and the therapy of established infection. The principles of prophylactic antibiotic therapy were discussed earlier in the section on wound infection. The next few paragraphs briefly outline the basic principles of antimicrobial therapy.

1. *There are certain indications for administration of antibiotics.* Such indications include prophylaxis (i.e., wound infections, endocarditis), therapy of established infection, and empiric therapy in the patient who exhibits signs or symptoms suggestive of infection. Clearly, not every patient who develops a fever or leukocytosis warrants antimicrobial therapy. Certainly if a patient has a defined infection such as pneumonia, urinary tract infection, or peritonitis, antibiotic therapy should be initiated. Although the specific pathogen(s) may not be identified, intelligent choices of antimicrobial agents can be made pending the results of the Gram stain and cultures of appropriate clinical specimens.

There are some instances when antimicrobial therapy should be initiated in the absence of a known focus of infection. This action is most appropriate when the patient is ill or appears to be developing a septic state. Patients who are neutropenic also warrant broad-spectrum empiric antibiotics when they develop a fever, even if no focus of infection is apparent.

2. *The antibiotic(s) administered must be active against the pathogen for which it is given.* At the onset of antibiotic therapy, the inciting pathogen(s) is frequently unknown, and antibiotic selection must be made empirically. Based on clinical and laboratory information, the most likely site(s) of infection must be defined and antibiotic therapy directed toward the organisms most likely to be involved. Consideration must also be given to host factors as well as whether the infection is hospital-acquired. For the treatment of hospital-acquired infections, it is essential to know the microbiology and typical antibiotic sensitivities of your institution. For instance, in

those hospitals where methicillin-resistant *Staphylococcus aureus* is a frequent pathogen, empiric therapy of presumed staphylococcal infections must include vancomycin rather than a semisynthetic penicillin or first-generation cephalosporin. Nosocomial pneumonia in some institutions are frequently due to *Legionella pneumophila,* whereas in others this organism is rarely seen.

To be most effective, empiric antimicrobial therapy must have a sufficiently broad spectrum to cover most clinical possibilities. The spectrum of antimicrobial coverage can always be narrowed after the etiologic agent(s) is more clearly defined.

Of course, the cornerstone of rationale utilization of antibiotics ultimately relies on the isolation and identification of the infecting microbial pathogen(s) with subsequent in vitro determination of its susceptibility to antimicrobial agents. Therefore every attempt should be made to obtain culture specimens from all likely sources.

3. *The antibiotic administered must be able to reach the area of infection.* For instance, although aminoglycosides are active against most gram-negative bacilli, in that they do not cross the blood-brain barrier, they are ineffective when administered intravenously for gram-negative meningitis. First and second generation cephalosporins, with the exception of cefuroxime, do not reach bactericidal levels in cerebrospinal fluid either and hence are similarly ineffective. Other organs into which antibiotics diffuse poorly include the prostate and the eye. Impairment of blood flow impedes delivery of antibiotics to the site of any infection. This is a particularly common problem when dealing with diabetic foot infections. Additionally, most antibiotics do not diffuse well into abscess cavities, frequently rendering antibiotic therapy of these infections ineffective unless combined with adequate drainage of the infected material.

4. *The antibiotic must maintain its activity once it reaches the site of infection.* Aminoglycoside activity is limited in a hypoxic or acidic environment. This point may be clinically significant during the treatment of abscesses or pulmonary infections where acidic, hypoxic environments are common. Similarly, β-lactam antibiotics may be inactivated by β-lactamases produced by microbial organisms. Of note is the phenomenon of indirect pathogenicity, whereby in a polymicrobial infection one bacterial species imparts antibiotic resistance upon another via production of a soluble antibiotic-degrading enzyme. This situation may result in treatment failure caused by organisms that had apparently been antibiotic-sensitive in vitro.

5. *Consideration must be given to the immune status of the host.* For the compromised host, one is more apt to begin empiric antimicrobial therapy early. For instance, in the neutropenic patient it is essential to initiate antibiotic therapy immediately when a fever develops. Patients with diabetes mellitus or those receiving chronic steroid therapy frequently exhibit blunted inflammatory responses. Signs and symptoms typical of catastrophic illness may hence be absent or minimal, making diagnosis difficult. In other immunocompromised hosts, the nature of the immunocompromised state may give clues to the etiology of the infection, as was previously discussed in the section on the immunocompromised patient.

6. *There are certain indications for bactericidal (versus bacteriostatic) antimicrobial therapy.* In general, agents that disrupt an organism's cell wall, e.g., penicillins, cephalosporins, aztreonam, imipenam, quinolones, and vancomycin, as well as aminoglycosides, are considered to be bactericidal agents. Bacteriostatic agents—those that principally inhibit the production of bacterial proteins—include clindamycin, erythromycin, sulfonamides, trimethoprim, tetracyclines, and chloramphenicol. At clinically achievable serum concentrations bacteriostatic agents merely inhibit bacterial growth, rather than killing the organism. In most clinical situations, bacteriostatic therapy is adequate if the host's immune system is intact.

Two infections for which bactericidal antibiotic therapy is essential for cure are endocarditis and meningitis. Although the successful utilization of chloramphenicol (a normally bacteriostatic agent) for childhood meningitis may thus appear paradoxical, it is in fact bactericidal at clinically achievable cerebrospinal fluid concentrations against common meningeal pathogens. For the therapy of osteomyelitis, it is also advantageous to utilize bactericidal antimicrobial combinations. In the immunocompromised patient, especially those with inadequate neutrophil number or function, bactericidal therapy is essential.

7. *There are certain indications for combination antimicrobial therapy.* Combination therapy is indicated only for certain defined infections: most infections due to *Pseudomonas aeruginosa,* certain other gram-nega-

tive pathogens, and *enterococcus* sp., where the synergistic activity of combination antimicrobial therapy has been shown to result in improved clinical outcomes. However, because of the high urinary concentrations achievable by active antibiotics, those infections limited to the urinary tract due to *P. aeruginosa* and the enterococcus may be successfully treated with single agents.

Synergism may also become an important treatment issue when dealing with "tolerant" strains of *Staphylococcus aureus*. The tolerance of these organisms often allows one to inhibit an infection without eradicating it, despite the use of "bactericidal" antibiotics. When dealing with staphylococcal infections that require bactericidal therapy, e.g., meningitis, endocarditis, and possibly osteomyelitis, the addition of a second agent active against *Staphylococcus,* such as rifampin or gentamicin, may help achieve cure.

Tuberculosis must be treated with combination therapy due to the rapid development of resistance when one agent is used alone. Infections due to *Cryptococcus neoformans* are probably best treated initially with the synergistic combination of amphotericin B and flucytosine.

The most common use of combination antibiotics is for empiric antimicrobial therapy. Selection of appropriate agents in this instance requires knowledge of the bacteriology of body spaces and the usual pathogens in various infections. In that single agents often do not provide coverage of all significant anticipated pathogens, the use of multiple agents is often necessary until a specific pathogen is implicated.

Although combination therapy often results in an enhanced antibacterial spectrum, as well as additive or synergistic killing of microbes, in some instances untoward effects may occur. For example, in vitro antagonism may occur, often in an unpredictable fashion. Other drawbacks to combination antimicrobial therapy include enhanced risk of adverse effects, alteration of the microecology, superinfection, and cost. Therefore multiple agents are not routinely recommended except in those circumstances described above.

8. *If all other factors are equal, the cost-effectiveness of an antibiotic should help guide decision-making.* During this era of cost-conscious medicine, financial considerations are becoming increasingly important. The thoughtful selection of antibiotics can often result in significant savings to the patient and hospital. However, the least expensive antibiotic is not necessarily the most cost-effective. For example, a more expensive antibiotic may be most cost-effective if it results in a shorter hospital stay or is associated with less toxicity. If a host has renal insufficiency, a renally eliminated antibiotic is often more favorable if it allows less frequent dosing without increased toxicity.

References

1. Stephen CR: Malignant hyperpyrexia. Annu Rev Med *28*:153–157, 1977.
2. Schlenker JD, Hubay CA: The pathogenesis of postoperative atelectasis: a clinical study. Arch Surg *107*:846–850, 1973.
3. Wynne JW, Modell JH: Respiratory aspiration of stomach contents. Ann Intern Med *87*:466–474, 1977.
4. Livelli FD, Johnson RA, McEnany MT, et al: Unexplained in-hospital fever following cardiac surgery: natural history relationship to postpericardiotomy syndrome, and a prospective study of therapy with indomethacin versus placebo. Circulation *57*:968–975, 1978.
5. Appleberg M: The value of the postoperative temperature chart as an aid to the diagnosis of deep vein thrombosis. S Afr Med J *50*:2149–2150, 1976.
6. Ottinger LW: Acute cholecystitis as a postoperative complication. Ann Surg *184*:162–165, 1976.
7. Green JW, Wenzel RP: Postoperative wound infection: a controlled study on the increased duration of hospital stay and direct cost of hospitalization. Ann Surg *185*:264–268, 1977.
8. Cruse PJE, Foord R: A five-year prospective study of 23,649 surgical wounds. Arch Surg *107*:206–210, 1973.
9. Shapiro M, Munoz A, Tager IB, et al: Risk factors for infection at the operative site after abdominal or vaginal hysterectomy. N Engl J Med *307*:1661–1666, 1982.
10. Balthazar ER, Colt JD, Nichols RC: Preoperative hair removal: a random, prospective study of shaving versus clipping. South Med J *75*:799–801, 1982.
11. Veterans Administration Ad Hoc Interdisciplinary Advisory Committee on Antimicrobial Drug Usage. Prophylaxis in surgery. JAMA *237*:1003–1007, 1977.
12. Antimicrobial prophylaxis in surgery. Med Lett Drug Ther *31*:105–108, 1989.
13. Nichols RL, Condon RE, Gorbach SL, et al: Efficacy of preoperative antimicrobial preparation of the bowel. Ann Surg *176*:227–232, 1972.
14. Bartlett P, Reingold AL, Graham DR, et al: Toxic shock syndrome associated with surgical wound infections. JAMA *247*:1448–1450, 1982.
15. Reingold AL, Dan BB, Shands KN, et al: Toxic shock syndrome not associated with menstruation. Lancet *1*:1–4, 1982.
16. Hampton AA, Sheretz RJ: Vascular-access infections in hospitalized patients. Surg Clin North Am *68*:57–71, 1988.
17. Tomford JW, Hershey CO, McClaren CE, et al: Intravenous therapy team and peripheral venous catheter-associated complications: a prospective controlled study. Arch Intern Med *144*:1191–1194, 1984.

18. Faubion WC, Wesley JR, Khalidin, et al: Total parenteral nutrition catheter sepsis: impact of the team approach. J Parent Enter Nutr *10*:642–645, 1986.

19. Levy RS, Goldstein J: Value of topical antibiotic ointment in reducing bacterial colonization of percutaneous venous catheters. J Albert Einstein Med Center *18*:67–70, 1970.

20. Maki DG, Band JD: A comparative study of polyantibiotic and iodophor ointments in prevention of catheter-related infection. Am J Med *70*:739–744, 1981.

21. Rusho WJ, Bair JN: Effect of filtration complications of postoperative intravenous therapy. Am J Hosp Pharm *36*:1355–1356, 1979.

22. Band JD, Maki DG: Safety of changing intravenous delivery systems at longer than 24-hour intervals. Ann Intern Med *91*:173–178, 1979.

23. Josephson A, Gombert ME, Sierra MF, et al: The relationship between intravenous fluid contamination and the frequency of tubing replacement. Infect Control *6*:367–370, 1985.

24. Shydman DR, Donnelly-Reidy M, Perry LK, et al: Intravenous tubing containing burettes can be safely changed at 72 hour intervals. Infect Control *8*:113–116, 1987.

25. Maki DG, Weise CE, Sarafin HW: A semiquantitative culture method for identifying intravenous-catheter-related infection. N Engl J Med *296*:1305–1309, 1977.

26. Sattler FR, Foderaro JB, Abner RC: Staphylococcus epidermidis bacteremia associated with vascular catheters: an important cause of febrile morbidity in hospitalized patients. Infect Control *5*:279–283, 1984.

27. Winston DJ, Dudnick DV, Chapin M, et al: Coagulase-negative staphylococcal bacteremia in patients receiving immunosuppressive therapy. Arch Intern Med *143*:32–36, 1983.

28. Dandalides PC, Rutula WA, Thomann CA, et al: Serious postoperative infections caused by coagulase-negative staphylococci: an epidemiological and clinical study. J Hosp Infect *8*:233–241, 1986.

29. Davies AJ, Stone JW: Current problems of chemotherapy of infections with coagulase-negative staphylococci. Eur J Clin Microbiol *5*:277–281, 1986.

30. Iannini PB, Crossley K: Therapy of Staphylococcus aureus bacteremia associated with a removable focus of infection. Ann Intern Med *84*:558–560, 1976.

31. Myloite JM, McDermott C: Staphylococcus aureus bacteremia caused by infected intravenous catheters. Am J Infect Control *15*:1–6, 1987.

32. Finkelstein R, Sobel JD, Nagler A, et al: Staphylococcus aureus bacteremia and endocarditis: comparison of nosocomial and community-acquired infections. J Med *15*:193–211, 1984.

33. Watanakunakorn C, Baird IM: Staphylococcus aureus bacteremia and endocarditis associated with a removable infected intravenous device. Am J Med *63*:253–256, 1977.

34. Rose HD: Venous catheter-associated candidemia. Am J Med Sci *275*:265–269, 1978.

35. Maki DG, Rhame FS, Mackel DC, et al: Nationwide epidemic of septicemia caused by contaminated intravenous products. Epidemiologic and clinical features. Am J Med *60*:471–485, 1976.

36. Philips I, Eykyn S, Laker M: Outbreak of hospital infection caused by contaminated autoclaved fluids. Lancet *1*:1258–1262, 1972.

37. Turck M, Stamm W: Nosocomial infection of the urinary tract. Am J Med *70*:651–654, 1981.

38. Garibaldi RA: Hospital acquired urinary tract infection. In Wenzel RP (ed): CRC Handbook of Hospital Acquired Infections. Boca Raton, CRC Press, 1981, pp. 513–537.

39. Haley RW, Culver DH, White JW, et al. The nationwide nosocomial infection rate: a new need for vital statistics. Am J Epidemiol *121*:182–205, 1985.

40. Dixon RE: Effect of infections on hospital care. Ann Intern Med *89*:749–753, 1978.

41. Berendt RF: Relationship of method of administration to respiratory virulence of Klebsiella pneumoniae for mice and squirrel monkey. Infect Immunol *20*:581–583, 1978.

42. Ansfield MJ, Woods DE, Johanson WG Jr: Lung bacterial clearance in murine pneumococcal pneumonia. Infect Immunol *17*:195–204, 1977.

43. Huxley EJ, Viruslav J, Cray WR, Pierce AK: Pharyngeal aspiration in normal adults and patients with depressed consciousness. Am J Med *64*:564–568, 1978.

44. Johanson WG Jr, Pierce AK, Sanford JP: Changing pharyngeal bacterial flora of hospitalized patients: emergence of gram-negative bacilli. N Engl J Med *281*:1137–1140, 1969.

45. Johanson WG Jr, Pierce AK, Sanford JP, Thomas GD: Nosocomial respiratory infections with gram-negative bacilli: the significance of colonization in the respiratory tract. Ann Intern Med *77*:701–706, 1972.

46. Langer M, Cigada M, Mandelli M, et al: Early onset pneumonia: a multicenter study in intensive care units. Intensive Care Med *13*:342–346, 1987.

47. Centers for Disease Control: National Nosocomial Infections Study Report, Annual Summary, 1984. MMWR *35*:17SS–29SS, 1986.

48. Klastersky J: Empiric treatment of infection in neutropenic patients with cancer. Rev Infect Dis *5*(suppl):S21–S31, 1983.

49. Hooten TM, Haley RW, Culver DH, et al: The joint associations of multiple risk factors with the occurrence of nosocomial infection. Am J Med *70*:960–970, 1981.

50. Driks MR, Craven PE, Celli BR, et al: Nosocomial pneumonia in intubated patients given sucralfate as compared with antacids or histamine type 2 blockers: the role of gastric colonization. N Engl J Med *317*:1376–1382, 1987.

51. Greenfield S, Teres D, Bushnell LS, et al: Prevention of gram-negative bacillary pneumonia using aerosol polymyxin as prophylaxis. J Clin Invest *52*:2935–2940, 1973.

52. Klastersky J, Huysmans E, Weerts D, et al: Endotracheally-administered gentamicin for the prevention of infections of the respiratory tract in patients with tracheostomy: a double blind study. Chest *65*:650–654, 1974.

53. Stoutenbeek CP, van Saene HKF, Miranda D, et al: The effect of selective decontamination of the digestive tract on colonization and infection rate in multiple trauma patients. Intensive Care Med *10*:185–192, 1984.

54. Unertl K, Ruckdeschel G, Selbmann HK, et al: Prevention of colonization and respiratory infections in long-term ventilated patients by local antimicrobial prophylaxis. Intensive Care Med *13*:106–113, 1987.

55. Machiedo G, LoVerme P, McGovern P, et al: Patterns of mortality in a surgical intensive care unit. Surg Gynecol Obstet *152*:757–759, 1981.

56. Wilson R: Etiology, diagnosis and prognosis of positive blood cultures. Am Surg *47*:112–115, 1981.

57. Bohnen J, Boulanger M, Meakins J, et al: Prognosis in generalized peritonitis: relation to cause and risk factors. Arch Surg *118*:285–290, 1983.

58. Bone RC, Fisher CJ, Clemmer TP, et al: A controlled trial of high dose methylprednisone in the treatment of severe sepsis and septic shock. N Engl J Med *317*:653–658, 1987.

58a. The Veterans Administration Systemic Sepsis Cooperative Study Group: Effect of high-dose glucocorticoid therapy on mortality in patients with clinical signs of systemic sepsis. N Engl J Med *317*:659–665, 1987.

59. Martin LF, Max MH, Polk HC: Failure of gastric pH control by antacids or cimetidine in the critically ill: a valid sign of sepsis. Surgery *88*:59–68, 1980.

60. Abraham E, Shoemaker WC, Bland RD, et al: Sequential cardiorespiratory patterns in septic shock. Crit Care Med *11*:799–803, 1983.

61. Parillo JE: The cardiovascular pathophysiology of sepsis. Annu Rev Med *40*:469–485, 1989.

62. Holloway WA, Reinhardt J: Septic shock in the elderly. Geriatrics *39*:48–54, 1984.

63. Dorff GJ, Geimer NE, Rosenthal DR, et al: Pseudomonas septicemia, illustrated evolution of its skin lesion. Arch Intern Med *128*:591–595, 1971.

64. Fisher KW, Berger B, Keusch GT: Subepidermal bullae secondary to Escherichia coli septicemia. Arch Dermatol *110*:105–106, 1974.

65. Altemeier WA, Fullen WO, McDonough JJ: Sepsis and gastrointestinal bleeding. Ann Surg *175*:759–770, 1972.

66. Moody FG, Cheung LY, Simons MA, et al: Stress and the acute gastric mucosal lesion. Am J Dig Dis Sci *21*:148–154, 1976.

67. Franson TR, Hierholzer WJ, LaBrecque DR: Frequency and characteristics of hyperbilirubinemia associated with bacteremia. Rev Infect Dis *7*:1–9, 1985.

68. Gutman RA, Striker GE, Gilliland BC, et al: The immune complex glomerulonephritis of bacterial endocarditis. Medicine (Baltimore) *51*:1–25, 1972.

69. Stickler GB, Shin MH, Burke EC, et al: Diffuse glomerulonephritis associated with infected ventriculoatrial shunt. N Engl J Med *279*:1077–1082, 1968.

70. Beaufils M: Glomerular disease complicating abdominal sepsis. Kidney Int *19*:609–618, 1981.

71. Galpin JE, Shinaberger JH, Stanley TM, et al: Acute interstitial nephritis due to methicillin. Am J Med *65*:756–765, 1978.

72. Ellis D, Fried WA, Yunis EJ, et al: Acute interstitial nephritis in children: a report of 13 cases and review of the literature. Pediatrics 6:862–870, 1981.

73. Zieve PD, Haghshenass M, Blanjs M, et al: Vacuolization of the neutrophil. Arch Intern Med *118*:356–357, 1966.

74. Malcolm ID, Flegel KM, Katz M: Vacuolization of the neutrophil in bacteremia. Arch Intern Med *139*:675–676, 1979.

75. Riedler GF, Straub PW, Frick PG: Thrombocytopenia in septicemia: a clinical study for the evaluation of its incidence and diagnostic value. Helv Med Acta *36*:23–38, 1971.

76. Oppenheimer L, Hryniuk WM, Bishop AJ: Thrombocytopenia in severe bacterial infections. J Surg Res *20*:211–214, 1976.

77. Corrigan JJ Jr, Ray WL, May N: Changes in the blood coagulation system associated with septicemia. N Engl J Med *279*:851–856, 1968.

78. Colman RW, Robboy SJ, Minna JD: Disseminated intravascular coagulation: a reappraisal. Annu Rev Med *30*:359–374, 1979.

79. Mant MJ, King EG: Severe, acute disseminated intravascular coagulation. Am J Med *67*:557–563, 1979.

80. Kreger BE, Craven DE, McCabe WR: Gram-negative bacteremia. IV. Re-evaluation of clinical features and treatment of 612 patients. Am J Med *68*:344–355, 1980.

81. Carrico CJ, Meakins JL, Marshall JC, et al: Multiple-organ failure syndrome. Arch Surg *121*:196–208, 1986.

82. Bell RC, Coalson JJ, Smith JD, Johanson WG Jr: Multiple organ system failure and infection in adult respiratory distress syndrome. Ann Intern Med *99*:293–298, 1983.

83. Jacobson MA, Young LS: New developments in the treatment of gram-negative bacteremia (medical progress). West J Med *144*:185–194, 1986.

84. Peters WP, Johnson MW, Friedman PA, et al: Pressor effect of naloxone in septic shock. Lancet *1*:529–534, 1981.

85. DeMaria A, Craven DE, Jeffeman JJ, et al: Naloxone versus placebo treatment of septic shock. Lancet *1*:1363–1367, 1985.

86. Rock P, Silverman H, Plump D, et al: Efficacy and safety of naloxone in septic shock. Crit Care Med *13*:28–32, 1985.

87. Jacob ER, Soulsby ME, Bone RC, et al: Ibuprofen in canine endotoxin shock. J Clin Invest *70*:536–541, 1982.

88. Cook JA, Wise WB, Halushka PV: Elevated thromboxane levels in the rat during endotoxic shock: protective effects of imidazole, 13-azaprostanoic acid or essential fatty acid deficiency. J Clin Invest *65*:227–230, 1980.

89. Ziegler EJ, McCutchan JA, Fiener J, et al: Treatment of gram negative bacteremia and shock with human antiserum to a mutant E. coli. N Engl J Med *303*:1225–1230, 1982.

90. Warren HS, Novitsky TJ, Bucklin A, et al: Endotoxin neutralization with rabbit antisera to Escherichia coli J5 and other gram-negative bacteria. Infect Immun *55*:1668–1673, 1987.

91. Siber GR, Kania SA, Warren HS: Cross-reactivity of rabbit antibodies to lipolysaccharides of Escherichia coli J5 and other gram-negative bacteria. J Infect Dis *152*:954–964, 1985.

92. Greisman SE, Johnston CA: Failure of antisera to J5 and R595 rough mutants to reduce endotoxic lethality. J Infect Dis *157*:54–64, 1988.

93. MacLean LD: Host resistance in surgical patients. J Trauma *19*:297–304, 1979.

94. Chandra RL: Nutrition, immunity, and infection: present knowledge and future directions. Lancet *1*:688–691, 1983.

95. Keusch GT: Host defense mechanisms in protein energy malnutrition. Adv Exp Med Biol *135*:183–209, 1981.

96. Smith D, Peter G, Ingram DL, et al: Responses of children immunized with the capsular polysac-

charide of Hemophilus influenzae type B. Pediatrics *52*:637–640, 1973.

97. Marodi L, Leijh PCJ, Braat A, et al: Opsonic activity of cord blood sera against various species of micro-organisms. Pediatr Res *19*:433–436, 1985.

98. Allen JC: The diabetic as a compromised host. *In* Allen JC (ed): Infection and the Compromised Host. Clinical Correlations and Therapeutic Approaches, 2nd ed. Baltimore, Williams & Wilkins, 1981, pp. 229–270.

99. Langhoff E, Ladefoged J: Cellular immunity in renal failure: depression of lymphocyte transformation by uraemia and methylprednisone. Int Arch Allergy Appl Immunol *74*:241–245, 1984.

100. Gloor HF, Nichols WK, Sorkin MI, et al: Peritoneal access and related complications in continuous ambulatory peritoneal dialysis. Am J Med *74*:593–598, 1983.

101. Schwartz PE, Sterioff S, Mucha P, et al: Post-splenectomy sepsis and mortality in adults. JAMA *284*:2279–2283, 1982.

102. Chilcote RR, Baehner RL, Hammond D: Septicemia and meningitis in children splenectomized for Hodgkin's disease. N Engl J Med *295*:798–800, 1976.

103. Weitzman S, Aisenberg AC: Fulminant sepsis after the successful treatment of Hodgkin's disease. Am J Med *62*:47–50, 1977.

104. DiPadova F, Dung M, Harder F, et al: Impaired antipneumococcal antibody production in patients without spleens. Br Med J *290*:14–16, 1985.

105. Johnston RB Jr, Newman LS, Struth AG: An abnormality of the alternate pathway of complement activation in sickle cell disease. N Engl J Med *288*:803–808, 1973.

106. Hand WL, King NL: Serum opsonization of Salmonella in sickle cell anemia. Am J Med *64*:388–395, 1978.

107. Weitzman SA, Aisenberg AC, Siber GR, et al: Immunity in treated Hodgkin's disease. N Engl J Med *297*:245–248, 1977.

108. Francis DP, Hadler SC, Prendergast TJ, et al: Occurrence of hepatitis A, B and non-A/non-B in the United States: CDC Sentinel County Hepatitis Study I. Am J Med *76*:69–74, 1984.

109. Hollinger FB, Khan NC, Oefinger PE, et al: Post-transfusion hepatitis type A. JAMA *250*:2313–2317, 1983.

110. Hadler SC, Webster HM, Erben JJ, et al: Hepatitis A in day-care centers: a community-wide assessment. N Engl J Med *302*:1222–1227, 1980.

111. Benenson MW, Takafuji ET, Bancroft WH, et al: A military community outbreak of hepatitis type A related to transmission in a child care facility. Am J Epidemiol *112*:471–481, 1980.

112. Hepatitis Surveillance Report No 49. Atlanta, Centers for Disease Control, January 1985.

113. Neefe JR, Gellis SS, Stokes J Jr: Homologous serum hepatitis and infectious (epidemic) hepatitis: studies in volunteers bearing on immunological and other characteristics of the etiological agents. Am J Med *1*:3–22, 1946.

114. Blumberg BS: Feasibility of controlling or eradicating the hepatitis B virus. Am J Med *87*(suppl 3A):2S–4S, 1989.

115. Seeff LB, Wright EC, Zimmerman HJ: Type B hepatitis after needle-stick exposure: prevention with hepatitis B immune globulin. Ann Intern Med *88*:285–293, 1978.

116. Dienstag JL: Non-A, non-B hepatitis. I. Recognition, epidemiology, and clinical features. Gastroenterology *85*:439–462, 1983.

117. Ziegler EJ, Fisher Jr EJ, Sprung CL, et al: Treatment of gram-negative bacteremia and septic shock with HA-1A human monoclonal antibody against endotoxin. N Engl J Med *324*:429–436, 1991.

118. Greenman RL, Schein RMH, Martin MA, et al: A controlled clinical trial of ES murine monoclonal IgM antibody to endotoxin in the treatment of gram-negative sepsis. JAMA *226*:1097–1102, 1991.

119. Alter MJ, Hadler SC, Margolis HS, et al: The changing epidemiology of non-A, non-B hepatitis in the United States: relationship to transfusions, abstracted. Transfusion Associated Infect Immune Response *3*:14, 1988.

120. Alter MJ, Gerety RJ, Smallwood LA, et al: Sporadic non-Α, non-B hepatitis: frequency and epidemiology in an urban U.S. population. J Infect Dis *145*:886–893, 1982.

121. Dienstag JL, Alter HJ: Non-A, non-B hepatitis: evolving epidemiologic and clinical perspectives. Semin Liver Dis *6*:67–81, 1986.

122. Alter HJ: The chronic consequences of non-A, non-B hepatitis. *In* Seeff LB (ed): Current Perspectives in Hepatology. New York, Plenum, 1989.

123. Revision of the CDC surveillance case definition for acquired immunodeficiency syndrome. Council of State and Territorial Epidemiologists; AIDS Program, Center for Infectious Disease. MMWR *36*(suppl 1):1S, 1987.

124. Curran JW, Jaffe HW, Hardy AM, et al: Epidemiology of HIV infection and AIDS in the United States. Science *239*:610–616, 1988.

125. Friedland GH, Klein RS: Transmission of the human immunodeficiency virus. N Engl J Med *317*:1125–1135, 1987.

126. Jaffe HW, Darrow WW, Echenberg DF, et al: The acquired immunodeficiency syndrome in a cohort of homosexual men: a six-year follow-up study. Ann Intern Med *103*:210–214, 1985.

127. Becker CE, Cone JE, Geberding J: Occupational infection with human immunodeficiency virus. Ann Intern Med *110*:653–656, 1989.

128. Glatt AE, Chirgwin K, Landesman SH: Treatment of infections associated with human immunodeficiency virus. N Engl J Med *318*:1439–1448, 1988.

129. CDC: Update: universal precautions for prevention of transmission of human immunodeficiency virus, hepatitis B virus, and other bloodborne pathogens in health care settings. MMWR *37*:377–388, 1988.

130. Peterman TA, Jaffe H, Feorino PM, et al: Transfusion-associated acquired immunodeficiency syndrome in the United States. JAMA *254*:2913–2917, 1985.

131. CDC: Provisional public health service inter-agency recommendations for screening donated blood and plasma for antibody to the virus causing acquired immunodeficiency syndrome. MMWR *34*:5–7, 1985.

132. Weiss SH, Goedert JJ, Sarngadharan MG, et al: Screening test for HTLV-III (AIDS agent) antibodies: specificity, sensitivity, and applications. JAMA *253*:221–225, 1985.

133. Sivak SL, Wormser GP: Predictive value of a screening test for antibodies to HTLV-III. Am J Clin Pathol *85*:700–703, 1986.

134. Update: serologic testing for antibody to human immunodeficiency virus. MMWR *36*:833–840, 845, 1988.

135. Burke DS, Brandt BL, Redfield RR, et al: Diagnosis

of human immunodeficiency virus infection by immunoassay using a molecularly cloned and expressed virus envelope polypeptide: comparison to Western Blot on 2707 consecutive serum samples. Ann Intern Med *106*:671–676, 1987.

136. Dawson GJ, Heller JS, Wood CA, et al: Reliable detection of individuals seropositive for the human immunodeficiency virus (HIV) by competitive immunoassays using Escherichia coli-expressed HIV structural proteins. J Infect Dis *157*:149–155, 1988.

137. Saladuddin SZ, Markham PD, Redfield RR, et al: HTLV III in symptom-free seronegative persons. Lancet *2*:1418–1420, 1984.

138. Imagawa DT, Lee MH, Wolinsky SM, et al: Human immunodeficiency virus type 1 infection in homosexual men who remain seronegative for prolonged periods. N Engl J Med *320*:1458–1462, 1989.

139. CDC: Update on hepatitis B prevention. MMWR *36*:353–366, 1987.

140. Hadler SC, Francis DP, Maynard JE, et al: Long-term immunogenicity and efficacy of hepatitis B vaccine in homosexual men. N Engl J Med *315*:209–214, 1986.

141. Fauci AS, Gallo RC, Koenig S, et al: Development and evaluation of a vaccine for human immunodeficiency virus infection. Ann Intern Med *110*:373–385, 1989.

142. Bond WW, Favero MS, Peterson NJ, et al: Survival of hepatitis B virus after drying and storage for one week. Lancet *1*:550–551, 1981.

143. Resnick L, Veren K, Salahuddin SZ, et al: Stability and inactivation of HTLV-III/LAV under clinical

and laboratory environments. JAMA *265*:1887–1891, 1986.

144. Spire B, Montagnier L, Barre-Sinoussi F, Chermann JC: Inactivation of lymphadenopathy-associated virus by chemical disinfectants. Lancet *2*:899–901, 1984.

145. CDC: Summary: recommendations for preventing transmission of HTLV-III/LAV in the workplace. JAMA *254*:3162–3168, 1985.

146. Martin LS, McDougal S, Loskoski SL: Disinfection and inactivation of the human T-lymphotrophic virus type III/lymphadenopathy-associated virus. J Infect Dis *152*:400–403, 1985.

147. Brown P, Gibbs CJ Jr, Amyx HL, et al: Chemical disinfection of Creutzfeldt-Jakob disease virus. N Engl J Med *306*:1279–1283, 1982.

148. Ruprecht RM, O'Brien LG, Rossoni LD, Nusinoff-Lehrman S: Suppression of mouse viraemia and retroviral disease by 3'-azido-3'deoxythymidine. Nature *323*:467–469, 1986. (letter).

149. Tavares L, Roneker C, Johnston K, et al: 3'-Azido-3'deoxythymidine in feline leukemia virus-infected cats: a model for therapy and prophylaxis of AIDS. Cancer Res *47*:3190–3194, 1987.

150. Henderson DK, Gerberding JL: Prophylactic zidovudine after occupational exposure to the human immunodeficiency virus. J Infect Dis *160*:321–327, 1989.

151. Fischl MA: Zidovudine: clinical experience in symptomatic HIV disease. *In* Volberding P, Jacobsen M (eds): AIDS Clinical Review 1989. New York, Marcel Dekker, 1989, pp. 221–242.

22 OBSTETRIC PATIENTS IN THE PACU AND ICU

RICHARD E. GELFAND

The post anesthetic care of the recently delivered mother or the pregnant woman having nonparturient surgery is a subject that deserves special attention. Although most of the post anesthetic care unit (PACU) and intensive care unit (ICU) considerations of these patients are similar to those for any other patient having similar surgery, the physiologic changes of pregnancy, the birthing process, and the newborn require additional attention.

This chapter first looks at the normal patient who has had an anesthetic for vaginal delivery or cesarean section. It then considers medical problems unique to the obstetric setting and the effects of anesthesia on the newborn and on breast feeding. Finally, the patient requiring an anesthetic and operation prior to delivery is discussed. This overview covers material adjunctive to the medical management by the anesthesiologist and obstetrician.

NORMAL POSTPARTUM PATIENT

There is a tendency to undermonitor and undertreat patients in the delivery room PACU. This tendency is partly because the obstetric patient is usually healthy and partly due to resistance by both patient and staff to interference with the interaction of the new family. The patient who has just delivered by cesarean section or complicated vaginal delivery is often surrounded by family members admiring the new baby in a room filled with other new families. Common sense, however, as well as the standards of the American Society of Anesthesiology (ASA) and the Harvard standards demand that she receive the same level of care in the delivery room PACU following general or major regional anesthesia as she would in the operating room PACU after similar procedures.[1–4] At the same time, though, consideration should be given to the

new family as they get to know each other and to the baby as he or she begins extrauterine life.

The PACU in the delivery room in each hospital must set its own routine care protocol. Table 22–1 contains one such plan. It provides for the basic monitoring of patients and provides backup for the PACU nurse should a problem be discovered. The procedures outlined must be supplemented with others for certain patients.

OBSTETRIC DISEASES

Problems following general or regional anesthesia may arise for the delivery room patient just as they do for the operating room patient. Some complications, e.g., aspiration and postdural puncture headache, are more frequent in the parturient than in the nonpregnant patient, but they are treated in the same way for both and are covered elsewhere in this book. The following sections discuss several pathophysiologic processes unique to the obstetric patient.

PREECLAMPSIA

Preeclampsia is defined as an acute onset of hypertension usually during the second or third trimester. It may occur, however, during the first 24 hours or more postpartum and so must be watched for in the PACU. Blood pressure of 140/90 mm Hg or a 30 mm Hg increase in systolic pressure or 15 mm Hg increase in diastolic pressure and either proteinuria or edema lead to the diagnosis. Severe preeclampsia involves a blood pressure reading of 160/110 mm Hg, 5 gm of proteinuria over a 24 hour period, or one of the other symptoms of end-organ injury, e.g., oliguria, epigastric or right upper quadrant pain, pulmonary edema,

TABLE 22–1. GUIDELINES FOR THE NORMAL POSTPARTUM PACU PATIENT: MINIMUM CARE[a]

Delivery/Surgery and Anesthesia	Report to PACU Nurse Given By	Physician Capable of Resuscitation Immediately Available	Specific Anesthesiologist Available for Consultation	Oxygen Given Routinely if SpO$_2$ ≥95	Monitoring		PACU Discharge Criteria Including PAR Score[5]
					Fundal No Color Check, BP, HR, RR Every 15 min for 1 hr then Every 30 min	ECG: Continuous Pulse Oximeter: on Admission and Discharge (if < 95, Continuous)	
Cesarean, postpartum tubal ligation GA	Anesthesiologist or anesthetist	Yes	Yes	Yes	Yes	Yes	Yes
D&C or other less common procedures after delivery							
Regional or MAC	Anesthesiologist or anesthetist	Yes	Yes	No	Yes	Yes	Yes
GA	Anesthesiologist or anesthetist	Yes	Yes	Yes	Yes	Yes	Yes
Regional or MAC	Anesthesiologist or anesthetist	Yes	Yes	No	Yes	Yes	Yes
Vaginal delivery							
Pudendal or local anesthesia after labor CLE has worn off	Obstetrician or labor nurse	Yes	Yes	No	Yes	No	Yes
Pudendal or local anesthesia without labor CLE	Obstetrician or labor nurse	Yes	No	No	Yes	No	No

[a] This outline is not intended to be a standard of care. The care of an individual patient is left to the discretion of the physicians caring for her.
GA = general anesthesia; MAC = monitored anesthesia care; CLE = continuous lumbar epidural; BP = blood pressure; HR = heart rate; RR = respiratory rate; PAR = post anesthesia recovery; SpO$_2$ = oxygen saturation determined by pulse oximeter.

or disseminated intravascular coagulation. Thus the signs of preeclampsia are hypertension, proteinuria, edema, and hyperreflexia.

Preeclampsia is more likely during a first pregnancy or after a previous preeclamptic pregnancy. It is also more common in the presence of chronic renal disease, chronic hypertension, fetal chromosomal anomalies, or conditions leading to an enlarged placenta, i.e., multiple gestations, polyhydramnios, diabetes, or fetal hydrops. The full preeclamptic disease process may fail to develop, leading to a curious nonhypertensive preeclamptic state. The HELP syndrome (hemolysis, elevated liver enzymes, and low platelet count), which may not include hypertension, has been described in association with preeclampsia.[6]

Hypertension is the usual presenting sign of preeclampsia. If diastolic blood pressure rises above 110 mm Hg, consideration of vasodilator therapy is warranted. In the PACU, nitroprusside is probably the initial drug of choice because of its effectiveness and quick onset and offset of action. After the blood pressure is controlled, other drugs, including hydralazine and labetalol, may be substituted. Invasive monitoring, including an arterial line and a central venous pressure (CVP) line, is helpful when the blood pressure requires that a vasodilator be given. The debate between CVP and pulmonary artery (PA) pressure monitoring continues.[7-9] The PA catheter allows more direct measurement of left heart filling pressures, cardiac output, and systemic vascular resistance, which in turn allows more precise vasodilator and fluid therapy to be prescribed.

With preeclampsia, total body water is increased but plasma volume is decreased compared to normal pregnancy, resulting in hemoconcentration and vasospasm. Urinary output is often decreased owing to either hypovolemia or kidney involvement. Intravenous fluids are indicated for dehydration but may lead to pulmonary edema in the patient with a renal injury. An initial gentle fluid challenge of a few hundred milliliters of crystalloid may be warranted. If this treatment is unsuccessful, a CVP monitor or PA pressure catheter is advisable before more aggressive therapy is attempted to improve urinary output.[10]

The choice of fluid for further therapy is controversial. Though crystalloid is most commonly used, the gentle use of albumin solutions may be warranted in the severely preeclamptic patient, as most of these patients have a low albumin and colloid osmotic pressure.[9]

The typical hemodynamic profile of a severe preeclamptic patient is low pulmonary capillary wedge pressure (PCWP), high or normal cardiac output, and high systemic vascular resistance. Consequently, increasing fluids is often required as the vasodilator is started so the preload, and consequently the cardiac output, does not decline dangerously.[10] An occasional patient, however, may have cardiac dysfunction and needs to be treated with vasodilator and fluid restriction.

Hyperreflexia and central nervous system irritability is seen in preeclamptic patients who are at increased risk for seizure. These problems are usually treated with a 4 to 6 gm intravenous bolus of magnesium sulfate followed by an infusion. The infusion rate is adjusted by following blood levels and deep tendon reflexes (Table 22–2). Should the patellar reflex disappear, the infusion is stopped and the obstetrician notified.

If a seizure occurs, eclampsia is diagnosed and the chance of death increases. The airway and ventilation must be ensured in such cases. Seizure activity usually stops spontaneously or can be easily treated with thiopental 50 to 75 mg. If this measure fails, diazepam 5 to 10 mg is given. Note that diazepam has been associated with neonatal problems (described below) and should be used with care. Once the seizure is terminated, magnesium sulfate loading and maintenance doses should be started. The patient's airway must be maintained and protected, which may require endotracheal intubation. The increased danger of aspiration in pregnant women is only partially alleviated by delivery.

The goals of therapy for the preeclamptic woman are a diastolic pressure of 100 mm Hg, normal preload and cardiac output, adequate urinary output, and avoidance of seizure. After delivery of the products of conception (the cause for the preeclamptic changes), the patient's status is expected to return to normal over the course of a day or two.

TABLE 22–2. MAGNESIUM THERAPY

Level (mg/dl)	Side Effect
1.5–2.0	Normal level—none
4–8	Therapeutic level—none
10–12	Loss of reflex muscle weakness
12–15	Hypoventilation
25–30	Cardiac depression

CARDIAC DISEASE

Cardiac disease in patients of childbearing age has been declining in prevalence and changing from nearly all rheumatic heart disease to include a much greater percentage of congenital and nonrheumatic heart disease. The normal physiologic changes of pregnancy include increased blood volume and increased cardiac output. In fact, cardiac output increases by 80 per cent above the pregnancy baseline during and immediately after delivery. Most of this massive increase is reversed during the next few hours, and the patient returns to prepregnancy levels over the next 6 to 8 weeks.[11,12]

Most New York Heart Association (NYHA) class I or II patients go through labor, delivery, and recovery without a problem. Class III and IV patients require continued care in the PACU and ICU as the altered cardiovascular state returns toward the prepregnancy values. If the patient has had a major conduction block for labor and delivery or cesarean section, she may require diuresis or vasodilatation as the sympathetic block regresses, decreasing the vascular space.

Whereas most heart disease manifests prior to the postpartum period, cardiomyopathy of pregnancy may manifest as late as 5 months postpartum. It is of unknown etiology and presents as cardiac failure with a hypocontractile and dilated left ventricle on echocardiogram and a high PCWP. Aggressive treatment with dopamine, digitalis, diuretics, and prolonged bed rest results in the best outcome, but even so mortality is still 40 to 50 per cent.[13]

Of increasing interest in the woman of childbearing age is coronary heart disease. The patient who has cardiac ischemia or a myocardial infarction while pregnant probably has more ischemia due to the increased cardiac demands of labor and delivery. She requires additional monitoring and epidural analgesia to reduce the cardiac stress of labor pain.[14] In the PACU and ICU, treatment of coronary disease is a logical continuation of the delivery room management and is similar to that for the nonpregnant patient (see Chapter 3).

POSTPARTUM HEMORRHAGE

All patients in the PACU must be observed for excessive postpartum bleeding and delayed relaxation of the uterus. Uterine atony accounts for most postpartum hemorrhaging in the PACU. The predisposing causes are variable and include rapid or precipitous delivery, prolonged labor, oxytocin induction or augmentation, magnesium therapy, chorioamnionitis, and conditions that cause an enlarged uterus, e.g., polyhydramnios. Retained products of conception may be a cause of delayed uterine atony and postpartum hemorrhage; and rarely an acquired or congenital coagulopathy is responsible (Table 22–3).

The management of postpartum hemorrhage starts with manual examination of the cervix and uterus. Uterine tone is examined, and lacerations and retained products are sought. Coagulation should be assessed if the initial findings and treatment are not successful.

The usual routine of using 20 U of oxytocin per liter of fluids for the first several hours

TABLE 22–3. POSTPARTUM HEMORRHAGE

Cause	Usual Time of Onset	Treatment
Uterine atony	Within 2 hours of delivery	Oxytocin by infusion; methergine or ergonovine by IM injection
Vaginal/cervical bleeding	Immediate	Surgical repair
Retained products of conception	Delayed up to a month postpartum	Manual removal or D&C
Disseminated intravascular coagulation	Usually immediate	Replace factors and platelets as needed for hemostasis
Von Willebrand syndrome	1–2 weeks postpartum	Cryoprecipitates: DDAVP (?)
Dilutional hypothrombocytopenia or decreased factors	Usually immediate	Replace platelets or factors

after delivery may serve to decrease blood loss.[16] If poor uterine tone is found to be the problem, additional oxytocin can be added to the fluids, or ergonovine or methylergonovine 0.2 mg IM may be given. An intravenous bolus of either drug should be avoided. Oxytocin may cause hypotension, and the ergots may cause severe hypertension. Prostaglandin $F_2\alpha$ given intramyometrially has been used.[15] These treatment decisions are typically made by the obstetrician.

At times the patient's survival depends on prompt blood replacement and surgical intervention, including possible hysterectomy. Platelets and other hemostatic factors may be diluted by transfusion of more than half the patient's blood volume and so may need to be replaced. When emergency surgery is required before the blood volume can be adequately restored, general anesthesia is preferable to epidural or spinal anesthesia in order to avoid the excessive hypotension that is likely to accompany the sympathetic blockade. Even though an epidural or spinal catheter is present, general anesthesia is used for hypovolemic patients unless the necessary anesthetic level is already present.

NEWBORNS: MATERNAL ANALGESIA AND BREAST FEEDING

The newborn in the PACU and nursery is observed for signs of difficulty adjusting to extrauterine life, including respiratory distress, cyanosis, abnormal temperature regulation, hypocalcemia, hypoglycemia, jitteriness, and feeding problems. Special concerns for the neonate related to maternal disease also must be kept in mind. Detailed discussion of such problems is beyond the scope of this chapter. The focus here is on the neonatal effects of maternal anesthesia and analgesia.

The neonate is affected in two ways by the anesthesia and analgesia the mother receives. Sedatives, narcotics, and local and general anesthetics cross the placenta and can be found in the newborn.

Secobarbital and other longer-acting barbiturates occasionally used for sedation during labor can cause drowsiness in the newborn that may last for days, especially if narcotics are also given.[17,18] The use of a small dose of promethazine or hydroxyzine does not appear to cause neonatal depression.[17]

The benzodiazepines may have significant neonatal effects. The fetal blood levels may exceed maternal levels, and enterohepatic recirculation and active metabolites are found in the newborn. These processes collaborate to produce neonatal sedation for several hours after the maternal dose is given.[17,19] Other neonatal problems include floppy baby syndrome (lethargy, hypotonia, and sucking difficulties), withdrawal syndrome, hypothermia, and hyperbilirubinemia.[20-22] If diazepam has been given during the first two trimesters, congenital anomalies including cardiac problems may occur and should be watched for in the PACU. Lorazepam may cause depressed neurobehavioral scores, feeding problems, and respiratory depression.[17] Midazolam, a water-soluble benzodiazepine, may be found to be safer for the neonate but has not yet been fully evaluated.

Narcotics given to the laboring patient may cause postdelivery respiratory depression and depressed neurobehavioral scores in the neonate.[23] Fentanyl appears to cause fewer problems than the more traditional narcotics,[24,25] but the baby requires close observation regardless of narcotic used.

After uncomplicated labor with epidural analgesia, no neonatal effects should be seen in the PACU, even on neurobehavioral scores[26-29] and even if fentanyl or sufentanyl has been used.[30-32] Hypotension may cause fetal and neonatal depression; but when treated promptly with fluids and ephedrine, no ill effects are seen.[17]

Inhalation analgesia for labor pain has been found to have minimal effects on the newborn.[33] General anesthesia for cesarean section may cause a transient sedative effect on the newborn. The resulting depressed Apgar scores can be eliminated with the use of modern anesthetic techniques and limiting the induction to delivery time to 10 minutes or less.[34-36] Neurobehavioral scores, however, may be mildly depressed for 24 hours. Regional anesthesia appears to have limited neurobehavioral effects on the newborn.[37,38]

The second way the neonate may be affected by maternal medications is through breast feeding. Breast feeding has both nutritional and emotional benefit for the newborn. Drugs must cross the blood-milk barrier, through the capillary wall and through the myothelial and alveolar cells, with much the same restriction to movement as is seen with the placental or blood-brain barriers. Once the drug is in the milk, the baby must ingest it and absorb it through the gastrointestinal tract before it can have any effect.[39]

The anesthetic drugs are all found in low

concentration in breast milk. The levels of thiopental, morphine, meperidine, and butorphanol are unlikely to have any significant effect especially during the first few days when less than 50 ml of colostrum is secreted per day.[20,40,41] In addition, these drugs are poorly absorbed orally. Such data are limited on fentanyl, hydromorphone, and related drugs but would be expected to be similar to those for other narcotics.

Sedatives are found in breast milk. Diazepam probably accumulates in breast milk and has been reported to cause neonatal lethargy and weight loss; it is therefore not recommended for breast-feeding mothers. There are no data on promethazine and midazolam in regard to breast-feeding. Hydroxyzine also has not been studied in breast milk but is apparently safe in reasonable doses during late pregnancy[42] and is probably also safe for breast-feeding mothers.

Large doses of atropine or antihistamine may or may not decrease milk production. Atropine may cause an anticholinergic effect in babies.[20,42]

Inhalational anesthetics are largely excreted by the lungs and are unlikely to be seen in significant concentrations in the milk. Muscle relaxants do not cross biologic barriers easily and would not be expected to cause problems in the newborn.

Vasodilator and β-blockers are occasionally used for preeclamptic patients. Nitroglycerine and sodium nitroprusside have not been studied. Hydralazine and α-methyldopa are found in breast milk but have not been found to have adverse effects. Labetalol and propranolol are in breast milk; and although no adverse effects have been seen, it is recommended that the baby be observed for bradycardia and hypotension. Esmolol has not been studied.[20]

NONPARTURIENT SURGERY DURING PREGNANCY

Elective surgery is not performed during pregnancy, so patients arriving in the PACU have had either urgent or emergent surgery. They require all of the observation and care required of other patients who have had such surgery as well as the care required by their pregnant state.

Supine position during the second and third trimesters may compromise blood flow to the placenta because of venocaval compression.[12] Positioning the pregnant patient in full left or right lateral or at least left pelvic tilt not only

minimizes this problem, it decreases the likelihood of pulmonary aspiration.

Preterm labor can occur during the immediate postoperative period. It is most common following certain types of surgery (that on the cervix, uterus, and ovaries).[12] Abdominal cramping, constant back pain or pelvic pressure, and increased or bloody vaginal discharge should alert the postoperative nurse to the possibility of preterm labor.[43] After 20 weeks' gestation an external tocodynamometer can be used to monitor uterine activity.

Fetal monitoring by external ultrasonic heart monitor can be done after 16 weeks' gestation.[12] The normal premature fetal baseline heart rate is higher than at term, and beat-to-beat variability is decreased or absent. After general anesthesia, beat-to-beat variability may be absent during the early postoperative period in older fetuses as well, until the baby emerges from the sedation of anesthesia. Monitoring the heart tones for fetal tachycardia or decelerations can alert the staff to maternal hypoventilation or decreased uterine perfusion.[44]

ACKNOWLEDGMENT. Thanks go to Dr. John Hobart for his input and help.

References

1. Anonymous: Standards for conduction anesthesia in obstetrics. Anesthesiol News April:22, 1989.
2. Anonymous: Standards for postoperative care. Anesthesiol News April:22, 1989.
3. Anonymous: Standards of Nursing Practice. Richmond, American Society of Post Anesthesia Nurses, 1986.
4. Eichhorn JH, Cooper JB, Cullen DJ, et al: Anesthesia practice standards at Harvard: review. J Clin Anesthesiol 1:55–65, 1988.
5. Aldrek JA, Kroulik D: Postanesthesic recovery score. Anesth Analg 49:924–934, 1970.
6. Weinstein L: Syndrome of hemolysis, elevated liver enzymes and low platelet count: a severe consequence of hypertension in pregnancy. Am J Obstet Gynecol 142:159–167, 1982.
7. Benedetti TL, Cotton DB, Read JC, Miller FC: Hemodynamic observations in severe pre-eclampsia with a flow-directed pulmonary artery catheter. Am J Obstet Gynecol 136:465–470, 1980.
8. Newsome LR, Bramwell RS, Curling PE: Severe preeclampsia: hemodynamic effects of lumbar epidural anesthesia. Anesth Analg 65:31–36, 1986.
9. Joyce TH, Loon M: Preeclampsia: effect of albumen 25% infusion. Anesthesiology 55:A313, 1981.
10. Kirshon B, Cotton DB: Invasive hemodynamic monitoring in the obstetric patient. Clin Obstet Gynecol 30:579–590, 1987.
11. Mangano DT: Anesthesia for the pregnant cardiac patient. In Shnider SM, Levinson G (eds): Anesthesia for Obstetrics. Baltimore, Williams & Wilkins, 1987, pp. 345–381.

12. Pedersen H, Finster M: Anesthetic risk in the pregnant surgical patient. Anesthesiology *51*:439–451, 1979.

13. Alder AK, Davis MR: Peripartum cardiomyopathy: two case reports and a review. Obstet Gynecol Surv *41*:675–682, 1986.

14. Roberts SL, Chestnut DH: Anesthesia for the obstetric patient with cardiac disease. Clin Obstet Gynecol *30*:601–610, 1987.

15. Hayashi RH: Hemorrhagic shock in obstetrics. Clin Perinatal *13*:755–764, 1986.

16. Newton M, Mosey LM, Egli GE, et al: Blood loss during and immediately after delivery. Obstet Gynecol *17*:9–18, 1961.

17. Shnider SM, Levinson G: Anesthesia for Obstetrics. Baltimore, Williams & Wilkins, 1987.

18. Shnider SM, Moya F: Effects of meperidine on the newborn infant. Am J Obstet Gynecol *89*:1009–1015, 1964.

19. Cree IE, Meyer J, Hailey DM: Diazepam in labour: its metabolites and effects on the clinical condition and thermogenesis of the newborn. Br Med J *4*:251–255, 1973.

20. Briggs G, Freeman RK, Yaffe SJ: Drugs in Pregnancy and Lactation. Baltimore, Williams & Wilkins, 1986.

21. Scanlon JW: Effects of benzodiazepines in neonates. N Engl J Med *292*:649, 1975 (letter).

22. Owen JR, Irani SF, Blair AW: Effect of diazepam administered to mothers during labour on temperature regulation of the neonate. Arch Dis Child *47*:107–110, 1972.

23. Kuhnert BR, Linn PL, Kennard MJ, Kuhnert PM: Effects of low doses of meperidine on neonatal behavior. Anesth Analg *64*:335–342, 1985.

24. Rayburn WF, Smith CV, Parriott JE, Woods RE: Randomized comparison of meperidine and fentanyl during labor. Obstet Gynecol *74*:604–606, 1989.

25. Rayburn W, Rathke A, Leuschen MP, et al: Fentanyl citrate analgesia during labor. Am J Obstet Gynecol *161*:202–206, 1989.

26. Wallis KL, Shnider SM, Hicks MD, Spivey HT: Epidural anesthesia in the normotensive pregnant ewe: effect on uterine blood flow and fetal acid-base status. Anesthesiology *44*:481–487, 1976.

27. Abboud TK, Sarkis F, Blikian A, et al: Lack of adverse neonatal behavioral effect of lidocaine. Anesth Analg *62*:473–475, 1983.

28. Abboud TK, Afrasiabi A, Sarkis F, et al: Continuous infusion epidural analgesia in parturients receiving bupivacaine, chloroprocaine, or lidocaine—maternal, fetal, and neonatal effects. Anesth Analg *63*:421–428, 1984.

29. Briggs G, Freeman RK, Yaffe SJ: Drugs in pregnancy and lactation: update. *1*:1–2, 1988.

30. Eisele JH, Wright R, Rogge P: Newborn and maternal fentanyl levels at cesarean section. Anesth Analg *61*:179–180, 1982.

31. Phillips GH: Epidural sufentanil/bupivacaine combinations for analgesia during labor: effect of varying sufentanil doses. Anesthesiology *67*:835–838, 1987.

32. Phillips G: Continuous infusion epidural analgesia in labor: the effect of adding sufentanil to 0.125% bupivacaine. Anesth Analg *67*:462–465, 1988.

33. Stefani SJ, Hughes SC, Shnider SM, et al. Neonatal neurobehavioral effects of inhalation analgesia for vaginal delivery. Anesthesiology *56*:351–355, 1982.

34. Datta S, Ostheimer GW, Weiss JB, et al: Neonatal effect of prolonged anesthetic induction for cesarean section. Obstet Gynecol *58*:331–335, 1981.

35. Hodges RJ, Tunstall ME: The choice of anesthesia and its influence on perinatal mortality in cesarean section. Br J Anaesth *33*: 572–588, 1961.

36. Ong BY, Cohen MM, Palahniuk RJ: Anesthesia for cesarean section—effects on neonates. Anesth Analg *68*:270–275, 1989.

37. Hodgkinson R, Bhatt M, Kim SS, et al: Neonatal neurobehavioral tests following cesarean section under general and spinal anesthesia. Am J Obstet Gynecol *132*:670–674, 1978.

38. Abboud TK, Nagappala S, Murakawa K, et al: Comparison of the effects of general and regional anesthesia for cesarean section on neonatal neurologic and adaptive capacity scores. Anesth Analg *64*:996–1000, 1985.

39. George DI, O'Tool TJ: A review of drug transfer to the infant by breast-feeding: concerns for the dentist. J Am Dent Assoc *106*:204–208, 1983.

40. Anderson LW, Ovist T, Hertz J, Mogensen F: Concentrations of thiopentone in mature breast milk and colostrum following induction dose. Acta Anesthesiol Scand *31*:30–32, 1987.

41. Quinn PG, Kuhnert BR, Kaine CJ, Syracuse CD: Measurement of meperidine and normeperidine in human breast milk by selected ion monitoring. Biomed Environ Mass Spectrom *13*:133–135, 1986.

42. Anderson PO: Drugs and breast feeding. Semin Perinatol *3*:271–278, 1979.

43. Creasy RK: Preterm labor. *In* Paverstein CJ (ed): Clinical Obstetrics. New York, Wiley, 1987.

44. Katz JD, Hook R, Barash PG: Fetal heart-rate monitoring in pregnant patients undergoing surgery. Am J Obstet Gynecol *125*:267–269, 1976

QUALITY ASSURANCE IN THE POST ANESTHESIA CARE UNIT

23

R. FRANCIS NARBONE

In response to the growing demands for public accountability, the Joint Commission on Accreditation of Hospitals (JCAH) initiated Quality Assurance (QA) programs as part of the surveying process and as part of its accreditation standards. The JCAH focused its attention on the quality and process of health care to establish standards by which to judge clinical performance and to define quality of care. Specifically, concern arose that the medical profession was not policing itself sufficiently to guarantee the implementation of necessary changes in medical care. The possibility also existed that potential problems might be ignored or remain undetected. Additionally, as health care resources have become scarcer, more information is being demanded by consumers on clinical performance and other dimensions of care quality. This demand is due in large part to the high cost of new technology and the restrictions placed on the health care industry by third party payers. Therefore the establishment of QA programs was mandated in hospitals across the country.

HISTORY OF QUALITY ASSURANCE

Quality assurance programs were originally designed to regain public trust through the use of standardized regulations to monitor systematically and objectively and to evaluate the quality and appropriateness of patient care in order to make changes where necessary. It has not always been easy for QA programs to gain the acceptance of many health care providers. This lack of acceptance has been attributed to the increased time and effort required to collect and analyze data, to implement any necessary changes in procedures or policies, and to follow up on the efficacy of

these changes. In an effort to focus the efforts of QA programs on the most significant areas of patient care, the JCAH developed 10 steps to monitor and evaluate the quality and appropriateness of hospital care (Tables 23–1 and 23–2).

ROLE OF RISK MANAGEMENT

Risk management programs usually coexist with QA programs, each using a different approach to minimize any adverse effects that could result from problems encountered in a health care institution. Risk management protects the legal and financial integrity of the health care institution and the health care providers by reducing the potential for adverse situations in the health care environment. Both risk management and QA programs address situations involving patients, visitors, and health care providers. Quality assurance not only addresses the risk, it evaluates the process by which the risk is reduced and measures the outcome. Problems encountered in reviews by risk management groups should be incorporated in QA investigations. These efforts protect the health and well-being of patients and others who come into contact with the health care delivery system.

ORGANIZATION AND OPERATION OF A QA PROGRAM IN THE PACU

Quality assurance programs are especially important in the post anesthesia care unit (PACU) because many interdependent elements of medical care are encountered there. This QA program is designed to complement the standards of excellence required in the

363

TABLE 23–1. MONITORING QUALITY ASSURANCE: JCAH STANDARDS

1. Assign responsibility for monitoring and evaluating activities.

2. Delineate the scope of care provided by the organization.

3. Identify the most important aspects of the care the organization provides.

4. Identify indicators (and appropriate clinical criteria) that can be used to monitor those important aspects of care.

5. Establish thresholds for the indicators at which further evaluation of care is triggered.

6. Collect and organize data for each indicator.

7. Evaluate the care when the thresholds are reached in order to identify the problems or opportunities to improve the care.

8. Take actions to correct identified problems or to improve care.

9. Assess the effectiveness of the actions and document improvement in care.

10. Communicate relevant information to other individuals, departments, or services and to the organization-wide quality assurance programs.

hospital operating room and extend them to the PACU. The need for such QA programs has been demonstrated by the number of anesthetized patients involved in PACU morbidity and mortality incidents. Approximately one third of anesthesia-related complications develop in the PACU; the other two thirds begin in the operating room and continue in the PACU. Therefore attention must be given to the care patients receive in the PACU to ensure an optimal outcome for their surgery.

The most important function of a QA program is to address the appropriateness and effectiveness of care. It is unfortunate that QA programs and their paperwork are often perceived as impositions on the limited time of the medical team. Moreover, QA programs are sometimes viewed as unwelcome watchdogs for regulating bodies or superiors.

It is imperative to stress the positive value of cooperating with QA requirements. Health care providers must possess a clear understanding of the public mandate that led to the establishment of QA programs, as developed and overseen by federal, state, and local governments in cooperation with the JCAH and third-party payers.

If clinicians are to view QA programs and their accompanying paperwork as valuable additions to the armamentarium of the medical team, they must be able to witness positive results for their time and cooperation. When used properly, QA programs can result in improved patient care and serve as one of the many tools that are now revolutionizing medical care. Full cooperation of all health care team members is integral to the success of a QA program. Without enthusiastic and intelligent participation, a QA program has a marginal chance for success.

TABLE 23–2. QUALITY ASSURANCE TERMINOLOGY

Quality assurance	Program for measuring the quality of work or the nature of service using set standards
Quality control	Mechanism that measures the accuracy of techniques, e.g., laboratory tests, sterilization controls
Value	Qualitative statement of outcome or outcome performance of a procedure
Standard	Quantitative statement of outcome or performance of a procedure
Policy	Statement or mandatory action
Procedure	Statement or outline of methodology
Audit tool	Document, usually a checklist, used to measure the quality of outcome or performance
Quality assurance report	Formal document containing a summary and analysis of data obtained through audits and other quality assurance mechanisms
Risk management	Identification and minimization of legal, financial, and medicolegal risks to the hospital

Concerns may already exist about certain areas of care. Although some information is available about these concerns, a mechanism to address them may not be in place. The goal of QA programs is to review these concerns and establish a comprehensive set of guidelines that address the delivery of appropriate patient care. Data must then be collected to evaluate and monitor these guidelines and their enforcement.

Without their intelligent participation, the QA process cannot function properly. Ideally, the QA team should include all participants in the care of the PACU patients: physicians, nurses, other PACU technicians, and individuals responsible for the unit's administration and equipment.

ROLE OF THE QA COMMITTEE

To carry out the duties of the QA mandate, members of the QA committee must assess care in the PACU. After deliberate and careful review of all pertinent activities, committee members must reach agreement on the major focal areas. In addition, a review of the literature is essential to find expert opinions about the areas of concern and introduce other areas that were not considered. In general, QA branches into three basic areas: structure, process, and outcome (Table 23–3).

Structure

Structure, in relation to QA programs, refers to the physical plant and equipment of the PACU, and the numbers and qualifications of the health care providers as they impact on patient care delivery. Sometimes PACU clinicians do not believe they are directly responsible for the structure of the PACU. They view these patient care features as the concern of "someone else." Structure, however, is essential to patient care. It is ideal if the entire team of health care providers feels actively involved in the selection and care of equipment used in the PACU. Thorough evaluations of all equipment by the members of the QA team ensures that all regulatory specifications concerning electrical or mechanical equipment are met. In addition, attendance should be required for ongoing in-service training. All equipment must be inspected thoroughly on a regular basis, and these safety inspections should be documented. "Structure" is not just the concern of "someone else." Quality care can be assured only when the entire health care team focuses on the importance of the PACU equipment. Strict adherence to QA structure guidelines protects patients and health care providers from "operator error" by thoroughly documenting the inspection, care, and use of all equipment in the PACU.

Process

Process refers to the important activities of the PACU and explains how these activities should be monitored. The health care providers in the PACU must reach consensus about the significance of activities. Priority must be given to those aspects of care that occur most frequently and affect the greatest number of patients. Top priority must also be given to procedures involving high risk patients who would suffer detrimental conse-

TABLE 23–3. ISSUES ADDRESSED THROUGH THE USE OF CLINICAL INDICATORS

Issue	Diagnosis	Treatment
Structure	Availability of resources (staff, equipment) for accurate diagnosis Diagnostic protocols	Availability of needed therapeutic resources Treatment plans
Process	Accuracy, timeliness, and technical skill when applying diagnostic protocols	Skill and technical quality of therapeutic interventions
Outcome	Correctness of diagnosis	Improvement in patient's functional or health status/; symptom remission

quences if inadequate or incorrect care was provided. It is difficult to anticipate all the care required by a postoperative patient. Careful deliberation about the numerous possibilities is necessary, however, and even this process may not reveal all of their potential needs in advance. Staff and patient inputs are needed to delineate any situations that may appear problematic.

Outcome

Outcome is the third integral component of quality care assessment. It is defined as the result of interaction between structure and process. In QA programs, a problem with outcome usually precipitates the need to review the structure and process of a certain activity. When an adverse outcome is identified, appropriate changes in structure or process should be considered. Change, however, is not always necessary. Current practice may need to be outlined more clearly in the Policy and Procedure Manual to ensure uniformity of practice. Structure and process are still worthy of study even if no adverse outcomes have surfaced. Each element of patient care—structure, process, and outcome—is studied by QA committee members, independently and in group review.

POLICY AND PROCEDURE MANUAL

Every clinician involved in patient care should be thoroughly familiar with the guidelines listed in the Policy and Procedure Manual, another product of the risk management process. The Policy and Procedure Manual, with its outline of activities in the PACU, should guide both the structure and process of activities in this area. The manual is a reference for all health care providers and should be the result of the collective input of all involved. Staff input and review are essential to guarantee a comprehensive understanding of policy and procedure. Cognizance of the QA process facilitates and maintains cooperation.

IMPLEMENTATION OF QA IN THE PACU

Cooperation between physicians and nursing personnel is the foundation on which a strong QA program thrives. Their unique but overlapping philosophies, experiences, and viewpoints regarding patient care, when incor-

porated into the QA program, ensure a depth of understanding that is not possible by either group independently. All members of the health care team need assurance that their input will be considered and integrated into the QA process. They must be confident that the time they take to think about the criteria in question is important, and that any time spent away from patient care to study QA concerns is worthwhile. Positive reinforcement for staff involvement is essential to the success of the QA team effort in the PACU. If positive results for their efforts are not evident, the participants will regard QA only as intrusive and unproductive paperwork.

The director of the PACU determines the duties of each member of the PACU team. In most cases, however, the chairperson of the PACU QA committees has overall responsibility for completion of the QA process. The chairperson must offer direction to the committee for accomplishing efficient data collection and competent data analysis. In addition, he or she must call regular meetings to review the data with committee members and other staff members who are involved.

The QA program consists in analysis of data about various aspects of structure, process, or outcome that surface as concerns in the PACU. These aspects are referred to as indicators. Indicators are identified for each element of care. They are measurable variables that facilitate collection of reliable data. To implement the monitoring and evaluation responsibilities of the QA team, a formal approach to the identification of indicators and a simple method of data collection are necessary.

When defining the scope of care available in the PACU, it is important to recognize the dual accountability that exists between the nursing staff and the medical staff. The nurses in the PACU have two sets of directives: One is derived from the nursing care plan as outlined by the nursing service, and the other is developed by the medical staff in cooperation with the PACU nurses. The first consideration of the QA committee when identifying indicators is to review both sets of nursing regulations so they complement one another. Analysis of elements of nursing structure and process, as well as an understanding of the desired outcome are required to provide the basis for study of indicators in the monitoring and evaluation process.

Two kinds of indicator can be discovered in the process of analysis: general and specific. General indicators may be as simple as hypothermia during the PACU stay or as severe as postoperative anesthesia-related death. Specific indicators include groups of specially focused questions. The general indicator airway complications may include such specific indicators as a loose tooth, cut lip, inadvertent endobronchial intubation, and accidental or premature extubation. The general indicator apparatus would include a specific indicator, e.g., breathing circuit disconnection during mechanical ventilation. The list of indicators resulting from the QA review process should be comprehensive but not so long as to be unmanageable. The quality of indicators is more important than their quantity.

The quality of an indicator can be assessed by its ease of measurement and familiarity to health care providers. The providers should reach consensus on a range of acceptable limits for the identification of each indicator. No yardstick to measure the accomplishment of an indicator should be dismissed by the majority of medical team members. Limits must guarantee that careful examination of a specific indicator will occur and will not be so restrictive or wide-ranging as to render itself inaccurate. For example, an indicator stating that any systolic blood pressure drop of less than 50 per cent need not be treated may create a negative perception of the QA process. It

would be more beneficial to state this indicator positively. To ensure valid collection of data about any indicator, it is essential to develop each indicator carefully. The QA program is only as good as the indicators chosen for monitoring and evaluation by the QA committee.

Data can be collected from many sources, e.g., patient records. Nursing notes, physician progress notes, consultation reports, and laboratory information are some of the sources available in the medical record. In the PACU, significant records are usually the preoperative anesthesia evaluation and the intraoperative anesthesia record(s). New data sources, however, may need to be identified after the QA committee organizes the final list of indicators.

Responsibility for data collection and its organization must be delegated to competent personnel (Fig. 23–1). Regular collection and organization of data deter the accumulation of unanalyzed information, which hinders the QA process. One member of the PACU staff usually performs these tasks. Clinicians often do not have the time required to fulfill this function, and for this reason the data collector can be a member of the support staff or even an individual who is hired outside the PACU, if the staff has no objections. Outside employees could be recommended by the hospital's

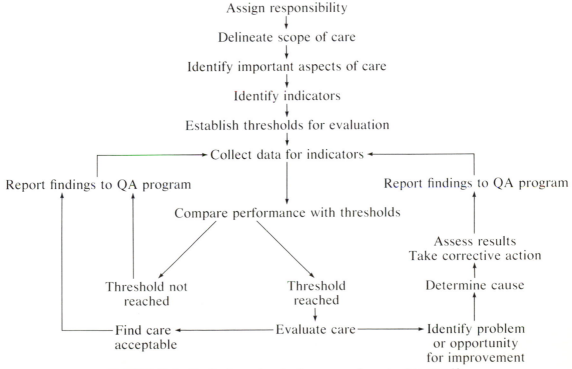

FIGURE 23–1. Monitoring and evaluation process from step 1 to step 10.

QA department. The most important consideration when choosing this employee is the need to ease any possible burden generated by QA data collection and, at the same time, to promote the efficient and productive analysis of the data.

Each chart should be examined for possible QA data. This task can be overwhelming unless a specified screening process is observed. Generic and occurrence screening are commonly used systems. *Generic screening* involves reviewing each particular case for data relevant to established indicators, a method of data gathering that results in a comprehensive review of the patient's experience and yields a broad spectrum of data. The *occurrence data collection* method involves self-reporting by members of the health care staff. Self-reporting emphasizes trust in staff members, stresses individual professionalism, and recognizes each member's desire to contribute to the success of the QA process.

All reports developed by staff members are accepted and considered confidential. An early review of the data gathered from self-reporting helps reassure all members involved that the effort is worth their time and continued participation. If self-reports are treated appropriately, they become an invaluable data source for revealing areas of concern shared by staff members. Both the generic and occurrence methods of data collection are effective, but self-reporting is most likely to engender the spirit of teamwork necessary for quality patient care. Teamwork between physicians and nurses is a key element of the QA program.

Evaluation of the data collected from numerous sources is another critical aspect of the QA process. Individuals responsible for data analysis must establish a framework for evaluating the structure, process, and outcome of patient care so that initial patterns and trends in patient care are evident. These patterns and trends are then studied further to examine their impact on patient care. In addition, discussions focus on the changes that may or may not be necessary in PACU policies and procedures.

After careful analysis of data and the establishment of trends and patterns, the QA committee must agree on possible interventions, if any are required. Following these discussions, members of the health care staff are notified of future changes and the reasons for their necessity. Those responsible for instituting changes in patient care structure, process, or outcome

are identified through the process of peer review. As with self-reporting, an atmosphere of respect and trust encourages the best results. Only those members of the staff who volunteer should be used as reviewers in the peer review process. These volunteers should demonstrate a clear understanding of the QA objectives and be ready to cooperate with the QA leadership. As a result of this cooperative teamwork, the success of the QA program can be guaranteed.

Analysis of data, peer review, and interactive discussions do not always result in changes made in PACU care. Such investigation can also reassure staff and leadership that the structure, process, and outcome are working well just as they are. Corrective measures, however, need to be established in advance, as a positive outcome is not always inevitable.

Several questions must be addressed when an intervention in a patient care area is necessary. What change is ideal? What alternative outcome do we want to achieve? How should the current policies and procedures be amended to facilitate this change? Those most responsible for patient care in the area to be improved would be likely candidates to formulate a framework for accomplishing the change. How much time will be given to make the change? Who will be involved? What specific differences in structure, process, or outcome are needed?

Both the physician and nursing teams must be assured that changes will occur as a result of their involvement in the QA process. More importantly, they must feel secure that changes can be implemented in ways that are appropriate and acceptable. Once changes are instituted, follow-up surveys must be conducted to determine whether outcomes have improved. Continued surveillance is necessary to ensure prolonged success of any QA program. If interventions do not result in sustained improvements in outcome, alternative plans for change must be considered.

SUMMARY

Quality assurance in the PACU is a process that demands the time and attention of both a committee and a team of health care providers. Both parties must be dedicated to monitoring and evaluating the three fundamental areas of patient care concern: structure, process, and outcome. The structure of care is the input available through the resources of equipment and the numbers and qualifications of the health care staff. The process of care is made up of those activities and functions performed by the health care practitioners, e.g., assessment of need and planning of care. The outcome of care involves any complications or adverse effects that occur in the PACU, with positive outcomes also being noted.

Quality assurance has sometimes been viewed as a negative review of patient care. Such a review demonstrates an incomplete understanding of the QA process. Although data collection and analysis may indicate the need for change in some areas, it is also possible that existing standards are adequate. In this case, it may be necessary only to rewrite standards listed in the existing Policy and Procedure Manual to reflect current policies. It is important for the PACU to identify its strengths as well as its weakness, thereby accentuating the positive aspects of the QA process.

Quality assurance is an essential component of current medical care. With the trust of patients and members of the medical health care team, the finest patient care available can be provided, and the future of our medical institutions can be guaranteed.

Bibliography

Agenda for Change Update: News about the Agenda for Change. News from the Joint Commission, September 1987.

Alternate care: push is on for ambulatory quality assurance. Hospitals 62:66, 1988.

Appendix B: Revisions Since the 1988 Division. Accreditation Manual for Hospitals. WX 15 A187, Chicago, 1989, pp. 289–292.

The ASA adopts two national standards. Anesthesiol News. American Society of Anesthesiology 53:22, 1989.

Brazil P: Cost effective care is better care. Hastings Center Rep 16:7–8, 1986.

Clemhagen C: Overcoming the barriers to QA: Dimensions (editorial). 64:6–7, 1987.

Cooper JB, Cullen DJ: Reply. Anesthesiology 68(6):68, 1988.

Cullen DJ: Recovery room care of the surgical patient. Int Anesthesiol Clin 18(3):39–52, 1980.

Eichhorn JH: Quality assurance. Curr Rev 11(17):133–140, 1989.

Goldman B: Quality assurance will play key role in reducing malpractice suits: CMPA. Can Med Assoc J 137:447–448, 1987.

A Guide to the Essentials of a Modern Medical Practice Act. Federation of State Medical Boards (FSMB). Fort Worth, Federation of State Medical Boards of the United States, 1985.

Illinois Administrative Code 77. Chapter 1 250.1240, 24402630, Subchapter b.

Kahn J: Quality assurance professionals: a national profile. Dimensions 63:14, 1986.

Knapp RM: Quality assurance: irrelevant data is never inexpensive enough. Anesthesiology 68:967, 1988. (letter to the editor).

Longo DR, Wilt JE, Laubenthal RM: Hospital compliance with Joint Commission standards: findings from 1984 surveys; Joint Commission forum. Quality Rev Bull 12:388–394, 1986.

Monitoring and evaluating the quality and appropriateness of care in a hospital: a hospital sample. Quality Rev Bull 12:326–330, 1986.

Norman DK, Randall RS, Hornsby BJ: Critical features of a curriculum in health care quality and resource management. Quality Rev Bull 16:317–36, 1990.

Quality Assurance (QA). Accreditation Manual for Hospitals. Joint Commission on Accreditation of Healthcare Organization, Chicago, 1989, pp. 219–223.

Quality Assurance. Joint Commission on Accreditation for Hospitals. Joint Commission on Accreditation of Healthcare Organization, Chicago, 1987.

Quality Assurance Support Service. Notes from Program on Hospital Accreditation Standards (PHAS). 1988.

Report of the Task Force on Medical Liability and Malpractice. Secretary of the Department of Health and Human Services (DHHS), 1987.

Shestowsky BJ: Quality assurance systems need a second look. Dimensions 65:28–29, 1988.

Stewart DJ: Experience with a hospital-wide quality assurance program in a teaching hospital. Presented to the Association of Canadian Teaching Hospitals, October 1984.

Stock R: Risk management: minimizing errors and liability. Dimensions 63:22–23, 1986.

Van Reenen JA: Quality assurance: introduction to terminology and literature. Hosp Trustee. 7(6):18, 1983.

Wallace P, Lowi M, Colton M: Practical QA program meets accreditation challenge. Dimensions 63:19–21, 1986.

White J: Five principles to simplify the QA process. Dimensions 63:15–17, 1986.

Index

Note: Page numbers in *italics* refer to illustrations, page numbers followed by t refer to tables.

Post anesthesia care unit, admission to (*continued*)
  narcotic analgesics in, 298–301
  nausea and vomiting in, 321–326
  obstetric patients in, 356–361
  pain management in, 296–298, 320–321
  pediatric, 256, 257t
  quality assurance in, 363–369
Postoperative care, problem-oriented approach to, 1–8
Postpartum hemorrhage, 359–360, 359t
Postpartum patient, in post anesthesia care unit, 356, 357t
Postural drainage, for bronchial hygiene, 115
Potassium metabolism, disorders of, 169, *170,* 171–173
Prednisone, for anaphylaxis, 248t
Preeclampsia, 356, 358
Pregnancy, nonparturient surgery during, 361
Premedication, for ambulatory surgery, 318–319
Procainamide, for arrhythmias, 43–44
Prochlorperazine (Compazine), as antiemetic, 17, 324t
Promethazine (Phenergan), as antiemetic, 17
Propofol, for ambulatory surgery, 319
Propranolol, anaphylaxis treatment complicated by, 241–242
  for arrhythmias, 44
  for hyperthyroidism, 223
Propylthiouracil, for hyperthyroidism, 223
Prostate, transurethral resection of, hyponatremia after, 161
Protamine, perioperative allergic reactions to, 249–250, *250*
Proteus infection, postoperative, 338
Pseudohypertension, 24
Pseudohyponatremia, 161
Pseudomonas infection, postoperative, 335, 336, 338, 341
Pulmonary artery catheterization, data from, evaluation of, 32t
  to evaluate renal function, 148
Pulmonary artery pressure monitoring, 67–71, *68–70*
Pulmonary dysfunction, altered consciousness and, 184
  hypothermia and, 209t
Pulmonary edema, postoperative, *88,* 88–90, 89t
  vasoconstrictor-induced, 290
Pulmonary embolism, after total hip arthroplasty, 275–276
  massive, as cause of hypotension, 31
  postoperative, 37, 91
Pulmonary pain, postoperative, causes of, 33t, 37–38
Pupillary response, examination of, 194–195, 194t
  in narcotic overdosage, 196
Pyridostigmine, for anesthetic reversal, 199

Quality assurance, in post anesthesia care unit, 363–369
Quality assurance terminology, 364t

Radial nerve, function of, 192t
Radio allergosorbent test, 245, 246
Radiocontrast medium, acute renal failure from, 144–145, 145t
  perioperative allergic reactions to, 247–248, 248t
Ranitidine, for anaphylaxis, 240t, 248t
Rash, morbilliform, 235t
Rebreathing mask, for oxygen delivery, 111
Rectal temperature, measurement of, 204t, 205
Red blood cell, storage of, 135
Red neck (red man's) syndrome, 245

Reflex hypotension, 120–121, 121t
Reflux esophagitis, 38
Regional anesthesia, classification of, 246t
  disadvantages of, 316–317
  effectiveness of, 306–307
  for ambulatory surgery, 315–318, 321
  intravenous, 318
  perioperative allergic reactions to, 246–247, 246t, 247t
  risks of, 197, 307–398
  side effects of, postoperative arrhythmias as, 42
  toxicity of, treatment of, 307
Renal disease, atheroembolic, 146
Renal dysfunction, after aortic reconstruction, 125, 125t
  altered consciousness and, 182t, 184
  hypothermia and, 209t
  in postoperative septic shock, 341
  pathogenesis of, 141–146
Renal failure, contrast medium-induced, 144–145
  fluid and electrolyte therapy for, 166
  hemodynamically mediated, 142–143, *143*
  incidence of, 141
  myoglobin-induced, 145, 145t
  nephrotoxic, 143–144
  nonoliguric, 146, 146t
  postoperative infection risk and, 343
  prevention of, 148
  seizures and, 185t
Renal function, in initial post anesthesia care unit assessment, 5
  laboratory evaluation of, 146–148
Renal injury, amphotericin-induced, 144
Renal replacement therapy, 149–153, 151t
Renin, in blood pressure control, 24
Respiratory alkalosis, acute, 99–101
  hypokalemia and, 171
Respiratory complications, 76–92
  after descending thoracoabdominal aneurysm surgery, 127–128
  effect of drugs on, 76–77
  following regional anesthetics, 316
  hypercarbia and, 90–91
  hypertension and, 26
  hypoxemia and, 81–90
  in anaphylaxis, 238, 239t
  of renal replacement therapy, 153
  of spinal narcotics, 305
  physical assessment of, 77–81
  with bacteremic shock, 341
Respiratory stimulants, narcotic interaction with, 310
Risk management, in post anesthesia care unit, 363
Roentgenography, renal, 147–148

Salicylate poisoning, 219
Saphenous nerve, injury of, prevention of, 193
Sciatic nerve, function of, 192t
  injury of, prevention of, 193
Scoliosis, anesthetic complications of, 278–279
Scopolamine (Hyoscine), as antiemetic, 15, 16
  postoperative agitation and, 11
Scoring systems, in post anesthesia care unit, 5–6, *6*
Secobarbital, maternal, effect of, on newborn, 360
Sedatives, sensitivity to, after carotid endarterectomy, 123, 124t
Seizures, conditions associated with, 185, 185t, 195
  in preeclampsia, 358
  treatment of, 199